FINANCIAL MANAGEMENT OF HEALTH CARE ORGANIZATIONS

FINANCIAL MANAGEMENT OF HEALTH CARE ORGANIZATIONS

An Introduction to Fundamental Tools, Concepts, and Applications

Third Edition

WILLIAM N. ZELMAN

MICHAEL J. McCUE

NOAH D. GLICK

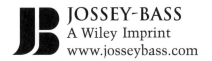

JOSSEY-BASS
A Wiley Imprint
www.josseybass.com

Published by Jossey-Bass
A Wiley Imprint
989 Market Street, San Francisco, CA 94103-1741—www.josseybass.com

Library of Congress Cataloging-in-Publication Data

ISBN 13: 978-0-4704-9752-4
ISBN 10: 0-4704-9752-1

Printed in the United States of America
THIRD EDITION
PB Printing   10 9 8 7 6 5

*To our families for their love and patience.
To our students and colleagues for their invaluable
insights and feedback.*

CONTENTS

EXHIBITS AND TABLES

PREFACE

This book offers an introduction to the most-used tools and techniques of health care financial management. It contains numerous examples from a variety of providers, including health maintenance organizations, hospitals, physician practices, home health agencies, nursing units, surgical centers, and integrated health care systems. The book avoids complicated formulas and uses numerous spreadsheet examples so that they can be adapted to problems in the workplace. For those desiring to go beyond the fundamentals, many chapters have additional information included in appendices. Each chapter begins with a detailed outline and concludes with a detailed summary, followed by a set of questions and problems. Answers to the questions and problems are available for download to instructors at http://www.josseybass.com/go/zelman3e. Finally, a number of perspectives are included in every chapter. Perspectives are intended to provide additional insight into the topic using examples from the real world.

The book begins with an overview of some of the key factors affecting the financial management of health care organizations in today's environment. Chapters Two, Three, and Four focus on the financial statements of the organization. Chapter Two presents an introduction to the financial statements of health care organizations. The financial statements are (perhaps along with the budget) the most important financial documents of a health care organization, and the bulk of the chapter is designed to help understand these statements.

Chapter Three provides an introduction to health care financial accounting. This chapter focuses on the relationship between the actions of health care providers and administrators and the financial condition of the organization, how the numbers on the financial statements are derived, the distinction between cash and accrual bases of accounting, and the importance of actually defining what is meant by "cost." By the time students complete Chapters Two and Three, they will have been introduced to a large portion of the terms used in health care financial management.

Building on Chapters Two and Three, Chapter Four focuses on interpreting the financial statements of health care organizations. Three approaches to analyzing statements are presented: horizontal, vertical, and ratio analysis. Great care has been taken to show how the ratios are computed and how to summarize the results.

Chapter Five focuses on the management of working capital: current assets and current liabilities. This chapter emphasizes the importance of cash management and provides many practical techniques for managing the inflows and outflows of funds through an organization, including managing the billing and collections cycle, and for paying off short-term liabilities.

Chapter Six introduces one of the most important concepts in long-term decision making: the time value of money. Chapter Seven builds on this concept, incorporating it into the investment decision by presenting several techniques to analyze investment decisions: the payback method, net present value, and internal rate of return. Examples are given for both not-for-profit and for-profit organizations.

Once an investment has been decided on, it is important to determine how the assets will be financed, which is the focus of Chapter Eight, Capital Financing. Whereas Chapter Five deals with issues of short-term financing, Chapter Eight focuses on long-term investments, with a particular emphasis on issuing bonds.

Chapters Nine through Twelve introduce topics typically covered in a managerial accounting course. Chapter Nine focuses on the concept of cost and using cost information for short-term decision making, including fixed cost, variable cost, and break-even analysis. In addition to covering the key concepts, it offers a set of rules to guide decision makers in making financial decisions. Chapter Ten explores budget models and the budgeting process. Several budget models are introduced, including program, performance, and zero-based budgeting. The chapter ends with an example of how to prepare each of the five main budgets: statistics budget, revenue budget, expense budget, cash budget, and capital budget. It also includes examples for various types of payors, including flat fee and capitation.

Chapter Eleven deals with responsibility accounting. It discusses the different types of responsibility centers and focuses on the performance measurement in general and budget variance analysis in particular. Chapter Twelve discusses methods used by health care providers to determine their costs, primarily focusing on the step-down method and activity-based costing. The book concludes with Chapter Thirteen, Provider Payment Systems. This chapter describes the evolution of the payment system in the United States and the specifics of various approaches to managing care and paying providers.

MAJOR CHANGES IN THE THIRD EDITION

As noted below, the major changes from the second edition involve:

- New sections to reflect changes in the health care environment
- Updated data used in examples
- Updated data used in problems
- New problems
- New perspectives

Chapter One: The Context of Health Care Financial Management

Changes to Chapter One, the introductory chapter, provide a more comprehensive view of the current health care setting. Enhancements include updated statistics for all of the pertinent exhibits as well as for those statistics embodied within the text. All perspectives have been replaced with recent events. The chapter also introduces numerous new terms and concepts, including new laws and regulations affecting the health care environment, as well as alternative health care methods.

Chapter Two: Health Care Financial Statements

Chapter Two has been expanded to include updated financial statements from investor-owned hospital management companies and expanded notes to the financial statements so students can see their importance to an overall balance sheet and statement of operations. All perspectives have been updated. In addition, problems 11 through 25 have been revised and updated.

Chapter Three: Principles and Practices of Health Care Accounting

In Chapter Three, the perspectives have been replaced with four new updated versions. Problems 11 through 20 have been changed and updated.

Chapter Four: Financial Statement Analysis

Several new ratios have been added, specifically operating revenue per adjusted discharge, operating expense per adjusted discharge, and salary expense as percentage of total operating expenses. Updated Thomson data have been used to expand the benchmarks. All chapter problems have been updated.

Chapter Five: Working Capital Management

In this chapter, the section on billing, collection, and disbursement policies and the concept of float have been condensed, and a new section on revenue cycle management has been added that covers registration, charge capture, coding, billing, payment, and methods to monitor accounts receivable management. All chapter problems have been revised and updated.

Chapter Six: The Time Value of Money

In Chapter Six, a discussion of the Excel function to compute the number of periods to pay off a loan has been added, and the problem sets have been updated.

Chapter Seven: The Investment Decision

In Chapter Seven, all perspectives have been updated, and problems 11 through 20 have been changed and updated.

Chapter Eight: Capital Financing for Health Care Providers

This chapter includes revisions to the debt financing section and added discussion on interest rate swaps and estimating a hospital's capacity to borrow. All the problems on lease financing and bond valuation have been revised, and new problems for measuring debt capacity have been added.

Chapter Nine: Using Cost Information to Make Special Decisions

The conceptual diagram and related explanation for understanding breaking even have been substantially revised, and all perspectives have been replaced with updated versions. Most problems have updated figures, and three new problems have been substituted.

Chapter Ten: Budgeting

Although the organization of the chapter remains essentially the same, the basic model on which this chapter is based has been almost totally revised. The new model is based on a hospitalist practice that has only two services, a simplification from the previous edition. The supplies budget has been dropped, but a discussion remains. All perspectives have been replaced with updated versions. The problems have been revised to reflect the new content, though the general format is the same.

Chapter Eleven: Responsibility Accounting

The discussion of cost centers has been modified slightly to recognize both service- and product-producing activities. A new section on compensation systems has been added.

Chapter Twelve: Provider Cost-Finding Methods

The old perspectives were dropped, and two new ones were added.

Chapter Thirteen: Provider Payment Systems

A discussion of evolving issues is presented regarding pay for reporting, pay for performance, medical errors, and consumer-directed health plans. A new update is presented on recent changes in Medicare related to the new diagnosis-related group (DRG) system called Medicare severity-adjusted DRGs (MSDRGs), and the Medicare Modernization Act, which allows prescription drug coverage for its beneficiaries as well as the option for them to enroll in a private health plan instead of the traditional fee-for-service Medicare program.

Glossary

The glossary has been updated and includes each term defined in the text as a marginal definition and key term.

THE AUTHORS

William N. Zelman is a full professor in the Department of Health Policy and Management, Gillings School of Global Public Health, University of North Carolina at Chapel Hill. He specializes in Health Care Financial Management, focusing on management-related issues, including measuring organizational performance and cost management. He has served as director of the Residential Master's Programs and is past chair of the Association of University Programs in Health Administration's Financial Management Task Force. He has authored or coauthored five books and numerous articles and has been an editorial board member, reviewer, or both, for a number of journals. He has extensive international experience, serving as a consultant to and presenting courses for academic, governmental, and international organizations primarily in South Asia and Central Europe.

Michael J. McCue is a professor of health administration within the Department of Health Administration at Virginia Commonwealth University in Richmond. Dr. McCue's research interests relate to corporate finance topics within the health care industry and the performance of hospitals, multihospital systems, and health plans. His previous research examines the determinants of hospital capital structure, factors influencing hospitals' cash flow and cash on hand, and the evaluation of hospital bond ratings. His current research examines the financial and operating performance of inpatient rehabilitation hospitals.

Noah D. Glick is currently a senior health care consultant for FTI Consulting in the corporate finance division, where he is engaged in physician strategy and health care analytics. Previously he was administrative director for Rehabilitation Medical Associates and the South Shore Hospitalist Group outside of Boston. He was a senior consultant for Integrated Healthcare Information Services in Waltham, Massachusetts, a staff member in the Department of Decision Support at the University of North Carolina Hospitals in Chapel Hill, and taught simulation modeling in the master's in health administration program at the University of North Carolina, where he also did health care research.

ACKNOWLEDGMENTS

We attempted throughout this book to challenge and enlighten. Quantitative as well as qualitative issues are presented in an effort to help readers better understand the wide range of issues considered under the topic *health care financial management*. We would like to thank the many students over the past several years who pointed out errors, offered suggestions and improvements, and provided new ways to solve problems. Particular thanks go to Daniel Bunow for his cooperation and excellent review of chapters and spreadsheets; the following students for their contributions to Chapters Nine, Ten, and Twelve: Leslie Ale, Megan Berlinger, Laura Dunlop, Danielle Doughman, Brad Heaton, Karoline Moon, Kavita Narayan, Meilike Ongen, Corrie Pointak, Cherry Poss, Ashley Purdy, Tina Rao, Bennett Thompson, Elizabeth Walker, Natilie Wilde, and Matt Womble; Yen-Ju Lin, Ph.D. and Tae Hyun Kim, Ph.D., for their review of the book; Reethi Iyengar for her help on the Perspectives; and Julie Peterman, CFA, vice president of BB&T Capital Markets, for her review and contributions to health care capital financing (Chapter Eight).

Most of all, we would like to thank our families for their encouragement and support and for their understanding during the countless hours we were not available to them.

The authors and publishers gratefully acknowledge permission to reproduce copyrighted material. Full source information has been given in the chapters.

The authors apologize for any errors or omissions in the citations in the chapters and would be grateful to be notified at ZMGText@gmail.com of any corrections that should be incorporated in the next edition or reprint of this book.

1

THE CONTEXT OF HEALTH CARE FINANCIAL MANAGEMENT

LEARNING OBJECTIVES

- Identify key factors that have led to rising health care costs
- Identify key approaches to controlling health care costs
- Identify key ethical issues resulting from attempts to control costs

Never before have health care professionals faced such complex issues and practical difficulties trying to keep their organizations financially viable (see Perspective 1–1). With turbulent changes taking place in payment, delivery, and social systems, health care professionals are faced with trying to meet their organization's health-related

---

Perspective 1–1   Health Care System in Distress

The Road to Economic Recovery: A Proposal to Support Health Care in America

The economic recession gripping this nation calls for immediate and swift action. The ripple effects of the financial market crisis, the subsequent rise in unemployment, and the loss of job-based health care coverage has impacted hospitals' ability to continue to serve their communities. This pressure, coupled with other payment pressures, is leading to a decline in hospitals' financial health at a time when demand for health care services is growing.

The American Hospital Association (AHA), through recent reports and surveys, has found

- The credit crunch has increased the costs of borrowing needed funds, making it more difficult for hospitals to find the money for needed facility and technology improvements. Hospitals saw interest payments on borrowed funds increase by an average of 15 percent from July to September 2008 versus the same period last year.

- Many hospitals are reconsidering or postponing investments in facilities or equipment that communities rely on for care. These include renovations or plans to increase capacity (56 percent), the purchase of clinical technology or equipment (45 percent), and investments in new information technology (39 percent).

- Many hospitals have noted an increase in the proportion of patients unable to pay for care. According to one AHA survey, uncompensated care increased 8 percent from July to September 2008 versus the same period last year.

- Among a sample of hospitals, total margins fell to *negative* 1.6 percent in the third quarter of 2008 versus *positive* 6.1 percent during the same period last year.

- Hospitals report that financial stress is forcing them to make or consider making cutbacks to meet their obligations. In one recent AHA survey, more than half of hospitals reported plans to reduce staff (53 percent) and more than a quarter of hospitals reported plans to reduce services (27 percent).

Source: Extract: American Hospital Association legislative proposal sent to Congress (January 2009) (http://www.aha.org/aha/content/2009/pdf/090106-economic-recovery-mo.pdf).

Exhibit 1-1 Organization of this chapter

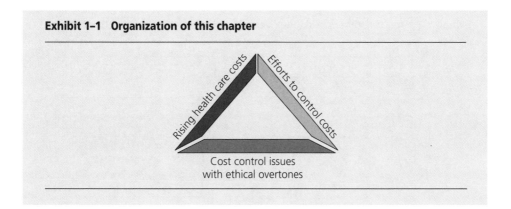

mission in an environment of extreme cost pressure. To provide a context for the topics covered in this text, this chapter highlights key issues affecting health care providers. It is organized into three sections: rising health care costs, efforts to control costs, and cost control issues with ethical overtones (see Exhibit 1–1).

RISING HEALTH CARE COSTS

Many factors have led to rising health care costs, which have increased faster than general inflation over the past decades (see Exhibit 1–2). Although the average life expectancy of the general population has risen by only approximately three years over this time period, the cost to keep people healthy has approximately doubled (Exhibit 1–3). The remainder of this section briefly discusses some of the key factors that have contributed to the higher cost of health care: the payment (reimbursement) system, technology, the aging population, prescription drug costs, chronic diseases, litigation, and the uninsured (see Exhibit 1–4).

The Payment System

The introduction of Medicare and Medicaid in 1965 in large part was designed to guarantee health care coverage to the country's most vulnerable populations: the poor and the elderly. Unfortunately, many officials at the time failed to recognize that these "Great Society" programs would become the impetus for two interrelated problems that have persisted ever since: health care costs rising far beyond those that were ever predicted and an increased expectation that access to a high level of affordable health care is a right for all citizens. For nearly fifty years, the health care payment system in the United States has undergone major changes, and the role of many providers has gradually shifted from price setter to price taker. The role of the federal government has changed from being a small participant before the mid-1960s to being a major

Exhibit 1–2   The consumer price index versus medical care inflation, 1990–2008

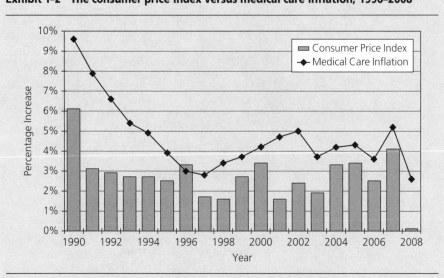

Source: U.S. Labor Department, Bureau of Labor Statistics (December, 2008).

Exhibit 1–3   Annual health care expenditures in the United States, 1997–2007

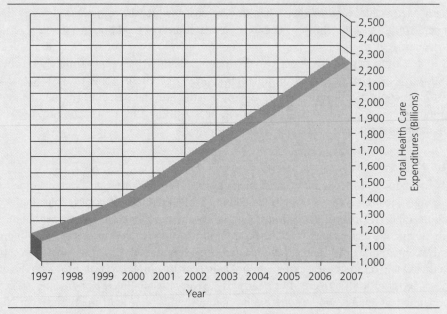

Source: Centers for Medicare and Medicaid Services, Office of the Actuary, 2008.

Exhibit 1–4   Selected factors contributing to the rising costs of health care

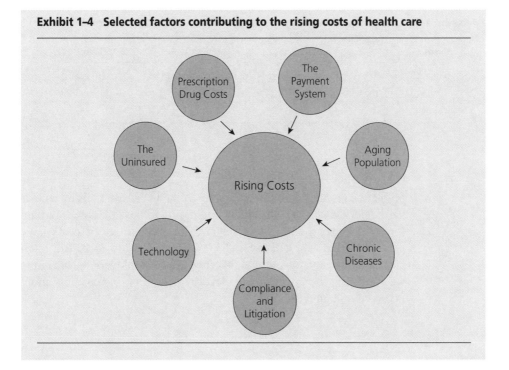

force in both setting amounts of payment and defining payment systems. As the federal government has attempted to control its costs, its inpatient payment systems have evolved from charge-based to cost-based to flat-fee, toward capitation, and now toward mixed systems that include a reversion to cost-based payments for critical access hospitals and an experimentation with performance-based systems (see Exhibit 1–5). In 2000 the federal government introduced a new payment system for outpatient services called *ambulatory payment classifications* (APCs), which changed the basis of payment for hospital outpatient services from a flat fee for individual services to fixed reimbursement for bundled services. A few years later, it helped to push the development of pay-for-performance (P4P) reimbursement methods, discussed later in this chapter. The federal government, of course, is not the only payor, but its policies and reimbursement amounts for services greatly influence the practices of other payors, including state governments.

As discussed in depth in Chapter Thirteen, in charge-based and cost-based systems, the provider plays a major role in setting prices. In flat-fee and capitated payment arrangements, the payor sets the prices and potentially has more control over its costs whereas the provider assumes an increased financial risk. However, a major

Ambulatory Payment Classifications (APCs) Enacted by the federal government in 2000, a prospective payment system for hospital outpatient services, similar to DRGs, which reimburses a fixed amount for a bundled set of services.

Exhibit 1–5 The introduction of new payment systems by Medicare since the 1960s

1960s	1980s	1990s	2000s
Fee-for-service and cost-based reimbursement	Prospective payment (DRGs)	Capitation and global payments	APCs and P4P

Cost-Shifting
When providers try to get one payor to pay for costs that have not been covered by another payor. A common example is a provider's trying to compensate for low Medicaid payments by increasing charges to a private insurer.

problem caused by individual payors' trying to control their own costs has been *cost-shifting*: providers attempting to pass on costs not paid for by one payor onto other payors. The private sector costs have nearly doubled over a decade: $533 billion in 1997 to $1.03 trillion in 2007.[1] As a result of these staggering costs, employers and insurers are following the government's lead by becoming increasingly more involved in managing care.

Technology

No one can deny the benefits of new and more sophisticated health care technologies, but the associated costs can be overwhelming. Premature infants and infants with gross birth defects, who would not have survived just a decade ago, can now survive, but can generate upward of half a million dollars in costs in the intensive care unit alone and possibly more afterward due to developmental disabilities. The total cost in the first year of life for a premature infant can easily surpass $1 million.

Transplants have saved countless lives, and procedure count more than doubled in number in twenty years, from 12,623 in 1988 to 27,961 in 2008 (U.S. Department of Health and Human Services, 2009). Many feel that it has not been the individual cost of a transplant but only the lack of donors that has limited the number of transplants performed. The rise in living-donor transplants (as opposed to cadaverous transplants) has led to more growth in this rapidly evolving field, but these procedures now involve two (or more) living patients who will be operated on, rather than just one. The use of other, more advanced technologies—and their associated costs—have significantly increased as well. For example, the number of magnetic resonance imagers (MRIs) per capita in the United States far exceeds the figure for any other country in the world, as do the figures for computerized axial tomography (CAT) scanners, cardiac catheterization procedures, and so forth. On the other hand, the United States has become a major destination for foreigners who do not have access to these types of advanced technologies in their own countries. Other countries are now entering this market, however, and a term, *medical tourism*, has entered the lexicon to describe this phenomenon (described more later on).

The Aging Population

Despite the increased costs and technological advances, the average life expectancy of Americans has risen only slightly over the past few decades: from 71.1 to 75.2 for men, and from 78.2 to 80.4 for women from 1985–2005.[2] In the meantime, the overall population has aged significantly, and there are more elderly Americans than ever before. In fact, by the mid-1990s, the age group 85 and older was the fastest-growing segment of the population, and the elderly tend to be the heaviest users of health care services. Whereas the leading causes of death in the early part of the last century typically were sudden illnesses (generally curable and/or preventable today), the current reasons for mortality include more chronic, long-term (and expensive) illnesses, such as heart disease and cancer (see Exhibit 1–6). If a person lives long enough, he or she has a relatively high probability of succumbing to a chronic illness.

The combination of age and technology has increased costs in other ways, too. For example, joint replacements to restore mobility are immensely popular among the elderly but can become very expensive, especially if complications arise. Although the benefit of such procedures is remarkable in human terms, these technologies have added costs to the system.

The increased need for long-term care for the elderly has also led to increased health care costs. As more working families find that they cannot take care of their aging parents' physical needs, the costs of long-term care become both their and society's burden. In fact, more than half of all Medicaid expenditures in the past decade went to elderly

Exhibit 1–6 Major causes of death and their approximate occurrences in 2005

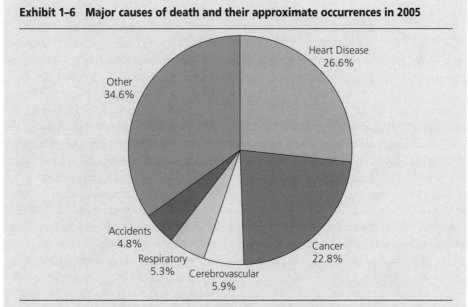

Source: Kung, K.; Hoyert, D. L.; Xu, J.; and Murphy, S. L., Division of Vital Statistics 2008. Deaths: final data for 2005, *National Vital Statistics Reports*, 56(10):5, Table B.

patients in nursing homes. In 2006 nursing home costs averaged about $200 per day. An alternative arrangement is home health and live-in nursing aides, but these options are not always covered by insurance and can be unaffordable to the average family: for example, as of 2006, home health aides were earning an average of $19 per hour.[3]

Prescription Drug Costs and Medicare Part D

A major reason why the population has aged and survived longer from debilitating chronic diseases has been the advent of increasingly effective—albeit costly—drugs. Drug manufacturers have received widespread criticism for stifling competition and raising prices, especially compared with the prices being offered in other countries. However, the manufacturers counter that they can spend hundreds of millions of dollars in research on drugs that reach the market, and that they need to recoup their investments (as well as their investments in numerous other failed drugs that never reached the market). Without the incentive to do research by being granted a patent on new medications (and thus monopoly control), drug manufacturers contend that they would not be able to bring as many promising new drugs to market. While the battle rages on, retail sales of prescription drugs in the United States have already nearly doubled since the turn of the new century, from $120.6 billion in 2000 to $227.5 billion in 2007.[4]

Medicare Part D
Prescription drug coverage for Medicare enrollees, begun in 2006, which offsets some of the out-of-pocket costs for medications. Enrollees pay an additional monthly premium for this supplemental benefit.

To help counter these rising prescription costs, in one of the few major changes to Medicare since its inception, Congress passed an optional prescription drug benefit program beginning in January 2006 for all Medicare enrollees, regardless of income, personal health, or other health insurance coverage: *Medicare Part D* for "drugs" (Medicare Part A covers facility charges; the optional Part B covers professional fees).

Although congressional supporters lauded the landmark legislation by stating that elderly Americans should never have to choose between paying for necessary medications at the expense of foregoing other basic needs, critics claimed that the legislation still did not provide sufficient coverage and that the bill was an unaffordable, open-ended obligation. Still others felt that the legislation did not go far enough to cap drug expenses by driving pharmaceutical companies into hard bargains with the government for lower prices. Last and most notably, many elderly consumers were left anxious and confused by the discreditable "doughnut hole," a gap in coverage in the middle cost range of annual drug expenditures that would leave many enrollees no better off than they were before. Indeed, many potential enrollees were forced into running complex calculations to determine if the added Part D premium was worth the benefit coverage depending on their expected level of drug usage and whether or not they would fall within the doughnut hole, which would require either additional out-of-pocket expenses or additional private insurance coverage. To add to the agitation, in an effort to avoid adverse selection, the program mandated that those who did not enroll early on would face significantly higher premiums if they waited, forcing many into making hasty decisions. While these issues have not all been resolved, the program spotlighted the problems facing many citizens of the cost to stay healthy, and it has provided some relief.

Chronic Diseases

Chronic diseases are often associated with the elderly, but long-term ailments may affect younger segments of the population as well. Sometimes these diseases can be cured, but at other times, only treated. The acquired immunodeficiency syndrome, or AIDS, became widespread in the 1980s, and despite a number of new medications to market, remains incurable. Average lifetime AIDS treatment costs exceed $600,000.[5] Other diseases, such as diabetes, liver failure, and cancer, can also affect younger people, who may end up needing expensive treatments for a lifetime. Still other conditions, such as mental illness or debilitating back pain, are expensive to treat and costly in terms of lost productivity: for example, the average lifetime cost for a patient with mental retardation surpassed $1 million early this century.[6]

Compliance and Litigation

Three interrelated factors have greatly contributed to the rise in health care costs:

- *Compliance*, which is the need to comply with governmental regulations, whether they be for the provision of care, billing, privacy, security, accounting standards, or the like. A noteworthy example of extraordinary compliance costs would be the *Health Insurance Portability and Accountability Act,* or *HIPAA* (discussed below and described in more detail in Chapter Five)
- *Increased insurance premiums* that providers have to pay insurers to cover the cost of defending against lawsuits and paying large jury awards
- The increased use of *defensive medicine* by practitioners: excessive tests and procedures, oftentimes unnecessary care, simply to ensure that nothing be overlooked should a lawsuit ever arise. And once a patient has undergone a test or procedure, the provider is liable to be aware of and to follow up on all the results, even if the original services were unnecessary.

Partially because of concerns over access to health care services as a result of cost-control measures by insurers, the federal government enacted HIPAA in 1996. HIPAA was introduced to:

- Improve the portability and continuity of health insurance coverage
- Ensure confidentiality in health care information storage and retrieval
- Combat waste, fraud, and abuse in the health insurance and delivery systems
- Promote the use of medical savings accounts
- Improve access to long-term care
- Simplify the administration of health insurance.

Compliance became mandatory for all health care institutions by 2005. Although individual state regulations can override HIPAA regulations if they more strictly ensure access to and coverage for health

Compliance
The need to abide by governmental regulations, whether they be for the provision of care, billing, privacy, accounting standards, security, or the like.

Health Insurance Portability and Accountability Act (HIPAA)
A set of federal compliance regulations enacted in 1996 to ensure standardization of billing, privacy, and reporting as institutions convert to electronic systems.

Defensive Medicine
The tendency of health care practitioners to do more testing and to provide more care for patients than might otherwise be necessary to protect themselves against potential litigation.

Sarbanes-Oxley Act
Federal legislation designed to tighten accounting standards in financial reporting and that holds top executives personally liable as to the accuracy and fairness of their financial statements.

care services, HIPAA imposes minimum standards that must be met by all institutions doing business in any state.

In 2002 Congress passed the *Sarbanes-Oxley Act* to help stem the rising tide of fraudulent corporate disclosures and ensuing bankruptcies, which had left many employees out of a job and which, without warning, had left investors with little or nothing to show for their investments. While extensive in length, the act enforces several notable key components to help prevent similar events from reoccurring:

- The corporate officers signing the financial statements must attest to the validity of the statements and to that of the organization's internal control processes

- All "off-balance sheet" obligations and liabilities must be accurately and transparently reported

- Any significant changes to the organization's financial statements must immediately become publicly available information to investors and employees; the corporate officers can be subject to prison terms and fines for willfully altering or providing misleading documentation about the true financial health of the organization

Although it applies only to large publicly traded organizations, many health care providers are voluntarily complying with Sarbanes-Oxley because they feel it represents business practices that should be implemented in any case.

Stark Law
Legislation enacted by CMS in 2005 to guard against providers' ordering self-referrals for Medicare or Medicaid patients directly to any settings in which they have a vested financial interest. Also referred to as "anti-kickback" legislation.

In addition, in 2006 the Centers for Medicare and Medicaid Services (CMS) added to what are commonly known as the *Stark Law* and related safe harbors to the Anti-Kickback Act Regulation. In essence, these regulations prevent self-referrals of Medicare and Medicaid patients for services to any entity in which the ordering provider has a vested financial interest.

The cost effects of litigation by patients and their families on health care providers cannot be directly measured, but they are generally believed to be significant. On the one hand, patients have a right to expect a reasonable and safe level of care dictated by medical necessity, not by profit margins. On the other hand, the definition of "reasonable" care seems open to debate, especially on a case-by-case basis. Under ever-tightening reimbursement, providers are forced or encouraged to restrict potentially unnecessary tests while opening themselves up to possible legal battles.

The Uninsured

Between 2000 and 2007, the number of uninsured rose and hovered around 45 million (see Exhibit 1–7). The high level of uninsured is due to several factors, including (1) health insurance premiums becoming too costly for many individuals, even if they were working; (2) individuals being screened out of insurance policies because of "preexisting conditions"; (3) employers, feeling they cannot afford to continue to provide health insurance as a benefit, either scaling back their benefits or eliminating them altogether by hiring part-time rather than full-time workers; (4) due to budget restrictions, the federal government and the states tightening Medicaid eligibility criteria, typically to a level too far below the official federal poverty level for most families to qualify; and (5) individuals voluntarily deciding not to purchase insurance for a variety of financial and nonfinancial reasons, including the assumption that they will not need care or that they will be taken care of by the "system" anyway. This puts a tremendous burden on health care facilities, especially community hospitals, to continue to provide indigent care because they can no longer pass on their costs as readily to other payors via cost-shifting (see Exhibit 1–8).

Exhibit 1–7 Number of uninsured, 2000–2007

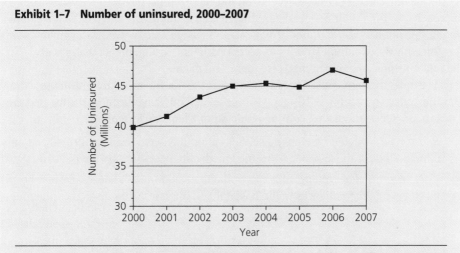

Source: U.S. Census Bureau, Current Population Survey, 2008, Annual Social and Economic Supplement.

Exhibit 1–8 Uncompensated care costs for the uninsured, 2000–2007

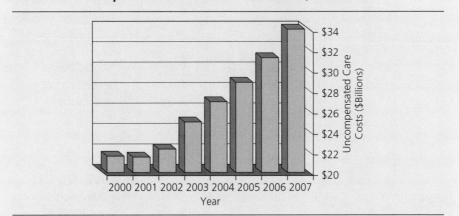

Source: Health Forum, American Hospital Association Annual Survey Data, 1980–2007 (November 2008).

EFFORTS TO CONTROL COSTS

Rising health care costs have had drastic consequences on the ability of providers to survive financially; hence, keen interest has been fostered by payors and providers to control this rise. Although the number of hospitals remains around 5,000, the number of surviving hospitals is significantly lower than it was two decades ago (see Exhibit 1–9). The following sections describe measures undertaken to control costs.

Efforts by Payors to Control Health Care Costs

Rising health care costs have forced private and public payors to try a variety of approaches to limit their financial risk. Increasingly, employers and payors have drawn on their position as the supplier of patients to manage care as well as payments. This has forced hospital administrators to accept payment arrangements that greatly affect the relationships among patients, providers, and payors.

The most commonly used methods by payors to control costs are introduced below and illustrated in Exhibit 1–10; many of these methods have been in use for decades. These approaches are discussed in more detail in Chapter Thirteen.

- *Retrospective review:* reviewing services after they have been performed and only reimbursing for those services deemed medically necessary by the payor
- *Concurrent review:* monitoring appropriateness and medical necessity of a hospital stay while the patient is in the hospital and implementing discharge planning

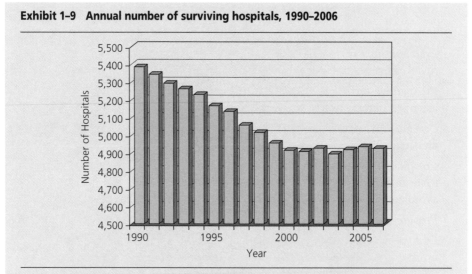

Exhibit 1–9 Annual number of surviving hospitals, 1990–2006

Source: Avalere Health Analysis of American Hospital Association Annual Survey Data, 2006, for Community Hospitals.

Exhibit 1–10   Selected methods implemented by payors to control costs

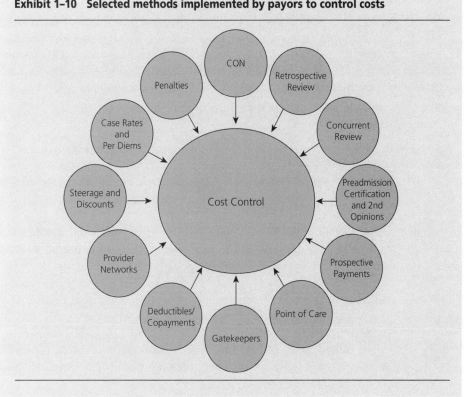

- *Preadmission certification and second opinions:* requiring prior approval or review of services to determine appropriateness of care
- *Prospective payments:* predetermining payments for services based on common use of resources for that service
- *Gatekeepers:* requiring a patient to obtain a referral from his or her primary care physician, the gatekeeper, before seeing a specialist
- *Certificate of need (CON):* requiring providers to have their capital expenditures (over a certain dollar amount) preapproved by an independent state agency to avoid unnecessary duplication of services (not implemented in all states)
- *Provider networks:* requiring a patient to select from a preapproved list of providers
- *Deductibles and copayments:* requiring patients to pay for part of their own care up to a given amount (deductible) or for a portion of each service they receive (copayment)
- *Steerage and discounts:* agreeing to send patients to providers in return for discounted services

- *Case rates and per diems:* setting reimbursement depending on the type of case (medical, surgical, maternity, etc.) or setting rates per inpatient day based on the type of case (per diems)

- *Penalties:* charging patients a penalty for seeking care outside the network without preapproval. Providers may also be penalized for not following managed care rules; such penalties include reducing or withholding incentive pay

- *Point of care:* allowing capitated patients to seek care outside the HMO for an increase in premium

Because of the enormity of their impact, two payment systems designed to control costs demand special attention: diagnosis-related groups (DRGs) and capitation. Other payment systems that have emerged, such as global payments, APCs, and pay-for-performance, are also discussed below.

Prospective Payment System (PPS)
The payment system used by Medicare to reimburse providers a predetermined amount. Several payment methods fall under the umbrella of PPS, including: DRGs (inpatient admissions), APCs (outpatient visits), resource-based relative value scale (RBRVS, professional services), and resource utilization groups (RUGs, skilled nursing home care). DRGs were the first category to fall under this type of predetermined payment arrangement.

DRGs In an effort to control Medicare inpatient costs, the Reagan administration introduced the *prospective payment* concept in 1984. Under this plan, the government created nearly 500 categories of illnesses called *diagnosis-related groups*, or DRGs, and reimbursed a fixed amount based on the patient's diagnosis. Since that time, DRGs have become more refined, and the total number is closer to 1,000; in addition, private payors using a DRG-based payment system have since added their own unique DRGs to include services typically not done on Medicare patients, such as obstetrics, neonatal, and pediatric care.

The goal of prospective payment was to shift the degree of responsibility to the provider to be more efficient because, with few exceptions (called *outliers*), the provider receives a fixed reimbursement for a patient in a particular DRG category, regardless of the services provided. Based on location, wage indices, and type of facility, providers receive a customized "weight" that affects the amount received, but the payment process remains the same across all institutions.

Several major problems arose from the DRG-based system, which led to searches for alternatives:

Reimbursement rates did not keep pace with health care inflation, which, despite having stabilized, has consistently exceeded the general rate of inflation, as noted earlier in this chapter. This trend caused some facilities to lose money on Medicare patients, which encouraged those facilities to steer Medicare patients to other providers.

Diagnosis-Related Groups (DRGs)
A system to classify inpatients based on their diagnoses, used by both Medicare and private insurers. In the most pervasive system, there are approximately 1,000 different diagnostic categories.

Providers began to engage in what became known as "DRG creep," a noticeable (possibly illegal) trend toward patients' being placed into higher-paying DRGs. This led to increased costs.

Many hospitals find fixed reimbursements to be inconvenient. For example, a patient is admitted for pneumonia, but during the patient's stay, the hospital discovers audiological-related problems. If the hospital performs audiologic services during the patient's inpatient stay (which would be convenient), the hospital would not get additional reimbursement for those services because the reimbursement amount is based only on the patient's principal diagnosis: pneumonia. To get compensated for audiologic services, the hospital must discharge the patient and then bring him or her back to the hospital later as an outpatient, which has a different and separate payment mechanism.

Capitation One of the alternative methods to control costs is *capitation*, whereby the provider receives a set payment to provide health care services to a population for a defined period. This type of engagement works best with large populations, sometimes referred to as *risk pools*, whereby risk can be spread out and managed better. Typically, the payment rate is set on a per member per month (PMPM) basis. Under this type of arrangement, the provider receives a fixed amount of money at the beginning of each month (based on the number of enrollees) and agrees to provide all covered services necessary for those enrollees during that month. Although there are various arrangements to limit financial risk, under a completely capitated arrangement, the burden of cost containment rests entirely on the provider.

Global Payments Under most of today's payment systems, each provider is paid separately. Under a *global payment* system, a single price is agreed on for several providers as a unit (i.e., the hospital, physicians, home health agency, etc.), who have bid a set price for a contract. Payors reduce risk by knowing in advance the amount that they will have to pay. Providers, on the other hand, are able to keep the profit if they can provide all services for less than the negotiated global payment. However, they are at risk for any loss. A particularly interesting problem arises in how the providing parties decide to split any profits or losses on the contract. Global pricing tends to increase the need for providers to cooperate and the need to scrutinize practice patterns. Regardless, it can be highly susceptible to unusually complicated or high-cost patients (outliers).

APCs APCs, or ambulatory payment classifications (referred to earlier), are similar to and based on the same concept as DRGs, but fixed amounts are reimbursed for bundled hospital-based outpatient services rather than for inpatient services. Implemented in 2000 as part of the Balanced Budget Act of 1997 (but modified according to the Balanced Budget

Capitation
A system that pays providers a specific amount in advance to care for defined health care needs of a population over a specific period. Providers are usually paid on a per member per month (PMPM) basis. The provider then assumes the risk that the cost of caring for the population will not exceed the aggregate PMPM amount received.

Risk Pools
A generally large population of individuals who are all insured under the same arrangement, regardless of working status. Health care utilization—and therefore cost—is more stable for larger groups than it is for smaller groups, which makes larger groups' costs more predictable for insurers and thus less of a risk.

Global Payments
A system to pay providers whereby the fees for all providers (i.e., hospitals, physicians, home health care agencies) are included in a single negotiated amount. This is sometimes called "bundling" of services. In non-global payment systems, each provider is paid separately.

Refinement Act of 1999), APCs were an effort by the government to control rising out-patient costs. With few exceptions, nearly all outpatient services and supplies are categorized into groupings, each with a fixed reimbursement based on a hospital's wage index. After a number of years' experience, APCs are now being extended into new areas, including imaging and emergency services.

Pay for Performance (P4P)
A recently instituted alternative payment arrangement that bases partial reimbursement creates additional reimbursement incentives, or both, for providers based on adherence to predefined standards for quality of care. Indicators include various patient outcomes and frequency and type of tests ordered and services performed.

Pay-for-Performance Insurers, including Medicare, have started to devise methods to tie pay into performance based on predetermined sets of quality-of-care-based indicators. Commonly referred to as *P4P* or pay-for-performance, the program does not simply withhold payments if performance criteria are not met, but rather creates financial incentives for providers to follow care guidelines and established treatment protocols so as to encourage preventive care, reduce unnecessary tests, prevent mistakes, and prevent unnecessary visits and re-hospitalizations. By creating a reward system in the early treatment of patients, the program hopes to avoid more costly expenditures later.

In addition, through P4P, providers have been encouraged to publicly report quality and outcomes data to lead to more personal accountability and to provide consumers a better opportunity to make informed choices about the quality and necessity of care that they receive. The Leapfrog Group, based in Washington, D.C., has taken a lead role in the P4P effort by providing a rewards-based program to voluntary participants who can demonstrate improved treatment methods.

Last, given increased access to better information through the Internet, consumers have taken advantage of other related online initiatives underway to grade the performance of providers. For example, data are available on morbidity and mortality rates for hospital-based procedures, while other Web sites, such as HealthGrades, incorporate consumer survey results from past patient experiences to use as a guide for expected care for the new patient. In brief, all of these initiatives including P4P serve to increase provider accountability and consumer awareness and are intended to lead to better and less-expensive patient care outcomes.

Cutting Delivery Costs

Faced with restrictions on payments, providers have become increasingly concerned with controlling costs. Some of the major trends that have resulted are the shift to outpatient services, new cost-accounting systems, improved information services technology, mergers and acquisitions, and reengineering or redesign.

Shift to Outpatient Services Many hospitals are offering an increasing number of services on an outpatient basis that have traditionally been performed on an inpatient basis, especially surgical services. In fact, a hospital today commonly performs more than half of all of its surgical cases on an outpatient basis, and stand-alone outpatient surgical centers have become commonplace. This has caused problems, however, for many hospitals that were primarily designed to provide inpatient surgical services, including inadequate preoperative and postoperative holding areas for extended time periods; inefficient processes for preoperative workup testing, as outpatients must find their own way to various departments throughout the hospital, such as labs and x-ray departments; and inefficient operating room operations because hospitals must rely on outpatients to arrive at the hospital on time in the early morning, instead of retrieving patients from their inpatient beds when requested. Other less-invasive outpatient procedures still have many of the same problems. This shift to outpatient services has forced hospitals to invest in facility enhancements to accommodate their changing needs, and many hospitals find themselves in a bind for funds as well as space.

Cost-Accounting Systems Many hospital accounting systems have a strong billing and collections component but a weak cost-accounting system. In fact, this is due in large part to the history of reimbursement. Financial incentives typically were in place to maximize reimbursement, not to control costs. Now that the environment has changed, providers have found it increasingly important to know their precise costs. As a result, there has been a major movement to separate cost-accounting systems from financial accounting systems and to move away from traditional allocation-based cost systems to activity-based cost systems (discussed in more depth in Chapter Twelve). Although an expensive endeavor, declining reimbursement is forcing hospitals to invest in more sophisticated cost-accounting systems.

Information Services Technology With the rapid advances in computer hardware and software applications, many institutions have invested in the information technologies in an effort to receive the most accurate information as quickly as possible. Most applications revolve around materials management, budgeting, accounts payable, payroll, patient registration, and human resource needs. It is essential for institutions to track the flow of materials through their organizations and to purchase and pay for supplies in the most cost-effective manner. Hospitals can keep funds longer and reduce inventory costs by incorporating "just-in-time" ordering techniques, and there is opportunity for cost savings by joining *group purchasing organizations (GPOs)* that can negotiate cost discounts through large volumes. If organizations can follow the flow of materials through their organization, they can better track costs and have better reporting and control over their budgets.

Group Purchasing Organizations (GPOs) Third-party entities that contract with multiple hospitals to offer cost savings in the purchase of supplies and equipment by negotiating large-volume discounted contracts with vendors.

Computerization of medical records and information security is also an evolving field requiring significant investments. Institutions are aware of the inefficiencies of trying to manually maintain paper records, and they will likely be forced by competition and by the federal government to resort to electronic systems. In conjunction with this notion come investments in telemedicine, the ability to perform services from a distance. Presumably, all these advancements are designed to save costs and to lead to better provision of services, but will involve investing many millions of dollars.

An *electronic health record* (EHR), or electronic medical record (EMR), is an electronic capture of all of a patient's encounters and health information over an extended period. These data may include patient demographics, past medical and immunization history, summary dictations and progress notes, laboratory and radiology results, and a medication history. This measure is intended not only to eliminate paper and create a more permanent and secure depository of information, but also to enable care providers from any location to access the information in a controlled environment on an as-needed basis for a mobile patient.

However, although these information technology advances are potentially time-saving and cost-saving enterprises, such ready access to information could lead to the temptation for personal financial gain. The availability of information in online electronic format has heightened the need for information security, as discussed in other sections of this introductory chapter.

Mergers and Acquisitions Many facilities have invested heavily in mergers and acquisitions under the premise that consolidation of services reduces costs. An acquisition could be as small as acquiring a physician group practice or as large as merging all the health care institutions in a specific market area. The financial impact of such measures can be tremendous, and health care professionals must have a keen understanding of the local markets and organizational cultures before engaging in such practices. Oftentimes mergers fail or lose money, such as the breakup of Stanford and the University of California, San Francisco, medical centers in San Francisco. Other acquisitions may be done inappropriately, which could result in forced breakups and penalties.

Reengineering or Redesign As a major measure to cut costs in the past decade and to operate more effectively and efficiently, facilities have been redesigning their work processes. Common techniques include: process analysis, layout redesign, work redesign, total quality management, *care mapping*, and layoff of unnecessary personnel.

One such method that has gained widespread attention is Six Sigma, including the related concept of Lean Sigma, which offers a systematic approach toward analysis and performance improvement. The five major components to the Six Sigma approach include define, measure, analyze, improve, and control, nicknamed DMAIC.

Alternative Forms of Care There is a large and growing movement toward complementary and alternative medicine, which has numerous roots, strong supporters, and strong detractors. As noted in Wikipedia, there is little agreement on even what constitutes alternative medicine, though Wikipedia begins by stating:

> The term *alternative medicine*, as used in the modern western world, encompasses any healing practice "that does not fall within the realm of conventional medicine." Commonly cited examples include naturopathy, chiropractic, herbalism, traditional Chinese medicine, Avurveda, meditation, yoga, biofeedback, hypnosis, homeopathy, acupuncture, and diet-based therapies, in addition to a range of other practices. It is frequently grouped with *complementary medicine*, which generally refers to the same interventions when used in conjunction with mainstream techniques, under the umbrella term *complementary and alternative medicine*, or CAM. Some significant researchers in alternative medicine oppose this grouping, preferring to emphasize differences of approach, but nevertheless use the term CAM, which has become standard
>
> Alternative medicine practices are as diverse in their foundations as in their methodologies. Practices may incorporate or base themselves on traditional medicine, folk knowledge, spiritual beliefs, or newly conceived approaches to healing.[7]

In an interesting development, a number of alternative approaches are now reimbursed by third parties.

Retail Health Care

Doctors' offices and hospitals are no longer the only setting where health care services are being provided. Given the tendency of consumers to use shopping malls, various retail outlets such as Wal-Mart, which already had been providing pharmacy services for years, have expanded by offering basic preventive health care services in some of their stores. These *retail health care* outlets hire licensed professionals, such as nurse practitioners, to offer flu shots and provide remedies for minor ailments like a sore throat and the common cold. These services tend to be popular among less-affluent and immigrant consumers, in part because the setting is familiar, it can be more accessible than a doctor's office, these patients may not have a personal physician, and the cost tends to be low because startup and operational costs to run such programs are minimal. The retailers also reap additional benefits by providing patients with convenient purchase options for medications there at the store. Critics, however, raise questions about quality of services provided.

Retail Health Care
Walk-in medical services provided in a retail outlet, such as a pharmacy, by a licensed care provider.

Medical Tourism
Patients who travel
to foreign countries to
obtain medical services
at a steep discount.
Even including a family
escort, who get the
added benefit of
foreign travel, the total
cost may be less than
what it would be at
home.

Medical Tourism

For years consumers have been traveling to neighboring countries like Canada and Mexico to purchase medications at lower rates than at home. To no surprise, then, consumers have started looking elsewhere for alternatives to more expensive and elaborate care, such as invasive procedures. Countries like India, Thailand, Brazil, and even Costa Rica, particularly where the dollar is strong, now host patients in a multibillion-dollar-a-year industry dubbed *medical tourism*. The cost to do an invasive procedure elsewhere can be as much as 80 percent less than that in the United States, and the patient and family member(s) may get the added benefit of a trip to a tourist destination for less than what it would cost to have the procedure done at home. Though foreign hospitals are increasingly seeking certification to U.S. standards, a number of critics continue to raise questions about potential risks.

Medical Home
A partnership between
primary care providers
(PCPs), patients, and
their families to deliver
comprehensive care
over the long-term in a
variety of settings.

Medical Home

Although the term may be considered somewhat of a misnomer, the *medical home* is a partnership between primary care providers (PCPs), the patients, and their families to deliver a coordinated and comprehensive range of services in all appropriate settings. The PCP takes full responsibility for the overall care of the patient from infancy into adulthood, including preventive care, acute and chronic care, and end-of-life support. The program is a patient-centered model using evidence-based medicine, care pathways, the latest in information technology, voluntary performance results, and open discussions to ensure the best possible care that is both necessary and understood.

COST CONTROL ISSUES WITH ETHICAL OVERTONES

Given the myriad efforts to control costs, health care administrators are increasingly faced with ethical dilemmas trying to balance cost with quality and access. Numerous studies have found a direct correlation among income, access, and health status. Administrators must keep in mind that they do not produce widgets but rather an essential service, often to vulnerable populations. There are literally hundreds of questions with ethical overtones that arise because of pressures to cut costs. The following are among the most common:

- How to control costs without cutting quality
- How to control costs, yet expand access to services, especially in remote or inner-city areas
- How to control costs and provide services to those who cannot pay
- How to control costs but offer expensive treatments to special populations, such as the terminally ill or premature infants

- How to control costs and still offer services that are typically reimbursed below cost, such as certain types of transplants or other special surgical procedures
- How to control costs and not over-restrict the use of specialty care
- How to ration health care services based on medical effectiveness
- How to weigh societal benefits against individual benefits when resources are limited.

In an effort to balance competing interests, financial and nonfinancial, some institutions have implemented a "balanced scorecard" approach. The actual measurements may vary across organizations, but the typical categories include finance (revenue and expense statistics), operations (clinical processes), community needs (patient and physician satisfaction), and employees (training, turnover).

SUMMARY

The health care administrator today and in the future will be faced with numerous complex issues to consider while making financial decisions. Many factors have led to the rise in health care costs: an aging population, increasingly "high-tech" care, prescription drug costs, chronic illnesses, compliance, legal concerns, and the ever-rising number of uninsured patients. Numerous efforts have been made to counter this rise: changes in reimbursement and shifting of risk to the providers, a shift toward greater use of outpatient services and shorter inpatient stays, more efficient administrative technologies, mergers and acquisitions, and redesign and reengineering of services in general. But the administrator must constantly maintain a high ethical standard in all decisions, not only for the obvious health and financial impacts, but also for myriad personal, professional, community, and societal implications.

The remainder of this text focuses on health care financial management topics such as how to analyze financial statements, manage internal funds, make sound business investments, borrow funds, analyze costs, and prepare a budget. It also provides more in-depth analyses of how regulations and restrictions affect how health care institutions must operate. Although this knowledge is essential in the financial decision-making process, health care administrators always need to carefully weigh nonfinancial factors as well.

KEY TERMS

a. Ambulatory payment classifications (APCs)
b. Capitation
c. Care mapping
d. Compliance

e. Cost-shifting
f. Defensive medicine
g. Diagnosis-related groups (DRGs)
h. Electronic health record (EHR)
i. Global payments

j. Group purchasing organizations (GPOs)
k. Health Insurance Portability and Accountability Act (HIPAA)
l. Medical home
m. Medical tourism
n. Medicare Part D
o. Pay-for-performance (P4P)
p. Prospective payment system
q. Retail health care
r. Risk pools
s. Sarbanes-Oxley Act
t. Stark Law

QUESTIONS

1. **Definitions.** Define the terms listed on the previous page and above.

2. **Increased Costs.** List several factors that have led to the rise in increased costs.

3. **Cost Control.** List several efforts that have been enacted by payors to control costs.

4. **Cost Control.** List several efforts that have been attempted by providers to control costs.

5. **Ethics.** What are some of the ethical issues that must be considered when making any financial decisions?

6. **Capitation.** Explain how and to whom capitation shifts the burden of risk.

7. **Litigation.** Explain the ramifications of allowing or disallowing an individual to be able to sue his or her HMO.

8. **Drugs.** Is the granting of patents good for the development of new drugs? Why or why not?

9. **Ethics.** If an uninsured individual needed expensive medical treatment and did not have the means to pay for it, should the treatment be provided? Would the answer be influenced by the financial status of the institution asked to provide the service? Would the answer be any different if the individual were uninsured voluntarily (e.g., "I'll take my chances and hope nothing happens") or involuntarily (e.g., "It's either health insurance or food for my children")?

10. **Ethics.** Should private for-profit institutions be forced to accept patients who will not reimburse satisfactorily? Why or why not?

NOTES

1. Personal health care expenditures, by source of funds: selected calendar years 1960–2007. *Health Care Financing Review*, 2008 statistical supplement.

2. *National Vital Statistics Reports*, Apr. 24, 2008, 56(10).

3. The MetLife Market Survey of Nursing Home & Home Care Costs, MetLife Mature Market Institute® in conjunction with LifePlans, Inc., Sept. 2006.

4. National Health Expenditure Data (http://www.cms.hhs.gov/NationalHealth ExpendData/downloads/nhe2007.zip), Centers for Medicare and Medicaid Services, January 2009.

5. Schackman, B. R., Gebo, K. A., Walensky, R. P., Losina, E., Muccio, T., Sax, P. E., Weinstein, M. C., Seage, G. R. 3rd, Moore, R. D., Freedberg, K. A. 2006 (Nov.). The lifetime cost of current human immunodeficiency virus care in the United States. *Medical Care 44*(11):990–997.

6. Centers for Disease Control and Prevention. 2004. Economic costs associated with mental retardation, cerebral palsy, hearing loss, and vision impairment— United States, 2003. *Mortality and Morbidity Weekly Report 53*:57–59.

7. Wikipedia: Alternative medicine (http://en.wikipedia.org/wiki/Alternative_ medicine). Date of access: Jan. 25, 2009.

2

HEALTH CARE FINANCIAL STATEMENTS

LEARNING OBJECTIVES

- Identify the four basic financial statements common to all organizations
- Identify and read the four basic financial statements particular to not-for-profit, business-oriented health care organizations: the balance sheet, the statement of operations, the statement of changes in net assets, and the statement of cash flows

Creditors, investors, and governmental and community agencies often require considerable information to make judgments about the financial performance of health care organizations. For instance, to decide whether to lend money to a home health agency, a lender may want to know how much debt the agency already has, how much cash it has available, and how much profit it is earning. Similarly, to make regulatory decisions, a governmental agency may want to know how much charity care is being offered or what the profit margin is for a group of providers. So that standardized financial information needed by outside parties is regularly available, almost all businesses are required to produce four financial statements at least annually.

■   Balance Sheet

■   Income Statement (or Statement of Operations)

■   Statement of Changes in Owners' Equity (or Statement of Changes in Net Assets)

■   Statement of Cash Flows

As shown in Perspectives 2–1 and 2–2, the financial statements are of interest not only internally, but also may be of general interest to outside parties. Although

Perspective 2–1   Strong Financials Result in Health Care System Credit Upgrade by Bond Rating Agencies

Trinity Healthcare System issued over $2.1 billion of outstanding debt and has issued roughly $200 million of long-term debt every year since the health care system was started in 2000. Fitch Ratings and Moody's Investors Services enhanced Trinity Healthcare System's credit rating, the fourth largest Catholic health care system in the country, to double-A in late 2007. In addition, Standard & Poor's raised its credit rating to AA from AA-minus in late 2007. Several factors contributed to the upgrade, ranging from a strong balance sheet, increased earnings, and a strong management team as well as a growing community benefit ministry.

Standard & Poor's also upgraded its taxable commercial paper to A1-plus—its highest short-term debt rating—from which Trinity plans to issue $150 million of commercial paper in 2008 to finance its working capital and other liquidity needs. The higher rating is validated by Trinity's higher operating cash flow margins of about 12 percent and its lower debt leverage of 31 percent. This access to debt capital helped finance over $2.4 billion in capital expenditures over the last five years. Future capital expenditures are projected to be $950 million a year for the next five years to help renovate and upgrade its hospitals over 29 states.

Source: Devitt, C. 2007. Michigan's bond-happy Trinity health gets another upgrade bond buyer. *New York Times* (Dec. 18), 362(32780): 4.

Perspective 2–2   Health Plans in Massachusetts Post Net Income but Incur Operating Losses

In June of 2007, three of the four largest health maintenance organizations (HMOs) in Massachusetts incurred operating losses. The underlying cause for these losses was higher medical costs. Fallon Community Health Plan incurred an operating loss of $3.2 million; however, $2 million in investment income did help reduce this loss. Fallon claimed that higher utilization rates for medical care, increased prescription drug costs, and rising inpatient hospital expenses were the underlying reasons for this poor performance. The health plan expects to manage its rising medical costs by making infrastructure investments that should enhance administrative efficiencies while expanding its service area and provider network.

Blue Cross and Blue Shield of Massachusetts HMO Blue Inc., the state's largest HMO, listed net income of $13.9 million; however, from operations, the plan incurred an operating loss of $9.2 million. The health plan's ability to earn positive returns from its investment enabled the health plan to generate a positive bottom line for the quarter. Higher claims were a contributing factor to this net loss position. Finally, Harvard Pilgrim Health Plan reported $700,000 of net income on revenues of $622 million for the second quarter. Similar to the previous plans, Harvard Pilgrim listed an operating loss of $7.6 million, which was offset by investment income of $8.3 million. Going forward, the Massachusetts Division of Insurance would pay closer attention to their financial condition.

Source: Kievra, B. 2007., "3 state HMOs seeing red in 2nd Q; Fallon, HMO Blue, Harvard post losses. *Telegram and Gazette* (Aug 16), Worcester, Mass.

the general format of these statements remains the same, they are often modified to reflect the idiosyncrasies of particular industries (e.g., transportation, energy, health care). In health care, four additional subsets of rules apply, depending on the type of organization: governmental entities; not-for-profit, business-oriented organizations; not-for-profit, non-business-oriented organizations; and investor owned. The focus of this text is primarily not-for-profit, business-oriented health care organizations, which are referred to hereafter as *not-for-profit health care organizations*. Other types of organizations have a high degree of overlap with the material presented here.

Exhibit 2–1 presents a comparison of the basic financial statements used by investor-owned and not-for-profit health care organizations.

The remainder of this chapter discusses the financial statements and terms used by health care organizations. A complete set of the financial statements discussed in

---

Exhibit 2–1   A comparison of generally used financial statements for investor-owned and not-for-profit health care organizations

Financial Statements Used by Investor-Owned Health Care Organizations	Financial Statements Used by Not-for-Profit Health Care Organizations
Balance sheet	Balance sheet
Income statement	Statement of operations
Statement of changes in owners' equity	Statement of changes in net assets
Statement of cash flows	Statement of cash flows

---

this chapter can be found in Appendix A, adapted from the American Institute of Certified Public Accountants' Audit and Accounting Guide: Health Care Organizations, 2007.

THE BALANCE SHEET

The balance sheet of investor-owned organizations presents a summary of the organization's assets, liabilities, and shareholders' equity (see Exhibit 2–2). Similarly, the balance sheet of a not-for-profit health care organization presents a summary of the organization's assets, liabilities, and net assets. (These terms and the relationship among them will be discussed in more detail shortly.) The balance sheet is similar to a snapshot of the organization, for it captures what the organization looks like *at a particular point in time*, usually the last day of the accounting period (i.e., quarter, half-year, fiscal year). Exhibit 2–3 presents an illustration of a balance sheet and serves as an overview of this section of the text.

As with all four financial statements, the balance sheet is organized into three major sections: heading, body, and notes (see Exhibit 2–2). At the top of the balance sheet (and each of the other financial statements) is a three-line *heading* that includes the name of the organization, the name of the statement, and two dates.

The *name of the organization* is important because it provides the reader with the name of the specific entity being summarized. This is not as trivial as it might seem. One health care organization may produce financial statements for more than one entity, depending on the degree of control, economic interest, or both. For example, a hospital may produce its own balance sheet or it may be included with other affiliated entities (e.g., managed care, outpatient services, home health). If more than one entity is being summarized, then the report is called a *consolidated* or *combined* balance sheet, and the names of the entities being summarized are in the notes.

Exhibit 2–2 Overview of the balance sheet sections of investor-owned and not-for-profit health care organizations

Heading	Name of Investor-Owned Organization Balance Sheet Dates	Name of Not-for-Profit Organization Balance Sheet Dates
Body	**Assets**	**Assets**
	Current assets	Current assets
	Noncurrent assets	Noncurrent assets
	Total assets	*Total assets*
	Liabilities	**Liabilities**
	Current liabilities	Current liabilities
	Noncurrent liabilities	Noncurrent liabilities
	Total liabilities	*Total liabilities*
	Shareholders' equity[a]	**Net assets**[a]
	Common stock	Unrestricted
	Retained earnings	Temporarily restricted
	Total shareholders' equity	Permanently restricted
	Total liabilities and shareholders' equity	*Total net assets*
		Total liabilities and net assets
Notes	Key pertinent information including:	Key pertinent information including:
	• Accounting policies	• Accounting policies
	• Payment arrangements with third parties	• Payment arrangements with third parties
	• Asset restrictions	• Asset restrictions
	• Property and equipment	• Property and equipment
	• Long-term debt	• Long-term debt
	• Pension obligations	• Pension obligations

[a]A major difference between the balance sheet of an investor-owned and a not-for-profit health care organization is in the owners' equity section. In an investor-owned organization, the section is organized to show the shareholders' ownership stake in the corporation. In a not-for-profit health care organization, the section is termed *net assets* and is organized to show the degree of donor restriction on the assets.

Below the name of the organization, the term *Balance Sheet* appears in the heading to differentiate it from the other financial statements. Finally, two *dates* are shown. As mentioned earlier, the balance sheet reports what the organization looks like *at a particular point in time*, usually the last day of the accounting period (i.e., quarter,

Exhibit 2-3 Annotated balance sheet for Sample Not-For-Profit Hospital (in thousands)

The balance sheet provides a snapshot of the organization's assets, liabilities and net assets as of a point in time.

1 **Title:** Gives the name of the organization, the name of the financial statement, and two dates for which the information is being provided.

2 **Assets:** The resources of the organizations which are eventually used to provide service and generate revenues.

3 **Current assets:** Assets which will be used or consumed within a year.
- **Cash and cash equivalents:** Coin, currency and checks held within the organization or in financial institutions such as banks.
- **Short-term investments:** Temporary investment accounts which allow the organization to earn interest and have ready access to cash.
- **Assets limited as to use:** The current portion of monies set aside for specific purposes, such as to insure debt repayment.
- **Patient accounts receivable net of estimated uncollectibles:** Money owed to the organization as a result of delivering service to patients, less an estimate of how much will not be collected.
  Uncollectibles: The amount owed to the organization which it expects it will probably not ever receive.
- **Other current assets:** A summary category which may contain smaller accounts.
  Inventory: The supplies used to run the organization and provide services.
  Prepaid expenses: Amounts the organization has paid in advance, such as rent, and insurance.

4 **Non-current assets:** Assets which will benefit the organization for periods longer than a year, such as major equipment and buildings.
- **Assets limited as to use:** Monies set aside for specific purposes such as to ensure debt repayment, less the amount needed this accounting period.
- **Long-term investments:** Investments, such as stocks, bonds and land, which the organization expects to realize a profit from over a period longer than one year.
- **Property and equipment, net:** The buildings and machinery (e.g., x-ray machine) of the organization, less the amount it has been depreciated ("used up") to date, called *accumulated depreciation*

Total assets: The sum of current and non-current assets.

5 **Liabilities:** The financial obligations of the organization to pay its creditors.
Current liabilities: The financial obligations which must be paid within one year.
- **Current portion of long-term debt:** That portion of multi-year debt which is due this year.
- **Accounts payable and accrued expenses:** Amounts due this year to suppliers, employees, and others for goods and services which have been received but not yet paid for.
- **Estimated third-party payor settlements:** An estimate of the amount which must be returned to third parties for overpayment of claims.
- **Other:** All other current liabilities not listed above. A major component may be *deferred revenue:* Money that has been received, but not yet earned (e.g., money received in advance from managed care organizations; it will be earned as time passes).

6 **Non-current liabilities:** The financial obligations which must be paid-off over a time period longer than one year (e.g. a capital leases).
- **Long-term debt, net of current portion:** The amount of multi-year debt due in future years.

7 **Net assets:** Assets - Liabilities. This section has traditionally been called *Stockholders' Equity* in investor-owned organizations and *Fund Balance* in not-for-profit organizations.
- **Unrestricted net assets:** The amount of the net assets which have no outside restrictions on them.
- **Temporarily restricted net assets:** Assets which have restrictions on their use which will be removed either with the passage of time or the occurrence of some event.
- **Permanently restricted net assets:** Assets which have restrictions on their use which will not be removed.

*An unannotated form of this statement can be found in Appendix A of this chapter.

Source: Reprinted with permission from the *Audit and Accounting Guide: Health Care Organizations*, copyright © 2007 by the American Institute of Certified Public Accountants, Inc.

Sample Not-For Profit Hospital
Balance Sheet
December 31, 20X1 and 20X0 (in '000)

	20X1	20X0
② Assets		
③ Current assets:		
Cash and cash equivalents	$4,758	$5,877
Short-term investments	15,836	10,740
Assets limited as to use	970	1,300
Patient accounts receivable, net estimated uncollectibles of $2,500 in 20X1 and $2,400 in 20X0	15,100	14,194
Supplies	2,000	2,000
Prepaid expenses	670	865
Total current assets	39,334	34,967
④ Non-current assets		
Assets limited as to use	18,949	19,841
Less amount required to meet current obligations	(970)	(1,300)
	17,979	18,541
Long-term investments	4,680	4,680
Long-term investments restricted for capital acquisition	320	520
Properties and equipment, net	51,038	50,492
Other assets	1,695	1,370
Total non-current assets	75,712	75,603
Total assets	$115,046	$110,570
⑤ Liabilities and net assets		
current liabilities		
Current portion of long-term debt	$1,470	$1,750
Accounts payable and accrued expenses	5,818	5,382
Estimated third-party payor settlements	2,143	1,942
Deferred revenues	1,969	2,114
Total current liabilities	11,400	11,188
⑥ Non-current liabilities		
Long-term debt, net of current portion	23,144	24,014
Other	3,953	3,166
Total non-current liabilities	27,097	27,180
Total liabilities	38,497	38,368
⑦ Net assets		
Unrestricted	70,846	66,199
Temporarily restricted	2,115	2,470
Permanently restricted	3,588	3,533
Total net assets	76,549	72,202
Total liabilities and net assets	$115,046	$110,570

half-year, fiscal year). Two dates are often shown so that the reader can compare two successive periods. This is called a comparative balance sheet.

 Key Point *The balance sheet reports what the organization's assets, liabilities, and equity are as of* a particular point in time, *usually the last day of the accounting period (i.e., quarter, half-year, fiscal year).*

The three major sections comprising the body of the balance sheet are *assets, liabilities,* and net assets (Exhibits 2–2 and 2–3). The balance sheet derives its name from the fact that the assets always equal the sum of the liabilities plus the owners' equity (called *shareholders' equity* in investor-owned health care organizations and *net assets* in not-for-profit health care organizations). The relationship among the three major sections of the balance sheet is expressed by the *basic accounting equation*:

$$\text{Assets} = \text{Liabilities} + \text{Owners' Equity}$$

In investor-owned organizations, the equation becomes:

$$\text{Assets} = \text{Liabilities} + \text{Shareholders' Equity}$$

In not-for-profit, business-oriented health care organizations, the equation becomes:

$$\text{Assets} = \text{Liabilities} + \text{Net Assets}$$

In Exhibit 2–3 for the year 20X1, the assets equal $115,046,000, and the liabilities plus the net assets also equal $115,046,000 ($38,497,000 plus $76,549,000). Incidentally, until mid-1996, not-for-profit health care organizations used the term *fund balance* instead of *net assets*, while governmental organizations such as states, cities, and local counties continue to use fund accounting.

Assets

The assets of an organization are the resources it owns. Assets are divided into two categories, current assets and noncurrent assets (see Exhibit 2–4).

Current Assets Current assets are assets that will be used or consumed within one year (see Exhibit 2–4). They help turn the capacity of the organization (i.e., buildings and equipment) into service. Current assets include:

■ Cash and cash equivalents

■ Short-term investments

Assets
Resources that the organization owns, typically recorded at their original costs.

Liabilities
The financial obligations of the organization (i.e., debts).

Net Assets
The difference between an organization's assets and liabilities (assets *minus* liabilities).

Basic Accounting Equation
Assets = Liabilities + Net Assets.

Fund Balance
A term used until 1996 for owners' equity by not-for-profit health care organizations. It was replaced with the current term, *net assets*, for nongovernmental, not-for-profit organizations.

Exhibit 2–4 Asset section of the balance sheet from Exhibit 2–3 with an emphasis on current assets (in thousands)

Assets	20X1	20X0
Current assets		
Cash and cash equivalents	$4,758	$5,877
Short-term investments	15,836	10,740
Assets limited as to use	970	1,300
Patient accounts receivable, net estimated uncollectibles	15,100	14,194
of $2,500 in 20X1 and $2,400 in 20X0		
Supplies	2,000	2,000
Prepaid expenses	670	856
Total current assets	39,334	34,967
Noncurrent assets		
Assets limited as to use	18,949	19,841
Less amount required to meet current obligations	(970)	(1,300)
	17,979	18,541
Long-term investments	4,680	4,680
Long-term investments restricted for capital acquisition	320	520
Properties and equipment, net	51,038	50,492
Other assets	1,695	1,370
Total noncurrent assets	75,712	75,603
Total assets	$115,046	$110,570

Source: Reprinted with permission from the *Audit and Accounting Guide: Health Care Organizations*, copyright © 2007 by the American Institute of Certified Public Accountants, Inc.

- Assets limited as to use
- Patient accounts receivable, net of estimated uncollectibles
- Supplies, prepaid expenses, and other current assets

Liquidity
A measure of how quickly an asset can be converted into cash.

How quickly an asset can be turned into cash is called its *liquidity*, and current assets are always listed in the order noted, which is based on their relative liquidity in the general business world. Although this order generally reflects the liquidity of many non-health care providers, a number of health care providers find that their patient accounts receivable (the money owed to them for services rendered to patients) is their least liquid current asset. Still, by convention, this generally accepted order is followed in the listing of current assets.

Because of their liquidity, current assets require special internal control procedures to ensure that they are handled appropriately and efficiently. For instance, a generally accepted internal control procedure in health care organizations is to have different people send out the bills, open the incoming mail, and record payments—a procedure that, if not followed, lends itself to considerable opportunities for mishandling of funds. Another internal control procedure is to restrict access to supplies and medicines. This leads to a discussion of each of the current asset accounts.

Cash and Cash Equivalents Cash and cash equivalents are the most liquid current assets (see Exhibit 2–4). This account is composed of actual money on hand as well as money equivalents, such as savings and checking accounts. It excludes cash that has restrictions regarding withdrawal or for use for other than current operations.

Key Point *Cash (or cash equivalents) is the most liquid asset on the balance sheet.*

Short-Term Investments Short-term investments include certificates of deposit, commercial paper, and treasury bills. These temporary investment accounts allow a health care facility to earn interest on idle cash and, at the same time, provide almost immediate access to cash for unexpected situations. Short-term investments are discussed in greater detail in Chapter Five.

Assets Limited as to Use The cash and short-term investments listed above in the current assets section are generally available for management to use to carry out its duties. In addition, a health care organization may have other cash, marketable securities, or other current assets that can be used only under special conditions. For example, in taking out a loan, a health care organization may agree to set aside an amount of funds equal to six months' worth of loan payments. Current assets that fall into this category are classified as *assets limited as to use* (see Exhibit 2–4). The assets limited as to use accounts for Sample Not-For-Profit Hospital's current assets are $1,300,000 in 20X0 and $970,000 in 20X1.

Patient Accounts Receivable, Net of Estimated Uncollectibles Gross *patient accounts receivable* is the amount owed the health care organization at full charges. However, many payors, such as Medicaid, insurance companies, large employers, and managed care organizations, are given discounts, called *contractual allowances*. By subtracting contractual allowances and *charity care discounts* from gross patient accounts receivable, what remains is patient accounts receivable. Patient accounts receivable represents the actual amount the health care organization has the right to collect.

Charity Care Discounts Discounts from gross patients accounts receivable given to those who cannot pay their bills.

Along with reporting patient accounts receivable (but not *gross* patient accounts receivable) on the balance sheet, health care organizations also present an estimate of how much of their patient accounts receivable they likely will not be able to collect. This estimate is called the *allowance for uncollectibles*.

Assuming gross patient accounts receivable were $24,800,000, discounts and contractual allowances were $7,200,000, and allowance for uncollectibles was $2,500,000, patient accounts receivable, net of uncollectibles for 20X1 would be $15,100,000, as shown in Exhibit 2–5.

By convention, the total amount of patient accounts receivable, in this case $17,600,000, is commonly omitted on the balance sheet because it can be derived by adding the allowance for uncollectibles and the patient accounts receivable, net of estimated uncollectibles.

Supplies, Prepaid Expenses, and Other Current Assets   Though presented separately here (see Exhibit 2–4), because of their relatively small size, in some organizations *supplies and prepaid expenses* may be grouped together with other assets under the title *other current assets*. Supplies include the day-to-day supplies used by the organization in the provision of health care services, including food, drugs, office, and medical supplies. Another name for supplies is inventory. A common mistake is to confuse supplies and equipment. *Supplies* refers to small-dollar items that will be "used up" or

Exhibit 2–5   Calculation of patient accounts receivable, net of estimated uncollectibles (in thousands)

Account Title	Amount	Explanation
Gross patient accounts receivable	$24,800	The amount owed to the organization, based on full charges; this amount is not reported on financial statements because it does not represent how much the health care organization is really owed because of discounts and allowances
– discounts and allowances	–7,200	Includes discounts given to third parties (large-scale purchasers of health care services) and discounts for charity care
Patient accounts receivable	17,600	Gross charges less discounts and allowances
– allowance for uncollectibles	–2,500	An estimate of how much of patient accounts receivable will likely *not* be collectible
Patient accounts receivable, net of estimated uncollectibles	$15,100	The amount expected to be collected

fully consumed within at least one year, such as pharmaceuticals and office supplies. *Equipment* refers to relatively expensive items that will be used over a long period, such as buildings and radiology equipment. *Prepaid assets*, also called *prepaid expenses*, includes items the health care organization has paid for in advance, such as rent and insurance. Although they are not tangible, they are still assets—in the form of rights the organization has purchased. For instance, by paying its rent in advance, the organization has a right to use a building for a specified period. To the extent that supplies and prepaid expenses are relatively large, they may be broken out and reported separately rather than grouped together.

Key Point *Supplies are sometimes called inventory.*

Noncurrent Assets Whereas current assets will be used or consumed within one year, noncurrent assets will be used or consumed over periods longer than one year (see Exhibit 2–6). Noncurrent assets are relatively costly items that allow the organization to deliver service over time. Whereas current assets require special management attention because of their liquidity and transportability, noncurrent assets require special attention because of their cost and the extensive time horizon it takes to plan, acquire, and manage them. Noncurrent assets are commonly organized into the following categories:

Noncurrent Assets
The resources of the organization that will be used or consumed over periods longer than one year.

- Assets limited as to use
- Long-term investments
- Property and equipment, net
- Other assets

Key Point *The terms* noncurrent *and* long-term *are often used interchangeably.*

Assets Limited as to Use With the exception of donor-restricted funds, which are reported elsewhere, this section reports the amount of the assets that have been set aside for long-term purposes and are thus not available for general use. The balance sheet presentation of assets limited as to use must separate internally designated and externally designated amounts either on the statements themselves or in the notes to the financial statements. In the case of Sample Not-For-Profit Hospital in 20X1, this category contains two items: the board has set aside $12,000,000 to purchase buildings or equipment, and as part of a loan agreement, the organization has placed with a trustee $6,949,000 that will be used to pay off the loan (see Exhibit 2–6). Notice that this category begins by presenting all assets limited as to use and then subtracts the amount required to meet current obligations, which is reported under current assets.

Exhibit 2–6   Asset section of the balance sheet from Exhibit 2–3 with an emphasis on noncurrent assets (in thousands)

Assets	20X1	20X0
Current assets		
Cash and cash equivalents	$4,758	$5,877
Short-term investments	15,836	10,740
Assets limited as to use	970	1,300
Patient accounts receivable, net estimated uncollectibles	15,100	14,194
of $2,500 in 20X1 and $2,400 in 20X0		
Supplies	2,000	2,000
Prepaid expenses	670	856
Total current assets	39,334	34,967
Noncurrent assets		
Assets limited as to use	18,949	19,841
Less amount required to meet current obligations	(970)	(1,300)
	17,979	18,541
Long-term investments	4,680	4,680
Long-term investments restricted for capital acquisition	320	520
Properties and equipment, net	51,038	50,492
Other assets	1,695	1,370
Total noncurrent assets	75,712	75,603
Total assets	$115,046	$110,570

Source: Reprinted with permission from the *Audit and Accounting Guide: Health Care Organizations*, copyright © 2007 by the American Institute of Certified Public Accountants, Inc.

Long-Term Investments *Long-term investments* are investments with a maturity of more than one year. *Securities* include various types of stocks and bonds and are discussed in more detail in Chapter Eight. Because long-term investments should be classified according to their intended purpose, $4,680,000 is shown in the general account "Long-term investments," and $320,000 is shown in the account "Long-term investments restricted for capital acquisition."

Properties and Equipment, Net This category of assets represents the major capital investments in the facility. Three types of assets are included in this category: land, plant, and equipment. *Plant* refers to buildings (fixed, immovable objects), *land* refers to property, and *equipment* includes a wide variety of durable items from beds to CAT scanners. Land, plant, and equipment are recorded on the organization's books at cost, and over time, plant and equipment (but not land!) are depreciated. *Depreciation* is an estimate of how much the plant or equipment has been "used up" during the accounting period.

The word *net* in *Properties and equipment, net* means that the total amount of depreciation taken up to this point in time has been subtracted from the original cost. To derive properties and equipment, net, the total amount of depreciation taken since the asset was put into use (called *accumulated depreciation*) is subtracted from the original cost of the asset (called *plant and equipment*). Assuming the original cost is $91,161,000 and accumulated depreciation is $40,123,000, properties and equipment, net would be calculated as shown in Exhibit 2–7.

By convention, plant and equipment are always kept on the books in their own accounts at their original cost until the assets are modified or sold. Similarly, the total amount of depreciation is kept in a separate account, accumulated depreciation. In this way, those looking at the balance sheet are always able to know (1) the original cost of the assets, (2) how much they have been depreciated, and (3) their current book value (original cost less depreciation).

Other Assets *Other assets* is a catchall account used for noncurrent assets not included in the other categories of noncurrent assets.

Liabilities

The preceding section focused on how assets are presented on the balance sheet. We now turn to a discussion of the liabilities of a health care organization. *Liabilities*

Depreciation
A measure of how much a tangible asset (such as plant or equipment) has been "used up" or consumed.

Accumulated Depreciation
The total amount of depreciation taken on an asset since it was put into use.

Exhibit 2–7 Calculation of properties and equipment, net (in thousands)

Account Title	Amount	Explanation
Properties and equipment	$91,161	The original cost of the land, plant, and equipment
Less: accumulated depreciation	− 40,123	An estimate of the amount the assets have been "used up," which is equal to the total amount of depreciation taken since the organization acquired the assets; by convention, plant and equipment depreciate, land does not
Properties and equipment, net	$51,038	The original cost minus the amount the assets have been depreciated (used up)

are the obligations of a health care provider to pay its creditors. As with assets, liabilities are divided into two categories: current and noncurrent (see Exhibit 2–8).

Current Liabilities Current liabilities are the financial obligations that, due to their contractual terms, will be paid within one year. Common account categories include:

- Current portion of long-term debt
- Accounts payable and accrued expenses
- Estimated third-party payor settlements
- Other current liabilities

Each of these accounts is discussed below.

Current Portion of Long-Term Debt This account contains the amount of the organization's long-term debt that is expected to be paid off within one year. For example, if a home health agency has executed a 5-year note payable, the principal amount due this year is reported in this account. The remainder is listed under noncurrent liabilities. This information is sometimes reported in the account *notes payable*, which reports the amount of short-term (less than one year) obligations for which a formal note has been signed.

Exhibit 2–8   Liabilities section of the balance sheet from Exhibit 2–3 (in thousands)

Liabilities and Net Assets	20X1	20X0
Current liabilities		
Current portion of long-term debt	$1,470	$1,750
Accounts payable and accrued expenses	5,818	5,382
Estimated third-party payor settlements	2,143	1,942
Deferred revenues	1,969	2,114
Total current liabilities	11,400	11,188
Noncurrent liabilities		
Long-term debt, net of current portion	23,144	24,014
Other	3,953	3,166
Total noncurrent liabilities	27,097	27,180
Total liabilities	$38,497	$38,368

Source: Reprinted with permission from the *Audit and Accounting Guide: Health Care Organizations*, copyright © 2007 by the American Institute of Certified Public Accountants, Inc.

Accounts Payable and Accrued Expenses *Accounts payable* are obligations to pay suppliers who have sold the health care organization goods or services on credit. *Accrued expenses* are expenses that arise in the normal course of business that have not yet been paid. Included in this category are salaries, wages, and interest. Sometimes accrued expenses are presented in separate accounts, such as:

- Salaries and wages payable
- Interest payable

Key Point *Accrued expenses are liabilities and are reflected in the balance sheet.*

Estimated Third-Party Payor Settlements This account represents an estimate of funds to be repaid to third-party payors. *Third-party payors* are organizations such as insurance companies and governmental agencies that pay on behalf of patients. This account is necessary because much of the payment process is done using estimates. For example, Medicare (actually, a contractor acting on its behalf) makes periodic payments to a hospital, based on the claims (i.e., bills) it has received and processed. However, the actual rate payable by Medicare to the hospital for some services may not be known until the hospital's fiscal year has been completed and a "cost report" has been submitted to Medicare. As Medicare and Medicaid become more and more fully prospective, settlements should diminish significantly. The amount that appears on the balance sheet under *estimated third-party payor settlements* is an estimate of how much the hospital will need to return to the third parties due to overpayments by the third parties. The estimate is based in large part on the history of such transactions. In addition to amounts based on claims submitted, estimated third-party payor settlements may also include advances from third parties to support the day-to-day needs of the organization (see Chapter Five). If the provider's experience indicates that third parties need to pay the organization instead, the account estimated third-party payor settlements would appear as a current asset similar to accounts receivable, rather than as a current liability.

> **Third-Party Payors**
> Commonly referred to as third parties, these are organizations that pay on behalf of patients.

Other Current Liabilities *Other current liabilities* includes all current liabilities not elsewhere presented in the current liabilities section. The accounts summarized in this category may be presented on their own lines or they may be detailed in the notes if they are material in amount. Increasingly, a major item in this account is *deferred revenues*.

Deferred revenues are fees that have been collected in advance. Although its name implies it is a revenue, it is in fact an obligation. For example, health care organizations receive capitation payments from managed care organizations. Capitated payments are often in the form of a specific amount per member per month (PMPM) and require that the health care organization receiving the capitated payment provide a range of services for the population covered by these payments. When the health care organization receives the capitated payment, it incurs an obligation to provide service. Thus, it records the amount received as an obligation (liability). After the obligation is satisfied (the time the payment covers has passed), the deferred revenue is taken out of the deferred revenue account and recorded as revenue.

Noncurrent Liabilities
The financial obligations not due within one year.

Noncurrent Liabilities *Noncurrent liabilitie*s are obligations that will be paid back over a period longer than one year. Most long-term liabilities fall into two categories: mortgages payable and bonds payable.

Net Assets

The final category of the balance sheet is *net assets* (see Exhibit 2–9). The term "net assets" is used to show the community's interest in the assets of the organization. In an investor-owned organization, it equals the stockholders' interest in the organization's assets. It is equal to the organization's assets minus its liabilities. Thus, in not-for-profit health care organizations, the terms in the basic accounting equation are rearranged to derive net assets as follows:

$$\text{Net Asset} = \text{Assets} - \text{Liabilities}$$

 Key Point *For not-for-profit health care providers, the net assets section of the balance sheet is analogous to the owner's equity section of a for-profit organization's balance sheet.*

Using the year 20X1 in Exhibit 2–3 as an example, by subtracting the amount of total liabilities ($38,497,000) from the value of the total assets ($115,046,000), net assets equals $76,549,000.

Exhibit 2–9   Net assets section of the balance sheet from Exhibit 2–3 (in thousands)

	20X1	20X0
Net assets		
Unrestricted	$70,846	$66,199
Temporarily restricted	2,115	2,470
Permanently restricted	3,588	3,533
Total net assets	$76,549	$72,202

Source: Reprinted with permission from the *Audit and Accounting Guide: Health Care Organizations*, copyright © 2007 by the American Institute of Certified Public Accountants, Inc.

Key Point *Although the terms* assets *and* liabilities *are used consistently, numerous names have been used for the third section of the balance sheet, including owners' equity, stockholders' equity, net assets, and fund balance. In any case, the amount reported is equal to the difference between assets and liabilities.*

In the presentation of net assets on the balance sheet, not-for-profit health care organizations must categorize net assets into three categories of restrictions:

- Unrestricted net assets
- Temporarily restricted net assets
- Permanently restricted net assets

All net assets *not* restricted by donors are considered *unrestricted net assets*. Net assets that are restricted by donors, on the other hand, must be shown on the balance sheet as temporarily or permanently restricted (see Exhibit 2–10 and Perspective 2–3). An example of a temporary restriction is the donation of land by the county with the provision that the hospital cannot sell it for five years. An example of a permanent restriction is an endowment that allows the health care organization to spend the interest, but never the principal.

Stockholders' Equity

Investor-owned health care organizations use a different form of presentation of the owners' equity section of the balance sheet (see Exhibit 2–11). The terms used in the shareholders' equity section (i.e., *par value of the stock, excess of par value*, and *retained earnings*) are technical and beyond the scope of this text.

 Key Point *Stockholders equity for investor-owned organizations represents the stock and retained earnings.*

Notes to Financial Statements

The *notes* to the balance sheet are grouped together with the notes of all other financial statements and presented after the financial statements. Although notes might be

---

Exhibit 2–10   Examples of types of restrictions on assets

Temporarily restricted
Donated land that cannot be sold for five years
Permanently restricted
An endowment in which only the interest can be spent

Perspective 2–3   Contribution Dollars Allocated Toward Buildings

Listed below are two examples of how hospitals still depend on contributions to help fund the building of a cancer center and new hospital. The first example is Hackensack University Medical Center, which will build a new $135 million four-story cancer center. Funding for the center was aided by a $10 million donation from a local member of the community. This contribution represents the second time in recent years this hospital has received a $10 million contribution. Given the fact that half the hospitals in New Jersey are losing money, this hospital has generated a surplus for the last 22 years. The CEO of Hackensack claims that higher volume and quality of care are the driving force behind these higher profits. The center's patient volume has more than doubled since 2003. The center has over 100,000 patient visits, which is the largest patient volume in the state, with 40,000 annual surgeries, and 30,000 annual radiology treatments

Source: McClatchy, M. J. L. 2008. Donation helps Hackensack University Medical Center break ground on facility. *Tribune Business News* (Apr. 16), Washington, D.C.

The second example demonstrates how Baylor College of Medicine in Houston depended on fundraising to help finance the building of a $568 million new teaching hospital and clinic. In addition, the new facility will purchase such cutting-edge technology as an electronic medical record system, advanced medical and surgical care, a variety of outpatient clinics, 300 faculty offices, and a 19,000-square-foot research area. Over the past three years, Baylor received $492 million in contributions through fundraising, which will account for more than 86 percent of the project's costs. The remaining funding source will come from a bond issuance and Baylor's building fund.

Source: Greene, J. 2007. From the ground up. *Modern Healthcare* (Aug 27), 37(34): 64.

Exhibit 2–11   Illustration of the owners' equity section of the balance sheet for an investor-owned health care organization (in thousands)

	20X1	20X0
Shareholders' equity		
Common stock, $10 par value; authorized 5,000 shares; issued and outstanding 3,500 shares	$35,000	$35,000
Excess of par value	35,000	35,000
Retained earnings	6,549	2,202
Total shareholders' equity	$76,549	$72,202

Source: Adapted from *AICPA Audit and Accounting Guide, Health Care Organizations* (new edition), American Institute of Certified Public Accountants, Inc., New York, May 1, 2007.

considered in texts to present somewhat superfluous information, they are an integral part of the financial statements. Because the information in the body of the statement is presented in summary form, additional key information must be presented in the notes. Notes often contain such information as the accounting policies followed by the health care organization, how charity care is determined, the composition of investments, which assets are restricted, the depreciation method used, the market value as well as the initial cost of investments, the maturity and interest rates of the long-term debt, the amount of professional liability insurance for malpractice, and whether there are suits filed against the organization that may adversely affect the financial position of the organization. Exhibit A–8 provides a detailed example of notes in a set of financial statements.

Notes to the Financial Statements Notes that follow the four financial statements and provide key information; notes for all four financial statements appear together after all four statements have been presented and are an integral part of the financial statements.

Policymakers, potential lenders, and bond credit rating agencies may want to know whether the health care organization's debt is tax-exempt or taxable, when the health care organization's debt comes due, and what interest rate it pays on its debt. The answers can be found in the notes to the financial statement. Exhibit A–8, Note 6, indicates that this health care organization has over $21 million in tax-exempt revenue bonds due in November 1, 20XX, and is paying at a rate of 7.25 percent. The provider also has over $2 million outstanding in a mortgage loan with a rate of 7.75 percent maturing in June 20XX and $1 million in a capital lease with an implied variable rate of 6.8 to 9.3 percent.

Policymakers and lenders would also want to know how much cash and investments are being designated for capital purchases. Note 3 in Exhibit A–8 indicates that this health care organization has $12 million designated for capital acquisitions as of December 31, 20X1, which is primarily invested in U.S. Treasury obligations.

THE STATEMENT OF OPERATIONS

As opposed to the balance sheet, which summarizes the organization's total assets, liabilities, and net assets at a particular *point in time*, the statement of operations is a summary of the organization's revenues and expenses over a *period of time* (see Exhibit 2–12). The period is usually the time between statements, such as a quarter, half-year, or fiscal year. The statement of operations is analogous to, but different from, an income statement of a for-profit organization (see Exhibit 2–13). Appendix A contains an example of the financial statements for a for-profit organization. Perspective 2–4 illustrates how improvement in a health care system's statement of operations contributed to a profitable turnaround.

The body of the income statement for investor-owned health care organizations is organized into five sections:

■ Operating income (the difference between revenues and expenses)

■ Non-operating income

Perspective 2–4 Improvement in Operations Contributes to a Profitable Turnaround for a Health Care System

Fitch rating agency confirms the A rating of Sisters of Charity Providence Hospitals (SCPH). SCPH is a two-hospital health care system with 314 operated acute care beds located in Columbia, South Carolina. The system is also owned by the Sisters of Charity of St. Augustine Health System (CSAHS), which is located in Cleveland, Ohio. SCPH's outstanding reputation for cardiac care has enabled the system to achieve a leading market share in cardiac surgery of approximately 65 percent and in cardiac catheterization procedures of approximately 55 percent.

Operationally, SCPH's profits have increased dramatically since a fiscal 2005 loss of $12.4 million. In 2006, CSAHS replaced SCPH's management team and as a result reduced its operating loss to $1.5 million and earned $5.0 million from operations through the nine-month period ended Sept. 30, 2007. Prior losses stem primarily from labor inefficiencies, poor revenue cycle and supply cost management, and an inability to control bad debt expense. Higher revenues were also generated by obtaining new disproportionate share (DSH) payments from Medicare/Medicaid that began in fiscal 2006 and totaled $5.7 million in federal fiscal 2006 and $7.5 million in federal fiscal 2007.

Source: 2008. Fitch affirms Sisters of Charity Providence Hospitals, South Carolina bonds. *Business Wire* (Jan. 17), New York.

Exhibit 2–12 Comparison of the time frame covered by the balance sheet and statement of operations

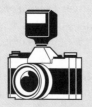

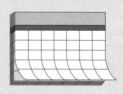

The balance sheet presents a snapshot of the organization as of a point in time.

The statement of operations presents a summary of revenues and expenses over a period of time.

Exhibit 2–13 Comparison of the heading and major sections of the body of the income statement for investor-owned and not-for-profit health care organizations

	Investor-Owned	Not-for-Profit
Title	Income statement	Statement of operations
Body	Revenues	Unrestricted revenues, gains, and other support
	– Expenses	– Expenses
	Operating income	*Operating income*
	+ Other income	+ Other income
	Operating earnings before income taxes	Excess of revenues, gains, and other support over expenses
	– Income taxes	+/– Other
	Net income	*Increase in unrestricted net assets*

- Income before taxes
- Provision for taxes
- Net income (the difference between revenues and expenses)

The body of the statement of operations for not-for-profit health care organizations includes the following major sections:

- Operating income
- Other income
- Excess of revenues, gains, and other support over expenses
- Other items
- Increase in unrestricted net assets

Exhibit 2–14 is an example of a statement of operations for a not-for-profit health care organization.

Key Point *The statement of operations uses the accrual basis of accounting, which summarizes how much the organization earned and the resources it used to generate that income during a period of time. It does not use the cash basis of accounting, which focuses on the cash that actually came in and went out. This is discussed in detail in the next chapter.*

This statement does not represent how much cash came into the organization or how much cash went out. Rather, it represents how much the organization earned, its gains and other sources of revenue and the resources it used during the accounting

Exhibit 2–14 Annotated statement of operations for Sample Not-For-Profit Hospital (in thousands)

1 The Statement of Operations (also called the *statement of activities*) provides a summary of the organization's revenues and expenses over a period of time.

1 Title: Gives the name of the organization, the name of the financial statement, and two periods of time for which information is being provided.

2 Unrestricted revenues, gains, and other support: The income of the organization derived from providing patient service, the sale of assets for more than their book value, contributions, appropriations and assets released from restriction.
- **Net patient service revenues:** Revenues earned from patient care minus the amounts the organization does not expect to collect because of contractual discounts.
- **Premium revenues:** Revenues earned from capitated contracts.
- **Other revenues:** Revenues derived from such sources as support services, investments, and certain contributions.
- **Net assets released from restriction:** funds formerly restricted by a donor, now available for general use to run the organization.

3 Expenses: Expenses are a measure of the resources used to generate revenue. (Those expenses listed which are self-evident have not been defined.)
- **Depreciation and amortization:** Measures of the use of long-lived assets during the accounting period.

4 • **Provision for bad debts:** An estimate of the amount of money owed the organization which it estimates will not be collected.
- **Other:** A catch-all category for miscellaneous expenses and losses including utilities, rent, telephone, travel, etc.

Operating income: Unrestricted Revenues, Gains, and Other Support minus Expenses and Losses. Traditionally, it is a measure of the income earned from healthcare-related endeavors.

5 Other income: Income earned from other than healthcare-related endeavors.

6 Excess of revenues over expenses: Operating Income plus Other Income. This is analogous to Net Income in for-profit entities.

7 Change in net unrealized gains and losses on other than trading securities: Changes in the fair value of assets other than trading securities.

8 Net assets released from restrictions used for purchase of property and equipment: Assets which were previously restricted by a donor, which must now be used to purchase property and equipment. Since they are for the purchase of long-lived assets, they are not considered revenue.

9 Contributions from sample hospital foundation for property acquisitions: Self explanatory. Since they are for the purchase of long-lived assets, they are not considered revenue.

10 Transfer to parent: Transfer of assets from a subsidiary to their parent company.

11 Extraordinary item: An extremely unusual and infrequent expense.

12 Increase in unrestricted net assets: The increase in unrestricted net assets during the period. It includes operating income, contributions of long-lived assets, transfers to parent and extraordinary items. Restricted revenues are not shown on this financial statement until they become unrestricted.

*An unannotated form of this statement can be found in Appendix A of this chapter.

Source: Reprinted with permission from the Audit and Accounting Guide: Health Care Organizations, copyright © 2007 by the American Institute of Certified Public Accountants, Inc.

Sample Not-For Profit Hospital
Statement of Operations
For the Years Ended December 31, 20X1 and 20X0 (in '000)

	20X1	20X0
② Unrestricted revenues, gains, and other support		
Net patient service revenue	$85,156	$78,942
Premium revenue	11,150	10,950
Other revenues	2,601	5,212
Net assets released from restriction used for operations	300	0
Total revenues, gains and other support	99,207	95,104
③ Expenses		
Salaries and benefits	53,900	49,938
Medical supplies and drugs	26,532	22,121
Insurance	8,089	8,526
Depreciation and amortization	4,782	4,280
Interest	1,752	1,825
④ Provision for bad debts	1,000	1,300
Other expenses	2,000	1,300
Total expenses	98,055	89,290
⑤ Operating income	1,152	5,814
⑥ Other income		
Investment income	3,900	3,025
Excess of revenues over expenses	5,052	8,839
⑦ Change in net unrealized gains and losses on other than trading securities	300	375
⑧ Net assets released from restrictions used for purchase of property and equipment	200	0
⑨ Contribution from sample hospital foundation for property acquisitions	235	485
⑩ Transfers to parent	(640)	(3,000)
Increase in unrestricted net assets, before extraordinary item	5,147	6,699
⑪ Extraordinary loss (debt extinguishment)	(500)	0
⑫ *Increase in unrestricted net assets*	$4,647	$6,699

period. The principle behind focusing on tracking cash and tracking resource use is discussed in detail in Chapter Three.

 Key Point *The statement of operations does not represent the cash flow of the organization. Instead, it represents how much the organization earned, its gains and other sources of revenue, and the resources it used during the accounting period.*

Unrestricted Revenues, Gains, and Other Support

This section of the statement of operations represents what most people think of as the revenues of the organization (see Exhibit 2–15). *Revenues* refers to the amounts earned by the organization, *gains* come about by selling assets for more than their value on the books (such as selling a building or other investment), and *other support* includes such items as appropriations from governmental organizations and unrestricted donations. Usually *net patient service revenue* and *premium revenue* make up the largest portion of unrestricted revenues, gains, and other support in not-for-profit business organizations.

 Key Point *As explained in detail in Chapter Three, revenues represent amounts earned by the organization, not the amount of cash it received during the period.*

Net Patient Service Revenues *Gross patient service revenues* is the amount the health care organization would have earned if everyone paid full price. However, as discussed under patient accounts receivable, many payors receive discounts, called *contractual allowances*. In addition, most health care organizations also provide some free care to indigent patients, called *charity care*. In reporting net patient service revenue, a health care organization must subtract amounts both for contractual allowances and for charity care. Thus, the amount reported on the statement of operations is net patient service revenue, which equals gross patient service revenues minus contractual allowances and charity care. For instance, assuming that gross patient service revenues were $130,284,000, contractual allowances $34,898,000, and charity care $10,230,000, then the net patient service revenue for 20X1 would be calculated as shown in Exhibit 2–16.

Premium Revenues *Premium revenues* are revenues earned from capitated contracts. They are not earned solely through the delivery of service, but rather through a combination of the passage of time (during which the organization is available to provide service when necessary) and actually delivering service as agreed to during the contract period.

Exhibit 2–15   Abbreviated statement of operations from Exhibit 2–14 emphasizing revenues, gains, and other support (in thousands)

	20X1	20X0
Unrestricted revenues, gains, and other support		
Net patient service revenue	$85,156	$78,942
Premium revenue	11,150	10,950
Other revenues	2,601	5,212
Net assets released from restriction used for operations	300	
Total revenues, gains, and other support	99,207	95,104
Expenses		
Salaries and benefits	53,900	49,938
Medical supplies and drugs	26,532	22,121
Insurance	8,089	8,526
Depreciation and amortization	4,782	4,280
Interest	1,752	1,825
Provision for bad debts	1,000	1,300
Other expenses	2,000	1,300
Total expenses	98,055	89,290
Operating income	1,152	5,814
Other income		
Investment income	3,900	3,025
Excess of revenues over expenses	$5,052	$8,839

Source: Reprinted with permission from the *Audit and Accounting Guide: Health Care Organizations*, copyright © 2007 by the American Institute of Certified Public Accountants, Inc.

Other Revenues   *Other revenues* are derived from four major sources: appropriations and grants, support services, income from investments, and revenues from contributions. Appropriations are monies provided by government agencies on an ongoing basis, usually for operating purposes. Grants are funds given to a health care organization for special purposes, usually for a limited time. Support services include such things as parking fees, cafeteria sales, and revenue from the gift shop and may be sometimes listed separately under an account called "Other operating revenue" because these services support the operations of patient care. Income from investments includes unrestricted interest, dividends, and gains from the sale of unrestricted investments. Although some health care organizations report their revenues from support services

Exhibit 2–16   Calculation of net patient service revenue (in thousands)

Account Title	Amount	Explanation
Gross patient service revenues	$130,284	The amount the health care organization earned at full retail price. It cannot be reported on financial statements because it does not recognize that all payors do not pay full charges
– Contractual allowances	–34,898	Discounts given to third parties (large-scale purchasers of health care services)
– Charity care discounts	–10,230	The amount of full charges the organization will not attempt to collect because the patient has been certified as unable to pay; usually reported only in the footnotes
Net patient service revenue	$85,156	Full price less contractual allowances and charity care discounts: this amount is reported on the financial statements for it is felt to be a more realistic estimate of how much revenue the health care organization has actually earned

and investments in this category, it is also possible to report them under "Other income," which is listed after "Operating income" (see Exhibit 2–15). This separates revenues earned through health care-related activities ("operating income") and those earned from other than health care-related activities ("non-operating income").

Net Assets Released from Restriction   *Net assets released from restriction* are funds transferred to unrestricted accounts from temporarily restricted net assets. The income earned from restricted investments and even the investments themselves may be released to unrestricted accounts as certain requirements are met. For example, a donor may stipulate that his or her contribution not be released until after the health care provider raises the required matching funds for a new service line. Net assets released from restrictions that are used to purchase capital items (plant and equipment) are not considered revenues, gains, or other support. They must be reported later in the statement of operations, below "excess of revenues over expenses."

Expenses

Although most of the expenses listed in Exhibit 2–17 are self-evident, several of them are discussed briefly.

Exhibit 2-17 Abbreviated statement of operations from Exhibit 2-14 emphasizing expenses (in thousands)

	20X1	20X0
Unrestricted revenues, gains, and other support		
Net patient service revenue	$85,156	$78,942
Premium revenue	11,150	10,950
Other revenues	2,601	5,212
Net assets released from restriction used for operations	300	
Total revenues, gains, and other support	99,207	95,104
Expenses		
Salaries and benefits	53,900	49,938
Medical supplies and drugs	26,532	22,121
Insurance	8,089	8,526
Depreciation and amortization	4,782	4,280
Interest	1,752	1,825
Provision for bad debts	1,000	1,300
Other expenses	2,000	1,300
Total expenses	98,055	89,290
Operating income	1,152	5,814
Other income		
Investment income	3,900	3,025
Excess of revenues over expenses	$5,052	$8,839

Source: Reprinted with permission from the *Audit and Accounting Guide: Health Care Organizations*, copyright © 2007 by the American Institute of Certified Public Accountants, Inc.

 Key Point *On the statement of operations, expenses are a measure of the amount of resources used or consumed in providing a service, not cash outflows. With this definition, assets are just expenses waiting to happen!*

Amortization
The allocation of the acquisition cost of debt to the period which it benefits.

Depreciation and Amortization Depreciation and amortization reflect the amount of a noncurrent asset used during the accounting period. Depreciation is a measure of how much a tangible asset (such as a building or equipment) has been "used up" during the accounting period. For example, if a facility buys new examining room equipment for $10,000 and expects it to last ten years, the accountant might record $1,000 depreciation each year on the assumption that one-tenth of the equipment is "used up" each year.

Amortization is a measure of how much of an intangible asset (such as debt issuance cost and goodwill) has been "used up" during the accounting period. Both expenses are noncash expenses.

Key Point *Depreciation and amortization are noncash expenses.*

Interest Interest is the cost to borrow money. If interest is 10 percent per year, then the cost to borrow $1,000 for one year is $100.

Provision for Bad Debts Just as a retail business considers bad debts a cost of doing business, so do not-for-profit health care organizations. *Provision for bad debts*, also called *bad debt expense* or *uncollectibles expense*, is the estimate of patient accounts receivable that will not be collected. It does not include charity care or contractual allowances, for they have already been deducted to derive patient accounts receivable.

Other Expenses *Other expenses* is a catchall category for miscellaneous operating expenses. This category includes all general and administrative expenses, rent, utilities, and contracted services not included in the other categories. Although they are grouped in this example, they may be reported separately.

Operating Income

Operating income is the income derived from the organization's main line of business: health care. It is calculated by subtracting expenses from unrestricted revenues, gains, and other support. In Exhibit 2–14, operating income of $1,152,000 in 20X1 is calculated by subtracting total expenses of $98,055,000 from unrestricted revenues, gains, and other support of $99,207,000.

> **Operating Income** Income derived from the organization's main line of business.

Other Income

Other income includes income earned from activities other than the organization's main line of business. Although there is discretion as to what constitutes operating and non-operating items, interest income, food sales to the public, and parking income are often considered non-operating.

Excess of Revenues Over Expenses

Excess of revenues over expenses is analogous to *net income* (profit) in a for-profit entity. However, not-for-profit business entities are prohibited from using the more common term, net income. This item, traditionally referred to as *the bottom line* in for-profit entities, is not actually the bottom line in the statement of operations because accounting rules favor treating not-for-profit, business-oriented health care entities more like traditional not-for-profit organizations than like their for-profit competitors. Thus, the emphasis is on the change in unrestricted net assets rather than what is traditionally called net income.

> **Net Income** Equivalent to excess of revenues over expenses.

Excess of revenues over expenses is derived by adding operating income and other income. In Exhibit 2–17, this is done by adding operating income of $1,152,000 and investment income of $3,900,000 to get an excess of revenues over expenses of $5,052,000.

Below-the-Line Items

In addition to the items that contribute to "Excess of revenues over expenses," several items must appear on the statement of operations below "Excess of revenues over

Exhibit 2–18 Statement of operations from Exhibit 2–14 emphasizing items that do not contribute to excess of revenues over expenses (in thousands)

	20X1	20X0
Expenses		
Salaries and benefits	$53,900	$49,938
Medical supplies and drugs	26,532	22,121
Insurance	8,089	8,526
Depreciation and amortization	4,782	4,280
Interest	1,752	1,825
Provision for bad debts	1,000	1,300
Other expenses	2,000	1,300
Total expenses	98,055	89,290
Operating income	1,152	5,814
Other income		
Investment income	3,900	3,025
Excess of revenues over expenses	5,052	8,839
Change in net unrealized gains and losses on other than trading securities	300	375
Net assets released from restrictions used for purchase of property and equipment	200	
Contribution from sample hospital foundation for property acquisitions	235	485
Transfers to parent	(640)	(3,000)
Increase in unrestricted net assets, before extraordinary item	5,147	6,699
Extraordinary loss (debt extinguishment)	(500)	
Increase in unrestricted net assets	$4,647	$6,699

Source: Adapted from *AICPA Audit and Accounting Guide, Health Care Organizations* (new edition). American Institute of Certified Public Accountants, Inc., New York, May 1, 2007.

expenses" (see Exhibit 2–18). These are generically referred to as *below-the-line items* and include:

- Change in net unrealized gains and losses on other than trading securities
- Net assets released from restrictions used for purchase of property and equipment
- Contributions to acquire long-lived capital assets
- Extraordinary loss

Change in Net Unrealized Gains and Losses on Other than Trading Securities
Although the guidelines pertaining to this item are complex, for most not-for-profit health care organizations the amount reported here is the change in equity interest in stocks that do not trade in the public market, such as venture capital funds or limited partnerships in a physician practice. It is called *unrealized* because until the asset is disposed of (i.e., sold), the gain or loss occurs only on the books. Once the investment is disposed of, the gain or loss becomes a *realized* gain or loss.

For example, assume that on the last day of last year, an organization purchased $1,000,000 of stock in a physician practice. One year later, the stock is worth $1,300,000. The organization must report a $300,000 *unrealized* gain. On the other hand, if the stocks were sold for $1,300,000 during the last year, the organization would report a $300,000 *realized* gain either under "Revenues, gains, and other support" or "Other income." Note that because of this, *realized* gains affect "Excess of revenues over expenses," whereas *unrealized* gains do not for non-publicly traded securities.

Increases in Long-Lived Unrestricted Net Assets
Most increases in unrestricted long-term assets resulting from donations are not considered increases in revenues, gains, and other support. Rather, they are reported below "Excess of revenues over expenses" in separate accounts. Two examples in the Sample Not-For-Profit Hospital case are net assets released from restrictions used for purchase of property and equipment and contributions for the acquisition of plant and equipment.

Key Point *Rather than being reported in "Revenues, gains, and other support," increases relating to the donation of unrestricted net assets for capital acquisitions are reported below "Excess of revenues over expenses."*

Transfers to Parent
Another item that affects net assets but not excess of revenues over expenses is the transfer of assets to corporate headquarters (*transfer to parent*). In 20X1, Sample Not-For-Profit Hospital transferred $640,000 to its parent corporation.

Extraordinary Items
Extraordinary items reflect unusual and infrequent gains or losses from such things as paying off loans early, and acts of nature such as hurricanes or earthquakes.

Increase in Unrestricted Net Assets
The final section of the statement of operations is *increase in unrestricted net assets*, which is derived by adding or subtracting the

Exhibit 2-19 Calculation of increase in unrestricted net assets (in thousands)

Excess of revenues over expenses	**$5,052**
+ Change in net unrealized gains and losses on other than trading securities	300
+ Net assets released from restrictions used for purchase of property and equipment	200
+ Contribution from sample hospital foundation for property acquisitions	235
– Transfers to parent	(640)
Increase in unrestricted net assets, before extraordinary item	5,147
– Extraordinary loss (debt extinguishment)	(500)
Increase in unrestricted net assets	**$4,647**

Source: Reprinted with permission from the *Audit and Accounting Guide: Health Care Organizations*, copyright © 2007 by the American Institute of Certified Public Accountants, Inc.

remaining items from net income as shown in Exhibit 2–19. There is a subtotal before the "Extraordinary items" so that readers of the financial statements can judge the organization's performance both before and after taking it into account.

THE STATEMENT OF CHANGES IN NET ASSETS

A third financial statement is the statement of changes in net assets. Its purpose is to explain why there was a change from one year to the next in the net asset section of the balance sheet (Exhibit 2–3). There are two major reasons why the net asset section of the balance sheet changes from year to year: increases (decreases) in unrestricted net assets (as shown on the statement of operations, Exhibit 2–14) and changes in restricted net assets, which are not included on the statement of operations. Thus, the statement of changes in net assets goes beyond the statement of operations by summarizing all the changes in net assets over the year.

 Key Point *The statement of changes in net assets repeats some of the information found on the statement of operations to explain changes in unrestricted net assets, but adds additional information about changes in restricted net assets.*

Like the other statements, the statement of changes in net assets has a descriptive heading, a body, and notes. The body of the statement of changes in net assets is organized to represent the changes in each of the three categories of restrictions of net assets: unrestricted, temporarily restricted, and permanently restricted (see Exhibit 2–20).

Exhibit 2–20 Statement of changes in net assets for Sample Not-For-Profit Hospital

Sample Not-For-Profit Hospital Statement of Changes in Net Assets for the Years Ended December 31, 20X1 and 20X0 (in thousands)

	20X1	20X0
Unrestricted net assets		
Excess of revenues over expenses	$5,052	$8,839
Net unrealized gains on investments other than trading securities	300	375
Contribution from sample hospital foundation for property acquisition	235	485
Transfers to parent	(640)	(3,000)
Net assets released from restrictions used for purchase of properties and equipment	200	
Increase in unrestricted net assets before extraordinary item	5,147	6,699
Extraordinary loss from extinguishment of debt	(500)	
Increase in unrestricted net assets	4,647	6,699
Temporarily restricted net assets		
Contributions for charity care	140	996
Net realized and unrealized gains on investments	5	8
Net assets released from restrictions	(500)	
Increase (decrease) in temporarily restricted net assets	(355)	1,004
Permanently restricted net assets		
Contributions for endowment funds	50	411
Net realized and unrealized gains on investments	5	2
Increase in permanently restricted net assets	55	413
Increase in net assets	4,347	8,116
Net assets, beginning of year	72,202	64,086
Net assets, end of year	$76,549	$72,202

Source: Reprinted with permission from the *Audit and Accounting Guide: Health Care Organizations*, copyright © 2007 by the American Institute of Certified Public Accountants, Inc.

The information in the first section, "Unrestricted net assets," summarizes the information from the statement of operations. The information in the remainder of the statement of changes in net assets reflects changes in restricted accounts.

To illustrate, the statement of changes in net assets explains how unrestricted net assets, temporarily restricted net assets, and permanently restricted net assets of Sample-Not-for-Profit-Hospital (see Exhibit 2–3) changed from 20X0 to 20X1.

Changes in Unrestricted Net Assets

Unrestricted net assets (see Exhibit 2–20) come directly from the statement of operations. During the year 20X1, Sample Not-For-Profit Hospital made $5,052,000, had an unrealized gain of $300,000 on its investments, received a $235,000 donation of funds to be used for property acquisitions, transferred $640,000 to its parent corporation, released from restriction $200,000 worth of temporarily restricted net assets to be used for the purchase of property and equipment, and lost $500,000 from debt extinguishment, producing an increase in unrestricted net assets of $4,647,000.

Key Point *The "unrestricted" section of the statement of changes in net assets shows how the various items on the statement of operations contributed to the changes in unrestricted net assets.*

Changes in Temporarily Restricted Net Assets

During 20X1 Sample Not-For-Profit Hospital received $140,000 in restricted contributions to pay for charity care, made $5,000 (net) in unrealized and realized gains on temporarily restricted investments, and released $500,000 from temporary restrictions. Because it is to be used for operations, $300,000 of the $500,000 is shown as an increase in "Unrestricted revenues, gains, and other support" on the statement of operations under the category "Net assets released from restriction used for operations" (Exhibit 2–14). The $200,000 is also shown below "Excess of revenues over expenses" in the "net assets released from restrictions used for purchase of properties an equipment" account because it is to be used for the acquisition of long-lived assets.

Changes in Permanently Restricted Net Assets

For Sample Not-For-Profit Hospital, the only two changes in permanently restricted net assets in 20X1 were an increase of $50,000 for a permanently restricted endowment and $5,000 (net) in unrealized and realized gains on permanently restricted assets (see Exhibit 2–20).

THE STATEMENT OF CASH FLOWS

The fourth and final major financial statement is the statement of cash flows, which answers the question, "Where did cash come from and where did it go?" Although the statement of operations (income statement) may be thought of to answer this question, it does not. As noted earlier, it answers the questions "How much was earned?" (not "How much cash came in?") and "What resources were used?" (not "How much cash went out?"). Hence, the statement of cash flows was developed to report the cash inflows and outflows.

Like the other statements, the statement of cash flows has a descriptive heading, a body, and notes (see Exhibit 2–21 and Exhibit A–4). The statement of cash flows covers the same time period as does the statement of operations and the statement of changes in net assets.

The body of the statement is organized into the following sections:

- Cash flows from operating activities
- Cash flows from investing activities
- Cash flows from financing activities
- Net increase (decrease) in cash and cash equivalents

The statement also discloses key noncash transactions such as the issuance of stock for debt payment or for the acquisition of a company. Although there are two alternative forms of this statement, the most common, called the *indirect method*, has been presented here. The other format is called the *direct method*. The first section of this statement is cash flows from operating activities.

Cash Flows from Operating Activities

This section identifies the cash inflows and outflows resulting from the normal operations of an organization. Because most organizations do not have this information readily available, they derive it by starting with the increase (decrease) in net assets from the statement of changes in net assets and then make adjustments to convert this accrual-based information into cash flows.

Assume for the purposes of illustration that the organization began with no assets or liabilities. During the first week in operation, only two transactions occurred: $150,000 worth of services rendered, and patients paid $50,000 of this amount. Thus, the balance sheet would show "Cash" of $50,000, "Patient accounts receivable" of $100,000, and "Net assets" of $150,000. Hence, the increase in net assets since the last period was $150,000 (see Exhibit 2–22).

 Key Point Cash flows from operating activities *identifies cash flow from normal operations of the organization.*

To estimate cash flows from operations, however, net assets must be adjusted for changes in accounts that really do not result in cash inflows or outflows. In this case, the $100,000 that is still owed from the $150,000 in changes in net assets is subtracted to determine how much cash actually came in ($150,000 – $100,000 = $50,000). This process occurs in order to convert the "Changes in net assets" account, which was derived using the accrual basis of accounting, into an estimate of actual cash flows: net cash provided from operating activities.

Exhibit 2-21   Annotated statement of cash flows for Sample Not-For-Profit Hospital (in thousands)

Sample Not-For-Profit Hospital
Statement of Cash Flows (Indirect Method)
For the Years Ended December 31, 20X1 and 20X0 (in '000)

	20X1	20X0
① Cash flows from operating activities		
Change in net assets	$4,347	$8,116
Adjustments to reconcile change in net assets to		
Net cash provided by operating activities:		
Extraordinary loss from debt extinguishment	500	
Depreciation	4,782	4,280
Net realized and unrealized gains on investments, other than trading	(450)	(575)
Transfers to parent	640	3,000
Provision for bad debt	1,000	1,300
Restricted contributions and investment income received	(55)	(413)
Increase (decrease) in:		
Patient accounts receivable	(1,906)	(2,036)
Trading securities	215	
Other current assets	186	(2,481)
Other assets	(325)	(241)
Increase (decrease) in:		
Accounts payable and accrued expenses	436	679
Estimated third-party payor settlements	201	305
Other current liabilities	(145)	(257)
Other liabilities	787	(128)
Net cash provided by operating activities	10,213	11,549
③ Cash flows from investing activities:		
Purchases of investment	(3,769)	(2,150)
Capital expenditures	(4,728)	(5,860)
Net cash used in investing activities	(8,497)	(8,010)
④ Cash flows from financing activities:		
Transfer to parent	(640)	(3,000)
Proceeds from restricted contributions and restricted investment income	55	413
Payments on long-term debt	(24,700)	(804)
Payments on capital lease obligations	(150)	(100)
Increase in long-term debt	22,600	500
Net cash used in financing activities	(2,835)	(2,991)
⑤ Net increase (decrease) in cash and cash equivalents	(1,119)	548
⑥ Cash and cash equivalents at beginning of year	5,877	5,329
⑦ Cash and cash equivalents at end of year	$4,758	$5,877
⑧ Supplemental disclosures and cash flow information:		

The Hospital entered into capital lease obligations in the amount of $600,000 for new equipment in 2001.
Cash paid for interest (net of amount capitalized) in 2001 and 2000 was $1,780,000 and $1,856,000 respectively.
See accompanying notes to financial statements.

---

① The Statement of Cash Flows provides a summary of the cash inflows and outflows form one year to the next.

① **Title:** Gives the name of the organization, the name of the financial statement and two periods for which the information is being provided.

② **Cash Flows from Operating Activities:** This section explains the changes in cash resulting from the normal operating activities of the organization. It begins by presenting the change in net assets from the *statement of changes in net assets*. However, since the *statement of changes in net assets* was prepared on the *accrual basis of accounting* to show revenues when earned, not when cash was received, and expenses when paid, the remainder of this section makes adjustments to convert the changes in current assets and liabilities and other operating accounts to actual cash flows. This is explained in more detail in the next chapter.

③ **Cash Flows from Investing Activities:** This section explains cash inflows and outflows of the organization resulting from investing activities such as purchasing and selling investments, or investing in itself such as purchasing or selling plant, property, or equipment.

④ **Cash Flows from Financing Activities:** This section explains cash inflows and outflows resulting from financing activities such as obtaining grants and endowments, or from borrowing or paying back long-term debt. It also includes transfers to and from the parent corporation.

⑤ **Net Increase (Decrease) in Cash and Cash Equivalents:** The total of cash flows from operating, investing and financing activities.

⑥ **Cash and Cash Equivalents at Beginning of Year:** The amount of cash and cash equivalents which the organization had at the beginning of the year.

⑦ **Cash and Cash Equivalents at End of Year:** The total of net increases in cash and cash equivalents at the end of the year. It is the same number that appears under this title on the balance sheet.

⑧ **Supplemental Information:** Additional information of use to the reader of the statement.

An unannotated form of this statement can be found in Appendix A of this chapter.

Source: Reprinted with permission from the *Audit and Accounting Guide: Health Care Organizations* copyright © 2007 American Institute of Certified Public Accountants, Inc.

Exhibit 2-22 Deriving net cash provided by operating activities by adjusting change in net assets for items that do not affect cash flows

Sample Not-For-Profit Hospital
Balance Sheet
January 7, 20X1, and January 1, 20X1

	1/7/20X1	1/1/20X1		1/7/20X1	1/1/20X1
Cash	$50,000	$0	Liabilities	$0	$0
Patient accounts receivable	100,000	0	Net assets	150,000	0
Total assets	$150,000	$0	Liabilities and net assets	$150,000	$0

Sample Not-For-Profit Hospital
Statement of Cash Flows
for the Period Ended January 7, 20X1

	1/7/20X1	1/1/20X1
Cash flows from operating activities		
Changes in net assets	$150,000	$0
Increase in patient accounts receivable	100,000	0
Net cash provided by operating activities	$50,000	$0

Cash Flows from Investing Activities

The second section of the statement of cash flows is *cash flows from investing activities*. This section shows cash inflows and outflows from such accounts as:

■ Purchase of plant, property, and equipment

■ Purchase of long-term investments

■ Proceeds from sale of plant, property, and equipment

■ Proceeds from sale of long-term investments

 Key Point *Investing by an organization includes investing in itself (such as when an organization buys new equipment).*

Information found in this section is derived from changes in the "Noncurrent assets" section of the balance sheet from one period to the next. It reports both the purchase or sale (or both) of outside investments and the purchase or sale (or both) of noncurrent assets, such as plant and equipment, which will be used to provide services. In the latter case, the organization is investing in itself.

Cash Flows from Financing Activities

In this section of the statement of cash flows, we identify the changes in cash flows resulting from financing activities. These include:

■ Transfers to parent

■ Proceeds from selected contributions

■ Proceeds from issuance of long-term debt

■ Repayment of long-term debt

■ Interest from restricted investments if interest income is also restricted

---

 Key Point *Repayment and issuance of long-term debt are identified in "Cash flow from financing activities" within the statement of cash flows.*

Cash and Cash Equivalents at the End of the Year

This is the "bottom line" of the statement of cash flows and is the same as the *cash and cash equivalents* amount that appears on the balance sheet. The latter is calculated by adding the net increase (decrease) in cash and cash equivalents for the year to the beginning balance of the cash and cash equivalents. The net increase (decrease) in cash and cash equivalents for the year on the statement of cash flows is computed by adding together the cash flows from the operating, investing, and financing activities, respectively. In Exhibit 2–21, the cash and cash equivalents at the end of 20X1 is $4,758,000.

SUMMARY

This chapter examined the four major statements of not-for-profit, business-oriented health care organizations: the balance sheet, the statement of operations, the statement of changes in net assets, and the statement of cash flows. Each of these statements is organized in the same way with a heading, a body, and notes. The notes are grouped together and presented after all four statements have been provided. They are considered an integral part of the financial statements.

The balance sheet presents a snapshot of the organization at a point in time (usually the last day of the year). The body of the balance sheet has three major sections: assets, liabilities, and net assets. The balance sheet is so named because *assets = liabilities + owners' equity*. This fundamental accounting equation is expressed as "assets = liabilities + shareholders' equity" in investor-owned health care organizations and "assets = liabilities + net assets" in not-for-profit, business-oriented health care organizations.

Assets are the resources of the organization, liabilities are the obligations of the organization to pay its creditors, and net assets are the difference between assets and liabilities. Assets are divided into two main sections: current and noncurrent. Current assets will be used or consumed within one year. Noncurrent assets will provide benefit to the organization for periods longer than one year. Assets limited as to use are noted separately from those without such restrictions.

Liabilities are also classified into current and noncurrent categories. Current liabilities are those that must be paid within one year. Noncurrent liabilities

will be due in more than one year. If part of a liability, such as a mortgage, is due within one year and the rest is due beyond one year, then the part due within one year is classified in the current section, and the remainder is presented under non-current liabilities. Revenues received in advance, such as capitated fees, are liabilities, classified as deferred revenues. They are considered liabilities because the organization has the obligation to deliver service. They are not recognized as revenues until they are earned.

Net assets are the owners' interest in the entity's assets. The owners of not-for-profit entities are generally assumed to be the community. Net assets are presented in three categories: unrestricted, temporarily restricted, and permanently restricted. Unrestricted net assets are not constrained by donors. Restricted net assets are funds that have limitations imposed on them by outside donors.

The statement of operations is analogous to, but not the same as, the traditional income statement. Rather than showing how much cash came in or went out, the body of the statement of operations summarizes the changes in unrestricted net assets during a period of time (usually a year). Excess of revenues over expenses is comparable to, but not the same as, the bottom line (net income) in for-profit health care organizations. It is determined by adding operating income and other (non-operating) income. Operating income comprises the organization's unrestricted revenues, gains, and other support less its expenses. Operating income is the income derived from the primary line of business, in this case health care-related services, whereas non-operating income is income from all other sources. In addition to the accounts that comprise excess of revenues over expenses, there are a number of "below-the-line" items that affect the change in unrestricted net assets but not excess of revenues over expenses. These generally relate to donations of long-lived assets, realized and unrealized gains or losses on other than trading securities, and transfers to parent. Occasionally there may be an extraordinary item.

The third financial statement is the statement of changes in net assets, which is called the statement of changes in owners' equity in for-profit entities. It summarizes why the net asset account changed during the period covered by the statement of operations by showing why each of the three main categories of net assets changed: unrestricted net assets, temporarily restricted net assets, and permanently restricted net assets.

The final financial statement of not-for-profit health care organizations is the statement of cash flows. Its purpose is to summarize where the organization's cash came from and how it was spent during the year. It summarizes cash flows in three major categories: cash flows from operating activities, cash flows from investing activities, and cash flows from financing activities. This statement is necessary because the statement of operations is based on the accrual basis of accounting and keeps track of earnings and resources when used, but not actual cash flows.

KEY TERMS

a. Accumulated depreciation
b. Amortization
c. Assets
d. Basic accounting equation
e. Charity care discounts
f. Current assets
g. Current liabilities
h. Depreciation
i. Fund balance
j. Liabilities

k. Liquidity
l. Net assets
m. Net income
n. Noncurrent assets
o. Noncurrent liabilities
p. Notes to the financial statements
q. Operating income
r. Owners' equity
s. Shareholders' equity
t. Third-party payors

KEY EQUATIONS

General accounting equation:

$$\text{Assets} = \text{Liabilities} + \text{Owners' Equity}$$

Basic accounting equation (not-for-profit entities):

$$\text{Assets} = \text{Liabilities} + \text{Net Assets}$$

Basic accounting equation (for-profit entities):

$$\text{Assets} = \text{Liabilities} + \text{Shareholders' Equity}$$

QUESTIONS AND PROBLEMS

1. **Definitions.** Define the terms listed on the previous page.

2. **Financial statement terminology.**

   a. What are each of the major financial statements commonly called in for-profit health care organizations and in not-for-profit health care organizations?

   b. Describe the three major sections common to all financial statements.

3. **Balance equation.** State the primary accounting equation that describes the balance sheet of a not-for-profit, business-oriented health care organization.

4. **Balance sheet.** The following questions relate to the balance sheet:

   a. What is the name of this statement in not-for-profit health care organizations?

   b. What are its main sections in investor-owned health care organizations?

   c. What are its main sections in not-for-profit health care organizations?

   d. What are patient accounts receivable?

   e. What is deferred revenue?

   f. What are restricted net assets?

5. **Statement of operations.** The following questions relate to the statement of operations of not-for-profit health care organizations.

   a. What is the analogous for-profit statement called? What are the main sections of the statement of operations?

   b. What are revenues, gains, and other support?

   c. What are expenses and losses?

   d. Funds released from restricted net assets to unrestricted net assets are presented in what section of the statement of revenue, expenses, and other activities?

6. **Statement of changes in net assets.** The following questions relate to the statement of changes in net assets.

   a. What is the traditional name for this statement?

   b. What is the purpose of this statement?

   c. What are the main sections of this statement?

   d. Discuss the difference between permanently restricted and temporarily restricted net assets.

7. **Statement of cash flows.** The following questions relate to the statement of cash flows of a not-for-profit health care organization.

   a. What are its main sections?

   b. What is the purpose of this statement?

8. **Financial statement element.** Where in the financial statements would there be important explanatory information?

9. **Financial statement element.** In what financial statement would one identify the purchase of long-term investments?

10. **Accounting methods.** How does the accrual basis of accounting differ from the cash basis of accounting?

11. **Balance sheet.** The following are account balances as of September 30, 20X1, for Zachary Hospital. Prepare a balance sheet at September 30, 20X1. (*Hint*: net assets will also need to be calculated.)

    Givens

Gross plant, property, and equipment	$20,000,000
Accrued expenses	$2,000,000
Cash	$2,000,000
Net accounts receivable	$8,500,000
Accounts payable	$6,000,000
Long-term debt	$15,000,000
Supplies	$1,000,000
Accumulated depreciation	$1,000,000

12. **Balance sheet.** The following are account balances as of September 30, 20X1, for White Stone Hospital. Prepare a balance sheet at September 30, 20X1. (*Hint:* net assets will also need to be calculated.)

    Givens

Gross plant, property, and equipment	$35,000,000
Cash	$4,000,000
Net accounts receivable	$9,700,000
Accrued expenses	$3,200,000
Inventory	$3,300,000
Long-term debt	$13,500,000
Accounts payable	$5,300,000
Accumulated depreciation	$18,500,000

13. **Statement of operations.** The following are annual account balances as of September 30, 20X1, for Homestead Hospital. Prepare a statement of operations for the 12-month period ending September 30, 20X1.

    Givens (in thousands)

Net patient revenues	$418,000
Transfer to parent corporation	$5,000
Net assets released from restriction for operations	$110,000
Depreciation expense	$35,000

Labor expense	$333,000
Interest expense	$8,000
Supply expense	$144,000

14. **Statement of operations.** The following are annual account balances as of September 30, 20X1, for Downtown Hospital. Prepare a statement of operations for the 12-month period ending September 30, 20X1.

Givens (in thousands)

Net patient revenues	$750,000
Supply expense	$145,000
Net assets released from restriction for operations	$25,000
Depreciation expense	$30,000
Transfer to parent corporation	$7,500
Interest expense	$8,000
Labor expense	$550,000

15. **Multiple statements.** The following are account balances as of September 30, 20X1, for Goshen Outpatient Center. Prepare (a) a balance sheet, (b) a statement of operations, and (c) a statement of changes in net assets for September 30, 20X1.

Givens

Insurance expense	$22,000
Cash	$45,000
Net patient revenues	$850,000
Net accounts receivable	$150,000
Ending balance, temporarily restricted net assets	$18,000
Wages payable	$25,000
Prepaid expenses	$3,000
Long-term debt	$150,000
Supply expense	$25,000
Gross plant, property, and equipment	$700,000
Net assets released from temporary restriction	$12,000
Depreciation expense	$11,000
General expense	$125,000
Transfer to parent corporation	$45,000
Beginning balance, unrestricted net assets	$176,000
Accounts payable	$65,000
Beginning balance, temporarily restricted net assets	$30,000
Interest expense	$8,000
Labor expense	$550,000
Accumulated depreciation	$350,000
Ending or beginning balance, permanently restricted net assets	$38,000
Ending balance, unrestricted net assets	$252,000

16. **Multiple statements.** The following are account balances (in thousands) on September 30, 20X1, for Marple Newton Medical Center. Prepare: (a) balance sheet, (b) statement of operations, and (c) statement of changes in net assets for September 30, 20X1.

Givens

Administrative expense	$25,000
Cash	$21,000
Net patient revenues	$345,000
Gross accounts receivable	$22,000
Ending balance, temporarily restricted net assets	$12,000
Wages payable	$12,000
Prepaid expenses	$11,000
Long-term debt	$295,000
Supply expense	$42,000
Gross plant, property, and equipment	$450,000
Net assets released from restriction for operations	$3,000
Uncollectibles in accounts receivable	$4,000
Inventory	$7,000
Premium revenues	$3,500
Long-term investments, unrestricted	$175,000
Depreciation expense	$22,000
General expense	$61,000
Transfer to parent corporation	$5,000
Beginning balance, unrestricted net assets	$135,700
Accounts payable	$14,000
Beginning balance, temporarily restricted net assets	$15,000
Interest expense	$6,500
Labor expense	$135,000
Accumulated depreciation	$145,000
Ending and beginning balance, permanently restricted net assets	$8,000
Ending balance, unrestricted net assets	$196,700
Accrued expense	$4,500
Temporary investments	$8,700
Other revenues	$6,000
Current portion of long-term debt	$3,500

17. **Statement of cash flows.** The following are account balances (in thousands) at December 31, 20X1, for Plainview Hospital. Prepare a statement of cash flows for the year ended December 31, 20X1. (*Hint:* the amounts have been stated as positive or negative numbers as they affect cash flow.)

Givens

Decrease in prepaid expenses	$1,500
Payments on long-term debt	($3,000)

Cash and cash equivalents at beginning of the year	$49,000
Increase in inventory	($1,800)
Increases in long-term debt	$125,000
Decrease in accrued expenses	($1,700)
Change in net assets	$4,500
Sale of long-term investments	$25,000
Increase in other current liabilities	$2,600
Depreciation	$8,500
Payments on capital lease	($5,500)
Purchases of equipment	($135,000)
Increase in net account receivables	($30,000)
Increase in accounts payable	$20,000

18. **Statement of cash flows.** The following are account balances (in thousands) at December 31, 20X1, for Sharon Hill Hospital. Prepare a statement of cash flows for the year ended December 31, 20X1. (*Hint:* the amounts have been stated as positive or negative numbers as they affect cash flow.)

Givens

Increase in prepaid expenses	($4,000)
Increase in accrued expenses	$7,000
Cash and cash equivalents at beginning of the year	$55,000
Proceeds from restricted contribution	$125,000
Change in net assets	$25,000
Increase in net account receivables	($12,000)
Sale of equipment	$85,000
Decrease in other current liabilities	($6,500)
Depreciation	$35,000
Increase in inventory	($8,000)
Purchase of long-term investments	($175,000)
Payments on long-term debt	($65,000)
Decrease in accounts payable	($15,000)

19. **Multiple statements.** The following are account balances (in thousands) for Aston Health Plan. Prepare (a) a balance sheet and (b) an income statement for the year ended December 31, 20X0.

Givens

Income tax benefit of operating loss	$12,000
Net property and equipment	$3,500
Physician services expense	$145,000
Premium revenue	$150,000
Marketing expense	$12,000
Compensation expense	$17,000
Interest income and other revenue	$5,000
Outside referral expense	$8,000

Medicare revenue	$125,000
Occupancy and depreciation expense	$4,000
Medical claims payable	$48,000
Accounts receivable	$6,500
Emergency room expense	$13,000
Inpatient services expense	$128,000
Interest expense	$3,000
Medicaid revenue	$15,000
Owners' equity	$55,500
Cash and cash equivalents	$95,000
Long-term debt	$1,500
Other administrative expense	$3,000

20. **Multiple statements.** The following are account balances (in thousands) at September 30, 20X1, for Ivy Health Plan. Prepare (a) a balance sheet and (b) an income statement.

Givens

Income tax expense	$825
Prepaid expense	$1,000
Physician services expense	$4,900
Premium revenues	$16,000
Cash and cash equivalents	$14,000
Marketing expense	$550
Compensation expense	$1,700
Other noncurrent assets	$2,800
Interest income and other revenue	$1,300
Accrued expense	$1,100
Outside referral expense	$4,500
Claims payable, medical	$13,000
Medicare revenues	$6,000
Occupancy and depreciation expense	$600
Owners' equity	$5,300
Emergency room expense	$1,600
Net property and equipment	$4,500
Premium receivables	$3,200
Inpatient service expense	$7,500
Notes payable	$1,200
Interest expense	$800
Unearned premium revenues	$1,500
Medicaid revenues	$2,000
Long-term debt	$3,400
Other administrative expense	$400

21. **Multiple statements.** The following are account balances (in thousands) at September 30, 20X1, for Edgemont Medical Center. Prepare (a) a balance sheet, (b) a statement of operations, and (c) a statement of changes in net assets for September 30, 20X1.

    Givens

Inventory	$5,000
Net patient revenues	$197,500
Gross plant, property, and equipment	$150,000
Net accounts receivable	$40,000
Ending balance, temporarily restricted net assets	$10,300
Wages payable	$11,500
Long-term debt	$87,000
Supply expense	$13,000
Net assets released from temporary restriction	($3,500)
Depreciation expense	$10,500
General expense	$55,000
Insurance expense	$12,000
Cash and cash equivalents	$8,800
Transfer to parent corporation	($1,300)
Beginning balance, unrestricted net assets	$50,000
Accounts payable	$18,000
Beginning balance, temporarily restricted net assets	$13,800
Interest expense	$8,500
Labor expense	$85,700
Accumulated depreciation	$70,000
Long-term investments	$58,000
Ending balance, unrestricted net assets	$65,000

22. **Multiple statements.** The following are account balances (in thousands) at September 30, 20X1, for Shively Medical Center. Prepare (a) a balance sheet, (b) a statement of operations, and (c) a statement of changes in net assets for September 30, 20X1.

    Givens

Inventory	$6,300
Net patient revenues	$284,000
Gross plant, property, and equipment	$410,000
Net accounts receivable	$52,000
Ending balance, temporarily restricted net assets	$6,000
Wages payable	$4,100
Long-term debt	$92,000
Supply expense	$41,000
Net assets released from temporary restriction	$12,000

Depreciation expense	$21,000
General expense	$85,000
Insurance expense	$4,500
Cash and cash equivalents	$13,500
Transfer to parent corporation	($2,500)
Beginning balance, unrestricted net assets	$239,400
Accounts payable	$12,500
Beginning balance, temporarily restricted net assets	$18,000
Interest expense	$4,200
Labor expense	$114,000
Accumulated depreciation	$225,000
Long-term investments	$121,000
Ending balance, unrestricted net assets	$263,200

23. **Multiple statements.** The following are account balances (in thousands) at September 30, 20X1, for El Paso Outpatient Center. Prepare (a) a balance sheet, (b) a statement of operations, and (c) a statement of changes in net assets for September 30, 20X1.

Givens

Insurance expense	$35,000
Cash	$44,000
Net patient revenues	$424,000
Net accounts receivable	$19,000
Ending balance, temporarily restricted net assets	$23,000
Wages payable	$3,400
Prepaid expense	$1,500
Long-term debt	$153,000
Supply expense	$44,000
Gross plant, property, and equipment	$335,000
Net assets released from temporary restriction	$13,700
Depreciation expense	$13,600
General expense	$88,000
Transfer to parent corporation	($11,000)
Beginning balance, unrestricted net assets	$203,400
Accounts payable	$41,000
Beginning balance, temporarily restricted net assets	$36,700
Interest expense	$5,400
Labor expense	$245,000
Accumulated depreciation	$110,000
Long-term investments	$130,000
Ending balance, unrestricted net assets	$199,100

24. **Multiple statements.** The following are account balances (in thousands) at September 30, 20X1, for Chester Springs Hospital. Prepare (a) a balance sheet, (b) a statement of operations, and (c) a statement of changes in net assets for September 30, 20X1.

Givens

Provision for bad debt expense	$10,200
Cash	$14,300
Net patient revenues	$198,700
Net accounts receivable	$26,400
Ending balance, temporarily restricted net assets	$4,100
Wages payable	$10,500
Inventory	$3,800
Long-term debt	$27,000
Supply expense	$25,000
Gross plant, property, and equipment	$130,000
Net assets released from temporary restriction	$1,200
Depreciation expense	$11,300
General expense	$48,000
Transfer to parent corporation	($1,400)
Beginning balance, unrestricted net assets	$160,600
Accounts payable	$4,800
Beginning balance, temporarily restricted net assets	$28,000
Interest expense	$1,400
Labor expense	$93,000
Accumulated depreciation	$40,000
Long-term investments, restricted	$104,800
Ending balance, unrestricted net assets	$192,900

25. **Multiple statements.** The following are account balances (in thousands) at September 30, 20X1, for Lower Merion Hospital. Prepare (a) a balance sheet, (b) a statement of operations, and (c) a statement of changes in net assets for September 30, 20X1.

Givens

Provision for bad debt expense	$23,800
Cash	$20,800
Net patient revenues	$242,400
Net accounts receivable	$38,600
Ending balance, temporarily restricted net assets	$4,700
Wages payable	$8,200
Inventory	$3,100
Long-term debt	$126,300
Supply expense	$67,000

Gross plant, property, and equipment	$220,000
Net assets released from temporary restriction	$7,800
Depreciation expense	$16,500
General expense	$17,500
Transfer to parent corporation	($3,500)
Beginning balance, unrestricted net assets	$246,100
Accounts payable	$11,300
Beginning balance, temporarily restricted net assets	$12,500
Interest expense	$6,000
Labor expense	$104,000
Accumulated depreciation	$55,000
Long-term investments	$181,000
Ending balance, unrestricted net assets	$258,000

APPENDIX A

FINANCIAL STATEMENTS FOR SAMPLE NOT-FOR-PROFIT AND FOR-PROFIT HOSPITAL, AND NOTES TO FINANCIAL STATEMENTS

Exhibit A-1   Balance Sheet for Sample Not-For-Profit Hospital

Sample Not-For-Profit Hospital
Balance Sheet
December 31, 20X1 and 20X0 (in thousands)

Assets	20X1	20X0
Current assets		
Cash and cash equivalents	$4,758	$5,877
Short-term investments	15,836	10,740
Assets limited as to use	970	1,300
Patient accounts receivable, net estimated	15,100	14,194
uncollectibles of $2,500 in 20X1 and $2,400 in 20X0		
Supplies	2,000	2,000
Prepaid expenses	670	856
Total current assets	39,334	34,967
Noncurrent assets		
Assets limited as to use	18,949	19,841
Less amount required to meet current obligations	(970)	(1,300)
	17,979	18,541
Long-term investments	4,680	4,680
Long-term investments restricted for capital acquisition	320	520
Properties and equipment, net	51,038	50,492
Other assets	1,695	1,370
Total noncurrent assets	75,712	75,603
Total assets	$115,046	$110,570
Liabilities and net assets		
Current liabilities		
Current portion of long-term debt	$1,470	$1,750
Accounts payable and accrued expenses	5,818	5,382
Estimated third-party payor settlements	2,143	1,942
Deferred revenues	1,969	2,114
Total current liabilities	11,400	11,188
Noncurrent liabilities		
Long-term debt, net of current portion	23,144	24,014
Other	3,953	3,166
Total non-current liabilities	27,097	27,180
Total liabilities	38,497	38,368
Net assets		
Unrestricted	70,846	66,199
Temporarily restricted	2,115	2,470
Permanently restricted	3,588	3,533
Total net assets	76,549	72,202
Total liabilities and net assets	$115,046	$110,570

Exhibit A–2 Statement of operations for Sample Not-For-Profit Hospital

Sample Not-For-Profit Hospital
Statement of Operations
For the Years Ended December 31, 20X1 and 20X0 (in thousands)

	20X1	20X0
Unrestricted revenues, gains, and other support		
Net patient service revenue	$85,156	$78,942
Premium revenue	11,150	10,950
Other revenues	2,601	5,212
Net assets released from restriction used for operations	300	
Total revenues, gains, and other support	99,207	95,104
Expenses		
Salaries and benefits	53,900	49,938
Medical supplies and drugs	26,532	22,121
Insurance	8,089	8,526
Depreciation and amortization	4,782	4,280
Interest	1,752	1,825
Provision for bad debts	1,000	1,300
Other expenses	2,000	1,300
Total expenses	98,055	89,290
Operating income	1,152	5,814
Other income		
Investment income	3,900	3,025
Excess of revenues over expenses	5,052	8,839
Change in net unrealized gains and losses on other than trading securities	300	375
Net assets released from restrictions used for purchase of property and equipment	200	
Contribution from sample hospital foundation for property acquisitions	235	485
Transfers to parent	(640)	(3,000)
Increase in unrestricted net assets, before extraordinary item	5,147	6,699
Extraordinary loss (debt extinguishment)	(500)	
Increase in unrestricted net assets	$4,647	$6,699

Source: Reprinted with permission from the *Audit and Accounting Guide: Health Care Organizations*, copyright © 2007 by the American Institute of Certified Public Accountants, Inc.

Exhibit A–3   Statement of changes in net assets for Sample Not-For-Profit Hospital

Sample Not-For-Profit Hospital
Statement of Changes in Net Assets
For the Years Ended December 31, 20X1 and 20X0 (in thousands)

	20X1	20X0
Unrestricted net assets		
Excess of revenues over expenses	$5,052	$8,839
Net unrealized gains on investments other than trading securities	300	375
Contribution from sample hospital foundation for property acquisition	235	485
Transfers to parent	(640)	(3,000)
Net assets released from restrictions used for purchase of properties and equipment	200	
Increase in unrestricted net assets before extraordinary item	5,147	6,699
Extraordinary loss from extinguishment of debt	(500)	
Increase in unrestricted net assets	4,647	6,699
Temporarily restricted net assets		
Contributions for charity care	140	996
Net realized and unrealized gains on investments	5	8
Net assets released from restrictions	(500)	
Increase (decrease) in temporarily restricted net assets	(355)	1,004
Permanently restricted net assets		
Contributions for endowment funds	50	411
Net realized and unrealized gains on investments	5	2
Increase in permanently restricted net assets	55	413
Increase in net assets	4,347	8,116
Net assets, beginning of year	72,202	64,086
Net assets, end of year	$76,549	$72,202

Source: Reprinted with permission from the *Audit and Accounting Guide: Health Care Organizations*, copyright © 2007 by the American Institute of Certified Public Accountants, Inc.

Exhibit A–4　Statement of cash flows for Sample Not-For-Profit Hospital

Sample Not-For-Profit Hospital
Statement of Cash Flows (Indirect Method)
December 31, 20X1 and 20X0 (in thousands)[a]

	20X1	20X0
Cash flows from operating activities		
Change in net assets	$4,347	$8,116
Adjustments to reconcile change in net assets to		
net cash provided by operating activities:		
Extraordinary loss from debt extinguishment	500	
Depreciation	4,782	4,280
Net realized and unrealized gains on investments	(450)	(575)
other than trading		
Transfers to parent	640	3,000
Provision for bad debt	1,000	1,300
Restricted contributions and investment income received	(55)	(413)
(Increase) decrease in:		
Patient accounts receivable	(1,906)	(2,036)
Trading securities	215	
Other current assets	186	(2,481)
Other assets	(325)	(241)
Increase (decrease) in:		
Accounts payable and accrued expenses	436	679
Estimated third-party pay or settlements	201	305
Other current liabilities	(145)	(257)
Other liabilities	787	(128)
Net cash provided by operating activities	10,213	11,549
Cash flows from investing activities		
Purchases of investment	(3,769)	(2,150)
Capital expenditures	(4,728)	(5,860)
Net cash used in investing activities	(8,497)	(8,010)
Cash flows from financing activities		
Transfer to parent	(640)	(3,000)
Proceeds from restricted contributions and restricted	55	413
investment income		
Payments on long-term debt	(24,700)	(804)
Payments on capital lease obligations	(150)	(100)
Increase in long-term debt	22,600	500
Net cash used in financing activities	(2,835)	(2,991)
Net increase (decrease) in cash and cash equivalents	(1,119)	548
Cash and cash equivalents at beginning of year	5,877	5,329
Cash and cash equivalents at end of year	$4,758	$5,877

Supplemental disclosures and cash flow information:
The Hospital entered into capital lease obligations in the amount of $600,000 for new equipment in 2001

[a]Cash paid for interest (net of amount capitalized in 20X1 and 20X0 was $1,780,000 and $1,856,000, respectively. See accompanying notes to financial statements in Exhibit A–8.)

Source: Reprinted with permission from the *Audit and Accounting Guide: Health Care Organizations*, copyright © 2007 by the American Institute of Certified Public Accountants, Inc.

Exhibit A–5   Consolidated income statement for LifePoint Hospitals Incorporated

LifePoint Hospitals Incorporated
Consolidated Income Statement
For the Years Ended December 31, 2006 and 2005 (in millions)

	2006	2005
Revenues	$2,439	$1,842
Operating expenses		
Salaries and benefits	961	740
Supplies	340	250
Other operating expenses	421	368
Provision for doubtful accounts	266	189
Depreciation and amortization	111	101
Interest expense	103	60
Total operating expenses	2,202	1,708
Income from continuing operations before minority interests	237	134
Minority interests in earnings of consolidated entities	1	1
Income from continuing operations before income taxes	236	133
Provision for income taxes	90	60
Net income	$146	$73

Source: LifePoint's 10-K report from Securities and Exchange Commission.

Exhibit A–6 Consolidated balance sheet for LifePoint Hospitals Incorporated

LifePoint Hospitals Incorporated
Consolidated Balance Sheet
December 31, 2006 and 2005 (in millions)

Assets	2006	2005
Current assets		
Cash and cash equivalents	$12	$30
Accounts receivable, less allowances	326	257
for doubtful accounts		
Inventories	67	57
Income taxes receivable	11	
Prepaid expenses	13	12
Other	185	77
Total current assets:	614	433
Property and equipment, at cost		
Land	80	64
Buildings	1,085	987
Equipment	610	540
Construction in progress	72	78
	1,847	1,669
Accumulated depreciation	(474)	(373)
Net Plant and equipment	1,373	1,296
Goodwill	1,581	1,449
Intangible assets	64	39
Other	109	35
Total assets	$3,741	$3,252
Liabilities and stockholders' equity		
Current liabilities		
Accounts payable	$109	$86
Accrued salaries	69	59
Other accrued expenses	125	72
Long-term debt due within one year	1	1
Total current liabilities	304	218
Long-term debt	1,770	1,515
Professional liability risks, deferred taxes and other liabilities	82	63
Deferred taxes	120	124
Minority interest in consolidated equities		
Stockholders' equity:		
Common stock $0.01 par; authorized 90,000,000 voting shares	1	1
Capital in excess of par value	1,044	1,053
Other		
Accumulated other comprehensive income		
Retained earnings	421	279
Total stockholders' equity	1,466	1,333
Total liabilities and stockholders' equity	$3,741	$3,252

Source: LifePoint's 10-K report from Securities and Exchange Commission.

Exhibit A–7   Consolidated statement of cash flows for LifePoint Hospitals Incorporated

LifePoint Hospitals Incorporated
Consolidated Statement of Cash Flows
For the Years Ended December 31, 2006 and 2005 (in millions)

	2006	2005
Cash flows from continuing operating activities		
Net income (loss)	$146	$73
Adjustments to reconcile net income (loss) to net cash provided by continuing operating activities		
Depreciation and amortization	111	101
Deferred taxes	45	(3)
Stock base compensation	22	19
Loss from discontinued operations	0	153
Increase (decrease) in cash from current assets and liabilities		
Accounts receivable	(52)	(26)
Inventories and other assets	(11)	(9)
Accounts payable and accrued expenses	21	23
Other	(36)	(30)
Net cash provided by continuing operating activities	246	301
Cash flows from investing activities		
Purchase of property and equipment	(199)	(169)
Acquisition of hospitals and health care entities	(281)	(963)
Discontinued operations	69	31
Other	(4)	0
Net cash provided by (used in) investing activities	(415)	(1,101)
Cash flows from financing activities		
Issuance of long-term debt	260	1,967
Proceeds from stock options	2	38
Repayment of long-term debt	(110)	(1,157)
Other	(1)	(37)
Net cash provided by (used in) financing activities	151	811
Change in cash and cash equivalents	(18)	11
Cash and cash equivalents at beginning of period	30	20
Cash and cash equivalents at end of period	$12	$30

Source: LifePoint's 10-K report from Securities and Exchange Commission.

Exhibit A–8 Abbreviated notes to financial statements for Sample Not-For-Profit Hospital December 31, 20X1 and 20X0

---

1. Description of Organization and Summary of Significant Accounting Policies

Organization. The Sample Not-For-Profit Hospital (the Hospital), located in [*city, state*], is a not-for-profit acute care hospital. The Hospital provides inpatient, outpatient, and emergency care services for residents of northeastern [*state*]. Admitting physicians are primarily practitioners in the local area. The Hospital was incorporated in [*state*] in 20X0 and is affiliated with the Sample Health System.

Use of estimates. The preparation of financial statements in conformity with generally accepted accounting principles requires management to make estimates and assumptions that affect the reported amounts of assets and liabilities, and disclosure of contingent assets and liabilities, at the date of the financial statements, and the reported amounts of revenues and expenses during the reporting period. Actual results could differ from those estimates.

Cash and cash equivalents. Cash and cash equivalents include certain investments in highly liquid debt instruments with original maturities of three months or less.

The Hospital routinely invests its surplus operating funds in money market mutual funds. These funds generally invest in highly liquid U.S. government and agency obligations.

Investments. Investments in equity securities with readily determinable fair values and all investments in debt securities are measured at fair value in the balance sheet. Investment income or loss (including realized gains and losses on investments, interest, and dividends) is included in the excess of revenues over expenses, unless the income or loss is restricted by donor or law. Unrealized gains and losses on investments are excluded from the excess of revenues over expenses, unless the investments are trading securities.

Assets limited as to use. Assets limited as to use primarily include assets held by trustees under indenture agreements, and designated assets set aside by the board of trustees for future capital improvements, over which the board retains control and may at its discretion subsequently use for other purposes. Amounts required to meet current liabilities of the hospital have been reclassified in the balance sheet at December 31, 20X1 and 20X0.

Property and equipment. Property and equipment acquisitions are recorded at cost. Depreciation is provided over the estimated useful life of each class of depreciable asset and is computed using the straight-line method. Equipment under capital lease obligations is amortized on the straight-line method over the shorter period of the lease term or the estimated useful life of the equipment. Such amortization is included in depreciation and amortization in the financial statements. Interest cost incurred on borrowed funds during the period of construction of capital assets is capitalized as a component of the cost of acquiring those assets.

(Continued)

Exhibit A–8   Abbreviated notes to financial statements for Sample Not-For-Profit Hospital December 31, 20X1 and 20X0 (Continued)

Gifts of long-lived assets such as land, buildings, or equipment are reported as unrestricted support and are excluded from the excess of revenues over expenses, unless explicit donor stipulations specify how the donated assets must be used. Gifts of long-lived assets with explicit restrictions that specify how the assets are to be used and gifts of cash or other assets that must be used to acquire long-lived assets are reported as restricted support. Absent explicit donor stipulations about how long those long-lived assets must be maintained, expirations of donor restrictions are reported when the donated or acquired long-lived assets are placed in service.

Temporarily and permanently restricted net assets. Temporarily restricted net assets are those whose use by the Hospital has been limited by donors to a specific time period or purpose. Permanently restricted net assets have been restricted by donors to be maintained by the Hospital in perpetuity.

Excess of revenues over expenses. The statement of operations includes excess of revenues over expenses. Changes in unrestricted net assets that are excluded from excess of revenues over expenses, consistent with industry practice, include unrealized gains and losses on investments other than trading securities, permanent transfers of assets to and from affiliates for other than goods and services, and contributions of long-lived assets (including assets acquired using contributions that by donor restriction were to be used for the purposes of acquiring such assets).

Net patient service revenue. The Hospital has agreements with third-party payors that provide for payments to the Hospital in amounts different from its established rates. Payment arrangements include prospectively determined rates per discharge, reimbursed costs, discounted charges, and per diem payments. Net patient service revenue is reported at the estimated net realizable amounts from patients, third-party payors, and others for services rendered, including estimated retroactive adjustments under reimbursement agreements with third-party payors. Retroactive adjustments are accrued on an estimated basis in the period the related services are rendered and adjusted in future periods as final settlements are determined.

Premium revenue. The Hospital has agreements with various health maintenance organizations (HMOs) to provide medical services to subscribing participants. Under these agreements, the Hospital receives monthly capitation payments based on the number of each HMO's participants, regardless of services actually performed by the Hospital. In addition, the HMOs make fee-for-service payments to the Hospital for certain covered services based on discounted fee schedules.

Charity care. The Hospital provides care to patients who meet certain criteria under its charity care policy without charge or at amounts less than its established rates. Because the Hospital does not pursue collection of amounts determined to qualify as charity care, they are not reported as revenue.

Donor-restricted gifts. Unconditional promises to give cash and other assets to the Hospital are reported at fair value at the date the promise is received. Conditional promises to give and indications of intentions to give are reported at fair value on the

Exhibit A–8 *(Continued)*

date the gift is received. The gifts are reported as either temporarily or permanently restricted support if they are received with donor stipulations that limit the use of the donated assets. When a donor restriction expires—that is, when a stipulated time restriction ends or purpose restriction is accomplished—temporarily restricted net assets are reclassified as unrestricted net assets and reported in the statement of operations as net assets released from restrictions. Donor-restricted contributions whose restrictions are met within the same year as received are reported as unrestricted contributions in the accompanying financial statements.

Estimated malpractice costs. The provision for estimated medical malpractice claims includes estimates of the ultimate costs for both reported claims and claims incurred but not reported.

Income taxes. The Hospital is a not-for-profit corporation and has been recognized as tax-exempt pursuant to Section 501(c)3 of the Internal Revenue Code.

2. Net Patient Service Revenue

The Hospital has agreements with third-party payors that provide for payments to the Hospital in amounts different from its established rates. A summary of the payment arrangements with major third-party payors follows:

Medicare. Inpatient acute care services rendered to Medicare program beneficiaries are paid at prospectively determined rates per discharge. These rates vary according to a patient classification system that is based on clinical, diagnostic, and other factors. Inpatient nonacute services, certain outpatient services, and defined capital and medical education costs related to Medicare beneficiaries are paid based on a cost-reimbursement method. The Hospital is reimbursed for cost-reimbursable items at a tentative rate with final settlement determined after submission of annual cost reports by the Hospital and audits thereof by the Medicare fiscal intermediary. Beginning in 20X0, the Hospital claimed Medicare payments based on an interpretation of certain "disproportionate share" rules. The intermediary disagreed and declined to pay the excess reimbursement claimed under that interpretation. Through 20X0, the Hospital has not included the claimed excess in net patient revenues pending resolution of the matter. In 20X1 the intermediary accepted the claims and paid the outstanding claims, including $950,000 applicable to 20X0 and $300,000 applicable to 20X1 and prior, which has been included in 20X0 net revenues.

Medicaid. Inpatient and outpatient services rendered to Medicaid program beneficiaries are reimbursed under a cost-reimbursement method. The Hospital is reimbursed at a tentative rate with final settlement determined after submission of annual cost reports by the Hospital and audits thereof by the Medicaid fiscal intermediary.

The Hospital also has entered into payment agreements with certain commercial insurance carriers, HMOs, and preferred provider organizations. The basis for payment to the Hospital under these agreements includes prospectively determined rates per discharge, discounts from established charges, and prospectively determined daily rates.

(Continued)

Exhibit A–8   Abbreviated notes to financial statements for Sample Not-For-Profit Hospital December 31, 20X1 and 20X0 *(Continued)*

3. Investments

Assets Limited as to Use. The composition of assets limited as to use at December 31, 20X1 and 20X0, is set forth in the following table. Investments are stated at fair value.

	20X1	20X0
Internally designated for capital acquisition		
Cash	$545,000	$350,000
U.S. Treasury obligations	11,435,000	12,115,000
Interest receivable	20,000	35,000
Total	12,000,000	12,500,000
Held by trustee under indenture agreement		
Cash and short-term investments	352,000	260,000
U.S. Treasury obligation	6,505,000	7,007,000
Interest receivable	92,000	74,000
	6,949,000	7,341,000
Total	$18,949,000	$19,841,000

Other Investments. Other investments, stated at fair value, at December 31, 20X1 and 20X0, include

	20X1	20X0
Trading:		
U.S. corporate bonds	$1,260,000	$1,475,000
Other		
U.S. Treasury obligations	19,266,000	14,233,000
Interest receivable	310,000	232,000
Total	20,836,000	15,940,000
Less		
Long-term investments	4,680,000	4,680,000
Long-term investments restricted for capital acquisitions	320,000	520,000
Total	$15,836,000	$10,740,000

Exhibit A–8 *(Continued)*

Investment income and gains for assets limited as to use, cash equivalents, and other investments are compiled on the following for the years ending September 30, 20X1 and 20X0:

	20X1	20X0
Income		
Interest income	$3,585,000	$2,725,000
Realized gains on sales of securities	150,000	200,000
Unrealized gains on trading securities	165,000	100,000
Total	3,900,000	3,025,000
Other changes in unrestricted net assets		
Unrealized gains on other than trading securities	$300,000	$375,000

4. Property and Equipment

A summary of property and equipment at September 30, 20X1 and 20X0, follows:

	20X1	20X0
Land	$3,000,000	$3,000,000
Land improvements	472,000	472,000
Buildings and improvements	46,852,000	46,636,000
Equipment	29,190,000	26,260,000
Equipment under capital lease obligations	2,851,000	2,752,000
Total	82,365,000	79,120,000
Less accumulated depreciation and amortization	34,928,000	30,661,000
	47,437,000	48,459,000
Construction in progress	3,601,000	2,033,000
Property and equipment, net	$51,038,000	$50,492,000

Depreciation expense for the years ended December 31, 20X1 and 20X0, amounted to approximately $4,782,000 and $4,280,000. Accumulated amortization for equipment under capital lease obligations were $689,000 and $453,000 at December 31, 20X1 and 20X0, respectively. Construction contracts of approximately $7,885,000 exist for the remodeling of Hospital facilities. At December 31, 20X1, the remaining commitment on these contracts approximated $4,625,000.

5. Charity Care

The amount of charges forgone for services and supplies furnished under the Hospital's charity policy aggregated approximately $4,500,000 and $4,100,000 in 20X1 and 20X0, respectively.

(Continued)

Exhibit A–8   Abbreviated notes to financial statements for Sample Not-For-Profit Hospital December 31, 20X1 and 20X0 (Concluded)

6. Long-Term Debt
A summary of long-term debt and capital leases at December 31, 20X1:

7.25% Tax-exempt revenue bonds principal maturing in varying amounts, due November 1, 20XX	$21,479,000
7.75% mortgage loan, principal maturing in varying amounts, due June 1, 20XX	$2,010,000
Capital lease obligations at varying rates of imputed interest from 6.8% to 9.3% collateralized by leased equipment	$1,000,000

Source: Adapted with permission from the *Audit and Accounting Guide: Health Care Organizations*, copyright © 2007 by the American Institute of Certified Public Accountants, Inc.

3

PRINCIPLES AND PRACTICES OF HEALTH CARE ACCOUNTING

LEARNING OBJECTIVES

- Record financial transactions
- Understand the basics of accrual accounting
- Summarize transactions into financial statements

The financial viability of a health care organization results from numerous decisions made by various people, including care givers, administrators, boards, lenders, community members, and politicians. These decisions eventually result in an organization's acquiring and using resources to provide services, to incur obligations, and to generate revenues. One of the major roles of accounting is to record these transactions and report the results in a standardized format to interested parties. This chapter shows how a series of typical transactions at a health center are recorded on the books and how these records are used to produce the four major financial statements for a not-for-profit, business-oriented health care organization. The recording and reporting process can be time-consuming, but changes are continually being made to automate it (see Exhibit 3–1 and Perspective 3–1).

THE BOOKS

As transactions of a health care organization occur (such as the purchase of supplies), they are recorded chronologically in a "book" called a *journal*. Today, this book is more likely to be a computer than a journal requiring manual entries. Periodically (simultaneously with most computer programs) these transactions are summarized by account (i.e., "Cash," "Equipment," "Revenues," etc.) into another book called a *ledger*. With these two books, the organization has both a chronological listing of transactions and the current balance in each account (see Exhibit 3–2). The totals for each account in the ledger are used to prepare the four financial statements. Although this procedure is simple to conceptualize, ensuring the financial statements are prepared accurately and in a timely manner is quite involved, as Perspective 3–1 shows.

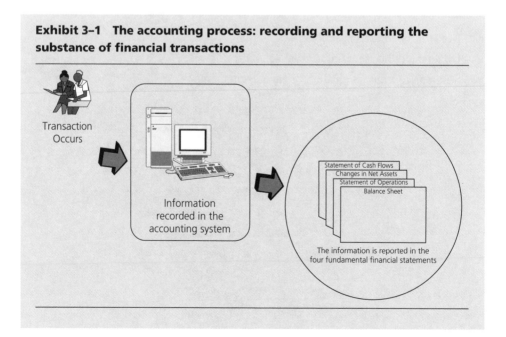

Exhibit 3–1   The accounting process: recording and reporting the substance of financial transactions

Transaction Occurs

Information recorded in the accounting system

Statement of Cash Flows
Changes in Net Assets
Statement of Operations
Balance Sheet

The information is reported in the four fundamental financial statements

Exhibit 3–2   Role of the journal and ledger in recording and reporting financial transactions

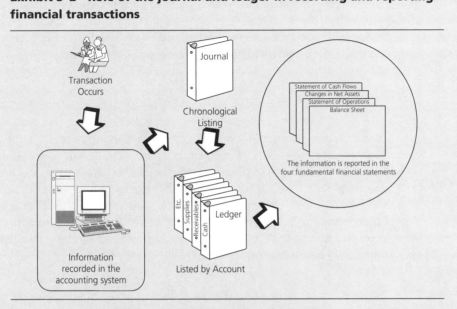

Perspective 3–1   Movement Toward Electronic Accounting Systems in Rural Hospitals

The rural setting of hospitals has created many obstacles in purchasing a health care IT [information technology] system. These barriers range from the insufficient resources to purchase the equipment, the inability to identify IT consultants to assist in the purchase of a quality IT system, and the challenge of being able to hire qualified and trained IT personnel to operate and maintain the IT system. However, the vast numbers of rural hospitals (over 2,100) and clinics (3,500) across the United States provide an opportunity to partner and pool resources among these providers. These partnerships have allowed them to share staff, hire IT consultants, and negotiate discounts in the purchasing of IT equipment. There are several examples of rural hospitals' pooling and partnering their IT services, especially with respect to accounting systems. In Duluth, Minnesota, a network of fourteen hospitals, including ten critical-access hospitals that share services, purchased an IT system that integrates across accounting, billing, and health records. In Illinois a 50-member critical access hospital network implemented an IT system that allowed its members access to electronic reporting of its financial records, along with electronically submitting more than 65 percent of its lab and x-ray results.

Source: Zigmond, J. 2006. Acting neighborly; rural hospitals share resources to advance use of IT. *Modern Healthcare*, April 17.

Cash Basis of Accounting
An accounting method that tracks when cash was received and when cash was expended, regardless of when services were provided or resources were used.

There is a fairly standard set of account categories used by all health care organizations, which is listed in a book entitled *chart of accounts*. The accounts that are used in the financial statements in Chapter Two comprise an important part of the standard set of account categories (though there may be subcategories in each one).

Cash and Accrual Bases of Accounting

Before introducing examples of recording and reporting transactions, the difference between cash and accrual accounting needs to be discussed. The *cash basis of accounting* focuses on the flows of cash in and out of the organization, whereas the *accrual basis of accounting* focuses on the flows of resources and the revenues those resources help to generate. This discussion begins with a focus on the cash basis of accounting, for it is more intuitive. The focus then turns to the accrual basis of accounting, which is the system the accounting profession applies to health care organizations.

Accrual Basis of Accounting
An accounting method that aligns the flow of resources and the revenues those resources helped to generate. It records revenues when earned and resources when used, regardless of the flow of cash in or out of the organization. This is the standard method in use today.

Cash Basis of Accounting The cash basis of accounting records transactions similarly to the way most people keep their personal checkbooks: revenues are recorded when cash is received, and expenses are recorded when cash is paid out (see Exhibit 3–3). For example, if an organization delivers a service to a patient, the revenue from that patient is recorded when received. Expenses are recorded as they are paid (such as when the staff are paid). The advantages of this method of accounting are that cash flows can be tracked, and it is simple. Its main disadvantages are that it does not match revenues with the resources used to generate those revenues and the financial reports under the cash basis of accounting are susceptible to managerial manipulation. Incidentally, one of the functions of auditors is to give assurance that the statements have been prepared according to generally accepted accounting principles (GAAP) (see Perspective 3–2).

Exhibit 3–3 Comparison of the cash and accrual bases of accounting

	Cash Basis of Accounting	Accrual Basis of Accounting
Revenues are recognized	when cash is received	when revenues are earned
Expenses are recognized	when cash is paid out	when resources are used

Perspective 3–2   Sarbanes-Oxley Has Motivated UPMC Health System to Improve Its Internal Audit Processes

University of Pittsburgh Medical Center, UPMC, a 19-hospital system, is the first not-for-profit health care organization in the nation to comply with the strict reporting and internal control requirements of the Sarbanes-Oxley Act of 2002, or SOX, which is the law that requires financial disclosures by publicly traded companies. Some non-profit hospitals voluntarily implement the standards that were enacted to control fraudulent public companies such as Enron Corp. Ernst & Young, a large accounting firm, projects that 80 percent of not-for-profit hospitals have implemented some sections of SOX, such as establishing an audit committee, changing lead audit partners, and preapproving nonaudit fees. Only 30 percent of hospitals are approving quarterly financial statements. However, fewer than 1 percent of the hospitals and health care systems are approving the most restrictive internal control standards, which is section 404 under SOX that requires management and external auditors to evaluate and assess the adequacy of the hospital's internal controls. UPMC health care system, which generates over $6 billion in revenues and employs more than 40,000 workers, decided to comply with SOX because "We consider ourselves a public company. We are not owned by shareholders but by the community. We are the stewards of public money, so we always want to be the best in class. This is an opportunity to hold ourselves up to the highest standard there is for internal controls and governance."

UPMC management projects that the cost for implementation is estimated to be over $6 million for a two-year period. In reality, the system will spend less than $2 million as most of the work was done internally. As part of SOX and its transparency, UPMC now lists its financial data on its Web site, http://www.upmc.com. Bond rating agencies contend that many of the regulations of SOX did not apply to hospitals; however, they also note that adding SOX to their health care organization will improve governance, raise accountability, and validate its financial statements.

Source: Becker, C. 2006. Transparent motives; UPMC blazes trail for not-for-profits in Sarbanes-Oxley compliance. *Modern Healthcare,* July 31.

Accrual Basis of Accounting   The accrual basis of accounting overcomes the disadvantages of the cash basis of accounting by recognizing revenues when they are earned and expenses when resources are used (see Exhibit 3–3). The advantages of the accrual basis of accounting are that (1) it keeps track of revenues generated and

Perspective 3–3   Application of Information Technology to Improve Financial Performance

St. Vincent's Medical Center decided on bankruptcy protection because it was unable to turn around its financial condition. A new management team was installed, and they valued the use of information technology, which could enhance its business operations. Operationally, the top priority of the medical center was to enhance the accuracy and reliability of the reported physician charges. The medical center installed a new mobile device, as part of a pilot program, to assist its physicians in the accurate reporting of inpatient charges for medical services. More than 24 physicians use the charge-capture device and now report nearly 100 percent of their charges and immediately submit them into the billing system. Three months after the implementation of this technology change, coupled with other process improvements, its physicians have been able to raise its collections by a significant amount.

Source: Anonymous. 2007. Going mobile: from square one. *Health Management Technology Atlanta, 28*(8): 26–27.

resources used as well as cash flows, (2) it matches revenues with the resources used to generate those revenues, and (3) the financial statements provide a broader picture of the provider's operation. Its main disadvantages are that it is more difficult to implement and it, too, is open to manipulation, often by bending accounting rules. Keeping track of revenues and resource use can be a technologically intensive endeavor (see Perspective 3–3).

AN EXAMPLE OF THE EFFECTS OF CASH FLOWS ON PROFIT REPORTING UNDER CASH AND ACCRUAL ACCOUNTING

Exhibit 3–4 illustrates how the cash basis of accounting is vulnerable to management's manipulation of revenues and expenses. Assume a health care organization earned $12,000 in revenues and had $4,000 in expenses. In scenario 1, management wants to show a high profit, so although it collects full payment of $12,000, it delays paying its bills until after the end of the accounting period; therefore, the reported profit is $12,000. In scenario 2, management wants to show low profit (perhaps so it can encourage more donations). In this case, management pays all of its bills, $4,000, but sends out its own bills late so that payment is not received from patients and third parties until after the end of the accounting period; reported profit under this scenario

---

Exhibit 3–4 Management manipulation under the cash basis of accounting

---

Situation: During the accounting period, a health care organization has earned $12,000 in revenues, and consumed $4,000 in resources.

Assume 3 scenarios:

1. Management wants to show a high profit, so although it collects full payment of $12,000, it delays paying its bills until after the end of the accounting period.
2. Management wants to show low profit, perhaps to encourage more donations. It pays the bills, $4000, but discourages patients and third parties from paying until after the end of the accounting period.
3. Accrual basis of accounting rules are followed, and the organization records revenues earned of $12,000 and resources used to generate those revenues of $4,000.

	Scenario 1	Scenario 2	Scenario 3
Revenues reported	$12,000	$0	$12,000
Expenses reported	$0	$4,000	$4,000
Profit reported	$12,000	($4,000)	$8,000

Points:

1. Management can manipulate reported profits through its payment and collection policies under the cash basis of accounting.
2. Revenues are not necessarily matched with the resources used to generate those revenues under the cash basis of accounting.

---

is –$4,000. Scenario 3 follows the accrual basis of accounting rules, and management records revenues earned of $12,000 and resources used to generate those revenues of $4,000, which shows a profit of $8,000. Thus, under accrual accounting, the organization cannot influence reported profit by accelerating or slowing cash inflows and outflows. Revenues *must* be recorded when they are earned and expenses recorded when resources are used. Perspective 3–4 shows the importance of accurate record keeping and how systems can go astray.

Generally accepted accounting principles recommend that health care organizations use the accrual basis of accounting. This does not mean that having information about cash flows is any less important than is having information about revenues and the resources used to generate those revenues.

Perspective 3–4   HealthSouth: A Case of Accounting Fraud

HealthSouth, a hospital management company of rehabilitation hospitals, reported a $440 million tax refund from the Internal Revenue Service. This accounting aberration stems from HealthSouth's tax payment on $2.7 billion of fraudulent income it reported to the IRS in 2003. In essence HealthSouth paid taxes on income that was not real.

Federal investigators found substantial accounting fraud within the company in 2003. Several senior executives pleaded guilty for their involvement in this accounting fraud case. However, HealthSouth's chief executive, Richard M. Scrushy, was not found guilty of these accounting fraud charges in 2005, although later Mr. Scrushy was sentenced to prison on an unrelated federal bribery conviction.

Although the company was profitable, the former chief financial officer of the company indicated that one of the major underlying motives for committing this accounting fraud was the financial pressure to show more profits so that the company could meet Wall Street's earnings' expectations. The irony of this accounting scheme is that the company's actual earnings were not high enough to pay taxes on the fraudulent profits. As a result, the company issued debt to help pay off the tax liability. In addition, this financial leverage position contributed to more than $3.6 billion in debt. Under new management, HealthSouth has lowered its outstanding debt to $1 billion, and it intends to use the tax refund to reduce this debt position even further.

Source: Whitemore, K. 2007. Profits aren't real, but the refund is. *New York Times*, October 21. *http://www.nytimes.com/2007/10/21/business/21suits.html*

RECORDING TRANSACTIONS

Assume Windmill Point Outpatient Center is a not-for-profit, business-oriented, health care organization that had the transactions summarized in Exhibit 3–5 during 20X1, its first year of operation. Exhibit 3–6 presents the journal and ledger entries to record the transactions listed in Exhibit 3–5. Because the transactions are recorded chronologically by row, the rows serve as the journal. Because each account has its own column summarized at the bottom, the columns serve as a ledger. These transactions are being recorded in part so that the four financial statements can be prepared. These statements allow interested parties to make informed judgments about the financial health of the organization.

Exhibit 3–5 Sample transactions for Windmill Point Outpatient Center, January 1, 20X1–December 31, 20X1

1. The center received $600,000 in unrestricted contributions.
2. The center obtained a $500,000 bank loan at 6 percent interest; $20,000 in principal is due this year.
3. The center purchased $450,000 of plant and equipment (P&E). It paid cash for the purchase.
4. The center purchased $100,000 of supplies on credit. The vendor expects payment within 30 days.
5. The center provided $500,000 of nondiscounted billable services to non-capitated patients. Payment has not yet been received.
6. On the first day of the year, the center received $250,000 in capitation payment from an HMO. This means an HMO paid the center $250,000 in advance on a per member per year (PMPY) basis to provide for the health care needs of its enrollees over the next year.
7. In the provision of services to all patients, the center incurred $300,000 in labor expenses, which it paid for in cash.
8. In the provision of services to all patients, the center used $80,000 of supplies.
9. The center paid $10,000 in advance for one year's insurance.
10. The center paid for $90,000 of the $100,000 of supplies purchased in transaction 4.
11. Patients or their third parties paid the center $400,000 of the $500,000 they owed (see transaction 5).
12. During the year, the center made a $50,000 cash payment toward its bank loan; $20,000 was for principal, and $30,000 was to pay the full amount of interest due.
13. The center transferred $25,000 to its parent corporation.

At the end of the year, the center recognized the following:
14. Since the last payday, employees have earned wages of $35,000.
15. Equipment has depreciated $45,000.
16. The $10,000 of insurance premium was for one year. That time has now expired.
17. The health center has fulfilled the health care service obligation it took on because the $250,000 in capitated payments for one year (transaction 6) has now expired. This revenue is now considered earned.
18. $20,000 of the note payable in transaction 2 is due within the next year.
19. Bad debt is estimated to be $5,000.
20. $60,000 is set aside for the beginning of the next fiscal year to be used toward purchase of new computer equipment.

Exhibit 3–6 Listing of financial transactions for Windmill Point Outpatient Center

Windmill Point Outpatient Center
Journal and Ledger
For the Period January 1 - December 31, 20X1.

Transaction	ASSETS									LIABILITIES			NET ASSETS				
	Cash	Assets Limited as to Use	Accounts Receivable	Allowance for Doubtful Accounts	Supplies	Prepaid Expenses	Long-term Investments	Plant & Equipment (P&E)	Accumulated Depreciation	Current Liabilities	Deferred Revenues	Non-Current Liabilities	Revenues, Gains and Other Support	Expenses	Transfer to Parent	Unrestricted Net Assets	Restricted Net Assets
Beginning Balance	$0	$0	$0	$0	$0	$0	$0	$0	$0	$0	$0	$0	$0	$0	$0	$0	$0
1 Contribution	600,000												600,000				
2 Long-term bank loan	500,000									20,000		480,000					
3 Purchased P & E with cash	-450,000							450,000									
4 Purchased supplies on credit					100,000					100,000							
5 Patient services on credit			500,000										500,000				
6 Received HMO capitation	250,000										250,000						
7 Paid labor	-300,000													-300,000			
8 Used supplies					-80,000									-80,000			
9 Prepaid insurance	-10,000					10,000											
10 Paid cash for supplies	-90,000									-90,000							
11 Patients paid accounts	400,000		-400,000														
12 Paid bank loan & interest	-50,000									-20,000				-30,000			
13 Transferred funds to parent	-25,000														-25,000		
14 Wages earned but not paid										35,000				-35,000			
15 Depreciation									-45,000					-45,000			
16 Expired insurance						-10,000								-10,000			
17 Capitation earned											-250,000		250,000				
18 Current portion of debt										20,000		-20,000					
19 Bad debt				-5,000										-5,000			
20 IS funds set aside	-60,000	60,000															
Balances after adjustments	765,000	60,000	100,000	-5,000	20,000	0	0	450,000	-45,000	65,000	0	460,000	1,350,000	-505,000	-25,000	0	0
Operating income													-505,000	505,000		845,000	
Closing income from operations to unrestricted net assets													845,000			845,000	
Transfer to parent																-25,000	
Ending balances	765,000	60,000	100,000	-5,000	20,000	0	0	450,000	-45,000	65,000	0	460,000	0	0	0	820,000	0
Balances with summarized net assets	$765,000	$60,000	$100,000	-$5,000	$20,000	$0	$0	$450,000	-$45,000	$65,000	$0	$460,000	$0	$0	$0	$820,000	$0

Summary:
Total Assets = 1,345,000
Liabilities + Net Assets = 1,345,000
Current Assets = 940,000
Non-Current Assets = 405,000

Rules for Recording Transactions

Two rules must be followed to record transactions under the accrual basis of accounting:

1. At least two accounts must be used to record a transaction.
   a. Increase (decrease) an *asset* account whenever assets are acquired (used).
   b. Increase (decrease) a *liability* account whenever obligations are incurred (paid for).
   c. Increase a *revenue, gain, or other support* account when revenues are earned, a gain occurs, or other support is received.
   d. Increase an *expense* account when an asset is used. Net assets increase when unrestricted revenues, gains, and other support increase, and net assets decrease when expenses occur.

There are additional rules that must be followed for donations; however, these rules can become complex and are beyond the scope of this text.

2. After each transaction, the fundamental accounting equation must be in balance:

Assets = Liabilities + Net Assets

The Recording Process

The following is an outline of the transactions listed in Exhibit 3–6.

1. The center received $600,000 in unrestricted contributions.
   a. Because cash was received, Cash (an asset) is increased by $600,000.
   b. Because an unrestricted contribution for operating purposes was received, Revenues, Gains, and Other Support is increased by $600,000. If Exhibit 3–6 were not constrained for space, the transaction would be more accurately recorded in a subcategory of Revenues, Gains, and Other Support, called *other revenue.*

Caution: Under accrual accounting, revenues are recognized when earned. Because the receipt of an unrestricted donation *that can be used for operating purposes* is not earned in the same sense that patient revenues are, such donations are recorded in the related account Other Revenue, under Revenue, Gains, and Other Support.

2. The center obtained a $500,000 bank loan at 6 percent interest; $20,000 in principal is due this year.
   a. Because cash was received, Cash (an asset) is increased by $500,000.
   b. Because the center borrowed $500,000, it must recognize this as a liability. The part due this year ($20,000) is a current liability. The part not due

this year ($480,000) is a noncurrent liability. Thus, Notes Payable under current liabilities is increased by $20,000, and Notes Payable under noncurrent liabilities is increased by $480,000.

Caution: Notice that although cash was received, no revenues were recognized. Under accrual accounting, revenues are recognized when they are earned. In this case, the cash received did not represent earnings, just the borrowing of funds. Also, this transaction involved three accounts, not just two: Cash and Notes Payable under both Current Liabilities and Noncurrent Liabilities. However, the fundamental accounting equation still remains in balance.

A common error is to record interest expense at this time. Because interest is a "usage" fee, interest is recognized when the borrower keeps the funds, not when the borrowing takes place. (This is shown in transaction 12.)

3. The center purchased $450,000 of properties and equipment. It paid cash for the purchase.
   a. Because cash was paid, Cash (an asset) is decreased by $450,000.
   b. Because properties and equipment were purchased, Properties and Equipment (an asset) is increased by $450,000.

Caution: Notice that although cash was paid, no expense was recognized. Under accrual accounting, expenses are recognized as assets are used, and the center has not yet used the plant and equipment. (This is shown in transaction 15.)

4. The center purchased $100,000 of supplies on credit. The vendor expects payment within 30 days.
   a. Because supplies increased, Supplies (an asset) is increased by $100,000.
   b. Because the vendor is owed $100,000, and the payment is due within 30 days, the current liability, Accounts Payable, is increased by $100,000.

Caution: Notice that although supplies were purchased, no supplies expense was recognized. Under accrual accounting, expenses are recognized when resources are used or consumed, and the center has not yet used the supplies. (This is shown in transaction 8.)

5. The center provided $500,000 of non-discounted billable services to non-capitated patients. Payment has not yet been received.
   a. Although the patients received services, they have not paid. Therefore, Accounts Receivable (an asset) is increased by $500,000 to show that the organization has a right to collect the money it is owed.
   b. Because revenue was earned by providing services, Patient Revenues, a net asset subaccount, is increased by $500,000.

Caution: Under accrual accounting, revenues are recognized when earned. Therefore, although no cash was received, revenues are increased because the service was performed.

6. On the first day of the year, the center received $250,000 in capitation pre-payment from an HMO. This means the HMO paid the center $250,000 in advance on a per member per year (PMPY) basis to take care of the medical needs of all its enrollees over the next year.
   a. Because cash was received, Cash (an asset) is increased by $250,000.
   b. The center has an obligation to provide services to the capitated patients. Therefore, Deferred Revenues (a liability) is increased by $250,000.

Caution: Under accrual accounting, revenues are recognized when they are earned. Although cash was received, the revenues will be earned only when the "coverage period" expires. (This is shown in transaction 17.)

7. In the provision of services to all patients, the center incurred $300,000 in labor expenses, which it paid for in cash.
   a. Because cash was paid out, Cash (an asset) is decreased by $300,000.
   b. Because labor, a resource, was used, Expenses, a net asset, is increased. Because expenses decrease net assets, it is recorded as a negative number.

Caution: Because cash was paid in recognition of the use of resources, expenses would have been recognized under either the cash or accrual bases of accounting.

8. In the provision of services to all patients, the center used $80,000 of supplies.
   a. The organization now has $80,000 less in supplies. Therefore, Supplies (an asset) is decreased by $80,000.
   b. Because $80,000 of supplies has been used, Supplies Expense is increased by $80,000. Because expenses decrease net assets, it is recorded as a negative number.

Caution: Although no cash was paid, the expense is recognized because resources have been used. Recall that no expense was recognized when the resource was purchased in transaction 4.

9. The center paid a $10,000 premium in advance for one year's insurance coverage.
   a. Because cash was paid out, Cash (an asset) is decreased by $10,000.
   b. $10,000 purchased the right to be covered by insurance for the entire year. Therefore, Prepaid Insurance (an asset) is increased by $10,000.

Caution: Under accrual accounting, expenses are recognized when assets are used. Thus, although cash has been paid out, no expense was recognized. The expense will be recognized as the right to be covered by insurance is "used up" (with the passage of time). (This is shown in transaction 16.)

10. The center paid for $90,000 of the $100,000 of supplies purchased in transaction 4.
   a. Because cash was paid, Cash (an asset) is decreased by $90,000.
   b. Because the center no longer owes $90,000 of the $100,000 liability, Accounts Payable (a liability) is decreased by $90,000.

Caution: Although cash has been paid out, no expense was recognized because no resources were used.

11. Patients or their third parties paid the center $400,000 of the $500,000 they owed (see transaction 5).
   a. Because cash was received, Cash (an asset) is increased by $400,000.
   b. Because payment has been received, the organization no longer has the right to collect this $400,000 from patients. Therefore, Accounts Receivable (an asset) is decreased by $400,000.

Caution: Notice that although cash was received, no revenues were recognized. Under accrual accounting, revenues are recognized when they are earned. The revenue was recognized when it was earned in transaction 5.

12. During the year, the center made a $50,000 cash payment toward its bank loan; $20,000 was for principal, and $30,000 was to pay the full amount of interest due.
    a. Because cash was paid out, Cash (an asset) is decreased by $50,000.
    b. Because $20,000 of the loan has been paid off, Notes Payable (a liability) is decreased by $20,000.
    c. Because the center paid $30,000 for the use of the $500,000 loan (6 percent interest rate), Interest Expense (a net asset) is increased by $30,000. Because expenses decrease net assets, it is recorded as a negative.

Caution: Remember, interest expense was *not* recognized when the loan was taken in transaction 2. Interest, the right to use someone else's money, is recognized over time, as the loan is outstanding.

---

13. The center transferred $25,000 to its parent corporation.
    a. Because cash was paid out, Cash (an asset) is decreased by $25,000.
    b. Because the organization now has $25,000 less assets, Transfer to Parent (a net asset) is decreased by $25,000. This is recorded as a negative because it has the effect of decreasing Unrestricted Net Assets (like expenses that are also recorded as negatives).

Caution: Although cash has been paid out, no expense is recognized because no resources were used.

---

14. Since the last payday, employees have earned wages of $35,000.
    a. Because the center owes its employees $35,000, it must recognize this obligation by increasing Wages Payable (a liability) by $35,000.
    b. Because the center used $35,000 of labor, it must increase Labor Expense (a liability) by $35,000. Because expenses decrease net assets, the increase in expenses is recorded as a negative number.

Caution: Although no cash was paid, the expense was recognized because labor resources have been used.

Contra-Asset
An asset that, when increased, decreases the value of a related asset on the books. Two primary examples are Accumulated Depreciation, which is the contra-asset to Properties and Equipment, and the Allowance for Uncollectibles, which is the contra-asset to Accounts Receivable. For example, by convention, the historical cost of a fixed asset is kept on the books in its own account under Properties and Equipment, and the amount of depreciation that has accumulated on that asset is kept in a related account called Accumulated Depreciation. To find the book value of the fixed asset, the Accumulated Depreciation is subtracted from the amount in Properties and Equipment. Patient Service Revenues (the asset) and Allowance for Uncollectibles (the contra-asset) work the same way.

15. Equipment has depreciated $45,000.
    a. To keep a cumulative record of the amount of depreciation taken on the assets, the center must increase Accumulated Depreciation (a *contra-asset account*) by $45,000. An increase in a contra-asset account results in a decrease in the value of the assets. Thus, the accumulated depreciation is subtracted from the amount in the equipment account to find the book value of the equipment.
    b. Because the organization has "used up" $45,000 of the equipment, it must increase Depreciation Expense (a net asset account) by $45,000. Because expenses decrease net assets, the increase in expenses is recorded as a negative number.

Caution: Although no cash was paid, the depreciation expense is recognized because resources have been used.

16. The $10,000 of insurance coverage was for one year. That time has now expired.
    a. Because the organization no longer has the $10,000 of insurance coverage it purchased, it must decrease Prepaid Insurance (an asset) by $10,000.
    b. Because the organization "used up" the right it purchased to be covered by insurance for one year, it must increase the Insurance Expense account by $10,000. The expense is recognized when the resource is used, not when the insurance is purchased (see transaction 9). Because expenses decrease net assets, the increase in expenses is recorded as a negative number.

Caution: Although no cash was paid, the insurance expense is recognized because the right to be covered by insurance has been "used up."

17. The center has fulfilled its health care service obligations under the $250,000 capitated arrangement in transaction 6. This revenue is now considered earned.
    a. The center no longer has the obligation to provide service to these HMO enrollees. Therefore, it must reduce Unearned HMO Revenues (a liability) by $250,000.
    b. By covering the health care needs of the HMO enrollees for one year, the center earned $250,000. Therefore, Revenues, Gains, and Other Support are increased by $250,000. The specific account that would be increased

under Revenues, Gains, and Other Support is Premium Revenues. Incidentally, note that revenue was not recognized when the cash was received (see transaction 6).

Caution: Although no cash was received, revenues are recognized when earned.

---

18. $20,000 of the note payable is due within the next year.
   a. Because the organization must pay $20,000 next year, the center must increase Notes Payable (a current liability) by $20,000.
   b. Because it no longer owes $20,000 over the long term, the center decreases Notes Payable (a noncurrent liability) by $20,000.

19. Bad debt is estimated to be $5,000.
   a. The estimate of how much of the accounts receivable will *not* be paid is placed in a contra-asset account called the Allowance for Uncollectibles. Therefore, the Allowance for Uncollectibles is increased by $5,000 and is recorded as a negative. By increasing the allowance for uncollectibles, Net Patient Accounts Receivable is decreased.
   b. By estimating uncollectibles, the organization is recognizing that there are certain patient accounts receivable it will not be able to collect. This is part of doing business. Essentially, the organization is "using up" the right to collect the funds without actually collecting anything. It recognizes this use of resources by increasing Bad Debt Expense by $5,000. Because expenses decrease net assets, the increase in expenses is recorded as a negative number.

Key Point *The terms* allowance for doubtful accounts, allowance for uncollectible accounts, *and* allowance for bad debt *are used interchangeably in practice. Similarly, the terms* provision for bad debt *and* bad debt expenses *are used interchangeably in practice. In this text, the terms* allowance for uncollectibles *and* bad debt expense *are used throughout.*

Caution: Although no cash was paid, the bad debt expense (Provision for Bad Debt) is recognized in the same time period as the earning occurred. If the organization did not recognize this expense at this time, it would be matching one year's bad debt with the revenues earned in a future year.

Key Point *If nothing else were done, the value of the Allowance for Uncollectibles would grow indefinitely. To avoid this, when deemed uncollectible, specific accounts are written off, and both the Allowance for Uncollectibles and Accounts Receivable are reduced by an equal amount.*

20. $60,000 is set aside by the board to be used next year to help purchase a new information system.
    a. Because cash was set aside, Cash (an asset) is decreased by $60,000.
    b. Because the board designated these funds for a specific use next year, Assets Limited as to Use (a current asset) is increased by $60,000.

Caution: Because no resource has been consumed, there is no expense.

DEVELOPING THE FINANCIAL STATEMENTS

Once the transactions have been analyzed and recorded, the organization can develop the four financial statements: the balance sheet, the statement of operations, the statement of changes in net assets, and the statement of cash flows.

The Balance Sheet

The balance sheet presents the assets, liabilities, and net assets for a health care provider (see Exhibit 3–7). To construct a balance sheet for Windmill Point Outpatient Center, the information from the transaction-recording sheet (Exhibit 3–6) is used to develop a snapshot of the organization's financial position at year's end.

Assets For Windmill Point Outpatient Center, Total Current Assets ($940,000) equals the sum of all Cash ($765,000), Assets Limited as to Use ($60,000), Net Accounts Receivable ($95,000: Accounts Receivable of $100,000 less the Allowance for Uncollectibles of $5,000), Supplies ($20,000), and Prepaid Assets ($0). The Properties and Equipment, Net is $405,000. This is computed by adding the original purchase of $450,000 and subtracting the $45,000 of accumulated depreciation. Thus, Total Assets are $1,345,000, which is the sum of current and noncurrent assets.

Liabilities Windmill Point Outpatient Center has a balance of $65,000 in current liabilities: $10,000 for supplies ($100,000 purchased – $90,000 paid for); $35,000 in wages payable; and $20,000, the current portion of the long-term debt. There are no deferred revenues, but there is $460,000 of the long-term portion of the loan remaining, which is a noncurrent liability. The sum of these accounts, $525,000, is the total liabilities.

Exhibit 3–7 Balance sheet for Windmill Point Outpatient Center

Windmill Point Outpatient Center Balance Sheet
for the Periods Ending December 31, 20X1 and 20X0

	12/31/20X1	12/31/20X0
Current assets		
Cash	$765,000	$0
Gross accounts receivable	100,000	0
(less allowance for uncollectibles)	(5,000)	0
Net accounts receivable	95,000	0
Supplies	20,000	0
Assets limited as to use	60,000	0
Prepaid expenses	0	0
Total current assets	940,000	0
Noncurrent assets		
Long-term investments (net)	0	0
Plant, property, and equipment	450,000	0
(less accumulated depreciation)	(45,000)	0
Net plant, property, and equipment	405,000	0
Total noncurrent assets	405,000	0
Total assets	$1,345,000	$0

	12/31/20X1	12/31/20X0
Current liabilities		
Accounts payable	$10,000	$0
Wages payable	35,000	0
Notes payable	20,000	0
Total current liabilities	65,000	0
Noncurrent liabilities	460,000	0
Total liabilities	525,000	0
Net assets		
Unrestricted	820,000	0
Temporarily restricted	0	0
Permanently restricted	0	0
Total net assets	820,000	0
Total liabilities and net assets	$1,345,000	$0

Net Assets Net assets equal $820,000. This net asset balance is computed by summing the beginning balance of $0, plus the increase in unrestricted net assets of $820,000 and $0 in temporarily restricted and permanently restricted net assets.

The Statement of Operations

As with the balance sheet, the information in Exhibit 3–6 is used to develop a statement of operations for Windmill Point Outpatient Center (see Exhibit 3–8). However, because the transactions that comprise this statement were recorded in an abbreviated form, it is necessary to refer also to the first column of Exhibit 3–6 to identify the specific nature of the transactions classified under Unrestricted Revenues, Gains, and Other Support as well as Expenses.

Exhibit 3–8   Statement of operations for Windmill Point Outpatient Center

Windmill Point Outpatient Center
Statement of Operations
for the Periods Ending December 31, 20X1 and 20X0

	12/31/20X1	12/31/20X0
Revenues		
Unrestricted revenues, gains, and other support		
Net patient revenue	$500,000	$0
Premium revenue	250,000	0
Other revenue	600,000	0
Total revenues	1,350,000	0
Expenses		
Labor expense	335,000	0
Supplies expense	80,000	0
Interest expense	30,000	0
Insurance expense	10,000	0
Provision for bad debt	5,000	0
Depreciation and amortization	45,000	0
Total expenses	505,000	0
Operating income	845,000	0
Excess of revenues over expenses	845,000	0
Contribution of long-lived assets	0	0
Transfers to parent	(25,000)	0
Increase in unrestricted net assets	**$820,000**	**$0**

Unrestricted Revenues, Gains, and Other Support The revenues of Windmill Point Outpatient Center are classified into three categories: net patient revenues earned from non-capitated patients, $500,000; premium revenue earned from capitated patients, $250,000; and unrestricted contributions, which are presented in the category Other Revenue, $600,000. These revenues total $1,350,000.

Operating Expenses *Operating expenses* are costs that are incurred in the day-to-day operation of the business. Exhibit 3–8 shows that the operating expense of $505,000 is made up of $335,000 Labor Expense ($300,000 paid for and $35,000 not yet paid for), $80,000 Supplies Expense, $30,000 Interest Expense, $10,000 Insurance Expense, $5,000 Provision for Bad Debt, and $45,000 Depreciation Expense.

Operating Income and Excess of Revenues over Expenses *Operating income* is the difference between Unrestricted Revenues, Gains, and Other Support and Expenses. For Windmill Point Outpatient Center, operating income is $845,000. Because there are no "non-operating income" items, this is also equal to *excess of revenues over expenses*, the net income of the organization.

Increase in Unrestricted Net Assets As shown in Exhibit 3–8, the increase in unrestricted net assets, $820,000, for Windmill Point Outpatient Center is calculated by adding operating income, $845,000, minus the transfers to parent ($25,000).

The Statement of Changes in Net Assets

The third financial statement is the statement of changes in net assets, or the statement of changes in owners' equity or stockholders' equity for a for-profit business. Its purpose is to explain the changes in net assets from one period to the next (see Exhibit 3–9). This statement reflects increases and decreases in net assets for both restricted and unrestricted net asset accounts. For Windmill Point Outpatient Center, the ending balance of net assets, $820,000, is the sum of the beginning total net asset account for the year, $0, plus the changes in unrestricted net assets for the year, $820,000 (from the statement of operations), plus contributions made to temporarily restricted net asset accounts, $0.

The Statement of Cash Flows

Because accrual accounting is used, the statement of operations provides information about how much revenue was generated and the amount of resources used to generate those revenues. However, the statement of operations does not tell how much cash came into the organization and how much went out. That is the purpose of the statement of cash flows (see Exhibit 3–10). The construction of the statement of cash flows is beyond this introductory text. Most standard introductory accounting texts can provide more detailed information.

This statement is organized into three major sections: cash flows from operating activities, cash flows from investing activities, and cash flows from financing

Exhibit 3–9   Statement of changes in net assets for Windmill Point Outpatient Center

Windmill Point Outpatient Center
Statement of Changes in Net Assets
for the Periods Ending December 31, 20X1 and 20X0

	12/31/20X1	12/31/20X0
Unrestricted net assets		
Excess of revenues over expenses	$845,000	$0
Contribution of long-lived assets	0	0
Transfers to parent	(25,000)	0
Increase in unrestricted net assets	820,000	0
Temporarily restricted net assets		
Restricted contribution	0	0
Increase in temporarily restricted net assets	0	0
Permanently restricted net assets		
Increase in permanently restricted net assets	0	0
Increase in net assets	820,000	0
Net assets, beginning of year	0	0
Net assets, end of year	**$820,000**	**$0**

activities. Whereas the sections on investing and financing activities are relatively straightforward, the section on cash flows from operating activities is not. The latter begins with changes in net assets and then makes adjustments required by the accrual basis of accounting.

Cash flows from investing activities include cash transactions involving the purchase or sale of properties and equipment, and the purchase or sale of long-term investments. Cash flows from financing activities include changes in noncurrent liability accounts, such as an increase or decrease in long-term debt (including the current portion), any increase in temporarily or permanently restricted assets, and the recognition of the transfer of cash funds to the parent corporation.

That Transfers to Parent appears twice in this statement can be confusing. It appears in the cash flows from operating activities section to show that there was $25,000 more cash available from operations than is shown in changes in net assets, which is the beginning point for calculating cash flows from operating activities. Because the inflow is included in the cash flows from operating activities, the cash outflow is then shown as a cash flow from financing activities.

Exhibit 3–10 Statement of cash flows for Windmill Point Outpatient Center

Windmill Point Outpatient Center
Statement of Cash Flows
for the Periods Ending December 31, 20X1 and 20X0

	12/31/20X1	12/31/20X0
Cash flows from operating activities		
Change in net assets	$820,000	$0
Depreciation expense	45,000	0
− Increase in temporarily restricted net assets	0	0
+ Transfers to parent	25,000	0
− Increase in net accounts receivable	(95,000)	0
− Increase in inventory	(20,000)	0
+ Increase in accounts payable	10,000	0
+ Increase in wages payable	35,000	0
Net cash provided by operating activities	820,000	0
Cash flows from investing activities		
Purchase of assets limited as to use	(60,000)	0
Purchase of plant, property, & equipment	(450,000)	0
Net cash flow used in investing activities	(510,000)	0
Cash flows from financing activities		
Transfers to parent	(25,000)	0
Increase in long-term debt	480,000	0
Net cash provided by financing activities	455,000	0
Net increase in cash & cash equivalents	765,000	0
Cash and cash equivalents, beginning of year	0	0
Cash and cash equivalents, end of year	**$765,000**	**$0**

SUMMARY

The financial viability of a health care organization is the result of numerous decisions made by a variety of people including caregivers, administrators, boards, lenders, community members, and politicians. These decisions eventually result in the organization's acquiring and using resources to provide services, incur obligations, and generate revenues. One of the major roles of accounting is to record these transactions in a standardized format and to report the results to interested parties. This chapter shows how a series of typical transactions of a health center are recorded on the books, and how these records are used to produce the four major financial statements of a not-for-profit, business-oriented health care organization.

Transactions are recorded using either the cash basis of accounting or the accrual basis of accounting. In the *cash basis* of accounting, revenues are recognized when cash is received, and expenses are recognized when cash is paid. In the *accrual basis* of accounting, revenues are recognized when earned, and expenses are recognized when resources are used. The accrual basis of accounting must be used by health care organizations.

Two rules must be followed to record transactions under the accrual basis of accounting:

1. At least two accounts must be used to record a transaction.
   a. Increase (decrease) an *asset* account whenever assets are acquired (used).
   b. Increase (decrease) a *liability* account whenever obligations are incurred (paid for).
   c. Increase a *revenue, gain, or other support* account when revenues are earned, a gain occurs, or other support is received.
   d. Increase an *expense* account when an asset is used. Net assets increase when unrestricted revenues, gains, and other support increase, and net assets decrease when expenses occur.
   There are additional rules that must be followed for donations; however, these rules can become complex and are beyond the scope of this text.

2. After *each* transaction, the fundamental accounting equation must be in balance:

Assets = Liabilities + Net Assets

KEY TERMS

a. Accrual basis of accounting
b. Cash basis of accounting
c. Contra-asset

QUESTIONS AND PROBLEMS

1. **Definitions.** Define the key terms in the list above.

2. **Accrual versus cash basis of accounting.** Explain the difference between the accrual basis of accounting and the cash basis of accounting. What are the major reasons for using accrual accounting?

3. **Accrual accounting.** How are revenues and expenses defined under accrual accounting?

4. **Journal versus ledger.** What are the purposes of a journal and a ledger?

5. **Adjustment of three accounts.** Give two examples of transactions that involve the adjustment of three accounts, rather than the usual two accounts.

6. **Contra-asset.** Give an example of a contra-asset, and explain how it is recorded on the ledger as a transaction.

7. **Prepaid expense.** Explain what a "prepaid expense" is and how it is recorded on the ledger as a transaction.

8. **Timing of transactions.** How would transactions differ if supplies were completely paid for and consumed in one period, or paid for in one period but not used until the next period?

9. **Timing of transactions.** Are transactions recorded on a fiscal-year basis or a calendar-year basis? Does it have to be one or the other; if so, why?

10. **For-profit versus not-for-profit transactions.** What are the major differences in recording transactions for a for-profit organization versus a not-for-profit, or are there any?

11. **Transactions plus multiple statements.** List and record each transaction for Claymont Outpatient Clinic under the accrual basis of accounting at December 31, 20X1. Then develop a balance sheet as of December 31, 20X1, and a statement of operations for the year ended December 31, 20X1.

   a. The clinic received an $8,000,000 unrestricted cash contribution from the community. (*Hint:* this transaction increases the unrestricted net assets account.)

   b. The clinic purchased $5,600,000 of equipment. The clinic paid cash for the equipment.

   c. The clinic borrowed $3,000,000 from the bank on a long-term basis.

   d. The clinic purchased $600,000 of supplies on credit.

   e. The clinic provided $9,400,000 of services on credit.

   f. In the provision of these services, the clinic used $300,000 of supplies.

   g. The clinic received $740,000 in advance to care for capitated patients.

   h. The clinic incurred $4,000,000 in labor expenses and paid cash for them.

   i. The clinic incurred $2,500,000 in general expenses and paid cash for them.

   j. The clinic received $7,300,000 from patients and their third parties in payment of outstanding accounts.

   k. The clinic met $540,000 of its obligation to capitated patients in transaction g.

   l. The clinic made a $300,000 cash payment on the long-term loan.

   m. The clinic also made a cash interest payment of $35,000.

   n. A donor made a temporarily restricted donation of $350,000, which is set aside in temporary investments.

o. The clinic recognized $380,000 in depreciation for the year.

p. The clinic estimated that $800,000 of patient accounts would not be received.

12. **Transactions plus multiple statements.** The following are the financial transactions for Family Home Health Care Center, a not-for-profit, business-oriented organization. Beginning balances at January 1, 20X1, for its assets, liabilities, and net asset accounts are shown in the list.

Givens:

Cash	$7,000
Accounts receivable	$75,000
Allowance for uncollectibles	$4,000
Supplies	$10,000
Long-term investments	$35,000
Properties and equipment	$900,000
Accumulated depreciation	$100,000
Short-term accounts payable	$35,000
Other current liabilities	$5,000
Long-term debt	$600,000
Unrestricted net assets	$273,000
Permanently restricted net assets	$10,000

List and record each transaction under the accrual basis of accounting. Then develop a balance sheet as of December 31, 20X1 and 20X0, and a statement of operations for the year ended December 31, 20X1.

a. The center purchased $3,000 of supplies on credit.

b. The center provided $390,000 of home health services on credit.

c. The center consumed $8,000 of supplies in the provision of its home health services.

d. The center provided $230,000 of home health services, and patients paid for services in cash.

e. The center paid cash for $6,000 of supplies in the provision of its home health services.

f. The center paid $20,000 in cash for supplies previously purchased on credit.

g. A donor established a $90,000 permanent endowment fund (in the form of long-term investments) for the center. (*Hint:* this transaction increases the permanently restricted net assets account.)

h. The center collected $300,000 from patients for outstanding receivables.

i. The center paid $325,000 in cash toward labor expense.

j. The center paid $85,000 in cash toward its long-term loan.

k. The center purchased $28,000 in small equipment on credit. Amount is due within one year.

l. The center incurred $48,000 in general expenses. The center used cash to pay for the general expenses.

m. The center incurred $9,000 in interest expense for the year. Cash payment of $9,000 was made to the bank.

n. The center made a $7,000 cash transfer to its parent corporation.

o. The center recognizes labor expense of $3,500 but does not incur a cash payment.

p. The center recognized depreciation expenses of $18,000.

q. The center estimated it would not collect $75,000 of the patient accounts receivable.

13. **Statement of Operations.** The following is a list of account balances for Krakower Healthcare Services, Inc. on December 31, 20X1. Prepare a statement of operations as of December 31, 20X1. (*Hint:* when net assets are released from restriction, the restricted account is decreased, and the unrestricted account is increased. It is recognized under revenues, gains, and other support).

Givens:

Supply expense	$75,000
Transfer to parent corporation	$13,000
Bad debt expense	$14,000
Depreciation expense	$30,000
Labor expense	$90,000
Interest expense	$8,000
Administrative expense	$49,000
Net patient service revenues	$243,000
Net assets released from restriction	$24,000

14. **Statement of Operations.** The following is a list of account balances (in thousands) for Kirkland County Hospital on September 30, 20X1. Prepare a statement of operations as of September 30, 20X1. (*Hint:* unrestricted donations are recognized under revenues, gains, and other support.)

Givens:

Labor expense	$13,400
Provision for bad debt	$3,000
Supplies expense	$4,300
Unrestricted cash donation for operations	$2,000

Net patient service revenues	$32,700
Professional fees	$9,150
Transfer to parent corporation	$1,400
Other revenues from cafeteria and gift shop	$1,200
Depreciation expense	$1,300
Income from investments (unrestricted investments)	$2,600
Administrative expense	$2,300

15. **Statement of Cash Flows.** The following is a list of account balances for Hover Hospital on June 30, 20X1. Prepare a statement of cash flows as of June 30, 20X1.

Givens:

Transfer to parent corporation	$34,000
Proceeds from sale of fixed equipment	$2,000,000
Principal payment on bonds payable	$700,000
Purchase of fixed equipment	$4,800,000
Beginning cash balance	$5,500,000
Cash from operating activities	$3,200,000
Principal payment on notes payable	$4,300

16. **Multiple statements.** The following is a list of accounts (in thousands) for St. Paul's Hospital on December 31, 20X1. Prepare a balance sheet and statement of operations as of December 31, 20X1. (*Hint:* unrestricted contributions increase the unrestricted net assets account, and they are a part of revenues, gains, and other support.)

Givens:

Interest expense	$1,200
Cash	$4,300
Gross accounts receivable	$38,400
Accrued expenses	$9,000
Long-term debt	$13,600
Labor expense	$75,600
Inventory	$2,700
Accumulated depreciation	$35,000
Net patient revenues	$116,100
Other noncurrent assets	$17,900
Professional expense	$2,300
Accounts payable	$10,600
Administrative and medical supplies expense	$26,000
Prepaid expenses	$1,950
Depreciation expense	$6,700
Non-operating gains	$1,200
Unrestricted contributions	$1,300

Temporary investments	$8,000
Other current liabilities	$1,900
Other revenues	$16,000
Gross plant and equipment	$75,000
Deferred revenue	$2,100
Bad debt expense	$11,100
Allowance for uncollectibles	$15,000

17. **Transactions plus multiple statements.** St. Catherine's Diagnostic Center had the following ending balances at December 31, 20X0, for its assets, liabilities, and net assets accounts.

Givens:

Cash and temporary investments	$240,000
Accounts receivable	$3,200,000
Allowance for uncollectibles	$230,000
Inventory	$134,000
Plant and equipment	$6,300,000
Accumulated depreciation	$300,000
Accounts payable	$230,000
Other short-term notes payable	$35,000
Long-term bonds payable	$450,000
Unrestricted net assets	$8,629,000
Temporarily restricted net assets	$0

List and record each 20X1 transaction under the accrual basis of accounting. Then develop a balance sheet for end-of-years 20X0 and 20X1, a statement of operations, and a statement of changes in net assets for the year ended December 31, 20X1.

a. The center collected $2,800,000 in cash from outstanding accounts receivable.

b. The center purchased $2,300,000 of inventory on credit.

c. The center provided $10,100,000 of patient services on credit.

d. The center incurred $5,500,000 of labor expenses, which it paid in cash.

e. The center consumed $2,100,000 of supplies from its inventory in the provision of its diagnostic services.

f. The center paid $32,000 in cash for outstanding short-term notes payable.

g. The center collected $7,300,000 in cash from outstanding accounts receivable.

h. The center paid $2,100,000 in cash for outstanding accounts payable.

i.   The center issued $4,000,000 in long-term bonds that it must pay back.

j.   The center purchased $3,200,000 in new equipment using a short-term note payable.

k.   The center incurred $45,000 in interest expense, which it paid in cash.

l.   The center incurred $1,300,000 in general expenses, which it paid in cash.

m. The center made a cash payment of $800,000 toward principal payment of its outstanding bonds.

n.   A local corporation gave an unrestricted $65,000 cash donation. (*Hint:* this transaction increases the unrestricted net assets account.)

o.   The center received in cash $5,000 in interest income from unrestricted temporary investments.

p.   The center transferred $530,000 in cash to its parent corporation.

q.   The center incurred an annual depreciation expense of $75,000.

r.   The center estimated that it incurred an additional $10,000 in its allowance for uncollectibles, which represented $10,000 in bad debt expenses.

18. **Transactions plus multiple statements.** Ambulatory Center, Inc. had the following ending balances for its assets, liabilities, and net assets accounts as of December 31, 20X0.

Givens:

Cash	$50,000
Accounts receivable	$85,000
Allowance for uncollectibles	$15,000
Inventory or supplies	$8,000
Prepaid insurance	$1,300
Long-term investments	$15,000
Plant, property, and equipment	$4,000,000
Accumulated depreciation	$2,000,000
Short-term accounts payable	$75,000
Accrued expenses	$22,000
Long-term debt	$1,300,000
Unrestricted net assets	$652,300
Permanently restricted net assets	$95,000

List and record each 20X1 transaction under the accrual basis of accounting. Then develop a balance sheet for end-of-years 20X0 and 20X1, a statement of operations, and a statement of changes in net assets for the year ended December 31, 20X1.

a. The center made a cash payment of $45,000 to pay off outstanding accounts payable.

b. The center received $10,000 in cash from a donor who temporarily restricted its use. (*Hint:* this transaction increases the temporarily restricted net assets account.)

c. The center provided $3,300,000 of services on credit.

d. The center consumed $6,000 of supplies in the provision of its ambulatory services.

e. The center paid off accrued interest expense of $18,500 in cash.

f. The center collected $2,800,000 in cash from outstanding accounts receivable.

g. The center incurred $22,000 in general expenses that it paid for in cash.

h. The center made a $300,000 cash principal payment toward its long-term debt.

i. The center collected $450,000 in cash from outstanding accounts receivable.

j. The center received $28,000 in cash from an HMO for future capitated services.

k. The center purchased $3,000 of supplies on credit.

l. The center earned, but did not receive, $3,500 in income from its restricted net assets. The income can be used for general operations. (*Hint:* this transaction increases interest receivable and is also recorded under revenues, gains, and other support.)

m. The center's temporarily restricted asset account released $2,500 from its restricted account to its unrestricted account for operations. (*Hint:* the transfer gets recorded under revenues, gains, and other support.)

n. The center incurred $6,000 in interest expense. The interest expense was recorded but not yet paid in cash.

o. The center incurred $2,700,000 in labor expenses, which it paid for in cash.

p. The center paid $3,200 in advance for insurance expense.

q. The center transferred $6,400 in cash to its parent corporation.

r. The center incurred $175,000 in depreciation expense.

s. The center's prepaid insurance of $3,400 expired for the year.

t. The center estimated $8,000 for bad debt expense for the year.

19. **Transactions plus multiple statements.** Happy Valley Hospital, Inc. had the following ending balances (in thousands) for its assets, liabilities, and net assets as of December 31, 20X0.

Givens:

Cash	$2,300
Accounts receivable	$39,000
Allowance for uncollectibles	$6,700
Inventory or supplies	$3,200
Prepaid insurance	$900
Long-term investments	$85,000
Plant, property, and equipment	$143,000
Accumulated depreciation	$66,000
Short-term accounts payable	$7,500
Accrued expenses	$14,000
Long-term debt	$41,000
Unrestricted net assets	$130,100
Temporarily restricted net assets	$7,100
Permanently restricted net assets	$1,000

List and record each 20X1 transaction under the accrual basis of accounting. Then develop a balance sheet for end-of-years 20X0 and 20X1, a statement of operations, and a statement of changes in net assets for the year ended December 31, 20X1.

a. The hospital made a cash payment of $3,300,000 toward outstanding accounts payable.

b. The hospital received $4,500,000 in cash from a donor who temporarily restricted its use. (*Hint:* this transaction increases the temporarily restricted net assets account.)

c. The hospital provided $120,000,000 of services on credit.

d. The hospital consumed $2,700,000 of supplies in the provision of its ambulatory services.

e. The hospital paid cash for incurred interest expense of $3,100,000.

f. The hospital collected $110,000,000 in cash from outstanding accounts receivable.

g. The hospital incurred $4,500,000 in general expenses that it paid for in cash.

h. The hospital made a $2,800,000 cash principal payment toward its long-term debt.

i. The hospital collected $22,000,000 in cash from outstanding accounts receivable.

j. The hospital purchased $32,000,000 of supplies on credit.

k. The hospital earned, but did not receive, $2,500,000 in income from its restricted net assets. The income can be used for general operations. (*Hint:* this transaction increases interest receivable and is also recorded under revenues, gains, and other support.)

l.   The hospital incurred $1,800,000 in interest expense but not yet paid in cash.

m. The hospital incurred $62,000,000 in labor expenses, which it paid for in cash.

n.   The hospital made a cash payment of $2,700,000 in advance for insurance expense.

o.   The hospital transferred $1,100,000 in cash to its parent corporation.

p.   The hospital incurred $8,700,000 in depreciation expense.

q.   The hospital's prepaid insurance of $3,100,000 expired for the year.

r.   The hospital estimated $600,000 for bad debt expense for the year.

20. **Transactions plus multiple statements.** Glenwood Hospital had the following ending balances (in thousands) for its assets, liabilities, and net assets accounts as of December 31, 20X0.

Givens:

Cash	$8,400
Accounts receivable	$48,000
Allowance for uncollectibles	$8,900
Inventory or supplies	$4,300
Prepaid insurance	$1,100
Long-term investments	$200,000
Plant, property, and equipment	$220,000
Accumulated depreciation	$98,000
Short-term accounts payable	$24,000
Accrued expenses	$7,700
Long-term debt	$155,000
Unrestricted net assets	$177,800
Temporarily restricted net assets	$4,900
Permanently restricted net assets	$5,500

List and record each 20X1 transaction under the accrual basis of accounting. Then develop a balance sheet for end-of-years 20X0 and 20X1, a statement of operations, and a statement of changes in net assets for the year ended December 31, 20X1.

a.   The hospital made a cash payment of $7,500,000 toward outstanding accounts payable.

b.   The hospital collected $44,000,000 in cash from outstanding accounts receivable.

c. The hospital provided $230,000,000 of services on credit.

d. The hospital consumed $3,800,000 of supplies in the provision of its ambulatory services.

e. The hospital paid cash for incurred interest expense of $4,500,000.

f. The hospital purchased $30,000,000 in long-term investments and used cash for this purpose.

g. The hospital incurred $8,700,000 in general expenses that it paid for in cash.

h. The hospital made a $3,100,000 cash principal payment toward its long-term debt.

i. The hospital collected $145,000,000 in cash from outstanding accounts receivable.

j. The hospital purchased $6,900,000 of supplies on credit.

k. The hospital earned, but did not receive, $300,000 in income from its restricted net assets. The income can be used for general operations. (*Hint:* this transaction increases interest receivable and is also recorded under revenues, gains, and other support.)

l. The hospital incurred $750,000 in interest expense, which it paid for in cash.

m. The hospital incurred $98,000,000 in labor expenses, which it paid for in cash.

n. The hospital made a cash payment of $700,000 in advance for insurance expense.

o. The hospital transferred $1,000,000 in cash to its parent corporation.

p. The hospital incurred $5,900,000 in depreciation expense.

q. The hospital's prepaid insurance of $600,000 expired for the year.

r. The hospital recognized $1,300,000 in bad debt for the year.

s. The hospital made a cash payment of $14,800,000 for radiology equipment.

4

FINANCIAL STATEMENT ANALYSIS

LEARNING OBJECTIVES

- Analyze the financial statements of health care organizations using horizontal analysis, vertical (common-size) analysis, and ratio analysis
- Calculate and interpret liquidity ratios, profitability ratios, activity ratios, and capital structure ratios

Perspective 4–1   Thomson Reuters Health Care Study Focuses on Financial and Quality of Care Measures

Every year Thomson Reuters identify the top 100 performing short-term acute-care hospitals across the United States by sampling 3,800 hospitals that have a bed size of over 25 beds. Health care facilities are then ranked into specific categories by bed size and teaching status. For example, there are three categories of community hospitals: large (250 or more beds), medium-size (100 to 249 beds), and small (25 to 99 beds). The selection criteria are developed from eight measures related to clinical quality, operating efficiency, and financial performance. For a hospital to be selected to the top 100, they are required to score higher than their peer hospitals on all eight measures. The results of these measures show that top hospitals had an average length of stay of 4.93 days relative to 5.48 days for comparison hospitals, and their risk-adjusted complication index was 0.85 relative to 0.99 for the comparison hospitals. In addition, the top 100 hospitals generated an operating margin of 10.13 percent relative to 3.29 percent for the comparison hospitals, incurred an operating expense per adjusted discharge of $4,775 relative to $5,503 for the comparison hospitals, and held a cash-to-total-debt ratio of 0.93 relative to 0.28 for comparison hospitals. However, the research analysts at Thomson Reuters note that there exists a wide variation between the top hospitals and their comparison within medium and small bed-size hospitals. The underlying reason for this disparity is the limited resources that affect hospitals within these bed-size categories to address quality-of-care issues.

Source: Wilson, L. 2008. Rising to the top. *Modern Healthcare* (Mar. 17) 38(11): 26–30.

The financial performance of health care organizations is of interest to numerous individuals and groups including administrators, board members, creditors, bondholders, community members, and government agencies (see Perspectives 4–1 and 4–2). Chapters Two and Three examined the four main financial statements of health care organizations and the accounting methods underlying the preparation of these statements. This chapter shows how to analyze the financial statements of health care organizations to help answer questions about the organization that produced them:

- Is the organization profitable? Why or why not?
- How effective is the organization in collecting its receivables?
- Is the organization in a good position to pay its bills?
- How efficiently is the organization using its assets?

Perspective 4–2 Use of Financial Ratios in Determining Bond Ratings

Fitch Credit Rating Agency rated the University of Maryland Medical System (UMMS) an A for its bond issue. A range of factors supported this assigned rating: upward profitability trends, greater state support, improving market position, constant utilization, positive rate increases, unique service mix, and increased capital expenditure for plant and equipment. Financially, in 2007 UMMS earned an operating profit margin of 2.5 percent and excess margin of 4.2 percent relative to Fitch A median benchmarks of 3.2 percent and 5.4 percent, respectively. Also, Fitch had a positive view of the system's continued reinvestment in its plant. More importantly, UMMS capital expenditures as a percentage of depreciation expenses were 198.3 percent and 208 percent in fiscal year 2006, which were higher than Fitch's A median benchmark of 158 percent.

However, Fitch had a negative view of UMMS's lower liquidity position, which was lowered from its capital outlays. In the future, the system is expected to invest $1.14 billion for facility upgrades including information technology, which Fitch views favorably for UMMS. The capital expenditure drains have reduced UMMS days-cash-on-hand ratio to 118 days of cash on hand, and 49.2 percent cash-to-debt ratio, which do not compare favorably with Fitch's median benchmarks of 188.6 days and 111.1 percent, respectively. UMMS has a high financial leverage position with a debt-to-total-capital ratio of 52.7 percent compared with Fitch's median benchmark of 41.7 percent.

Source: Editors. 2007. Fitch rates University of Maryland Medical System (Maryland) $140MM 2007 underlying revs "A." *Biotech Business Week via NewsRx.com* (Aug. 20), 402.

- Are the organization's plant and equipment in need of replacement?
- Is the organization in a good position to take on additional debt?

Three approaches are commonly used to analyze financial statements: horizontal analysis, vertical analysis, and ratio analysis. Each of these approaches is examined using the financial statements shown in Exhibit 4–1, Newport Hospital's statement of operations and balance sheet. For simplicity, the statement of operations contains only operating items.

Caution: The financial statements presented in this chapter have been simplified from those presented in Chapter Two to facilitate the application of the tools and techniques presented in this chapter.

Exhibit 4–1   Statement of operations and balance sheet for Newport Hospital

**Newport Hospital Statement of Operations
for Years Ended December 31, 20X1 and 20X0**

	20X1	20X0
Operating revenues		
Net patient revenues	$10,778,272	$10,566,176
Other operating revenues	233,749	253,517
Total operating revenues	11,012,021	10,819,693
Operating expenses		
Salaries and benefits	5,644,880	5,345,498
Supplies	1,660,000	1,529,680
Insurance	1,536,357	1,551,579
Depreciation & amortization	383,493	420,238
Interest	500,000	276,379
Bad debt	456,289	365,678
Other operating revenues	500,093	276,455
Total operating expenses	10,681,112	9,765,507
Operating income	330,909	1,054,186
Non-operating revenue	185,000	165,000
Excess of revenues over expenses	515,909	1,219,186
Increase (decrease) in unrestricted net assets	**$515,909**	**$1,219,186**

Newport Hospital Balance Sheet for Years Ended December 31, 20X1 and 20X0

	20X1	20X0
ASSETS		
Current assets		
Cash and marketable securities	$363,181	$158,458
Patient accounts receivables net of uncollectible accounts	1,541,244	1,400,013
Inventories	346,176	316,875
Prepaid expenses	163,734	78,788
Other current assets	100,000	0
Total current assets	2,514,335	1,954,134

Exhibit 4–1   *(Continued)*

Noncurrent assets		
Gross plant, property, and equipment	7,088,495	6,893,370
(less accumulated depreciation)	(2,781,741)	(2,398,248)
Net plant, property, and equipment	4,306,754	4,495,122
Long-term investments	3,414,732	4,525,476
Other assets	640,915	340,853
Total noncurrent assets	8,362,401	9,361,451
Total assets	**$10,876,736**	**$11,315,585**
LIABILITIES AND NET ASSETS		
Current liabilities		
Accounts payable	$387,646	$166,600
Salaries payable	135,512	529,298
Notes payable	500,000	2,359,524
Current portion of long-term debt	372,032	338,996
Total current liabilities	1,395,190	3,394,418
Long-term liabilities		
Bonds payable	6,938,891	6,009,484
Total long-term liabilities	6,938,891	6,009,484
Total liabilities	8,334,081	9,403,902
Net assets		
Unrestricted	1,901,739	1,570,830
Temporary restricted	328,000	40,853
Permanently restricted	312,916	300,000
Total net assets	2,542,655	1,911,683
Total liabilities and net assets	**$10,876,736**	**$11,315,585**

HORIZONTAL ANALYSIS

Horizontal and vertical analyses are two of the most commonly used techniques to analyze financial statements; each is based on percentages. *Horizontal analysis* looks at the percentage change in a line item from one year to the next. A horizontal analysis of Newport Hospital's statement of operations and balance sheet is presented in Exhibit 4–2 and serves as the basis for the discussion in this section. Horizontal analysis uses the formula:

Horizontal Analysis
A method of analyzing financial statements that looks at the percentage change in a line item from one year to the next. It is computed by the formula: (subsequent year – previous year)/ previous year.

$$\left(\frac{\text{subsequent year} - \text{previous year}}{\text{previous year}} \right) 100 = \text{percentage change}$$

Exhibit 4–2   Horizontal analysis of the statement of operations and balance sheet for Newport Hospital

Newport Hospital Statement of Operations for the Years Ended December 31, 20X1 and 20X0

	20X1	20X0	Percentage Change 20X1–20X0
Operating revenues			
Net patient revenues	$10,778,272	$10,566,176	2.0%
Other operating revenues	233,749	253,517	−7.8%
Total operating revenues	11,012,021	10,819,693	1.8%
Operating expenses			
Total operating expenses	10,681,112	9,765,507	9.4%
Operating income	330,909	1,054,186	−68.6%
Non-operating revenue	185,000	165,000	12.1%
Excess of revenues over expenses	515,909	1,219,186	−57.7%
Increase (decrease) in unrestricted net assets	**$515,909**	**$1,219,186**	**−57.7%**

Newport Hospital Balance Sheet December 31, 20X1 and 20X0

	20X1	20X0	Percentage Change 20X1–20X0
Assets			
Current assets	$2,514,335	$1,954,134	28.7%
Non-current assets	8,362,401	9,361,451	−10.7%
Total assets	**$10,876,736**	**$11,315,585**	**−3.9%**
Liabilities			
Current liabilities	$1,395,190	$3,394,418	−58.9%
Long-term liabilities	6,938,891	6,009,484	15.5%
Total liabilities	8,334,081	9,403,902	
Net assets			
Total net assets	2,542,655	1,911,683	33.0%
Total liabilities and net assets	**$10,876,736**	**$11,315,585**	**−3.9%**

The goal is to answer the question, "What is the percentage change in a line item from one year to the next year?" For example, from Newport Hospital's statement of operations in Exhibit 4–2, the change in operating income from 20X0 (where 20X0 is the base year) to 20X1 using horizontal analysis would be:

$$\left(\frac{\$330,909 - \$1,054,186}{\$1,054,186} \right) 100 = -68.6 \text{ percent}$$

Key Point *Three approaches to analyze financial statements: horizontal analysis, vertical analysis, and ratio analysis.*

A problem with horizontal analysis is that percentage changes can hide major dollar effects. For example, there is an 80.9 percent change in interest expense from the statement of operations, which was the result of a $223,621 change from 20X0 to 20X1 ($500,000 – $276,379) (Exhibit 4–1); on the other hand, the 9.4 percent change in total operating expenses was a $915,605 change (Exhibit 4–2).

Key Point *When using horizontal analysis: (1) small percentage changes can mask large dollar changes from one year to the next, and (2) large percentage changes from year to year may be relatively inconsequential in terms of dollar amounts. This usually occurs when the base year is a small dollar amount.*

Horizontal analysis is also often used to compare changes from one year to the next over several years. The following example analyzes five consecutive years of Newport Hospital's operating income (not shown in the Exhibits):

	20X0	20X1	20X2	20X3	20X4
Operating income	$1,054,186	$330,909	$500,098	$1,232,565	$1,453,567
Percentage change from previous year		−68.6%	51.1%	146.5%	17.9%

Note: The year 20X0 in the above table and ensuing discussion represents the first year of the next decade. The change from 20X1 to 20X2 is calculated as follows:

$$\left(\frac{\$500,098 - \$330,909}{\$330,909} \right) 100 = 51.1 \text{ percent}$$

This analysis shows how successful the organization was in increasing operating income from one year to the next. A disadvantage of this approach is that it does not answer the question, "How much overall change has there been since 20X0?" Trend analysis supplies an answer to this question.

TREND ANALYSIS

Trend Analysis
A type of horizontal analysis that looks at changes in line items compared with a base year.

Instead of looking at single-year changes, *trend analysis* compares changes over a longer period of time by comparing each year with a base year. The formula for a trend analysis is:

$$\left(\frac{\text{any subsequent year} - \text{base year}}{\text{base year}} \right) 100$$

Applying this formula to operating income for the same 5-year period used to illustrate horizontal analysis yields the following results:

	20X0	20X1	20X2	20X3	20X4
Operating income	$1,054,186	$330,909	$500,098	$1,232,565	$1,453,567
Percentage change from 20X0		−68.6%	−52.6%	16.9%	37.9%

Vertical Analysis
A method to analyze financial statements that answers the general question: What percentage of one line item is another line item? Also called common-size analysis because it converts every line item to a percentage, thus allowing comparisons among the financial statements of different organizations. Because all items are stated as percentages, this method can be used to compare several different organizations to determine, for example, "Which organization has the highest percentage of its assets as current assets?"

For instance, the change from 20X0 to 20X4 is calculated as follows:

$$\left(\frac{\$1,453,567 - \$1,054,186}{\$1,054,186} \right) 100 = 37.9 \text{ percent}$$

Thus, from 20X0 (the base year) to 20X4, operating income rose 37.9 percent. Note that the average annual increase of 9.5 percent (37.9 percent / 4 years) is different from that of simply averaging the increases or decreases each year.

VERTICAL (COMMON-SIZE) ANALYSIS

The purpose of *vertical analysis* is to answer the general question, "What percentage of one line item is another line item?" The formula to use in this case is:

$$\left(\frac{\text{line item of interest}}{\text{base line item}} \right) 100$$

For instance, Newport Hospital might want to know if net patient revenues has increased as a percentage of total operating revenues or, similarly, what percentage of its operating revenues are the operating expenses. The top of Exhibit 4–3 computes all line items for Newport Hospital's statement of operations as a percentage of total operating revenues. In 20X0, total operating expenses were 90.3 percent of total operating revenues [($9,765,507 / $10,819,693) × 100], but by 20X1, they had increased to 97 percent of total operating revenues [($10,681,112 / $11,012,021) × 100]. This information provides some insight as to why Newport Hospital experienced the 68.6 percent decrease in operating income observed in the horizontal analysis.

Although the focus up until now has been on the statement of operations, vertical analysis is useful for analyzing the balance sheet as well, as shown in the bottom of Exhibit 4–3, which presents all line items as a percentage of total assets. By using total assets as a base, the reader can ask such questions as: "Has the composition of the balance sheet changed appreciably from 20X0 to 20X1?" In this example, total liabilities decreased from 83.1 percent of total assets in 20X0 to 76.6 percent in 20X1.

Two points can be noted from this information: In 20X1, debt was used to finance 76.6 percent of Newport Hospital's assets, whereas in 20X0 it was used to finance over 83 percent; and the use of long-term debt to finance assets grew from 53.1 percent of total assets in 20X0 to 63.8 percent in 20X1. In other words, Newport is more highly leveraged in 20X1 than it was in 20X0.

Key Point *Vertical analysis is also called common-size analysis because it converts every line item to a percentage, thus allowing comparisons of the makeup of the financial statements of different-sized organizations.*

Exhibit 4–4 presents common-size financial statements for a small community hospital and a large community hospital. The larger facility has a smaller percentage of its assets, 75 percent, in plant and equipment compared with 88 percent for the smaller facility. However, the smaller facility has a lower proportion of its capital structure, 58 percent, in total debt compared with 70 percent for the larger facility. The larger facility also has a higher percentage of its revenues from net patient revenues (97 percent) than does the smaller facility (83 percent). Although there are no benchmarks to compare these percentages with, they can elicit questions as to why the differences exist.

Financial Leverage The degree to which an organization is financed by debt.

RATIO ANALYSIS

Although horizontal and vertical analyses are easy to calculate and commonly used, ratio analysis is the preferred approach to gain an in-depth understanding of

Exhibit 4–3   Vertical (common-size) analysis for the statement of operations and balance sheet for Newport Hospital

Newport Hospital
Statement of Operations
For Years Ended December 31, 20X1 and 20X0

	20X1	Percentage of Total Revenues	20X0	Percentage of Total Revenues
Operating revenues				
Net patient revenues	$10,778,272	97.9%	$10,566,176	97.7%
Other operating revenues	233,749	2.1%	253,517	2.3%
Total operating revenues	11,012,021	100.0%	10,819,693	100.0%
Operating expenses				
Total operating expenses	10,681,112	97.0%	9,765,507	90.3%
Operating income	330,909	3.0%	1,054,186	9.7%
Non-operating revenue	185,000	1.7%	165,000	1.5%
Excess of revenues over expenses	515,909	4.7%	1,219,186	11.3%
Increase (decrease) in unrestricted net assets	**$515,909**	**4.7%**	**$1,219,186**	**11.3%**

Newport Hospital
Balance Sheet
For Years Ended December 31, 20X1 and 20X0

	20X1	Percentage of Total Assets	20X0	Percentage of Total Assets
Assets				
Current assets	$2,514,335	23.1%	$1,954,134	17.3%
Noncurrent assets	8,362,401	76.9%	9,361,451	82.7%
Total assets	**$10,876,736**	**100.0%**	**$11,315,585**	**100.0%**
Liabilities				
Current liabilities	$1,395,190	12.8%	$3,394,418	30.0%
Long-term liabilities	6,938,891	63.8%	6,009,484	53.1%
Total liabilities	8,334,081	76.6%	9,403,902	83.1%
Net assets				
Total net assets	2,542,655	23.4%	1,911,683	16.9%
Total liabilities and net assets	**$10,876,736**	**100.0%**	**$11,315,585**	**100.0%**

Exhibit 4-4 Common-size financial statements for a small and a large hospital

Small Community Hospital
Balance Sheet December 31, 20X0[a]

		Percentage of Total Assets
Current assets	$1,000	10%
Net plant and equipment	9,000	88%
Other assets	200	2%
Total assets	10,200	100%
Current liabilities	900	9%
Long-term debt	5,000	49%
Total liabilities	5,900	58%
Net assets	4,300	42%
Total liabilities and net assets	$10,200	100%

Small Community Hospital
Statement of Operations December 31, 20X0[a]

		Percentage of Total Revenues
Net patient revenues	$10,000	83%
Investment income	2,000	17%
Total operating revenues	12,000	100%
Operating expenses	10,000	83%
Income from operations	2,000	17%
Excess of revenues over expenses	2,000	17%
Increase in net assets	$2,000	17%

Large Community Hospital Balance Sheet
December 31, 20X0[a]

		Percentage of Total Assets
Current assets	$15,000	22%
Net plant and equipment	50,000	75%
Other assets	2,000	3%
Total assets	67,000	100%
Current liabilities	12,000	18%
Long-term debt	35,000	52%
Total liabilities	47,000	70%
Net assets	20,000	30%
Total liabilities and net assets	$67,000	100%

Large Community Hospital
Statement of Operations December 31, 20X0[a]

		Percentage of Total Revenues
Net patient revenues	$68,000	97%
Investment income	2,000	3%
Total operating revenues	70,000	100%
Operating expenses	65,000	93%
Income from operations	5,000	7%
Excess of revenues over expenses	5,000	7%
Increase in net assets	$5,000	7%

[a]Note: All figures other than percentages are expressed in thousands.

Ratio
An expression of the relationship between two numbers as a single number.

financial statements. A *ratio* expresses the relationship between two numbers as a single number. For instance, the current ratio expresses the relationship between current assets and current liabilities. This provides an indication of the organization's ability to cover current obligations with current assets (the ability to pay short-term debt).

$$\text{Current Ratio} = \frac{\text{Current Assets}}{\text{Current Liabilities}}$$

Categories of Ratios

Ratios are generally grouped into four categories: liquidity, profitability, activity, and capital structure.

- *Liquidity ratios* answer the question, "How well is the organization positioned to meet its short-term obligations?"
- *Profitability ratios* answer the question, "How profitable is the organization?"
- *Activity ratios* answer the question, "How efficiently is the organization using its assets to produce revenues?"
- *Capital structure ratios* answer the questions, "How are the organization's assets financed?" and "How able is the organization to take on new debt?"

Exhibit 4–5 shows what the ratios would be for Newport Hospital and compares them with industry norms. The remaining sections of this chapter will describe how these results were derived.

Key Point *Industry norms vary by hospital size. For purposes of the example used throughout this chapter, Newport is assumed to be a small hospital of fewer than 100 beds. Ratios for facilities of various sizes can be found at the end of the chapter in Exhibit 4–16a.*

Key Point *The term "benchmark" is used to indicate the desired level of performance an organization wishes to compare itself with.*

Key Point *The latest data available from Thomson Reuters and the Centers for Medicare and Medicaid Services are used as benchmarks in the remainder of the chapter.*

Exhibit 4-5 Newport Hospital ratios for 20X0 and 20X1, and Thomson and CMS median ratio values

Ratios	Benchmark Small Hospitals' Thomson and CMS Median Ratio[a]	Newport Ratios 20X1	Newport Ratios 20X0	Desired Position	Current Year Position[c]	Trend Position
Liquidity ratios						
Current ratio	2.20	1.80	0.58	Above	−18% Unfavorable	Increasing
Quick ratio[b]	1.66	1.36	0.46	Above	−18% Unfavorable	Increasing
Acid test ratio	0.37	0.26	0.05	Above	−30% Unfavorable	Increasing
Days in accounts receivable	53	52	48	Below	−2% Favorable	Increasing
Days cash on hand[b]	80	134	183	Above	67% Favorable	Decreasing
Average payment period	50	49	133	Below	−1% Favorable	Decreasing
Revenue, expense and profitability ratios						
Operating revenue per adjusted discharge	$5,679	$4,235	$4,704	Above	−25% Unfavorable	Decreasing
Operating expense per adjusted discharge	$5,497	$4,108	$4,246	Below	−25% Favorable	Decreasing
Salary and benefit expense as a percentage of operating expense	49%	53%	55%	Below	7% Unfavorable	Decreasing
Operating margin	0.03	0.03	0.10	Above	5% Favorable	Decreasing
Non-operating revenue[b]	0.05	0.02	0.02	Varies	−66% Unfavorable	Increasing
Return on total assets	0.04	0.05	0.11	Above	25% Favorable	Decreasing
Return on net assets[b]	0.06	0.20	0.64	Above	244% Favorable	Decreasing
Activity ratios						
Total asset turnover ratio	1.07	1.01	0.96	Above	−5% Unfavorable	Increasing
Net fixed assets turnover ratio	2.80	2.56	2.41	Above	−9% Unfavorable	Increasing
Age of plant ratio	10.17	7.25	5.71	Below	−29% Favorable	Increasing
Capital structure ratios						
Long-term debt to net assets ratio	0.21	2.73	3.14	Below	1,193% Unfavorable	Decreasing
Net assets to total assets ratio[b]	0.54	0.23	0.17	Above	−57% Unfavorable	Increasing
Times interest earned ratio[b]	2.73	2.03	5.41	Above	−26% Unfavorable	Decreasing
Debt service coverage ratio	3.73	2.00	4.02	Above	−46% Unfavorable	Decreasing

[a]Because Newport Hospital has fewer than 100 beds, the Thomson benchmark ratio values for bed size of less than 100 is used.

(Continued)

Exhibit 4–5 Newport Hospital ratios for 20X0 and 20X1, and Thomson and CMS median ratio values (Continued)

bThese values were obtained from the Centers for Medicare and Medicaid Services (CMS) Hospital Cost Report information system files for financial statements ending in 2004 and Thomson's 2006 median values. *The Comparative Performance of U.S. Hospitals: The Sourcebook 2007.* Thomson Healthcare Publications, 2008.

cAll ratios presented here are rounded for ease of reading, but the percentages for the current year position are computed on the basis of the unrounded numbers in the cells. Therefore, current-year position percentages calculated manually may vary slightly from those shown here.

Liquidity Analysis: Newport's liquidity is improving, though several ratios are still considered unfavorable relative to the desired benchmark positions. The current and quick ratios are both 18 percent below standard, while the most stringent acid test ratio is 30 percent below standard. This suggests potential difficulty in being able to pay off immediate debt obligations, such as monthly payments, without having to tap into a reserve fund. For the current ratio to be at the 2.20 benchmark with given current liabilities, Newport would need an additional $555,000 in liquidity. However, on the other hand, Newport does have a favorable days in accounts receivable, suggesting good control in collecting funds; its days cash on hand is still comfortably high; and the favorable average payment period shows that, so far, Newport has been able to pay all of its bills in a timely manner.

Revenue, Expense, and Profitability Analysis: Whereas Newport's operating expense per adjusted discharge has decreased slightly and remains well below the norm, of concern is the declining operating revenue per adjusted discharge. This could arise from lower payor payment rates or possibly poor medical record documentation, leading to an inability to code discharges appropriately at higher levels to generate additional income. Lower expenditures could be due to better control over labor and supply costs, though overall operating expense devoted to salary and benefit costs remains too high. Newport's operating margin is currently at benchmark but has dropped precipitously over the past year. Returns on total assets and on net assets have also dropped precipitously, yet both remain above benchmark. Newport's low non-operating revenue suggests that it needs to do a better job investing its money and generating income from sources other than simply direct patient care revenues.

Activity Analysis: The total asset turnover and net fixed assets turnover ratios for Newport have both increased slightly over the past year but still reside below benchmark. This implies that the hospital is not using its assets effectively to generate income. The age of plant ratio remains comfortably below benchmark, which indicates that Newport does not have a pressing need to upgrade its facilities but only to make better use of its existing assets.

Capital Structure Analysis: As indicated above, Newport fortunately does not need to upgrade its facilities in the near future because it is highly leveraged, as evidenced by the long term debt to net assets ratio. The ratio of 2.73 means that for every $1.00 in net assets, Newport has $2.73 in long-term debt, whereas the desired position is the inverse of this situation. Though net assets have increased (from approximately $1.9 million to over $2.5 million in the past year; see Exhibit 4–1), this amount as a proportion of total assets remains too low. On a similar note, the hospital's times interest earned and debt service coverage ratios have both plummeted below benchmark for similarly sized institutions, which makes potential creditors nervous about Newport's ability to take on additional debt if need be. This risk in turn would raise the cost of capital for Newport, should it need to look to the market to borrow funds.

Overall Analysis: Although Newport is able to hold its own at this point, the trends generally are not favorable. Receivables are being collected, and bills are being paid in a timely manner right now, but this may not persist, and Newport has little margin if cash gets tight. The facility is not collecting as much as it could be in patient care revenues, and it has not fared well trying to generate income from other sources. Fortunately, Newport does not have pressing need to upgrade its facilities, but these assets currently are not being used as effectively now as they could be to generate much-needed income. The hospital is also already highly leveraged at this point and not in a good position to borrow if need be. In summary, Newport needs to be operating more efficiently with the resources available because other alternative options are limited at this point.

Key Points to Consider When Using and Interpreting Ratios

1. *No one ratio is necessarily better than any other ratio.* It is often useful to use more than one ratio to help answer a question.

2. *Each ratio's terms offer clues about how to fix a problem.* For example, if the current ratio (current assets/current liabilities) is too low, it can be improved by increasing the numerator (current assets), decreasing the denominator (current liabilities), or both. However, changing the conditions to improve one ratio may affect other ratios as well.

3. *Most ratios are interpreted as follows: "There are* n *dollars in the numerator for every dollar in the denominator."* Thus, a current ratio of 2.00 indicates that there is $2 in current assets for every $1 in current liabilities.

4. *A ratio can best be interpreted relative to a benchmark.* The benchmark may be the organization's past performance, a goal set by the organization, a comparison group (such as similar organizations), or some combination thereof. For example, a current ratio of 2.00 probably would be interpreted favorably if the industry benchmark were 1.75; however, it probably would be interpreted unfavorably if the industry benchmark were 2.50.

5. *There are several problems with using benchmarks for comparison in the health care industry.* Two of the most prominent are the availability and reliability of the data:

   - *Finding appropriate data.* Not all segments of the health care industry have data available that can be used for benchmarks. For example, there are no complete, national-level ratio data on health departments or mental health centers. On the other hand, certain segments of the industry have excellent data. Ingenix and Thomson Reuters Healthcare both provide excellent ratio information on hospitals on both a national and regional basis. Alternatively, individual providers may join together to develop their own benchmarks.

   - Even if data are available, it is important to *compare an organization with similar organizations.* It might be highly inappropriate for a small rural hospital in North Dakota to use the ratios of large academic medical centers in Boston for comparison. Services such as Thomson Reuters Healthcare can provide data by size and location. The data are presented by both median and percentile, which means that an organization can set its own benchmarks relative to what it considers an appropriate comparison group.

   - *The reliability of the data.* The same ratio may be calculated differently by different organizations, different sources of industry benchmarks, or both. For example, in calculating the days in accounts receivable, one organization may use the ending balance in accounts receivable, whereas another organization may use the average daily balance. *Therefore, when comparing organizations with one another or with benchmarks, it is necessary to make sure the same formula is being used* (see Perspective 4–3). There may be differences in practices and procedures among organizations that may not be immediately apparent to those using the information. For example, hospitals

Perspective 4–3   Formulas Hospitals Report Using to Calculate Net Days in Accounts Receivable

Hospital	Formula
Hospital 1	Gross Accounts Receivable − Uncollectibles / [(Gross Charges − Deductions) / Number of Days in Period]
Hospital 2	Net Patient Accounts Receivable / (Net Patient Service Revenue / 365)
Hospital 3	Net Accounts Receivable / Net Charges per Day
Hospital 4	Net Accounts Receivable / [(Gross Patient Service Revenue − Charity − Contractual Allowances − Bad Debt) / 365]
Hospital 5	Accounts Receivable + Reserve For Bad Debt + Contractual Adjustments / (Net Patient Revenue / Number of Days in the Period)
Hospital 6	Accounts Receivable / (Revenue Available / Days in Current Year)
Hospital 7	Net Patient Revenue / Operating Margin
Hospital 8	Net Accounts Receivable / (Net Revenue Past 3 Months / Days in Period)

Source: Contributed by Denise R. Smith, Data Analyst, Columbia Cape Fear Memorial Hospital.

may use different depreciation or inventory valuation methods. This could have a profound effect on certain ratios.

6. *In general, a ratio should be neither too high nor too low relative to the benchmark.* For example, the acid test ratio [(cash + marketable securities) / current liabilities] looks at an organization's ability to meet its short-term debt. Although an organization would like to have this ratio above the benchmark, a value too high may indicate too much cash on hand, which likely could be better invested elsewhere.

7. *Not only should a ratio be compared with a benchmark, but also the trend of the ratio can help to interpret how well an organization is doing.* For example, an organization would feel differently if a ratio were at the benchmark and declining versus being at the benchmark and rising over the past five years.

8. *Because ratios are usually relatively small, relatively small differences may indicate large percentage deviations from the benchmark.* For example, if the organization's current ratio were 1.5 and the industry benchmark 2.0, although this is only a 0.5 difference, the organization would be 25 percent below benchmark.

Caution: When comparing organizations with one another or with benchmarks, it is necessary to make sure the same formula is being used.

The remainder of this chapter uses ratio analysis to analyze the statement of operations and balance sheet for Newport Hospital (see Exhibit 4–1) using industry benchmarks for small hospitals.

LIQUIDITY RATIOS

Liquidity ratios answer the question, "How well is the organization positioned to meet its current obligations?" Six key ratios fall into this category: the current ratio, quick ratio, acid test ratio, days in accounts receivable, days cash on hand, and average payment period (Exhibit 4–6). Incidentally, by convention, the current ratio, quick ratio, and acid test ratio all have the word "ratio" in their title, but the other three do not.

Each of these liquidity ratios provides a different insight into Newport Hospital's liquidity. Notice that the first three ratios focus only on the balance sheet, each giving a little more stringent picture of the organization's ability to pay off its current liabilities. The last three ratios use information from both the statement of operations and the balance sheet to look at different aspects of liquidity: the ability of the organization to turn its receivables into cash, the actual amount of cash it has on hand to meet its short-term obligations, and how long it takes the organization to pay its bills.

 Key Point Liquidity ratios *measure a facility's ability to meet short-term obligations, collect receivables, and maintain a cash position.*

Current Ratio

The current ratio (Current Assets / Current Liabilities) is one of the most commonly used ratios. The *current ratio* is the proportion of all current assets to all current liabilities. Values above the benchmark indicate either too many current assets, too few current liabilities, or both. Values below the benchmark indicate either too few current assets, too many current liabilities, or both. To calculate the current ratio (see Exhibit 4–6a):

Step 1. Identify the dollar amount of current assets on the balance sheet.

Step 2. Identify the dollar amount of current liabilities on the balance sheet.

Step 3. Divide the current assets by the current liabilities.

Newport Hospital's current ratio increased from 0.58 in 20X0 to 1.80 in 20X1. The benchmark used for comparison is 2.20. Although the 20X1 value is still below the industry median, this dramatic increase in Newport's current ratio reflects a major improvement in liquidity according to this measure.

Quick Ratio

The *quick ratio* [(Cash + Marketable Securities + Net Accounts Receivable) / Current Liabilities] is commonly used in industries in which net accounts receivable is

Exhibit 4–6 Selected liquidity ratios

Ratio	Formula	Benchmark[a]	Desired Position
Current ratio	$\dfrac{\text{Current assets}}{\text{Current liabilities}}$	2.20	Above
Quick ratio	$\dfrac{\text{Cash + marketable securities + net receivables}}{\text{Current liabilities}}$	1.66	Above
Acid-test ratio	$\dfrac{\text{Cash + marketable securities}}{\text{Current liabilities}}$	0.37	Above
Days in accounts receivable	$\dfrac{\text{Net patient accounts receivable}}{\text{Net patient revenues / 365}}$	53	Above
Days cash on hand	$\dfrac{\text{Cash + marketable securities + long-term investments}}{\text{(Operating expenses – depreciation \& amortization expenses) / 365}}$	80	Above
Average payment period (days)	$\dfrac{\text{Current liabilities}}{\text{(Operating expenses – depreciation and amortization expenses) / 365}}$	50	Organizationally Dependent

[a]Based upon Thomson 2006 approximate hospital median values.

Exhibit 4–6a   Newport's current ratio for 20X0 and 20X1

Year	Current Ratio[a]	=	Current Assets	/	Current Liabilities
20X1	1.80	=	$2,514,335	/	$1,395,190
20X0	0.58	=	$1,954,134	/	$3,394,418

[a]Benchmark = 2.20.

Exhibit 4–6b   Newport's quick ratio for 20X0 and 20X1

Year	Quick Ratio[a]	=	(Cash + Marketable Securities	+	Net Accounts Receivable)	/	Current Liabilities
20X1	1.36	=	$363,181	+	$1,541,244	/	$1,395,190
20X0	0.46	=	$158,458	+	$1,400,013	/	$3,394,418

[a]Benchmark = 1.66.

relatively liquid. Traditionally, this has not been the case in health care organizations. To compute the quick ratio (see Exhibit 4–6b):

Step 1.   Identify the dollar amount of cash, marketable securities, and net accounts receivable on the balance sheet.

Step 2.   Identify the dollar amount of current liabilities on the balance sheet.

Step 3.   Divide the sum of cash, marketable securities, and net accounts receivable by current liabilities.

As with the current ratio, Newport Hospital's quick ratio improved from 20X0 to 20X1, but it is still approximately 18 percent below the industry benchmark of 1.66. To improve this ratio, Newport Hospital must either increase its current assets or decrease its current liabilities or both.

Acid Test Ratio

The *acid test ratio* [(Cash + Marketable Securities) / Current Liabilities] provides the most stringent test of liquidity. It looks at how much cash is on hand or readily available from marketable securities to pay off all current liabilities. This ratio is particularly useful if current liabilities contain a high percentage of accounts that must be

Exhibit 4–6c   Newport's acid test ratio for 20X0 and 20X1

Year	Acid Test Ratio[a]	=	(Cash + Marketable Securities)	/	Current Liabilities
20X1	0.26	=	$363,181	/	$1,395,190
20X0	0.05	=	$158,458	/	$3,394,418

[a]Benchmark = 0.37.

paid off soon (such as wages payable), if collections of accounts receivable are slow, or both. To compute the acid test ratio (see Exhibit 4–6c):

Step 1. Identify the dollar amount of cash and marketable securities on the balance sheet.

Step 2. Identify the dollar amount of current liabilities on the balance sheet.

Step 3. Divide the sum of cash and temporary investments by current liabilities.

Key Point *The* current ratio, quick ratio, *and* acid test ratio *all measure the relationship of various current assets to current liabilities.* The acid test ratio *provides the most stringent test of liquidity of the three.*

Newport's acid test ratio increased from 0.05 to 0.26 from 20X0 to 20X1. In this case, there is a favorable trend, but a concern might be raised because Newport is still below the industry benchmark of 0.37. This means that Newport needs to increase its cash and marketable securities or decrease its current liabilities to meet the target figure.

Days in Accounts Receivable

The *days in accounts receivable ratio* [Net Patient Accounts Receivable / (Net Patient Revenues / 365)] provides an indication of how quickly a hospital is converting its receivables into cash. By dividing net patient accounts receivable by an average day's revenue (Net Patient Revenues / 365), this ratio provides an estimate of how many days' revenues have not yet been collected. Values above the benchmark indicate problems relating to credit collection policies, or both. To calculate the days in accounts receivable ratio (see Exhibit 4–6d):

Step 1.   Identify the dollar amount of net patient revenues on the statement of operations.

Exhibit 4–6d Newport's days in accounts receivable ratio for 20X0 and 20X1

Steps 1, 2

Year	Average Net Patient Revenues per Day	=	Net Patient Revenues	/	365 Days
20X1	$29,530	=	$10,778,272	/	365 days
20X0	$28,948	=	$10,566,176	/	365 days

Steps 3, 4

Year	Days in Accounts Receivable[a]	=	Net Patient Accounts Receivable	/	Average Net Patient Revenues per Day
20X1	52	=	$1,541,244	/	$29,530
20X0	48	=	$1,400,013	/	$28,948

[a]Benchmark = 53 days.

Step 2. Divide net patient revenues by 365 to compute average net patient revenues per day.

Step 3. Identify the dollar amount of net patient accounts receivable on the balance sheet.

Step 4. Divide net patient accounts receivable by average net patient revenues per day.

Key Point *The term* average collection period *can also be used interchangeably with* days in accounts receivable.

Although it took 4 days longer on average to collect receivables in 20X1 than it did in 20X0 (48 days vs. 52 days), Newport Hospital is below the benchmark of 53 days for both years. This generally indicates excellent performance in this area.

Days Cash on Hand

The *days cash on hand ratio* {(Cash + Marketable Securities + Long-Term Investments) / [(Operating Expenses − Depreciation and Amortization Expenses) / 365]} provides an indication of the number of days' worth of expenses an organization can cover with its most liquid assets: cash and marketable securities. The denominator [(operating expenses − depreciation and amortization expenses) / 365] measures an

Exhibit 4–6e   Newport's days cash on hand ratio for 20X0 and 20X1

Year	Operating Expense per Day	=	(Operating Expenses	–	Depreciation & Amortization Expenses)	/ 365 Days
20X1	$28,213 / day	=	$10,681,112	–	$383,493	/ 365 days
20X0	$25,603 / day	=	$9,765,507	–	$420,238	/ 365 days

(Cash + Marketable Securities

Year	Days Cash on Hand[a]		+ Long-term Investments)	/	Operating Expense per Day
20X1	134 days	=	$3,777,913	/	$28,213
20X0	183 days	=	$4,683,934	/	$25,603

[a]Benchmark = 80 days.

average day's cash outflow. Depreciation and amortization are subtracted from operating expenses in the denominator because these are operating expenses but require no cash outflow. To compute the days cash on hand ratio (see Exhibit 4–6e):

Step 1.   Identify the dollar amount of operating expenses and depreciation and amortization expenses on the statement of operations.

Step 2.   Divide operating expenses minus depreciation and amortization expenses by 365 days to compute average cash operating expense per day.

Step 3.   Identify the dollar amount of cash, marketable securities, and long-term investments on the balance sheet. In addition, any long-term investments that are under "Assets limited as to use" or "Board-designated" accounts should also be included as well.

Step 4.   Divide cash and marketable securities and long-term investments by the average cash operating expense per day (from Step 2).

Newport Hospital has lowered its day's cash on hand from 183 days (20X0) to 134 days (20X1). Although this is still 54 days above the benchmark, it is viewed as unfavorable because these days are declining. This decline may stem from either decreasing its cash, marketable securities, and long-term investments or from increasing its operating expenses. When examining a hospital's days cash on hand ratio, be aware that system-affiliated hospitals may keep a low balance of cash on hand because they may transfer a large portion of cash to their parent organization each day. If an unusual amount of cash is needed, the parent will transfer back the needed amount. By doing this, the parent organization has larger amounts of cash available for investment purposes and in many cases is in a better position to invest cash than are the subsidiaries. In such cases, a low days cash on hand ratio of the subsidiary organization is not indicative of a problem.

Average Payment Period

The *average payment period ratio* {Current Liabilities / [(Total Operating Expenses − Depreciation and Amortization Expenses) / 365]} is the counterpart to the days in accounts receivable ratio. It is a measure of how long, on average, it takes an organization to pay its bills. Because the denominator is a measure of an average day's payments for bills, dividing current liabilities by an average day's payment provides a measure of how many days' bills have not been paid. To develop a creditworthy relationship and goodwill with vendors and suppliers, health care organizations should attempt to pay their bills on time. To calculate the average payment period ratio (see Exhibit 4–6f):

Step 1.   Identify the dollar amount of total operating expenses and depreciation and amortization expenses on the statement of operations.

Step 2.   Divide total operating expenses minus depreciation and amortization expenses by 365 days to compute average cash expense per day.

Step 3.   Identify the dollar amount of current liabilities on the balance sheet.

Step 4.   Divide the current liabilities by average cash expense per day.

Exhibit 4–6f   Newport's average payment period ratio for 20X0 and 20X1

Steps 1, 2

Year	Average Cash Expense per Day	=	(Operating Expenses	−	Depreciation & Amortization Expenses)	/ 365 Days
20X1	$28,213 / day	=	($10,681,112	−	$383,493)	/ 365 days
20X0	$25,603 / day	=	($9,765,507	−	$420,238)	/ 365 days

Steps 3, 4

Year	Average Payment Period Days[a]		Current Liabilities	/ Average Cash Expense per Day
20X1	49 days	=	$1,395,190	/ $28,213 / day
20X0	133 days	=	$3,394,418	/ $25,603 / day

[a]Benchmark = 50 days.

In the period of one year, Newport Hospital has decreased its average payment period from 133 days to 49 days and is now below the industry benchmark of 50 days.

 Key Point Days in accounts receivable, cash on hand, *and* average payment period *are all liquidity ratios that give an insight into how quickly cash is flowing in and out of the organization.*

Liquidity Summary

From 20X0 to 20X1, Newport Hospital improved its ability to meet current obligations with current assets as indicated by its current, quick and acid-test ratios, and average payment period, although the first three are still considerably below their benchmarks (Exhibit 4–7). In terms of the relative amount of cash actually available, a mixed picture emerges. On the one hand, the acid-test ratio, which indicates the amount of cash and marketable securities available to meet current liabilities, is below its desired position of being at the benchmark. Newport has a favorable position on its days in accounts receivable, which (see Exhibit 4–8) indicates that the organization is performing well in turning its receivables into cash. This higher cash position may have increased its days cash on hand, which now is 50 days above its benchmark.

In regard to collecting money owed and paying its bills, Newport's days in accounts receivable is increasing toward the benchmark (which means that revenues will be converted to cash more slowly), while it has greatly decreased its average payment period (which will likely be well received by its suppliers). Fortunately, days cash on hand is still favorable, which should create some relief for the organization.

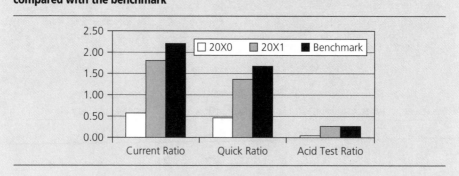

Exhibit 4–7 Newport Hospital's current, quick, and acid test ratios in 20X0 and 20X1 compared with the benchmark

Exhibit 4–8 Newport Hospital's days in accounts receivable, days cash on hand, and average payment period ratios for 20X0 and 20X1 compared with the benchmark

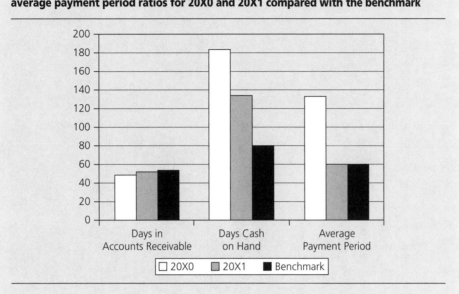

REVENUE, EXPENSE, AND PROFITABILITY RATIOS

There are several revenue, expense, and profitability ratios, each providing a different insight into the ability of a health care organization to produce a profit. The most commonly used ratios include operating revenue per adjusted discharge, operating expense per adjusted discharge, salary and benefit expense as a percentage of total operating expenses, operating margin, non-patient-service revenue, return on net assets, and return on total assets (see Exhibit 4–9 and Perspective 4–4).

Operating Revenue per Adjusted Discharge

The *operating revenue per adjusted discharge* ratio (Total Operating Revenue / Adjusted Discharge) measures total operating revenues generated from the organization's patient care line of business based on its adjusted inpatient discharges. The adjusted discharge attempts to transform all of the health care provider's revenue, including outpatient revenue, into units representing inpatient care services. Discharges are adjusted by multiplying hospital total discharges by a factor defined as *gross patient revenue* divided by *gross inpatient revenue*. Other adjustments can be also made for case complexity (by dividing by case-mix index) and geographic wage differences (wage index); however, this textbook adjusts only for inpatient care services. The ratio measures the

Exhibit 4-9 Selected revenue, expense, and profitability ratios

Ratio	Formula	Benchmark[a]	Desired Position
Operating revenue per adjusted discharge	$\dfrac{\text{Total operating revenue}}{\text{Adjusted discharges}^{b}}$	$5,679	Above
Operating expense per adjusted discharge	$\dfrac{\text{Total operating expenses}}{\text{Adjusted discharges}^{b}}$	$5,497	Below
Salary and benefit expense as a percentage of operating expense	$\dfrac{\text{Salary and benefit expenses}}{\text{Total operating expenses}}$	49%	Below
Operating margin	$\dfrac{\text{Operating income}}{\text{Total operating revenues}}$	0.03	Above
Non-operating revenue ratio	$\dfrac{\text{Non-operating revenues}}{\text{Total operating revenues}}$	0.05	Organizationally Dependent
Return on total assets[c]	$\dfrac{\text{Excess of revenues over expenses}}{\text{Total assets}}$	0.04	Above
Return on net assets[d]	$\dfrac{\text{Excess of revenues over expenses}}{\text{Net assets}}$	0.06	Above

[a] Based upon Thomson 2006 approximate hospital median values.
[b] Adjusted discharges = (adjustment factor) x (total discharges).
 Adjustment factor = (total gross patient revenues) / (total gross inpatient revenues).
 The adjustment factor expresses healthcare organizations' revenue activities in terms of inpatient acute-care services.
[c] Called return on assets in for-profit health care organizations and calculated as: (net income) / (total assets).
[d] Called return on equity in for-profit health care organizations and calculated as: (net income) / (owners' equity).

Perspective 4–4   Key Profitability Ratios for Hospitals

Thomson HealthCare promotes three profitability ratios: operating profit margin, total profit margin, and cash flow margin. Operating profit margin ratio measures operating income earned from patient care services. Total profit margin includes non-operating income sources, such as interest income and realized gains from investments and private contributions and any other income earned from non-operating sources. Cash flow margin ratio measures income earned before depreciation, interest, and taxes and includes non-operating income sources that are earned during the accounting period. Declining operating income from operations and reliance on investment income to fund operations will reduce a hospital's ability to borrow and lower its liquidity position. Fewer cash and investment reserves, coupled with a hospital's inability to access debt borrowings, will create a capital shortage to fund the replacement of its plant and equipment.

Source: Thomson Healthcare. 2007. *The Comparative Performance of US Hospitals: The Sourcebook 2007*, 20th edition. Evanston, Ill.: Thomson.

Exhibit 4–9a   Newport's operating revenue per adjusted discharge for 20X0 and 20X1

Year	Operating Revenue per Adjusted Discharge[a]	=	Total Operating Revenue	/	Adjusted Discharges
20X1	$4,235	=	$11,012,021	/	2,600
20X0	$4,704	=	$10,819,693	/	2,300

[a]Benchmark = $5,679.

amount of operating revenue generated from its patient care services. To compute the operating revenue per adjusted discharge (see Exhibit 4–9a):

Step 1.   Identify operating revenue on the statement of operations.

Step 2.   Identify adjusted discharges from utilization data.

Step 3.   Divide operating revenue by adjusted discharges.

In 20X0, Newport Hospital was moderately below the industry benchmark ($4,704 vs. $5,679). However, the operating revenue per adjusted discharge has decreased further to $4,235 in 20X1, reflecting the fact that total operating revenues related to patient care services have decreased during this time.

Operating Expense per Adjusted Discharge

The *operating expense per adjusted discharge ratio* (Total Operating Expense / Adjusted Discharge) measures total operating expenses incurred from providing its patient care services, and it is adjusted for inpatient discharges where adjusted discharges are calculated the same as for the previous ratio. To compute the operating expense per adjusted discharge (see Exhibit 4–9b):

Step 1. Identify total operating expenses on the statement of operations.

Step 2. Identify adjusted discharges from utilization data.

Step 3. Divide total operating expenses by adjusted discharges.

In 20X0, Newport Hospital's operating expense per adjusted discharge ratio was considerably below the industry benchmark ($4,246 vs. $5,497). However, this ratio has decreased slightly to $4,108 in 20X1, indicating that Newport has lowered its operating costs during this period.

Key Point *The* operating revenue per adjusted discharge *measures the amount of operating revenues generated from the organization's patient care line of business patient, and the* operating expense per adjusted discharge *measures operating expenses incurred from providing its patient care services.*

Salary and Benefit Expense as a Percentage of Total Operating Expense

The *salary and benefit expense as a percentage of total operating expense ratio* (Total Salary and Benefit Expenses / Total Operating Expenses) measures the percentage of

Exhibit 4–9b   Newport's operating expense per adjusted discharge for 20X0 and 20X1

Year	Operating Expense per Adjusted Discharge[a]	=	Total Operating Expense	/	Adjusted Discharges
20X1	$4,108	=	$10,681,112	/	2,600
20X0	$4,246	=	$9,765,507	/	2,300

[a]Benchmark = $5,497.

total operating expenses that are attributed to labor costs. Labor costs are a major expense in the operation of a health care facility. To compute the salary and benefit expense as a percentage of total operating expenses (see Exhibit 4–9c):

Step 1. Identify the total salary and benefit expenses on the statement of operations.

Step 2. Identify the total operating expenses on the statement of operations.

Step 3. Divide the total salary and benefit expenses by the total operating expense.

In 20X0, Newport Hospital was well above the industry benchmark (55 percent vs. 49 percent). However, the salary and benefit expenses as a percentage of total operating expenses has decreased to 53 percent in 20X1, reflecting the fact that Newport has lowered its labor costs during this period relative to its other costs.

Operating Margin

The *operating margin ratio* (Operating Income / Total Operating Revenues) measures profits earned from the organization's main line of business. The margin indicates the proportion of profit earned for each dollar of operating revenue—that is, the proportion of profit remaining after subtracting total operating expenses from operating revenues. To compute the operating margin (see Exhibit 4–9d):

Exhibit 4–9c **Newport's salary and benefit expense as a percentage of total operating expense for 20X0 and 20X1**

Year	Salary and Benefit Expense as a Percentage of Total Operating Expense[a]	=	Salary and Benefit Expense	/	Total Operating Expense
20X1	53%	=	$5,644,880	/	$10,681,112
20X0	55%	=	$5,345,498	/	$9,765,507

[a]Benchmark = 49%.

Exhibit 4–9d **Newport's operating margin ratio for 20X0 and 20X1**

Year	Operating Margin[a]	=	Operating Income	/	Total Operating Revenues
20X1	0.03	=	$330,909	/	$11,012,021
20X0	0.10	=	$1,054,186	/	$10,819,693

[a]Benchmark = 0.03.

Step 1. Identify the operating income on the statement of operations.

Step 2. Identify the total operating revenues on the statement of operations.

Step 3. Divide the operating income by total operating revenues.

In 20X0, Newport Hospital was considerably above the industry benchmark (10 percent vs. 3 percent). Unfortunately, the operating-margin ratio has decreased to 3.0 percent in 20X1, reflecting the fact that total operating expenses have increased faster than have total operating revenues.

Non-Operating Revenue Ratio

The purpose of the *non-operating revenue ratio* (Non-operating Revenues / Total Operating Revenues) is to find out how dependent the organization is on patient-related net income. The higher the ratio, the less the organization is dependent on direct patient-related income and the more it is dependent on revenues from other non-operating sources. This ratio is becoming increasingly difficult to use to compare health care organizations because under recent accounting rules, there is considerable discretion as to what is classified as operating or non-operating revenues.

This results in two potential problems: to the extent that the ratio for any one organization is not calculated in exactly the same way as the benchmark, a comparison with the benchmark may be inappropriate; and when multiple organizations are being compared, to the extent they did not classify various items (such as interest expense) in exactly the same way, the comparisons may be invalid. Non-operating revenue may include such accounts as interest income, dividends, gains from investment activities, and assets released from restricted investment accounts (see Exhibit 4–9e):

Step 1.   Identify the non-operating revenues on the statement of operations.

Step 2.   Identify the total operating revenues on the statement of operations.

Step 3.   Divide the non-operating revenues by the total operating revenues.

Newport's non-operating revenue ratio is 2 percent for both 20X1 and 20X0, which is below the national benchmark of 5 percent. An increase in contributions and greater investment portfolio performance could raise its ratio value.

Return on Total Assets

In not-for-profit organizations, the *return on total assets ratio* is calculated as (Excess of Revenues Over Expenses / Total Assets). In for-profit organizations, it is called *return on assets* and is calculated as (Net Income / Total Assets). It measures how much profit is earned for each dollar invested in assets. To compute the return on total assets ratio (see Exhibit 4–9f):

Step 1.   Identify the excess of revenues over expenses on the statement of operations.

Exhibit 4–9e Newport's non-operating revenue ratio for 20X0 and 20X1

Year	Non-Operating Revenue Ratio[a]	=	Non-Operating Revenues	/	Total Operating Revenues
20X1	0.02	=	$185,000	/	$11,012,021
20X0	0.02	=	$165,000	/	$10,819,693

[a]Benchmark = 0.05.

Exhibit 4–9f Newport's return on total assets ratio for 20X0 and 20X1

Year	Return on Total Assets[a]	=	Excess of Revenues Over Expenses	/	Total Assets
20X1	0.05	=	$515,909	/	$10,876,736
20X0	0.11	=	$1,219,186	/	$11,315,585

[a]Benchmark = 0.04.

Step 2. Identify total assets on the balance sheet.

Step 3. Divide the excess of revenues over expenses by total assets.

Newport Hospital's return-on-total-assets ratio declined significantly over this time period (11 percent to 5 percent) and is currently only slightly above the benchmark of 4 percent in 20X1. One reason for this decrease could be that Newport's expenses have increased faster than its revenues, thereby reducing the excess of revenues over expenses. To improve this ratio, Newport could increase operating revenues, decrease expenses, or decrease total assets (or all three).

Return on Net Assets

In not-for-profit organizations, this ratio is called *return on net assets* (Excess of Revenues Over Expenses / Net Assets). In for-profit organizations, it is called *return on equity* and is calculated using the formula (Net Income / Owners' Equity). In for-profit organizations, it measures the rate of return for each dollar in owners' equity. In not-for-profit health care organizations, it measures the rate of return for each dollar in net assets. To calculate the return on net assets ratio (see Exhibit 4–9g):

Step 1. Identify the excess of revenues over expenses on the statement of operations.

Exhibit 4–9g Newport's return on net assets ratio for 20X0 and 20X1

Year	Return on Net Assets[a]	=	Excess of Revenues Over Expenses	/	Net Assets
20X1	0.20	=	$515,909	/	$2,542,655
20X0	0.64	=	$1,219,186	/	$1,911,683

[a]Benchmark = 0.06.

Step 2. Identify the net assets on the balance sheet.

Step 3. Divide excess of revenues over expenses by net assets.

As in the case for the return on total assets ratio, the return on net assets ratio also decreased (from 64 percent in 20X0 to 20 percent in 20X1). Expenses growing faster than revenues contributed to this decrease. However, the return on net assets in 20X1 is still considerably above the industry benchmark of 6 percent.

It is important to note that the return on net assets ratio is magnified by the amount of debt financing. The higher the level of debt relative to net assets, the greater the return on net assets is affected for a given level of profit or loss. Exhibit 4–10 provides an example of this phenomenon.

In Case 1, the organization earns a profit (excess of revenues over expenses) of $100,000. Because there is no debt, the return on net assets is 10 percent ($100,000 / $1,000,000). However, in Case 2, the assets are financed with 50 percent debt and 50 percent equity. Thus, the return to the owners is doubled (20 percent) because they have only half as much invested ($500,000 instead of $1,000,000), the remainder of the assets being financed by debt. Although it results in higher returns when there is a profit (as in both Cases 1 and 2), there is a greater loss in return on net assets when the organization is unprofitable (as illustrated in Cases 3 and 4). As previously noted, financial leverage reflects the proportion of debt used within the organization's capital structure. Thus, these cases show that debt increases the financial risk to the owners of a health care organization. It magnifies positive returns when there is a profit but negative returns when there is a loss. It also carries the added burden of fixed interest payments.

 Key Point *Higher debt increases financial risk by magnifying the returns on net asset or equity.*

Exhibit 4–10 Example of how increased debt magnifies gains and losses when computing return on net assets

In Case 1, the organization has no debt. In Case 2, the organization has 50 percent of its assets financed by debt. In both cases, the organization makes a $100,000 profit, but the return on net assets is twice as high in Case 2.

Case 1: $100,000 Excess of revenues over expenses; no debt

Balance Sheet				Statement of Operations	
Assets	$1,000,000	Debt	$0	Excess of revenues over expenses	$100,000
		Net assets	$1,000,000		

Return on net assets = $100,000 / $1,000,000 = 0.10

Case 2: $100,000 Excess of revenues over expenses; 50 percent debt

Balance Sheet				Statement of Operations	
Assets	$1,000,000	Debt	$500,000	Excess of revenues over expenses	$100,000
		Net assets	$500,000		

Return on net assets = $100,000 / $500,000 = 0.20

In Case 3, the organization has no debt. In Case 4, the organization has 50 percent of its assets financed by debt. In both cases, the organization incurs a $100,000 loss, but the negative return on net assets is twice as much in Case 4.

Case 3: ($100,000) Excess of revenues over expenses; no debt

Balance Sheet				Statement of Operations	
Assets	$1,000,000	Debt	$0	Excess of revenues over expenses	($100,000)
		Net assets	$1,000,000		

Return on net assets = −$100,000 / $1,000,000 = −0.10

Case 4: ($100,000) Excess of revenues over expenses; 50 percent debt

Balance Sheet				Statement of Operations	
Assets	$1,000,000	Debt	$500,000	Excess of revenues over expenses	($100,000)
		Net assets	$500,000		

Return on net assets = −$100,000 / $500,000 = −0.20

Point: Increased debt magnifies both gains and losses when computing return on net assets.

Revenue, Expense, and Profitability Summary

Newport Hospital has a favorable position with three of the five revenue and profitability ratios in 20X1 at or above the benchmark. For its two expense ratios, operating expense per adjusted discharge ratio is the only one below the benchmark position, which reflects a desirable position. However, it has also shown a decline from 20X0 to 20X1 in six of the seven revenue, expense, and profitability ratios (see Exhibits 4–11a and 4–11b). This raises concerns about the control of revenues and expenses.

ACTIVITY RATIOS

In general, activity ratios (see Exhibit 4–12) ask the question, "For every dollar invested in assets, how many dollars of revenue (not excess of revenues over expenses) are being generated?" Most ratios in this category take the general form:

$$\frac{\text{Revenues}}{\text{Assets}}$$

Thus, the more revenue generated, the higher the ratio.

Key Point *Because many of the activity ratios ask the general question, "How many dollars in revenue (the numerator) are being generated relative to [specific] assets (the denominator)?" activity ratios are also called efficiency ratios. The higher the ratio, the more efficiently the assets are being used.*

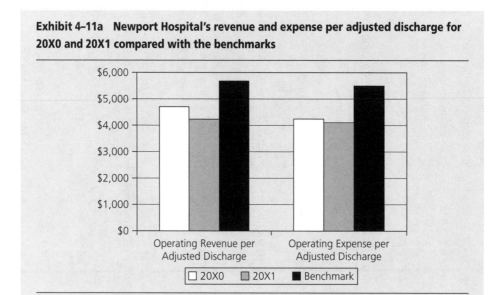

Exhibit 4–11a   Newport Hospital's revenue and expense per adjusted discharge for 20X0 and 20X1 compared with the benchmarks

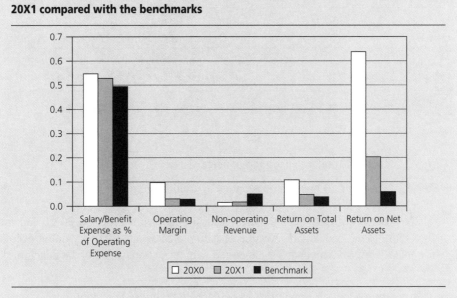

Exhibit 4–11b Newport Hospital's expense and profitability ratios for 20X0 and 20X1 compared with the benchmarks

Exhibit 4–12 Selected activity ratios

Ratio	Formula	Benchmark[a]	Desired Position
Total asset turnover ratio	$\dfrac{\text{Total operating revenues}}{\text{Total assets}}$	1.07	Above
Fixed asset turnover ratio	$\dfrac{\text{Total operating revenues}}{\text{Net plant and equipment}}$	2.80	Above
Age of plant ratio	$\dfrac{\text{Accumulated depreciation}}{\text{Depreciation expense}}$	10.17	Below

[a] Based on Thomson 2006 median values.

Total Asset Turnover

The *total asset turnover ratio* (Total Operating Revenues / Total Assets) measures the overall efficiency of the organization's assets to produce revenue. It answers the question, "For every dollar in assets, how many dollars of operating revenue are being generated?" To calculate the total asset turnover ratio (see Exhibit 4–12a):

Step 1.   Identify total operating revenues on the statement of operations.

Exhibit 4–12a   Newport's total asset turnover ratio for 20X0 and 20X1

Year	Total Asset Turnover[a]	=	Total Operating Revenues	/	Total Assets
20X1	1.01	=	$11,012,021	/	$10,876,736
20X0	0.96	=	$10,819,693	/	$11,315,585

[a]Benchmarket = 1.07.

Step 2.   Identify total assets on the balance sheet.

Step 3.   Divide total operating revenues by total assets.

For Newport Hospital, the ratio increased slightly from 20X0 to 20X1 and has remained close to the benchmark. A value of 1.00 indicates that for every dollar of total assets, one dollar of total revenues is generated, which is approximately the benchmark.

 Key Point *Asset accounts reflect values at a specific point in time, which in turn can fail to account for seasonal changes in asset accounts. To deal with this problem, some analysts use an average of the beginning and ending year values for the fixed asset or current asset accounts. That convention, however, is not used in this text.*

Fixed Asset Turnover

The *fixed asset turnover ratio* (Total Operating Revenues / Net Plant and Equipment) aids in the evaluation of the most productive assets, plant and equipment. To calculate the fixed asset turnover ratio (see Exhibit 4–12b):

Step 1.   Identify total operating revenues on the statement of operations.

Step 2.   Identify net plant and equipment assets on the balance sheet.

Step 3.   Divide total operating revenues by net plant and equipment (fixed) assets.

 Key Point *The* fixed asset turnover ratio *is a measure of how productive the fixed assets of the organization are in generating operating revenues.*

Newport's fixed asset turnover ratio increased from 20X0 to 20X1 (2.41 to 2.56) but is still below the benchmark of 2.80. The fixed asset turnover value of 2.56 indicates that for every dollar of fixed assets, only $2.56 of operating revenues is being generated.

Exhibit 4–12b   Newport's fixed asset turnover ratio for 20X0 and 20X1

Year	Fixed Asset Turnover[a]	=	Total Operating Revenues	/	Net Plant and Equipment
20X1	2.56	=	$11,012,021	/	$4,306,754
20X0	2.41	=	$10,819,693	/	$4,495,122

[a]Benchmarket = 2.80.

Key Point *Asset turnover ratios have an interesting property because of accrual accounting. When revenues (the numerator) stay the same, the ratio will continually increase from year to year because asset values (the denominator) decrease each year due to depreciation. This will occur until the assets are fully depreciated. To check how old the assets are, the age of plant ratio is used.*

Caution: Note that this text uses excess of revenues over expenses in the numerator for the profitability ratios *return on total assets* and *return on net assets*, and it uses total operating revenues in the numerator for the activity ratios *total asset turnover ratio* and *net asset turnover ratio*.

Age of Plant Ratio

The *age of plant ratio* (Accumulated Depreciation / Depreciation Expense) provides an indication of the average age of a hospital's plant and equipment. This ratio complements the fixed asset turnover ratio. High fixed asset turnover ratios may be an indication of a lack of investment in fixed assets. If the average age of plant is high, it may indicate that the organization needs to replace its fixed assets shortly. If so, it would be important to look at other ratios to see how well positioned the organization is to finance the purchase of new assets. To compute the age of plant ratio (see Exhibit 4–12c):

Step 1.   Identify the accumulated depreciation on the balance sheet.

Step 2.   Identify the depreciation expense on the statement of operations.

Step 3.   Divide the accumulated depreciation by the depreciation expense.

Newport Hospital's average age of plant ratio has increased by over one and one-half years (5.71 to 7.25), but it is still more than 3 years below the industry benchmark of 10.17.

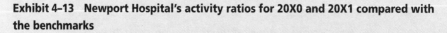

Exhibit 4–12c Newport's age of plant ratio for 20X0 and 20X1

Year	Age of Plant[a]	=	Accumulated Depreciation	/	Depreciation Expense
20X1	7.25	=	$2,781,741	/	$383,493
20X0	5.71	=	$2,398,248	/	$420,238

[a] Benchmarket = 10.17.

Exhibit 4–13 Newport Hospital's activity ratios for 20X0 and 20X1 compared with the benchmarks

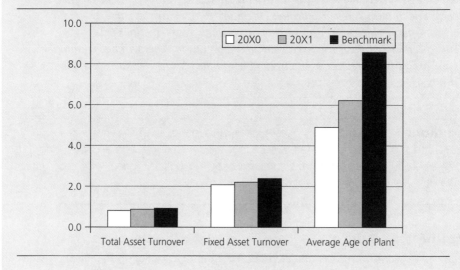

Activity Summary

Newport Hospital is below the benchmark on both its total asset turnover ratio and its fixed asset turnover ratio but shows improvement from 20X0 to 20X1 for both ratios (see Exhibit 4–13). Its average age of plant is still well below the benchmark of 10.17 years, which indicates that the hospital has newer assets relative to the benchmark of small hospitals. Thus, because of the fixed asset ratio, a question should be raised regarding how efficiently the fixed assets are being used to generate revenue.

CAPITAL STRUCTURE RATIOS

Capital structure ratios answer two questions: "How are an organization's assets financed?" and "How able is this organization to take on new debt?" In many cases, a greater understanding of these ratios (and answers to these questions) can be gained by examining the statement of cash flows to see if significant long-term debt has been acquired or paid off, or if there has been a sale or purchase of fixed assets. Capital structure ratios include long-term debt to net assets, net assets to total assets, times interest earned, and debt service coverage (see Exhibit 4–14).

Key Point Capital structure ratios *measure how an organization's assets are financed and how able the organization is to pay for the new debt.*

Key Point *One might also want to measure capital structure ratios by using the unrestricted net asset account rather than the combined restricted and unrestricted net asset values. The unrestricted net asset account represents the claim on assets that the provider could sell to meet debt payments.*

Long-Term Debt to Net Assets

The *long-term debt to net assets ratio* (Long-Term Debt / Net Assets) measures the proportion of debt to net assets. In for-profit organizations, this ratio is called the *long-term debt to equity ratio* and is calculated by the formula: (Long-Term Debt / Owners' Equity). Although most organizations certainly want to finance a portion of their assets with debt,

Exhibit 4–14 Selected capital structure ratios

Ratio	Formula	Benchmark[a]	Desired Position
Long-term debt to net assets ratio	$\dfrac{\text{Long-term debt}}{\text{Net assets}}$	0.21	Below
Net assets to total assets ratio	$\dfrac{\text{Net assets}}{\text{Total assets}}$	0.54	Above
Times interest earned ratio	$\dfrac{\text{(Excess of revenues over expenses + interest expense)}}{\text{Interest expense}}$	2.73	Above
Debt service coverage ratio	$\dfrac{\text{(Excess of revenues over expenses + interest expense + depreciation and amortization expenses)}}{\text{(Interest expense + principal payments)}}$	3.73	Above

[a] Based on Thomson 2006 median values.

at a certain level an organization takes on too much debt and may find itself in a precarious position where it has difficulty both paying back its existing debt and borrowing additional funds. To calculate the long-term debt to net assets ratio (see Exhibit 4–14a):

Step 1. Identify noncurrent debt on the balance sheet.

Step 2. Identify net assets on the balance sheet.

Step 3. Divide noncurrent debt by net assets.

Key Point Long-term debt to net assets ratio *measures the proportion of assets that are financed by debt relative to those that are not.*

For Newport Hospital, despite an increase in noncurrent debt, the long-term debt to net assets ratio actually decreased from 20X0 to 20X1 due to the increase in net assets. Still, the 20X1 ending value (2.73) is over 10 times the industry benchmark (0.21).

Net Assets to Total Assets

The *net assets to total assets ratio* (Net Assets / Total Assets) reflects the proportion of total assets financed by equity. In for-profit organizations, this ratio is called the equity to total asset ratio and is calculated by the formula: Owners' Equity / Total Assets. Creditors desire a strong equity position with sufficient funds to pay off debt obligations. A high net asset or equity position is enhanced either through the retention of earnings or through private contributions from the community. In investor-owned facilities, the retention of earnings and issuance of stock increase the equity. To calculate the net assets to total assets ratio (see Exhibit 4–14b):

Step 1. Identify net assets on the balance sheet.

Step 2. Identify total assets on the balance sheet.

Step 3. Divide net assets by total assets.

Exhibit 4–14a   Newport's long-term debt to net assets ratio for 20X0 and 20X1

Year	Long-term Debt to Net Assets[a]	=	Long-term Debt	/	Net Assets
20X1	2.73	=	$6,938,891	/	$2,542,655
20X0	3.14	=	$6,009,484	/	$1,911,683

[a]Benchmarket = 0.21.

In 20X1, this ratio was less than half the industry benchmark (0.54), but it did increase from 0.17 (20X0) to 0.23 (20X1). With this thin equity state, creditors probably would be cautious about lending funds to this facility in the future.

Times Interest Earned

The *times interest earned ratio* [(Excess Of Revenues Over Expenses + Interest Expense) / Interest Expense] enables creditors and lenders to evaluate a hospital's ability to generate earnings necessary to meet interest expense requirements. In for-profit organizations, the ratio is calculated by the formula: [(Net Income + Interest Expense) / Interest Expense]. The ratio answers the question, "For every dollar in interest expense, how many dollars are there in profit?" Interest expense is added back into the numerator so that the numerator reflects profit *before* taking interest into account. To calculate the times interest earned ratio (see Exhibit 4–14c):

Step 1. Identify excess of revenues over expenses on the statement of operations.

Step 2. Identify interest expense on the statement of operations.

Step 3. Add together excess of revenues over expenses and interest expense and divide the total by interest expense.

Exhibit 4–14b Newport's net assets to total assets ratio for 20X0 and 20X1

Year	Net Assets to Total Assets[a]	=	Net Assets	/	Total Assets
20X1	0.23	=	$2,542,655	/	$10,876,736
20X0	0.17	=	$1,911,683	/	$11,315,585

[a]Benchmark = 0.54.

Exhibit 4–14c Newport's times interest earned ratio for 20X0 and 20X1

Year	Times Interest Earned[a]	=	(Excess of Revenues over Expenses	+	Interest Expense)	/	Interest Expense
20X1	2.03	=	($515,909	+	$500,000)	/	$500,000
20X0	5.41	=	($1,219,186	+	$276,379)	/	$276,379

[a]Benchmark = 2.73

Unfortunately, Newport's times interest earned ratio decreased precipitously from 20X0 (5.41) to 20X1 (2.03), falling below the benchmark of 2.73. A continued decline in the times interest earned ratio may affect Newport's ability to borrow in the future.

Debt Service Coverage

A more robust measure of ability to repay a loan is the *debt service coverage ratio* [(Excess of Revenues Over Expenses + Interest Expense + Depreciation and Amortization Expenses) / (Interest Expense + Principal Payments)]. In for-profit organizations, it is calculated as [(Net Income + Interest Expense + Depreciation and Amortization Expenses) / (Interest Expense + Principal Payments)]. It answers the question, "For every dollar the organization has to pay on debt service (Principal + Interest), what is its approximate cash inflow during the year?" This ratio is used extensively by investment bankers and bond rating agencies to evaluate a facility's ability to meet its total loan requirements, principal payments plus interest. Principal payments are usually presented in the statement of cash flows. Because it is not provided, assume that Newport's principal payments are $200,000 per year. Interest expense and depreciation expense are added to the excess of revenues over expenses to develop an indication of cash flow before interest expense. To compute the debt service coverage ratio (see Exhibit 4–14d):

Step 1.   Identify excess of revenues over expenses on the statement of operations.

Step 2.   Identify interest expense on the statement of operations.

Step 3.   Identify principal payments on the statement of cash flows.

Step 4.   Add the excess of revenues over expenses, interest expense, and depreciation and amortization expense from the statement of operations.

Step 5.   Divide the sum from step 4 by the sum of interest expense and principal payments.

Key Point Debt service coverage ratio *is a critical ratio used by investment bankers because it reflects what proportion of the cash flow payments are being used to pay off debt.*

Reconfirming the outcome of the times interest earned ratio, Newport also has placed itself in a precarious position in terms of meeting its interest and principal payments. It is considerably below the benchmark of 3.73 and has dropped in half from 20X0 (4.02) to 20X1 (2.00). It currently has a cash flow before principal and interest payments of only 2.00 times its debt service payments. If this condition continues, Newport likely would find itself in technical default on its long-term obligations.

Exhibit 4–14d   Newport's debt service coverage ratio for 20X0 and 20X1

Steps 1–4

Year	Cash Flow before Interest	=	(Excess of Revenues over Expenses	+	Interest Expense	+	Depreciation Expense)
20X1	$1,399,402	=	($515,909	+	$500,000	+	$383,493)
20X0	$1,915,803	=	($1,219,186	+	$276,379	+	$420,238)

Steps 5

Year	Debit Service Coverage[a]	=	Cash Flow before Interest	/	(Interest Expense	+	Principal Payments)
20X1	2.00	=	$1,399,402	/	($500,000	+	$200,000)
20X0	4.02	=	$1,915,803	/	($276,379	+	$200,000)

[a]Benchmark = 3.73.

Capital Structure Summary

Newport Hospital decreased its debt position from 20X0 to 20X1; however; this amount of debt is still well above the industry benchmark. This is reflected in the capital structure ratios, which show that its proportion of debt to net assets is still too high, albeit decreasing. More troublesome for Newport is its ability to pay its debt: both the times interest earned and debt service coverage ratios fell considerably below the benchmark in 20X1 (see Exhibit 4–15).

Summary of Newport Hospital's Ratios

Newport Hospital's ratios cause some concern. Most problematic are the capital structure ratios, which indicate that Newport Hospital is above the benchmark in debt and considerably below the benchmark in ability to pay it off. Though improving in liquidity from 20X0 to 20X1, it is still below the benchmark in its ability to meet current obligations with current assets, except with its ability to collect on its receivables. Most of Newport's profitability ratios are above benchmark, but they are falling precipitously, indicating potential problems in its ability to pay off its short-term obligations. Although Newport Hospital seems to be using its assets more efficiently as indicated by most of the activity ratios, this is likely due to the increasing age of plant. Newport's capital structure ratios raise serious concerns about its ability to pay off current debt or to increase debt financing if needed to replace properties and equipment in the near future.

Although this chapter has introduced commonly used financial ratios, there are many others. Perspective 4–5 presents some used by HMOs.

Exhibit 4–15   Newport Hospital's capital structure ratios for 20X0 and 20X1 compared with the benchmarks

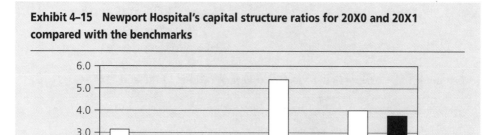

Perspective 4–5   The Financial Performance of Large Health Plans in California

The key financial ratios that are employed to assess and evaluate the financial performance of health plans include medical loss, sometimes called "medical benefit" ratio, the administrative cost ratio, and total profit margin ratio. The medical loss ratio is defined as medical expenses divided by insurance premium revenue and measures the amount of the insurance revenues paid out as medical expenses. Blue Cross has the lowest and indicates that only 78.9 percent of its insurance premiums are paid out as medical expenses. Kaiser's higher medical loss ratio may stem from reallocation of its administrative costs to medical costs. For example, Kaiser may allocate the cost of its computer system in its clinic to its medical costs.

Administrative cost measures the percentage of its total revenues including investment income that is paid for by administrative costs such as employee labor costs, marketing, and office expenses. Aetna and Blue Cross paid out over 10 percent of their revenue, whereas Kaiser paid out only 4 percent. In terms of total profit margin ratio, Aetna generated 7.3 percent of its total revenue as earnings, whereas Blue Cross and Kaiser earned 6 percent and 3 percent, respectively.

Key Ratios 2005	Aetna Health Plan, %	Blue Cross, %	Kaiser, %
Medical loss	81.4	78.9	93.9
Administrative cost	10.0	11.9	4.1
Total profit margin	7.3	6.0	3.0

Source: Baumgarten, A. 2007. *California health care market report 2006.* California Healthcare Foundation, http://www.chcf.org/topics/view.cfm?itemID=131345

SUMMARY

The financial performance of health care organizations is of interest to numerous individuals and groups, including administrators, board members, creditors, bondholders, community members, and government agencies. This chapter presented three ways to analyze the financial statements of health care organizations: horizontal analysis, vertical analysis, and ratio analysis.

Horizontal analysis examines year-to-year changes in the line items of the financial statements. It answers the question, "What is the percentage change from one year to the next in a particular line item (such as cash, long-term debt, patient accounts receivable)?" The formula for horizontal analysis is [(Subsequent Year – Base Year) / Base Year] × 100 = percentage increase (decrease) between years.

A variant of horizontal analysis is trend analysis. Instead of comparing one line item with that of the previous year, trend analysis compares a line item from any subsequent year with that of the base year. Trend analysis answers the question, "What is the percentage change from a base year?" For example: "How much have net patient service revenues increased between 20X4 and 20X0?" The formula for trend analysis is [(Any Subsequent Year – Base Year) / Base Year]. As the name suggests, trend analysis is most useful when data for multiple periods are available. Generally, there are no recognized national benchmarks for either horizontal or trend analysis.

Vertical analysis compares one line item with another line item for the same period. It answers the question, "What percentage of one line item is another line item?" For example: "What percentage of current assets is cash?" or "What percentage of operating revenues are operating expenses?" Vertical analysis is also called common-size analysis because it allows comparison of different-sized organizations by converting all items to percentages. As with horizontal analysis, there are no nationally recognized benchmarks.

Ratio analysis is the preferred approach for a detailed analysis of the financial statements of health care organizations. Ratio analysis asks the question, "What is the ratio of one line item to another?" For example: "How many dollars are there in current assets compared with current liabilities?" Because ratios are not limited to just one financial statement at a time, they may combine and compare items from several different financial statements. The four categories of ratios are liquidity, profitability, activity, and capital structure.

- *Liquidity ratios* answer the question, "How well is an organization positioned to meet its short-term obligations?"

- *Revenue, expense, and profitability ratios* answer the two questions, "How profitable is an organization?" and "How effective is it in controlling its operating costs and increasing its operating revenues?"

- *Activity ratios* answer the question, "How efficiently is an organization using its assets to produce revenues?"

- *Capital structure ratios* answer two questions: "How are an organization's assets financed?" and "How able is this organization to take on new debt?"

Once calculated, these ratios are generally compared with some meaningful benchmark (historical, industry, etc.). Such comparisons yield clues as to how well an entity is functioning and how it might improve its operational performance and financial position. Exhibit 4–16a presents financial ratios for U.S. hospitals overall and by bed-size categories. Exhibit 4–16b presents a summary of key financial ratios and their formulas.

KEY TERMS

a. Financial leverage
b. Horizontal analysis
c. Ratio
d. Trend analysis
e. Vertical analysis

KEY EQUATIONS

See Exhibit 4.16b

Exhibit 4–16a   Financial ratios for all U.S. hospitals by bed size

Ratio	Thomson and CMS Median Ratio[a] Hospital Industry	1–99 Beds	100–249 Beds	250–399 Beds	400 + Beds	Desired Position[b]
Liquidity ratios						
Current ratio	2.02	2.20	1.98	1.96	1.88	Above
Quick ratio	1.65	1.66	1.60	1.65	1.58	Above
Acid test ratio	0.31	0.37	0.28	0.28	0.29	Above
Days in accounts receivable	52	53	52	52	50	Below
Days cash on hand	84	80	90	98	103	Above
Average payment period, days	52	50	52	52	57	Below
Revenue, expense, and profitability ratios						
Operating revenue per adjusted discharge	$7,590	$5,679	$7,609	$9,394	$11,771	Above
Operating expense per adjusted discharge	$7,267	$5,497	$7,324	$8,954	$11,353	Below
Salary and benefit expense as a percentage of operating expense	47%	49%	46%	45%	44%	Below
Operating margin	0.03	0.03	0.03	0.04	0.04	Above
Non-operating revenue	0.05	0.05	0.05	0.06	0.07	Varies
Return on total assets	0.04	0.04	0.04	0.04	0.05	Above
Return on net assets	0.08	0.06	0.08	0.08	0.09	Above
Activity ratios						
Total asset turnover ratio	1.02	1.07	1.06	0.93	0.94	Above
Net fixed assets turnover ratio	2.69	2.80	2.51	2.45	2.49	Above
Age of plant ratio	10.43	10.17	10.26	11.12	11.28	Below
Capital structure ratios						
Long-term debt to net assets ratio	0.38	0.21	0.48	0.56	0.64	Below
Net assets to total assets ratio	0.54	0.54	0.50	0.53	0.50	Above
Times interest earned ratio	3.16	2.73	4.30	5.39	4.31	Above
Debt service coverage ratio	4.55	3.73	4.57	5.23	5.62	Above

[a]These values were obtained from: *The CMS Hospital Cost Report Information System Files* for financial statements ending in 2004 and Thomson Benchmark's 2006 median values. *The Comparative Performance of U.S. Hospitals: The Sourcebook 2007.*

[b]These are true to a certain point. For example, in general the higher the better for the current ratio, but after a certain point, the organization might be better off investing some of the excess cash.

Exhibit 4–16b Formulas for key financial ratios

Liquidity ratios

	Formula
Current ratio	Current Assets / Current Liabilities
Quick ratio	(Cash + Marketable Securities + Net Receivables) / Current Liabilities
Acid test ratio	(Cash + Marketable Securities) / Current Liabilities
Days in accounts receivable	Net Patient Accounts Receivables / (Net Patient Revenues / 365)
Days cash on hand	(Cash + Marketable Securities + Long-term investments) / [(Operating Expenses – Depreciation and Amortization Expenses) / 365]
Average payment period, days	Current Liabilities / [(Operating Expenses – Depreciation and Amortization Expenses) / 365]

Revenue, expense, and profitability ratios

	Formula
Operating revenue per adjusted discharge[a]	Total Operating Revenue / Adjusted Discharges
Operating expense per adjusted discharge[a]	Total Operating Expense / Adjusted Discharges
Salary expense as a percentage of operating expense	Total Salary Expense / Total Operating Expenses
Operating margin	Operating Income / Total Operating Revenues
Non-operating revenue ratio	Non-operating Revenues and Other Income / Total Operating Revenues
Return on total assets[b]	Excess of Revenues Over Expenses / Total Assets
Return on net assets[c]	Excess of Revenues Over Expenses / Net Assets

Activity ratios

	Formula
Total asset turnover ratio	Total Operating Revenues / Total Assets
Net fixed assets turnover ratio	Total Operating Revenues / Net Plant and Equipment
Age of plant ratio	Accumulated Depreciation / Depreciation Expense

Capital structure ratios

	Formula
Long-term debt to net assets ratio[d]	Long-Term Debt / Net Assets
Net assets to total assets ratio[e]	Net Assets / Total Assets
Times interest earned ratio[f]	(Excess of Revenues Over Expenses + Interest Expense) / Interest Expense
Debt service coverage ratio[g]	(Excess of Revenues Over Expenses + Interest Expense + Depreciation and Amortization Expenses) / (Interest Expense + Principal Payments)

[a] Adjusted discharges = (total gross patient revenue / total gross inpatient revenues) x total discharges.
[b] In for-profit health care organizations, calculated as: net income / total assets.
[c] Called the *return on equity* in for-profit health care organizations, and calculated as: net income / owners' equity.
[d] Called *long-term debt to equity* in for-profit health care organizations and calculated as: long-term debt / owners' equity.
[e] Called *equity to total assets* in for-profit health care organizations and calculated as: owners' equity / total assets.
[f] In for-profit health care organizations, calculated as: (net income + interest expense) / interest expense.
[g] In for-profit health care organizations, calculated as: (net income + interest expense + depreciation & amortization expenses) / (interest expense + principal payments).

QUESTIONS AND PROBLEMS

1. **Definitions.** Define the key terms in the list on the previous page.
2. **Horizontal and vertical analyses.** Compare horizontal and vertical analyses, including trend analysis. How are they used?
3. **Vertical analysis.** Explain common-sized analysis.
4. **Ratio analysis.** What is the purpose of ratio analysis? What are the four benchmark categories of ratios?
5. **Medians.** Explain why an industry median may not be an appropriate benchmark with which a particular organization wants to compare itself.
6. **Ratio interpretation.** How do the current, quick, and acid test ratios differ from the average payment period ratio? To what categories do these ratios belong?
7. **Ratio interpretation.** How do capital structure ratios and liquidity ratios differ in providing insight into an organization's ability to pay debt obligations? Identify two situations where an organization might have increasing activity ratios but declining profitability.
8. **Ratio interpretation.** What is the difference between the operating margin ratio and a return on total assets ratio? What is the difference between operating revenue per adjusted discharge ratio and operating expense per adjusted discharge ratio? To what categories of ratios do these belong?
9. **Ratio interpretation.** What capital structure ratio measures the ability to pay debt service payments?
10. **Ratio interpretation.** Discuss the plant and equipment status of a health care provider with an increasing age of plant ratio.
11. **Profitability analysis.** Compare the profitability ratios for Glen Hall Hospital with its industry benchmarks. During this time period, Glen Hall has increased its patient volume, negotiated higher rates for its managed care contracts, and lowered its labor expenses by outsourcing several support services (see Exhibit 4–17).

Exhibit 4–17   Selected ratios for Glen Hall Hospital and the industry benchmarks

Revenue, Expense, and Profitability Ratios	Industry Benchmark	Glen Hall Hospital
Operating revenue per adjusted discharge	$4,900	$5,250
Operating expense per adjusted discharge	$4,833	$4,300
Salary and benefits as a percentage of total operating expense	50%	45%
Operating margin	0.02	0.06
Return on total assets	0.03	0.09
Non-operating revenue ratio	0.04	0.15

12. **Ratio analysis.** Compare the capital structure ratios for Buxton Hospital against industry benchmarks (see Exhibit 4–18). Note that during this time period, Buxton has refinanced its fixed rate debt with lower variable rate debt.

13. **Ratio analysis.** The balance sheet and statement of operations for Dogwood Community Hospital for the years ended 20X0 and 20X1 are shown in Exhibits 4–19a and 4–19b. Compute the following ratios for both years: current, acid test, days in accounts receivable, average payment period, long-term debt to net assets, net assets to total assets, total asset turnover, fixed asset turnover, operating revenue per adjusted

Exhibit 4–18   Selected ratios for Buxton Hospital and the industry benchmarks

Capital Ratios	Industry Benchmark	Buxton Hospital (20X1)	Buxton Hospital (20X0)
Debt service coverage	2.50	3.90	2.90
Times interest earned	2.20	2.90	2.00
Net assets to total assets	0.45	0.60	0.60
Long-term debt to net assets	0.71	0.40	0.40

Exhibit 4–19a   Statement of operations for Dogwood Community Hospital

Dogwood Community Hospital Statement of Operations (in thousands)
for the Years Ended December 31, 20X1 and 20X0

	20X1	20X0
Revenues		
Net patient service revenue	$52,000	$53,000
Other revenue	751	781
Total operating revenues	52,751	53,781
Expenses		
Salaries and benefits	33,000	30,000
Supplies	10,200	10,550
Depreciation	2,900	3,100
Provision for bad debt	5,500	6,200
Total operating expenses	51,600	49,850
Operating income	1,151	3,931
Excess of revenues over expenses	1,151	3,931
Increase (decrease) in net assets	**$1,151**	**$3,931**

Exhibit 4–19b   Balance sheet for Dogwood Community Hospital

Dogwood Community Hospital Balance Sheet (in thousands)
for the Years Ended December 31, 20X1 and 20X0

	20X1	20X0
Current assets		
Cash and cash equivalents	$2,590	$3,150
Net patient receivables	9,600	10,194
Prepaid expenses	1,200	1,300
Total current assets	13,390	14,644
Noncurrent assets		
Plant, property, and equipment		
Gross plant, property, and equipment	22,000	24,000
(less accumulated depreciation)	(1,500)	(1,300)
Net plant, property, and equipment	20,500	22,700
Construction in progress	2,000	3,000
Total assets	**$35,890**	**$40,344**
Current liabilities		
Accounts payable	$4,800	$4,600
Salaries payable	3,200	2,200
Total current liabilities	8,000	6,800
Long-term liabilities		
Bonds payable	17,000	16,000
Total long-term liabilities	17,000	16,000
Net assets	10,890	17,544
Total liabilities and net assets	**$35,890**	**$40,344**

discharge, operating expense per adjusted discharge, salary and benefits as a percentage of total operating expense, return on total assets, and operating margin. After calculating the ratios, comment on Dogwood's liquidity, efficient use of assets or activity ratios, revenue, expense and profitability, and capital structure relative to its industry benchmarks for its respective bed size listed in Exhibit 4–16a. Cite at least two meaningful ratios per category. Assume that Dogwood is a 250-bed facility for the analysis and its adjusted discharges were 6,300 for 20X0 and 6,400 for 20X1.

14. **Ratio analysis.** Exhibits 4–20a and 4–20b show the statement of operations and balance sheet for Maryville Community Hospital for the years ended 20X0 and 20X1.

Exhibit 4–20a Statement of operations for Maryville Community Hospital

**Maryville Community Hospital Statement of Operations (in thousands)
for the Years Ended December 31, 20X1 and 20X0**

	20X1	20X0
Revenues		
Net patient service revenue	$16,000	$18,000
Net assets released from restriction	500	1,000
Total operating revenues	16,500	19,000
Expenses		
Salaries and benefits	12,000	9,000
Supplies and other expenses	5,000	6,000
Depreciation	1,000	1,000
General services	200	100
Total operating expenses	18,200	16,100
Operating income	(1,700)	2,900
Non-operating income	1,000	1,500
Excess of revenues over expenses	(700)	4,400
Increase (decrease) in net assets	($700)	$4,400

Exhibit 4–20b Balance sheet for Maryville Community Hospital

**Maryville Community Hospital Balance Sheet (in thousands)
for the Years Ended December 31, 20X1 and 20X0**

	20X1	20X0
Current assets		
Cash and cash equivalents	$137	$589
Net patient receivables	3,600	2,746
Inventory	850	750
Total current assets	4,587	5,250
Noncurrent assets		
Plant, property, and equipment		
Gross plant, property, and equipment	23,500	22,600
(less accumulated depreciation)	(14,900)	(13,800)
Net plant, property, and equipment	8,600	8,800
Board-designated funds	12,000	16,000
Total assets	$25,187	$30,050
Current liabilities		
Accounts payable	$1,500	$1,400
Accrued expenses	900	750
Total current liabilities	2,400	2,150
Long-term liabilities		
Bonds payable	10,500	7,520
Total long-term liabilities	10,500	7,520
Net assets	12,287	20,380
Total liabilities and net assets	$25,187	$30,050

Compute the following ratios for both years: current, quick, acid tests, days in accounts receivable, days cash on hand, average payment period, operating revenue per adjusted discharge, operating expense per adjusted discharge, salary and benefits as a percentage of total operating expense, operating margin, non-operating revenue, return on total assets and net assets, total asset turnover, fixed asset turnover, age of plant, long-term debt to net assets, and net assets to total assets. Comment on Maryville's liquidity, efficient use of assets, revenue, expense and profitability, and capital structure, citing at least one ratio per category. Use the national hospital industry benchmarks listed in Exhibit 4–16a for 100 beds, and assume that its adjusted discharges were 2,200 for 20X0 and 2,400 for 20X1.

15. **Ratio analysis.** Exhibit 4–21 lists the financial ratios for 227-bed Hollywood Community Hospital. Assess the revenue, expense, profitability, liquidity, activity,

Exhibit 4–21 Selected financial ratios for Hollywood Community Hospital

Ratio	20X1	20X0
Liquidity ratios		
Current ratio	4.05	2.29
Acid test ratio	0.96	0.20
Days in accounts receivable	49	64
Days cash on hand	132	84
Average payment period, days	60	53
Revenue, expense, and profitability ratios		
Operating revenue per adjusted discharge	$8,087	$7,009
Operating expense per adjusted discharge	$6,934	$7,168
Salary and benefit as a percentage of total operating expense	43%	50%
Operating margin	0.05	(0.01)
Non-operating revenue	0.15	0.04
Return on net assets	0.13	0.04
Activity ratios		
Total asset turnover ratio	1.15	0.95
Fixed asset turnover ratio	3.02	2.10
Age of plant	8.49	10.56
Capital structure ratios		
Debt service coverage ratio	4.40	2.47
Long-term debt to net assets (equity)	0.48	3.06
Net assets to total assets	0.55	0.38

and capital structure of Hollywood for 20X1. Explain why these financial measures changed between 20X0 and 20X1.

16. **Ratio analysis.** McGill Healthcare System, an 800-bed institution, is located in a highly competitive, urban market area. Using the financial ratios from Exhibit 4–22 for the current and previous years, evaluate McGill's financial condition, focusing on revenue, expense, profitability, liquidity, activity, and capital structure ratios.

Exhibit 4–22   Selected financial ratios for McGill Healthcare System

Ratio	20X1	20X0
Liquidity ratios		
Current ratio	1.99	1.52
Quick ratio	1.70	0.89
Acid test ratio	0.45	0.30
Days in accounts receivable	70	55
Days cash on hand	140	111
Average payment period, days	66	45
Revenue, expense, and profitability ratios		
Operating revenue per adjusted discharge	$12,232	$11,123
Operating expense per adjusted discharge	$12,697	$10,508
Salary and benefit as a percentage of total operating expense	43%	45%
Operating margin	(0.02)	0.02
Non-operating revenue	0.18	0.10
Return on assets	0.06	0.04
Activity ratios		
Total asset turnover ratio	1.17	1.10
Fixed asset turnover ratio	2.62	2.52
Age of plant	12.75	11.18
Capital structure ratios		
Long-term debt to equity	0.60	0.65
Equity to total assets	0.51	0.43
Debt service coverage ratio	4.70	3.55

17. **Ratio analysis, unknown bed size.** Compare Hope Community Hospital's liquidity, revenue, expense and profitability, activity, and capital structure ratios with its national industry benchmarks using the data from Exhibits 4–16a and 4–23.

Exhibit 4–23   Selected financial ratios for Hope Community Hospital

Ratio	20X1	20X0
Liquidity ratios		
Current ratio	1.78	1.81
Quick ratio	1.29	1.39
Acid test ratio	0.18	0.25
Days in accounts receivable	82	60
Days cash on hand	60	70
Average payment period, days	50	50
Revenue, expense, and profitability ratios		
Operating revenue per adjusted discharge	$7,500	$7,300
Operating expense per adjusted discharge	$6,700	$6,800
Salary and benefit as a percentage of total operating expense	44%	45%
Operating margin	0.04	0.03
Non-operating revenue	(0.01)	0.01
Return on total assets	0.02	0.03
Return on net assets	0.04	0.05
Activity ratios		
Total asset turnover ratio	1.07	0.84
Fixed asset turnover ratio	2.70	1.46
Age of plant	9.26	11.08
Capital structure ratios		
Long-term debt to net assets	0.47	0.95
Net assets to total assets	0.48	0.44
Times interest earned	2.90	3.20
Debt service coverage ratio	3.20	3.70

18. **Ratio analysis, unknown bed size.** In Exhibit 4–24 are the financial ratios for St. Jude Hospital. Compare its liquidity, revenue, expense, profitability, activity, and capital structure ratios against national industry benchmarks for all hospitals.

Exhibit 4–24   Selected financial ratios for St. Jude Hospital

Ratio	20X1	20X0
Liquidity ratios		
Current ratio	1.70	1.85
Acid test ratio	0.15	0.19
Days in accounts receivable	65	53
Days cash on hand	60	75
Average payment period, days	55	50
Revenue, expense, and profitability ratios		
Operating revenue per adjusted discharge	$7,500	$7,200
Operating expense per adjusted discharge	$6,500	$6,700
Salary and benefit as a percentage of total operating expense	44%	47%
Operating margin	0.04	0.03
Return on total assets	0.06	0.05
Activity ratios		
Total asset turnover ratio	1.04	0.99
Fixed asset turnover ratio	2.80	2.10
Age of plant	8.34	10.89
Capital structure ratios		
Long-term debt to equity	0.60	0.35
Equity to total assets	0.45	0.60
Debt service coverage ratio	4.75	4.50

19. **Ratio analysis.** Swayze Community Hospital, a 265-bed facility, is a sole provider hospital in small, rural New England serving a large area. Recently, a wealthy philanthropist made a major contribution to the hospital's long-term investment fund. Assess Swayze's profitability, liquidity, activity, and capital structure ratios. Using the financial ratios from Exhibit 4–25 for the current and previous years, evaluate Swayze's financial condition.

Exhibit 4–25   Selected financial ratios for Swayze Community Hospital

Ratio	20X1	20X0
Liquidity ratios		
Current ratio	3.12	1.95
Quick ratio	2.12	1.45
Acid test ratio	0.89	0.25
Days in accounts receivable	81	50
Days cash on hand	245	48
Average payment period, days	50	56
Profitability ratios		
Operating margin	(0.01)	0.01
Non-operating revenue	0.35	0.05
Return on assets	0.15	0.04
Activity ratios		
Total asset turnover ratio	0.80	0.90
Fixed asset turnover ratio	1.90	2.10
Age of plant	12.92	11.04
Capital structure ratios		
Long-term debt to net assets	0.45	0.60
Net assets to total assets	0.60	0.35
Debt service coverage ratio	4.50	2.25

20. **Ratio analysis.** Avon Community Hospital is a small 95-bed hospital. The hospital just completed a major renovation of its facility, which has helped to attract new physicians and patients to the hospital. Assess Avon's revenue, expense, profitability, liquidity, activity, and capital structure ratios. Using the financial ratios from Exhibit 4–26 for the current and previous years, evaluate Avon's financial condition.

Exhibit 4–26   Selected financial ratios for Avon Community Hospital

Ratio	20X1	20X0
Liquidity ratios		
Current ratio	2.50	1.60
Acid test ratio	0.44	0.20
Days in accounts receivable	53	63
Days cash on hand	90	70
Average payment period, days	55	75
Revenue, expense, and profitability ratios		
Operating revenue per adjusted discharge	$5,114	$4,926
Operating expense per adjusted discharge	$4,885	$5,467
Salary and benefit as a percentage of total operating expense	50%	55%
Operating margin	0.02	(0.01)
Return on assets	0.04	0.03
Activity ratios		
Total asset turnover	1.20	0.95
Fixed asset turnover	2.95	2.20
Age of plant	7.85	11.52
Capital structure ratios		
Long-term debt to equity	1.47	0.51
Equity to total assets	0.30	0.44
Debt service coverage ratio	2.08	3.02

21. **Horizontal, vertical, and ratio analyses.** Exhibits 4–27a and 4–27b show the statement of operations and balance sheet for 270-bed Lake Community Hospital for 20X0 and 20X1. Adjusted discharges for 20X0 and 20X1 are 19,000 and 20,000, respectively

   a. Perform a horizontal analysis on both statements.

   b. Perform a vertical analysis on both statements relative to 20X0.

   c. Compute all the selected ratios listed in Exhibit 4–16a, and compare them with the industry benchmarks.

   Using these financial performance measures, evaluate the financial state of Lake Community. The debt principal payments each year are $5.5 million, whereas adjusted discharges are 19,000 in 20X0 and 20,000 in 20X1.

Exhibit 4–27a   Statement of operations for Lake Community Hospital

Lake Community Hospital Statement of Operations (in thousands)
for the Years Ended December 31, 20X1 and 20X0

	20X1	20X0
Revenues		
Net patient service revenue	$197,000	$184,000
Other operating revenue	6,400	5,700
Total operating revenues	203,400	189,700
Operating expenses		
Salaries and benefits	101,600	93,500
Supplies and other expenses	70,100	61,000
Depreciation	12,000	11,300
Provision for bad debts	9,173	9,167
Interest	1,413	1,433
Total operating expenses	194,286	176,400
Income from operations	9,114	13,300
Non-operating income		
Investment income/contributions	9,500	8,500
Excess of revenues over expenses	18,614	21,800
Net income	**$18,614**	**$21,800**

Exhibit 4–27b   Balance sheet for Lake Community Hospital

Lake Community Hospital Balance Sheet (in thousands) for the Years Ended December 31, 20X1 and 20X0

	20X1	20X0
Current assets		
Cash and cash equivalents	$40,500	$15,500
Net patient accounts receivables	29,500	26,400
Inventories	3,800	4,000
Other current assets	10,500	5,200
Total current assets	84,300	51,100
Plant, property, and equipment		
Gross plant, property, and equipment	115,000	200,500
(less accumulated depreciation)	(65,000)	(107,000)
Net property, plant and equipment	50,000	93,500
Funded depreciation/board-designated funds		
Cash and short-term investments	185,000	110,000
Total assets	**$319,300**	**$254,600**
Current liabilities		
Accounts payable	$9,500	$8,500
Salaries payable	4,500	3,500
Notes payable	4,300	4,500
Total current liabilities	18,300	16,500
Long-term liabilities		
Bonds payable	54,000	27,500
Total long-term liabilities	54,000	27,500
Net assets	247,000	210,600
Total liabilities and net assets	**$319,300**	**$254,600**

22. **Horizontal, vertical, and ratio analyses.** Exhibits 4–28a and 4–28b show the statement of operations and balance sheet for 375-bed Pine Island Regional Medical Center for 20X0 and 20X1.

   a. Perform a horizontal analysis on both statements.

   b. Perform a vertical analysis on both statements relative to 20X0.

   c. Compute all the selected ratios listed in Exhibit 4–16a, and compare them with the benchmark.

   Using these financial performance measures, evaluate the financial state of Pine Island. The debt principal payments each year are $4,500,000, and adjusted discharges are 11,500 for 20X0 and 12,000 for 20X1.

Exhibit 4–28a   Statement of operations for Pine Island Regional Medical Center

Pine Island Regional Medical Center Statement of Operations (in thousands) for the Years Ended December 31, 20X1 and 20X0

	20X1	20X0
Revenues		
Net patient service revenue	$96,500	$85,600
Other operating revenue	2,100	2,300
Total operating revenues	98,600	87,900
Expenses		
Salaries and benefits	42,300	44,300
Supplies and other expenses	34,500	32,300
Depreciation	5,500	4,500
Provision for bad debts	2,500	1,000
Interest	1,200	1,300
Total operating expenses	86,000	83,400
Operating income	12,600	4,500
Non-operating revenue	1,500	2,500
Excess of revenues over expenses	14,100	7,000
Increase (decrease) in net assets	**$14,100**	**$7,000**

Exhibit 4–28b   Balance sheet for Pine Island Regional Medical Center

Pine Island Regional Medical Center Balance Sheet (in thousands) for the Years Ended December 31, 20X1 and 20X0

	20X1	20X0
Current assets		
Cash and cash equivalents	$9,800	$14,300
Net patient receivables	18,919	17,032
Inventory	1,840	1,800
Prepaid expenses	750	800
Total current assets	**31,309**	**33,932**
Plant, property, and equipment		
Gross plant, property, and equipment	72,000	65,000
(less accumulated depreciation)	(37,000)	(32,000)
Net property, plant, and equipment	35,000	33,000
Long-term investments	38,000	32,000
Total assets	**$104,309**	**$98,932**
Current liabilities		
Accounts payable	$6,200	$6,800
Salaries payable	5,400	4,300
Total current liabilities	11,600	11,100
Long-term liabilities		
Bonds payable	55,000	65,000
Total long-term liabilities	55,000	65,000
Net assets	37,709	22,832
Total liabilities and net assets	**$104,309**	**$98,932**

23. **Horizontal, vertical, and ratio analyses.** Exhibits 4–29a and 4.29b show the statement of operations and balance sheet for Rocky Mountain Resort Hospital for 20X1 and 20X0. The debt principal payments each year for Rocky Mountain Resort is $1,300,000, and its adjusted discharges are 6,500 for 20X0 and 5,500 for 20X1.

   a. Perform horizontal and vertical analyses using the statement of operations.

   b. Perform horizontal and vertical analyses using the balance sheet.

   c. Compute all the selected ratios listed in Exhibit 4–16a.

Evaluate the financial state of Rocky Mountain Resort Hospital, a 60-bed facility, using all of the above measures. Make the basis for the vertical analyses the year 20X0.

Exhibit 4–29a   Statement of operations for Rocky Mountain Resort Hospital

Rocky Mountain Resort Hospital Statement of Operations (in thousands) for the Years Ended December 31, 20X1 and 20X0

	20X1	20X0
Revenues		
Net patient service revenue	$23,500	$25,500
Other operating revenue	2,600	2,500
Total operating revenues	26,100	28,000
Expenses		
Salaries and benefits	15,200	14,500
Supplies and other expenses	11,400	10,500
Depreciation	700	700
Provision for bad debts	425	275
Interest	250	375
Total operating expenses	27,975	26,350
Operating income	(1,875)	1,650
Non-operating revenue	2,500	1,200
Excess of revenues over expenses	$625	$2,850

Exhibit 4–29b   Balance sheet for Rocky Mountain Resort Hospital

**Rocky Mountain Resort Hospital Balance Sheet (in thousands)
for the Years Ended December 31, 20X1 and 20X0**

	20X1	20X0
Current assets		
Cash and cash equivalents	$1,500	$2,500
Net patient receivables	5,300	4,500
Inventory	400	350
Prepaid expenses	350	250
Total current assets	7,550	7,600
Plant, property, and equipment		
Gross plant, property, and equipment	16,700	17,400
(less accumulated depreciation)	(15,700)	(15,000)
Net property, plant, and equipment	1,000	2,400
Long-term investments	6,500	8,500
Total assets	**$15,050**	**$18,500**
Current liabilities		
Accounts payable	$4,300	$2,800
Salaries payable	1,000	900
Total current liabilities	5,300	3,700
Long-term liabilities		
Bonds payable	1,200	2,500
Total long-term liabilities	1,200	2,500
Net assets	8,550	12,300
Total liabilities and net assets	**$15,050**	**$18,500**

24. **Horizontal, vertical, and ratio analyses.** Exhibits 4–30a and 4–30b show the balance sheet and income statement for 660-bed Williamson Academic Medical Center for the years 20X0 and 20X1.

   a.   Perform full horizontal and vertical analyses on the balance sheet.

   b.   Perform full horizontal and vertical analyses on the income statement.

c.   Calculate every ratio described in the chapter for both years compared with the benchmark. (*Note:* Assume that principal payments each year are $4,500,000 and that its adjusted discharges are 65,000 for 20X0 and 64,000 for 20X1.)

Discuss Williamson's current financial position and future outlook based on these results. Make the basis for the vertical analyses the year 20X0.

Exhibit 4–30a   Balance sheet for Williamson Academic Medical Center

Williamson Academic Medical Center Balance Sheet (in thousands) for the Years Ended December 31, 20X0 and 20X1

	20X1	20X0
Current assets		
Cash and cash equivalents	$26,300	$23,500
Patient accounts receivables, net	165,000	145,000
Inventories	9,500	12,000
Other current assets	3,000	2,400
Total current assets	203,800	182,900
Plant, property, and equipment		
Gross plant, property, and equipment	640,000	576,000
(less accumulated depreciation)	(254,000)	(226,000)
Net property, plant, and equipment	386,000	350,000
Long-term investments	195,000	175,000
Total assets	**$784,800**	**$707,900**
Current liabilities		
Accounts payable	$87,200	$85,000
Salaries payable	23,000	20,000
Notes payable	3,200	3,000
Other current liabilities	2,100	2,000
Total current liabilities	115,500	110,000
Noncurrent liabilities		
Bonds payable	136,500	141,000
Total noncurrent liabilities	136,500	141,000
Owners' equity	532,800	456,900
Total liabilities and equity	**$784,800**	**$707,900**

Exhibit 4–30b   Income statement for Williamson Academic Medical Center

Williamson Academic Medical Center Income Statement (in thousands)
for the Years Ended December 31, 20X0 and 20X1

	20X1	20X0
Revenues		
Net patient revenues	$745,300	$735,200
Other operating revenues	37,000	35,600
Total operating revenues	782,300	770,800
Expenses		
Salaries and benefits	315,000	325,000
Supply expenses	112,400	105,000
Depreciation	33,000	32,800
Purchased services	88,000	84,000
Provision for bad debt	55,000	45,000
Other expenses	24,500	32,000
Interest	12,700	12,500
Total operating expenses	640,600	636,300
Income from operations	141,700	134,500
Non-operating income		
Investment income and contributions	21,000	19,000
Total income before taxes	162,700	153,500
(less income taxes)	(65,080)	(61,400)
Net income (loss)	**$97,620**	**$92,100**

NOTE

1. In the case of Newport's depreciation and amortization expense account, the hospital did not incur any amortization expense for this time period; therefore, the entire account represents depreciation expense.

5

WORKING CAPITAL MANAGEMENT

LEARNING OBJECTIVES

- Define working capital
- Understand working capital management strategies
- Construct a cash budget
- Understand receivables and payables management

Working Capital
Current assets and
current liabilities.

Net Working Capital
The difference between
current assets and current
liabilities.

Although noncurrent assets provide the capability to provide services, it is the combination of current assets and current liabilities that turns that capability into service. For example, an x-ray machine is useless without an adequate supply of film on hand or cash to pay the radiation technologists. This chapter begins with a discussion of working capital and then focuses on the management of two primary components of working capital in the health care industry: cash and accounts receivable.

The term *working capital* refers to both current assets and current liabilities. A related term, *net working capital*, refers to the *difference* between current assets and current liabilities. That is:

Net working capital = current assets − current liabilities

WORKING CAPITAL CYCLE

In the day-to-day operations of an organization, an ongoing series of cash inflows and outflows pays for day-to-day expenses (such as supplies and salaries). The organization must have sufficient funds available to pay for these items on a timely basis. This is particularly problematic in health care, where it is not unusual for payments to be received more than two months after the patient or third party has been billed for the provided services.

Ideally, a health care organization would earn and receive sufficient funds from providing services to enable it to meet its current obligations with available cash. To do this requires managing the four phases of the working capital cycle (see Exhibit 5–1):

- Obtaining cash
- Turning cash into resources, such as supplies and labor, and paying bills
- Using these resources to provide services
- Billing patients for the services and collecting revenues so that the cycle can be continued.

In regards to cash, managing the working capital cycle involves not only ensuring that total cash inflows cover cash outflows but also managing the timing of these flows. To the extent that payments come due before cash is available, the organization has to obtain cash from sources other than existing revenues, such as from investments or through short-term borrowing. To illustrate, suppose an organization starts the month of September with no working capital (see Exhibit 5–2). During the month, it delivers $20,000 worth of services but must pay $9,000 in staff salaries every fifteen days and $2,000 for supplies every thirty days. Situation No. 1 assumes that the full amount owed is collected during the month but is not received until the end of the month. Situation No. 2 assumes that the organization also collects the full amount owed but in two equal payments of $10,000 each, the first payment arriving after fifteen days and the second payment after thirty days.

Exhibit 5–1 The working capital cycle: the importance of timing in managing working capital

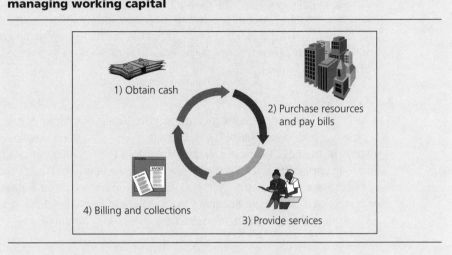

1) Obtain cash

2) Purchase resources and pay bills

3) Provide services

4) Billing and collections

Exhibit 5–2 The effects of timing on working capital needs

	Situation No. 1				Situation No. 2			
	Account	Cash Inflows	Cash Outflows	Balance	Account	Cash Inflows	Cash Outflows	Balance
Day 1				$0				$0
Day 15	Revenues				Revenues	$10,000		
	Salaries		$9,000	($9,000)	Salaries		$9,000	$1,000
Day 30	Revenues	$20,000			Revenues	$10,000		
	Salaries		$9,000		Salaries		$9,000	
	Supplies		$2,000	$0	Supplies		$2,000	$0

In both cases, cash inflows ($20,000) equal cash outflows ($20,000). However, whereas in situation No. 2 there is always sufficient cash on hand to meet the payments when due, in situation No. 1 the organization would not be able to meet its first $9,000 payroll on day 15. To meet this obligation, it either must take cash out of existing reserves or borrow. However, even in situation No. 2, there is little margin for error. How much extra working capital an organization determines it must keep as a cushion is called its *working capital strategy*.

Working Capital Strategy
How much extra working capital an organization determines it must keep as a cushion.

Asset Mix
The amount of working capital an organization keeps on hand relative to its potential working capital obligations.

Financing Mix
How an organization chooses to finance its working capital needs.

Liquidity
A measure of how easily an asset can be converted into cash.

WORKING CAPITAL MANAGEMENT STRATEGIES

Working capital management strategy has two components: asset mix and financing mix. *Asset mix* is the amount of working capital an organization keeps on hand relative to its potential working capital obligations. *Financing mix* refers to how an organization chooses to finance its working capital needs.

Asset Mix Strategy

A health care provider's asset mix strategy falls on a continuum between aggressive and conservative (see Exhibit 5–3). Under an *aggressive approach*, the health care organization attempts to maximize returns by investing excess funds in expectedly higher-earning non-liquid assets such as buildings and equipment; yet, it does so at the risk of lower *liquidity* with increased chances of inventory stock-outs, lost customers from stringent credit policies, and lack of cash to pay employees and suppliers.

 Key point *A health care organization that utilizes an aggressive asset mix strategy seeks to maximize its returns by investing in non-liquid assets but faces the risk of lower liquidity.*

Conversely, under a *conservative approach*, a health care organization seeks to minimize its risk of having insufficient short-term funds by maintaining higher liquidity. However, it does so at the cost of receiving lower returns because short-term investments typically earn a lower return than do long-term investments.

Financing Mix Strategy

Financing mix refers to how the organization chooses to finance its working capital needs. Temporary working capital needs result from short-term fluctuations, whereas permanent working capital needs arise from more ongoing factors, such as a permanent increase in patient volume. Borrowing short-term at lower interest costs for short-term needs under normal conditions leads to a higher profit because working capital is

Exhibit 5–3   Working capital management strategies

	Aggressive Strategy	Conservative Strategy
Goal	Maximize returns	Minimize risk
Liquidity	Low	High
Risk	High	Low
Return	High	Low

otherwise being invested optimally (everything else being equal), but this places the facility at risk because of possible higher debt payments if the need to borrow arises. If the organization has long-term working capital financing needs, it is better off financing those needs with long-term financing under normal conditions. Facilities borrowing long term at higher interest costs to support ongoing working capital needs face lower earnings because they are paying higher interest than with low-cost short-term borrowing. Exhibit 5–4 compares the key characteristics of short-term and long-term borrowing. Overall, an aggressive working capital strategy involves maintaining a relatively low amount of working capital on hand and financing working capital shortfalls with short-term debt. For example, a hospital could follow an aggressive strategy by maintaining less cash and inventory on hand and increasing access to low-interest, short-term debt to cover shortfalls. This aggressive strategy expectedly would generate higher returns for the hospital because it would invest a smaller proportion of its total assets in low-return current assets, and a higher proportion of its debt in low-interest, short-term debt. However, the risk to this greater return is lower liquidity because there would be an increased chance of not having the working capital available to meet short-term financing needs. For instance, hospitals may not have enough cash and inventory on hand to pay any unexpected current obligations that may come due, nor sufficient supplies to support a sudden increase in demand for hospital services. Another risk is that in a tight credit market, the cost to borrow short-term may suddenly rise higher than would be expected, as occurred during the 2008–2009 recession.

In reality, the health care market and the risk tolerance of the health care provider may influence its working capital strategy. A health care provider located in a market with little competition and a high degree of stability for services might consider a more aggressive approach, since it would be better able to forecast its working capital needs, especially in regards to cash and inventory (see Perspectives 5–1 and 5–2). On the other hand, a provider in a competitive, unsettled market with fluctuating demand for services should choose a more conservative approach to working capital management. Unpredictable patient volume makes it difficult to estimate future needs for cash on hand and inventory, and to estimate how much revenue will be tied up in patient

Exhibit 5–4 Comparison of key characteristics of short- and long-term borrowing under normal conditions

	Short-term	Long-term
Interest rate[a]	Lower	Higher
Interest cost	Lower	Higher
Profit	Higher	Lower
Volatility risks	Variable	Fixed

[a]Short-term rates are typically lower than long-term rates.

Perspective 5–1　New Mexico Bank's Loan Gives Boost to Hospital in Rural Oklahoma

Aug. 11: A New Mexico bank's loan has given a rural Oklahoma hospital a financial shot in the arm. Farmers and Stockmans Bank of Clayton loaned Cimarron Memorial Hospital $300,000, to be repaid by a sales tax expected to bring in $22,000 a month, according to the Aug. 4 edition of the *Boise City News*. Rod Burrus, the hospital's administrator, said the loan is a one-shot deal.

Burrus said the loan will give the hospital breathing room to get through the summer when the number of patients declines because people are away and the incidence of illness drops. Many rural hospitals need loans to get through summer months when few patients are hospitalized. Since May 26, when he began, there were "several weeks" with no one in the twenty-bed hospital.

The hospital has no long-term debt but faces a short-term debt of $350,000, he said, confirming the data in the newspaper that reported liabilities of $129,000 to suppliers, $34,000 in back wages, and $135,000 in contingency funds.

"[Employees] have gone with their paychecks being late," he said. "We have gone with employees who have not received their paychecks for sometimes up to a month and a half just to help out this hospital and sustain the hospital."

Source: Schwarz, G. 2004. Bank loan gives boost to hospital, *Amarillo Globe-News Texas-News* (August 11).

accounts receivable. Therefore, a provider may resign itself to having all these current asset accounts being higher than it would like, leaving a smaller proportion of long-term assets to generate the higher rates of return.

 Key point *Three rules to follow under normal conditions to decide between short-term and long-term borrowing to finance working capital needs: (1) finance short-term working capital needs with short-term debt; (2) finance long-term working capital needs with long-term financing; and (3) when an organization has fluctuating needs for working capital, employ a mixed strategy by financing a certain base amount with long-term financing, and as short-term situations arise, finance those with short-term debt.*

CASH MANAGEMENT

In general, the term *cash* refers not only to coin and currency but also to *cash equivalents*, such as interest-bearing savings and checking accounts. There are three major reasons for a health care provider to hold cash:

Perspective 5–2   Accounts Receivable Funding

Accounts receivable funding allows health care providers to obtain cash infusion derived from its accounts receivable to finance its working capital. This form of financing reduces a hospital's dependency on debt-incurring bank loans and lines of credit as their sole forms of financing. It provides a predictable and steady cash stream and the amount of funding.

This cash-flow solution for working capital is not only debt-free, it also grows as patient volume and claims increase, and it boosts liquidity by utilizing currently available assets while maintaining debt capacity. It increases purchasing power and provides working capital needed to meet payroll and overhead, reduce debt, and cut costs by using cash discounts. Health care providers can also use this cash infusion to purchase new equipment, upgrade systems and software, enhance employee development, expand existing facilities, or fund the construction or purchase of a new building.

Sun Capital HealthCare, Inc. (SCH) is a respected leader in this form of financing to each provider's requirements. SCH's funding program can provide cash within twenty-four to forty-eight hours of submission of claims. For example, SCH provided funding to Chino Valley Medical Center in Chino, California, which "maxed out" its bank credit limit and could not secure additional capital to fulfill payroll and operating expenses. According to its financial advisor for the 126-bed hospital, "Sun's initial funding provided debt-free cash to pay off the existing asset-based line of credit, plus additional short-term working capital to keep census going, and support management's ultimate financial strategy to position the hospital for purchase."

Source: Anonymous. 2007 (May). Medical accounts receivable funding propels provider growth and profitability. *Hospitals & Health Networks*, 81(5): 21.

- Daily operations
- Precautionary purposes
- Speculative purposes.

Daily operations refers to holding cash to pay day-to-day bills. *Precautionary purposes* refers to holding cash to meet unexpected demands, such as unforeseen maintenance. *Speculative purposes* refers to holding cash to take advantage of unexpected opportunities, such as buying a competing group practice that has decided to sell.

Key point *There are three major reasons to hold cash: daily operations, precautionary measures, and speculative needs.*

SOURCES OF TEMPORARY CASH

Although it would be favorable to always have excess short-term funds available to invest, health care organizations often find that they need to borrow funds for short periods to meet their maturing obligations. The two primary sources of short-term funds include:

- Bank loans
- Extension of credit from suppliers (i.e., trade payables).

Normal Line of Credit
An agreement established by a bank and a borrower that establishes the maximum amount of funds that could be borrowed, and the bank may loan the funds at its own discretion.

Revolving Line of Credit
An agreement established by the bank and the borrower that legally requires the bank to loan money to the borrower at any time requested up to the pre-negotiated limit.

Bank Loans

There are two major types of *unsecured* (not backed by an asset) short-term loans offered by banks: lines of credit, and transaction notes. The interest expense associated with these alternatives is a function of economic conditions and the credit background of the borrower.

Lines of Credit There are two types of lines of credit: a normal line of credit and a revolving line of credit. A *normal line of credit* is an agreement established by the bank and the borrower that establishes the maximum amount of funds that could be borrowed, but the bank is not legally obligated to fulfill the borrower's credit request. On the other hand, a *revolving line of credit* legally requires the bank to fulfill the borrower's credit request up to a pre-negotiated limit.

 Key point *A revolving line of credit differs from a normal line of credit in that the revolving line of credit legally requires a bank to fulfill the borrower's credit request up to the pre-negotiated limit.*

Commitment Fees In addition to the interest rate on a line of credit, financial institutions are also compensated through either commitment fees, compensating balances, or both. A *commitment fee* is a percentage of the *unused* portion of the credit line that is charged to the potential borrower. The annual fee, often between 0.25 percent and 0.50 percent, is a function of the credit risk of the borrower and the reason for the line of credit. For example, assume a health care organization has a line of credit of $4 million and borrows on average $2.5 million during the year. If the commitment fee rate were 0.25 percent, then the borrower would pay an annual fee of $3,750 [($4 million − $2.5 million) × 0.0025] to have the right to borrow the full $4 million essentially on demand. Sometimes an organization can negotiate with a bank to reduce or eliminate a commitment fee for a line of credit, especially if it has a favorable long-standing history with the lending institution.

Commitment Fee
A percentage of the unused portion of a credit line that is charged to the potential borrower.

Compensating Balance
A designated dollar amount on deposit with a bank that a borrower is required to maintain.

Compensating Balances Under a *compensating balance*, the borrower is required to maintain a designated dollar amount on deposit with the bank. The balance requirement generally is a percentage (perhaps 10 to 20 percent) of the total credit line or a percentage of the unused portion of the credit line. The effect of the compensating balance is to increase the true or *effective interest rate* that the borrower must pay. The effective interest rate is calculated using the following formula:

Effective Interest Rate The true interest rate that a borrower pays.

$$\text{Effective Interest Rate} = \frac{(\text{Interest Expense on Amount Borrowed} + \text{Total Fees})}{(\text{Amount Borrowed} - \text{Compensating Balance})}$$

Assume Community Healthcare Provider borrowed $600,000 during the year on a credit line of $1 million with an interest rate of 9 percent with no fees. Using this formula, the interest expense in the numerator is $54,000 (9 percent × $600,000). The amount borrowed in the denominator is $600,000, and the compensating balance is 10 percent of the unused portion of the line of credit (0.10 × $400,000), or $40,000. Thus, the effective interest rate is 9.64 percent [($54,000 + $0) / ($600,000 − $40,000)].

$$9.64\% = \frac{(\$54,000 + \$0)}{(\$600,000 - \$40,000)}$$

Transaction Notes The second type of bank loan commonly used for short-term borrowing by health care providers is a transaction note. A *transaction note* is a short-term, unsecured loan made for some specific purpose, such as financing inventory purchases. Transaction notes have compensating balance requirements. The borrower obtains the loan by signing a promissory note or IOU. The terms of transaction (maturity and cost) are similar to that for the line of credit.

Transaction Note A short-term unsecured loan made for some specific purpose.

Trade Credit or Payables

Instead of relying solely on an external lending source to obtain cash, an organization can generate cash by controlling its outflow, but the health care organization must have strict cash disbursement policies and procedures in effect. When a health care organization buys on credit, it is in fact using the supplier's money to pay for the purchase up until the time it pays the supplier the amount owed. These credit obligations are called *trade payables* (often referred to as accounts payable). Thus, one of the most important areas to address in cash management is that of either accepting or rejecting discounts offered by suppliers for early payment. These discounts are often stated as:

Trade Credit Short-term credit offered by the supplier of a good or service to the purchaser.

Trade Payables Short-term debt that results from supplies purchased on credit for a given length of time. This allows an organization to use the supplier's money to pay for the purchase up until the time it pays the supplier the amount owed.

2/10 net 30

This means that full payment is due within thirty days ("net 30"), but a 2 percent discount is offered if the payment is made within ten days after the sale ("2/10") (see Exhibit 5–5). Although at first glance it may seem optimal to delay payment for thirty days to retain cash on

Exhibit 5–5 Explanation of commonly used discount terms

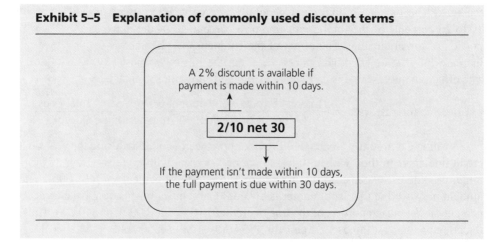

A 2% discount is available if payment is made within 10 days.

2/10 net 30

If the payment isn't made within 10 days, the full payment is due within 30 days.

hand, in fact, depending on the credit terms, it is usually in the best interests of an organization to pay early and take the discount.

To compare the financial implications of taking a discount versus not doing so, assume an organization receives an invoice for $1,000 with terms of 2/10 net 30. If the organization pays within ten days, it receives a 2 percent discount worth $20 (0.02 × $1,000) and therefore only has to pay $980 ($1,000 – $20). If the payment isn't made until thirty days, the health care organization has to pay the full $1,000. Although clearly if the organization takes the discount, it is paying less than it would by holding onto its cash longer, the true cost of paying late may not be so apparent. To understand this involves switching perspectives.

Key point *Depending on a health care organization's credit terms for its trade payables, it is usually in the best interest of an organization to pay early and take the discount.*

Approximate Interest Rate
The annual interest rate incurred by not taking advantage of a supplier's discount offer to pay bills early. The formula in this chapter gives an approximate annual interest rate. A more precise method of calculation can be found in more advanced texts.

A common way to approach this situation would be to think that paying $1,000 by thirty days would be the "normal" management action, and paying $980 early would be the alternative action. From this perspective, the savings from taking the discount is $20 (see Exhibit 5–6). However, a better way to approach this decision would be to consider the discounted price ($980) within ten days as the "real" price, and the full price paid by thirty days ($1,000) as being a penalty price with a supplemental interest charge for not paying within the discount period. In other words, the organization would be paying $20 in interest ($1,000 – $980) to keep the $980 for an extra twenty days (the time between day 10 and day 30).

To determine the *approximate interest rate* the health care organization would pay to keep $980 for an extra 20 days, use the formula given in Exhibit 5–7.

Exhibit 5–6   Two approaches to conceptualize the cost associated with not taking a discount

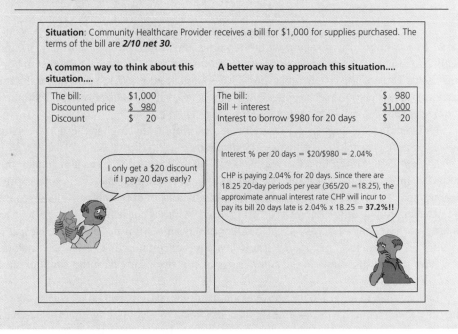

Situation: Community Healthcare Provider receives a bill for $1,000 for supplies purchased. The terms of the bill are **2/10 net 30.**

A common way to think about this situation....

The bill:	$1,000
Discounted price	$ 980
Discount	$ 20

I only get a $20 discount if I pay 20 days early?

A better way to approach this situation....

The bill:	$ 980
Bill + interest	$1,000
Interest to borrow $980 for 20 days	$ 20

Interest % per 20 days = $20/$980 = 2.04%

CHP is paying 2.04% for 20 days. Since there are 18.25 20-day periods per year (365/20 =18.25), the approximate annual interest rate CHP will incur to pay its bill 20 days late is 2.04% x 18.25 = **37.2%!!**

Exhibit 5–7   Calculating the approximate interest rate associated with not taking trade discounts

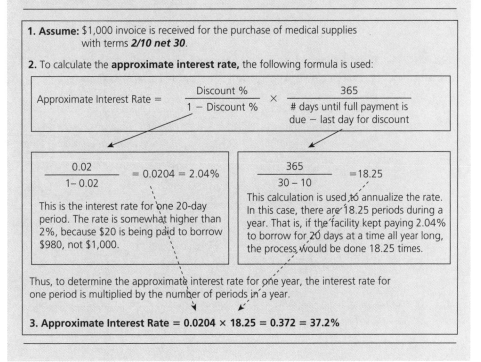

1. Assume: $1,000 invoice is received for the purchase of medical supplies with terms **2/10 net 30**.

2. To calculate the **approximate interest rate,** the following formula is used:

$$\text{Approximate Interest Rate} = \frac{\text{Discount \%}}{1 - \text{Discount \%}} \times \frac{365}{\text{\# days until full payment is due} - \text{last day for discount}}$$

$$\frac{0.02}{1 - 0.02} = 0.0204 = 2.04\%$$

This is the interest rate for one 20-day period. The rate is somewhat higher than 2%, because $20 is being paid to borrow $980, not $1,000.

$$\frac{365}{30 - 10} = 18.25$$

This calculation is used to annualize the rate. In this case, there are 18.25 periods during a year. That is, if the facility kept paying 2.04% to borrow for 20 days at a time all year long, the process would be done 18.25 times.

Thus, to determine the approximate interest rate for one year, the interest rate for one period is multiplied by the number of periods in a year.

3. Approximate Interest Rate = 0.0204 × 18.25 = 0.372 = 37.2%

The calculation shows that the approximate annual interest rate is 37.2 percent. Thus, by not taking the discount within ten days and waiting to pay until day 30, the health care organization is paying the annual equivalent of 37.2 percent interest to borrow $980. Thus, if the organization has the $980, it should take the discount unless it can earn this much by investing the $980 elsewhere, or it should borrow the $980 on a short-term basis if it can do so at a rate less than 37.2 percent.

Incidentally, the higher the discount being offered, the higher the approximate interest rate for not taking (or losing) the discount.

Exhibit 5–8 shows that the approximate interest rate decreases the longer the period of time after the discount date increases until the bill is paid. Therefore, a prudent approach is to pay as late as possible within the discount period or, if the discount is not taken, to pay at the end of the "net" period. Although it is true that the effective interest costs seem to decrease as the number of days the bill is not paid increases, at a certain point after the "net" period, new costs are encountered. These costs include late fees, loss of discounts in the future, loss of priority status with the supplier, and so forth.

Incidentally, in regard to the above example, organizations that do weekly processing may find it virtually impossible to take advantage of a contract with terms such as "2/10 net 30." In such cases, an organization may try to negotiate terms such as "2/15 net 35" to give itself enough time to process the invoice and still meet the early payment deadline.

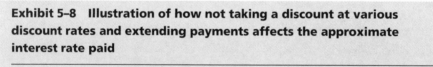

Exhibit 5–8   Illustration of how not taking a discount at various discount rates and extending payments affects the approximate interest rate paid

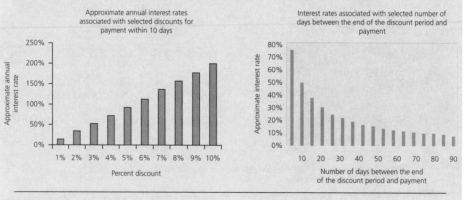

REVENUE CYCLE MANAGEMENT

The success of cash management is driven by the billing process. Ideally, a hospital bill is composed of a list of delivered services; therefore, at discharge, or even at any point during the service delivery process, the patient's bill reflects all services received. However, assembling the final bill can be a problem for many health care organizations, which for some may take weeks. Several hindrances can delay the billing process and collection of cash, for instance:

- Patients who use more than one name or name changes
- Address changes or no address or phone number on file
- Lack of clarity as to who is responsible to pay the bill, or outdated insurance information
- Specific requirements demanded by various insurers, such as retrospective review.

A typical example may be an incoherent patient who is accepted into the emergency department for treatment. In its effort to turn around beds quickly to make room for the next patient, the hospital could discharge the first patient when medically cleared but before complete billing information has been gathered. Or an uninsured patient may intentionally provide an expired insurance card or go under the name of an insured relative or friend to avoid payment. By the time the hospital realizes the problem, the claim has been denied and the patient is unreachable.

As a result, in recent years, health care providers have implemented revenue cycle management techniques developed to help overcome billing-related problems. An essential component of an effective billing process is to have systematic, up-to-date, well-utilized billing policies and procedures in place, with the clear objective of ensuring fair, timely, and accurate invoicing. These management techniques define the goals, roles and responsibilities, and procedures to be used at various stages in the billing process. The revenue cycle includes several key processes, which are presented in Exhibit 5–9 and detailed below.

Scheduling or Preregistration

The normal revenue cycle begins with the patient's phone call to schedule an appointment. The preregistration screening process begins with gathering and verifying demographic and billing-related information before the patient enters the providing organization. Preregistration and admission screenings are important because they help the health care organization determine a patient's ability to pay, including the verification of name, address, employment status, and insurance coverage. Also in this process, the health care organization can make financial arrangements for patients who are unable to pay and can inform patients at the time of registration what they are responsible to pay under their insurance plans.

Exhibit 5–9   The revenue cycle management process

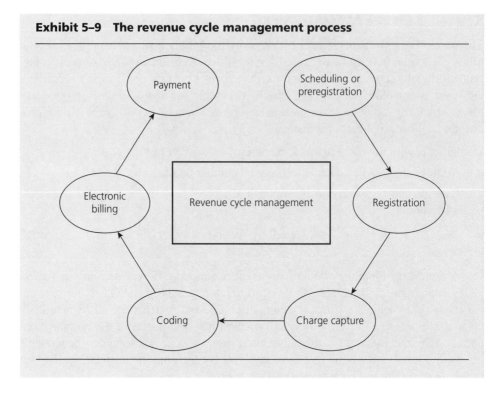

Registration

For patients who did not preregister (for example, an emergency room patient), hospitals need to try to follow the same processes of preregistration activities in terms of insurance verification and ability to pay. Preregistered patients will encounter either a shortened registration process or, for some facilities, bypass the registration process altogether and report directly to the clinical area.

Charge Capture

The integration of a patient's financial and clinical information is critical to the revenue cycle. Correctly identifying the diagnostic and procedural codes when providing patient services is a critical step toward capturing charges and identifying billing items. The health care provider's management information system should allow easy interface among admissions or visits, patient accounts, and medical records in a process that gathers and submits charge data in an accurate and timely manner. The primary objective among these systems is the accurate, timely, and seamless transfer of data and information.

Coding

The primary objective of internal claims processing is to avoid claims denials. This involves the proper conduct of utilization review: preadmission certification and second opinions to verify medical necessity, verification of patient insurance, appropriate record-keeping and patient classification, and the like. An important area to address is improper or incomplete medical record documentation and coding, which can result in delays and lost charges. For instance, failure of the medical staff to assign final diagnoses to the patient's medical record or to sign it can delay the timeliness of the billing submission process and hence the receipt of payment. Similarly, miscoding a diagnosis can also affect the funds the organization receives. Perspective 5–3 lists key reasons behind denied claims. The health care provider bylaws should state the responsibility of physicians to fulfill these obligations.

Electronic Billing

Electronic billing is a process whereby bills are sent electronically to third parties through electronic data interfacing (EDI). This not only accelerates the transmission of bills but also provides an editing function (often called *claims scrubbing*) that reduces the number of processing errors and subsequent audits, ultimately decreasing turn-around time (see Perspective 5–4).

Perspective 5–3 Reasons for Denial of Medical Claims

Relative to the cost to process a clean electronic claim, it costs more to process a paper claim, and even more to process delayed claims on the back end which have been denied. Claims denials also slow reimbursement, which can place stress on an organization's cash flow. (As a way to delay payment, insurers may only provide one denial reason at a time, rather than give all denial reasons at once.) Claims can be denied for a variety of reasons, including:

- Incorrect policy number (name and policy number do not match insurer files)
- Beneficiary is not covered by the insurer (either the insurance coverage has lapsed, or else a dependent is not a covered member on the policy)
- The provided service is deemed not reasonable or medically necessary
- The service provided is not a covered service under the patient's insurance policy
- Duplicate billing
- Unbundled services (trying to bill separately for a procedure which is part of a global payment)
- Procedure code modifier not provided
- Diagnosis code does not match service provided
- Procedure code does not match patient's gender, is inconsistent with the modifier used, or is inconsistent with the place of service
- Diagnosis code is inconsistent with age, gender, procedure, and so forth.

Source: Amy Buttell, *"Taking the Offensive Against CLAIMS DENIALS."* Hospitals & Health Networks, May 2007, Vol. 81, Issue 5, 46–50

Perspective 5–4   Reduce Health Care Costs Through More Efficient Payment Process

One of the recent findings from an E-health study was that the electronic medical claims and payment process could lower health care costs in the United States and benefit patients. Based on a telephone survey that contacted 150 senior managers from U.S. hospitals, health systems, and insurance organizations from January to February 2006, the following results were found:

INDUSTRY COST SAVINGS AND IMPROVED PATIENT CARE

- 50 percent of the hospital executives and 40 percent of the insurance executives indicated that efficiencies in billing and payment processes could save at least $1 million and as much as $10 million a year in expenses related to these processes.
- 75 percent of the responding hospital executives indicated that these cost savings would be passed on directly to patients while 66 percent indicated they would use these funds to pay for care to the uninsured.

BILLING AND PAYMENT PROBLEMS

- 91 percent of hospital executives surveyed indicated they must resubmit claims one or more times before they are paid, while 20 percent indicated they must resubmit claims over six times, and 5 percent of all hospital claims are never paid.
- Insurance executives estimate they need to go back to the health care providers an average of six times for information necessary to pay a claim. Patient ineligibility is the primary reason given by both hospitals (84 percent) and insurance executives (80 percent) for the delay and denial of claims.

POTENTIAL PATIENT BENEFITS

- E-Health study findings also indicate that hospitals can gain the greatest financial benefit from adopting electronic data interchange (EDI) and electronic funds transfer (EFT) standards. For those hospitals that indicated that they have implemented an EDI/EFT system in place:
  - 84 percent found higher cash flow.
  - 80 percent found significant cost savings.
  - 60 percent were able to reduce their bad debt.

Source: Anonymous. 2006 (March). Hospitals would use savings from automation to benefit patient care. *PRNewswire-FirstCall.*

Payment

Payment of the claim, especially if it is paid electronically, can speed up the cash flow payments. Electronic fund transfers directly into designated bank accounts also provide a more secure and reliable process for hospitals to receive their cash. The major obstacle health care providers face is reconciling payments with the electronic remittance advice, which provides details on how the claims were paid by the third-party payer (i.e., insurer), why they were denied, or both.

Key point *To achieve timely collection of billing, health care providers need to assess its management revenue cycle process, which includes the areas of scheduling, preregistration, charge capture, coding, electronic billing, and payment.*

Claims Scrubbing
The process of ensuring that billing claims contain all information required by an insurer before it will submit payment. This includes accurate patient demographics, consistency between coding and diagnoses, and preauthorization verification for the services provided. Good information systems can complete most of this work automatically and electronically.

COLLECTING CASH PAYMENTS

Because health care providers primarily depend on third-party health plans to pay for patient bills, they constantly try to upgrade and improve their revenue cycle management processes to ensure timely and accurate cash collections. However, because more of the payment responsibility is now being shifted to patients through higher deductible health plans, health care providers also need to more proactively implement policies regarding timely receipts for services from the patients. Cash payment should occur at the first encounter with a patient, especially for elective procedures and in cases where insurance coverage cannot be validated. For non-elective procedures and services for non-charity care cases, health care providers should be encouraged to develop cash payment programs at the time of discharge. Accordingly, proper internal controls must be implemented to ensure accurate recording and depositing of cash payments. Finally, providers should utilize banking services to accept online credit card payments over the Internet and debit or credit card accounts for high-deductible health plans. By electronically accepting cash payments, health care providers can avoid the cost of billing and carrying accounts receivable. Health care providers can also employ other techniques to assist in collecting their payments, such as:

- Decentralized collection centers and concentration banking
- Lockboxes
- Wire transfers.

Decentralized Collection Centers and Concentration Banking

Decentralized collection centers and *concentration banking* allow health care providers to establish collection centers so that payors send their payment to a location near themselves (thus reducing mail float, the time spent in the mail before the payment reaches its destination). These collection centers deposit the payments they have received in the provider's local bank. Finally, the funds are transferred to a concentration bank where the health care provider can draw on the cash for payments. This procedure is designed to help a health care provider reduce its mail and processing time, but there is a trade-off between the number of collection centers and the savings they provide versus the costs incurred to maintain accounts at a number of different financial institutions.

Lockboxes

Lockbox
A post office box located near a Federal Reserve Bank or branch that for a fee will pick up and process checks quickly.

Under the *lockbox* form of collection, a payor sends payments to a post office box located near a Federal Reserve Bank or branch. The bank picks up the payments from the box and at various times during the day deposits these funds into the health care provider's account, processes the checks, and sends the facility a list of the payors and payments. Having the bank perform these duties enables the facility to reduce its mail and processing time. The decision to invest in the lockbox approach depends on whether the interest earned from the acceleration of funds exceeds the cost of having a lockbox. Lockboxes usually have a fixed fee and a variable rate based on a per check basis. To offset the costs to establish a lockbox, an organization may be able to save money by freeing up internal staff who perform some of the functions that the bank would be taking over.

Wire Transfers

Wire transfers eliminate mail and transit float. They are generally operated two ways: third parties electronically deposit payments into the health care organization's bank; and banks of multi-provider systems electronically transfer cash from their local branches to the corporate headquarters' bank, from where all payments are disbursed. This minimizes the "excess cash" kept at subsidiaries and maximizes the amount at headquarters, which is responsible to invest all cash. However, this approach can be expensive because banks often charge $2 to $4 per transfer. One large central bank account may draw a better overall return than would several smaller accounts, and there is an increased likelihood that working capital funds would be available as needed, with less need to borrow. Related techniques are zero-balance accounts and sweep accounts, whereby the bank automatically removes any excess cash from subsidiaries and places it in the account of the parent corporation.

Key point *Decentralized collection centers, concentration banking, lockboxes, and wire transfers are methods to reduce collection and transit float.*

INVESTING CASH ON A SHORT-TERM BASIS

After an organization has gone through the effort to collect its cash, it wants to ensure that the money is invested appropriately to generate a favorable return. Myriad short-term investment instruments exist, including treasury bills, certificates of deposit, commercial paper, and money market mutual funds. Some of the key attributes of these short-term investments are summarized in Exhibit 5–10.

Treasury Bills

Treasury bills (T-bills) are financial instruments purchased for a short term. Normally, they have maturities of thirteen, twenty-six, or fifty-two weeks and are sold in units of $10,000, $15,000, $50,000, $100,000, $500,000, and $1 million. Because they are

Exhibit 5–10 Key characteristics of selected short-term investments

Investment	Denominations	Term	Where Purchased	Comments
Treasury bills	$10,000, $15,000, $50,000, $100,000, $500,000, or $1,000,000	Usually 13, 26, or 52 weeks	Banks, government	Most liquid and default free; purchased at a discount and redeemed at face value
Certificates of deposit (CDs)	Large: $100,000 to $1,000,000 + Small: $500 to $10,000	Usually 2 weeks to 18 months	Banks	Higher risk and higher yield than treasury bills; smaller amounts have lower returns than larger amounts
Commercial paper	$100,000+	1 to 270 days	Broker, dealer, or corporation	Higher risk and higher yield than CDs
Money market mutual funds	Varies; typically >$1,000+	Varies (can be bought and sold on the market)	Mutual fund, broker, or bank	Highly liquid; higher risk and higher yield than commercial paper

issued by the government and are part of an active secondary market to buy and sell these securities, they are considered default-free and the most liquid short-term investment available. Instead of earning interest directly, T-bills are purchased at a discount and redeemed at face value when they mature. The discount represents the difference between the purchase price and the face value at time of maturity. Typically, the face value is presented on a $100 maturity value basis. If the discount price is $3, the purchase price is $97. Being virtually risk free and short-term, T-bills offer low rates of return.

Negotiable Certificates of Deposit

Certificates of deposit (CDs) are issued by commercial banks as negotiable, interest-bearing, short-term certificates. In other words, when the deposit matures, the investor receives the interest earned plus the amount deposited. The maturities of CDs usually range from fourteen days to eighteen months. Small-value CDs are normally issued in $500 to $10,000 denominations. Large-value CDs are normally issued in $100,000 to $1 million denominations. Because of their size, large-value CDs earn a higher return than do small-value CDs. Negotiable CDs means the investor may sell the certificate to someone else before maturity. Non-negotiable CDs are offered in smaller denominations. CDs are not as liquid as T-bills and have a higher risk because they are issued by banks rather than the federal government. Because of their risk and illiquidity, investors demand a higher yield or return on CDs than they do on T-bills.

Commercial Paper

Commercial paper is a negotiable promissory note issued at a discount by large corporations (usually publicly traded) that need to raise internal capital. This instrument is issued for maturities of 1 to 270 days through a bank or a dealer that specializes in selling short-term securities. Commercial paper is sold in denominations of $100,000 or more. Because of the possibility of default from a major corporation, this security carries a higher credit risk than do T-bills or CDs and, therefore, requires a higher yield.

Money Market Mutual Funds

These funds, which have a minimum investment of $1,000, represent a pooling of investors' funds for the purchase of a diversified portfolio of short-term financial instruments, such as CDs, T-bills, and commercial paper. This pooling of funds allows small investors, such as rural health care facilities, to earn short-term money market rates on their investments. Furthermore, most money market funds offer an investor a high degree of liquidity by allowing withdrawals by check, telephone, and wire transfer.

 Key point *Some of the primary instruments for health care organizations to invest in on a short-term basis include treasury bills, certificates of deposit, commercial paper, and money market funds.*

FORECASTING CASH SURPLUSES AND DEFICITS: THE CASH BUDGET

To minimize costs and plan ahead to finance deficits and invest excess cash, a health care organization needs to clearly identify the timing of its cash inflows and outflows. The main vehicle to project cash inflows and outflows is a cash budget. Depending on the decision at hand, it may show inflows on a daily, weekly, monthly, quarterly, semi-annual, annual, or multi-year basis. For instance, forecasts about weekly inflows and outflows are not needed for long-range planning, but monthly planning may require forecasting on a weekly or even daily basis. Much of the information about preparing the cash budget comes from the operating and capital budgets (see Chapter Ten on budgeting).

To illustrate cash inflows and outflows, a monthly cash budget for January through March, 20X7, for Community Health Organization (CHO) is illustrated in Exhibit 5–11.

Cash Inflows

Cash inflow estimates are generally derived from patient revenues; other operating revenues; proceeds from borrowing, stock issuances, or both (for investor-owned organizations); and non-operating contributions. To estimate cash receipts from patient revenues for the month, CHO needs to estimate the amount of revenues and when they will be received in cash. Assume that CHO forecasts the following revenues for 20X7 based on 20X6 data:

Actual Patient Revenues, 20X6		Estimated Patient Revenues, 20X7	
October	$400,000	January	$500,000
November	$500,000	February	$600,000
December	$300,000	March	$700,000

From its historical records, CHO estimates that it will collect 50 percent of revenues earned in the month of service, 40 percent the following month, and 10 percent two months after service has been delivered. All other revenues, such as contributions, appropriations, cash from sale of investments and used equipment, and interest income are expected to total $44,000, $55,000, and $52,000 in January, February, and March, respectively.

Based on this information, CHO can calculate cash inflows. For instance, February's cash inflows of $585,000 are composed of 50 percent of February's revenue ($600,000 × 0.50 = $300,000), 40 percent of January's revenue ($500,000 × 0.40 = $200,000), 10 percent of December's revenue ($300,000 × 0.10 = $30,000), plus the other revenues for February ($55,000) given above.

Key point *The cash budget is the major budgetary tool to forecast an organization's cash surplus and deficits over a given period of time.*

Exhibit 5–11 Cash budget for Community Health Organization (CHO) for three months beginning January 20X7

Givens

1 Revenues:

Actual Patient Revenues, 20X6		Estimated Patient Revenues, 20X7	
October	$400,000	January	$500,000
November	$500,000	February	$600,000
December	$300,000	March	$700,000

2 Funds are received as follows: 50 percent within the month of service, 40 percent one month after service, and 10 percent two months after service.

3 "Other revenues" includes interest earned and are forecasted to be $44,000 in January, $55,000 in February, and $52,000 in March.

4 Cash outflows are forecasted to be $350,000, $450,000, $600,000, and $500,000 in January, February, March, and April, respectively.

5 "Cash outflows" are for the current month.

6 The ending cash balance for December was $50,000.

7 CHO desires a required cash balance of 40 percent of the following month's forecasted cash outflows.

CHO Cash Budget for the Quarter Ending March 31, 20X7

	Item	Formula	January	February	March	Total
	Cash inflows					
A	From October	Givens 1, 2	$0	$0	$0	$0
B	From November	Givens 1, 2	50,000	0	0	50,000
C	From December	Givens 1, 2	120,000	30,000	0	150,000
D	From January	Givens 1, 2	250,000	200,000	50,000	500,000
E	From February	Givens 1, 2	0	300,000	240,000	540,000
F	From March	Givens 1, 2	0	0	350,000	350,000
G	Other revenues	Given 3	44,000	55,000	52,000	151,000
H	Net cash inflows	Sum A:G	464,000	585,000	692,000	1,741,000
I	Forecasted cash outflows	Givens 4, 5	350,000	450,000	600,000	1,400,000
J	**Monthly or quarterly net cash flow**	H − I	114,000	135,000	92,000	341,000
K	Beginning balance	a	50,000	180,000	240,000	50,000
L	**Cash before borrowing or investing**	J + K	164,000	315,000	332,000	391,000
M	Required cash balance	b	180,000	240,000	200,000	200,000
N	Surplus (deficit)	L − M	(16,000)	75,000	132,000	191,000
O	Investment of surplus in short-term investments	c	0	(75,000)	(132,000)	(207,000)
P	Short-term borrowing	d	16,000	0	0	16,000
Q	Ending cash balance	M + N + O + P	$180,000	$240,000	$200,000	$200,000

[a] January: Given 6: February/March: Row Q, previous month.

[b] (Givens 4, 7) x (Row I), next month.

[c] (− Row N), but only if there is a surplus.

[d] (− Row N), but only if there is a deficit.

Cash Outflows

Cash outflows are estimated at $350,000, $450,000, $600,000 and $500,000 for January through April, respectively (Exhibit 5–11, Given 4). These outflows include such operating items as salaries and benefits, supplies, interest, capital expenditure outflows for equipment and land, and debt payments.

Ending Cash Balance

By subtracting cash outflows from net cash inflows, CHO can derive its monthly net cash flow. To this amount, it adds the beginning cash balance to calculate the cash available before borrowing or investing. For instance, in January there were net cash inflows of $464,000 and cash outflows of $350,000 that resulted in a $114,000 net cash inflow for the month (Row J). When this is added to the $50,000 available at the beginning of the month (Row K), CHO had $164,000 in cash before borrowing or investing (Row L).

Although this number represents how much cash is available at the end of the month as a result of the normal cash flows during the month plus the beginning balance, many health care organizations are required to end a month (actually, begin the next month) with a certain minimum balance, called a *required cash balance*. If they are below this amount, they must borrow money, and if they are above, they invest the excess. In the case of CHO, the required cash balance is 40 percent of the next month's forecasted cash outflows (Row M, January, and Row I, February: $180,000 / $450,000 = 0.40).

To illustrate this process, CHO had $164,000 in January's cash before borrowing or investing (Row L), but the required cash balance is $180,000 (0.40 × $450,000, February's cash outflows). Therefore, it must borrow $16,000 to make up the difference (Row P). This results in an ending cash balance of $180,000 (Row Q). If there had been a surplus, as in February (Row N), CHO would have invested the excess funds (Row O). Last, note that February's ending cash balance is higher than in January (Row Q), $240,000 versus $180,000. This is because March's projected cash outflows are $600,000, whereas February's projected cash outflows are only $450,000 (Row I), and 40 percent of the next month's projected cash outflows must be available at the end of each current month.

Required Cash Balance The amount of cash an organization must have on hand at the end of the current period to ensure that it has enough cash to cover the expected outflows during the next forecasting period.

ACCOUNTS RECEIVABLE MANAGEMENT

Accounts receivable, most of which comes through third-party payors, constitutes approximately 75 percent of a health care provider's current assets. Unfortunately, having a large dollar amount tied up in accounts receivable means lost returns in other investment opportunities. Because third-party payors are volume purchasers of health care services, health care providers continuously face the problem of trying to externally control the timely payment of accounts. To expedite collections, health care provider management does hold some degree of control with respect to processing payments internally. The earlier discussion introduced several ways to reduce float, including pre-admission and admission screenings, computerized information systems, electronic billing, and billing and collection policies and procedures. These methods also reduce receivables because bringing cash in more quickly reduces the amount outstanding.

Methods to Monitor Accounts Receivable

Because most payments for services come well after the services have been provided, it is imperative that an organization closely monitor its outstanding balances. The tracking of outstanding accounts is often carried out through an analysis similar to that presented in Exhibit 5–12.

Net accounts receivable (row B) presents the total amount of receivables outstanding, both in total and by month. Thus, at the end of the first quarter, there are $6.4 million in receivables outstanding, of which $3.6 million are aged 1–30 days (row B), $2.0 million are aged 31–60 days, and $0.8 million are aged 61–90 days. For simplicity, assume that each month has thirty days and that all accounts are written off as bad debt after ninety days.

Aging Schedule
A table that shows the percentage of receivables outstanding by the month they were incurred. This is oftentimes also called an *age trial balance*, or ATB.

This information leads to an *aging schedule*, as shown in row C. Thus, at the end of the first quarter, of the $6.4 million in receivables outstanding, 56.3 percent was generated in the third and most recent month ($3.6M / $6.4M), 31.3 percent in the second month ($2.0M / $6.4M), and 12.5 percent in the first month ($0.8M / $6.4M). Row D in each quarter shows the revenues recorded during each of the three months of the quarter and for the quarter as a whole. Row E is the average daily patient revenue (monthly revenue / 30 days, and total quarterly revenue / 90 days).

The information combined from rows A, B, and D yields two new measures: days in accounts receivable (row F) and receivables as a percentage of revenue (row G). Days in accounts receivable is calculated by dividing the net accounts receivable (row B) by the average daily patient revenue for the quarter (row E). For the first quarter, the average daily net revenue was $15.0 million / 90 days = $166,667 per day, whereas the net accounts receivable is $6.4 million; therefore, the days in accounts receivable (row F) at the end of the quarter is $6,400,000 / $166,667 = 38.4 days. This same procedure can be applied to each month to show the number of days of outstanding receivables attributable to each month (using the quarter's average daily net revenue as the denominator).

The final item, receivables as a percentage of revenue (row G), is computed by dividing net accounts receivable (row B) for each thirty-day period by that month's net patient revenue (row D). For example, at the end of the first quarter, 60 percent of the third month's revenues ($3.6 / $6.0), 40 percent of the second month's revenues ($2.0 / $5.0), and 20 percent of the first month's revenues ($0.8 / $4.0) are all receivables outstanding (dollar figures expressed in millions). A similar analysis follows throughout for Quarter 2 (rows H through N).

Exhibit 5–12   Key measures to monitor accounts receivable

		Formula	Quarter 1 (in thousands)			
			Mar	Feb	Jan	Total
A	Days old at the end of the quarter[a]	Given	1–30	31–60	61–90	1–90
B	Net accounts receivable	Given	$3,600	$2,000	$800	$6,400
C	Aging schedule	(Row B) (month) / (row B) (total)	56.3%	31.3%	12.5%	
D	Net patient revenues	Given	$6,000	$5,000	$4,000	$15,000
E	Average daily patient revenue	(Row D) / No. of days in period (row A)	$200	$167	$133	$167
F	Days in accounts receivable	B / E				38.4
G	Receivables as a percentage of revenue	B / D	60%	40%	20%	

		Formula	Quarter 2 (in thousands)			
			Jun	May	Apr	Total
H	Days old at the end of the quarter[a]	Given	1–30	31–60	61–90	1–90
I	Net accounts receivable	Given	$6,900	$1,000	$200	$8,100
J	Aging schedule	(Row I) (month) / (row I) (total)	85.2%	12.3%	2.5%	
K	Net patient revenues	Given	$11,500	$2,500	$1,000	$15,000
L	Average daily patient revenue	(Row K) / No. of days in period (row H)	$383	$83	$33	$167
M	Days in accounts receivable	I / L				48.6
N	Receivables as a percentage of revenue	I / K	60%	40%	20%	

[a]For simplicity, each month is assumed to be 30 days.

Receivables as a percentage of revenues is a better measure than days in accounts receivable to judge management's success in collecting revenues. In the example, it may appear as if collections are worsening because days in accounts receivable rose from 38.4 days for the first quarter to 48.6 days for the second quarter. However, receivables as a percentage of revenue shows that collections as a percentage of revenue for each 30-day period remain the same for both quarters: 60 percent, 40 percent, and 20 percent. The reason for the discrepancy is that during the first quarter, a higher percentage of revenues came in the early months than did revenues in the second quarter, when most of the patient revenues occurred in the last month of the quarter. Thus, the reason that the days in accounts receivable went up is not because collection efforts have changed, but rather because the timing of the revenues varied (total revenues are $15,000,000 in each quarter). Because patient revenues are higher in the earlier months of the first quarter, fewer receivables are outstanding later into the quarter. In turn, this outcome reduces the days in accounts receivable to 38.4 days as well as the percentage of older receivables outstanding.

 Key point *A common mistake is to infer that because days in accounts receivable is decreasing, collections are improving. This is not necessarily the case.*

Methods to Finance Accounts Receivable

In addition to trying to improve its cash and receivables collections, an organization has two other options to bring funds in to meet cash needs: selling its accounts receivable, called "factoring," and using receivables as collateral.

 Key point *Factoring and using receivables as collateral are two ways to receive cash advances from outstanding accounts receivable.*

Factoring
Selling accounts receivable at a discount, usually to a financial institution. The latter then assumes the responsibility of trying to collect on the outstanding payment obligations.

Factoring *Factoring* is the selling of accounts receivable, usually to a bank, at a discount. There are two main reasons why a health care organization would decide to factor its accounts: it needs the cash currently tied up in receivables and cannot afford to wait to collect that money from patients and third parties, and it predicts that the benefits of selling the receivables at a discount would outweigh the possible returns it would receive by holding onto the accounts and trying to manage the collections process.

Typical discounts involved in factoring transactions range from 5 to 10 percent. In addition, the financing institution may impose a factoring fee equal to 15 to 20 percent of the value of the receivables. Under this arrangement, the financing institution purchasing the receivables assumes the risk and control over the collection of the receivables from the health care provider. The more risky the collection of the accounts receivable, the higher the discount demanded by the bank and the higher the fees.

It is important to recognize that when a health care organization sells its receivables, another institution takes over the collections process. The potential ill will that may be generated to collect these funds by this other institution should receive serious consideration before factoring is undertaken. By law, Medicaid accounts receivable cannot be factored.

Pledging Receivables as Collateral As noted earlier, health care organizations can negotiate a line of credit with a financial institution to cover temporary cash shortfalls. In such instances, the amount of receivables outstanding can be used as *collateral*. The cost of a line of credit is typically one to two percentage points above the prime rate, unless an organization has an excellent credit history, in which case it can negotiate for the prime rate or even slightly below it.

Collateral
A tangible asset that is pledged as a promise to repay a loan. If the loan is not paid, the lending institution as legal recourse may seize the pledged asset.

METHODS TO MONITOR REVENUE CYCLE PERFORMANCE

Previously mentioned accounts receivable methods are tailored to senior management because they are interested in more highly aggregated numbers. However, personnel involved in the day-to-day operation and evaluation of revenue cycle management, such as the director of patient financial services and service-line managing directors, may have an interest in more detailed measures related to the revenue cycle. Cost to collect is viewed by these managers as a "key" revenue cycle performance indicator because it measures the costs of all the departments involved in managing the revenue cycle processes. The majority of these costs relate to staff (salary, training, and benefits), information technology costs (technology hardware, software, and support), and telecommunications (call center and long distance service). These operating costs are measured as a percentage of the actual cash collected during a given period (monthly, quarterly, or annually).

Exhibit 5–13 lists the key components of the cost to collect in two parts: unadjusted and adjusted. Net patient revenues (row A) present the total amount of net revenues for the year, while revenue collected as cash during the year is presented in row B. Thus, 90 percent ($90M /$100M) of the net patient revenues is collected as cash during the year. This health care provider incurred $3 million (row D) in operating costs to manage the revenue cycle processes; hence, the provider had a cost-to-collect ratio of 3.3 percent ($3M / $90M, row E). For a reference statistic, the hospital industry's cost-to-collect benchmark, provided in row L, is 2 percent. Part of the reason for this provider's higher cost to collect compared with the industry standard may relate to longer duration of a claim. For example, this provider may have a large proportion of claims outstanding for more than one hundred twenty days, which requires a heavier investment of resources to track and collect than do claims outstanding for sixty days. In addition, this provider may have fewer cleaner and more accurate claims that

Exhibit 5–13   Cost-to-collect method to monitor revenue cycle management

	Cost-to-Collect Accounts Receivable: Unadjusted	Formula	(in millions)
A	Net patient revenues	Given	$100
B	Cash collections	Given	$90
C	Cash as a percentage of net patient revenues	B / A	90%
D	Costs incurred in collection	Given	$3
E	Cost to collect ratio	D / B	3.3%
	Cost to collect accounts receivable: Adjusted for human intervention		
F	Cash collections incurring just EDI costs	Given	$45
G	Cash collections incurring human intervention	Given	$45
H	Costs incurred in collection	Given	$3
I	Less EDI costs	Given	($0.3)
J	Revised costs incurred in collection	H – I	$2.7
K	Cost to collect for high-cost claims	J / G	6.0%
L	Health care industry cost-to-collect standard	Given	2.0%

Source: Healthcare Financial Management Association. 2006 (January). *Understanding Your True Cost to Collect*.

consume less resource time to collect. Finally, this provider may need to invest in more up-front resources, both people and technology, to improve its efficiency in the revenue cycle process and lead to more efficient cash collections.

Health care providers should also conduct a more detailed analysis of the cost-to-collect ratio by separating out clean claims or claims collected using only electronic services without human intervention. For example, in the lower half of Exhibit 5–13, row F shows the cash collected from claims needing only EDI, $45M, whereas row G presents the balance of cash collections from row B that involved human intervention as also $45M. The total cost to collect is $3M (row H), but after excluding the EDI costs of $300,000 (row I), the revised cost to collect involving human intervention is $2.7M (row J). The adjusted cost to collect then becomes 6 percent (row K), which is the $2.7M in row J divided by $45M from row G. This presents a much different picture, that of the high cost to collect claims needing human intervention.

The cost to collect should be trended over time as well as compared with an industry benchmark, which is typically around 2 percent to 3 percent. If the cost to collect is rising, potential sources may be: higher staff turnover; higher information technology costs in hardware, software, and personnel; outsourcing costs in billing or collections, or both; or other inefficiencies in the revenue cycle processes. Other key revenue cycle metrics are presented in Perspective 5–5.

Perspective 5–5   Key Revenue Cycle and Accounts Receivable Metrics

Key Revenue Cycle Performance Area	Relevant Metrics
Scheduling / Pre-registration	Physician referral compliance Percentage of pre-registered accounts (inpatient and outpatient)
Registration	Percentage of insurance cards copied and on file Turn-around time until receipt of pre-certification from insurance company Inpatient admissions error rate Outpatient registration error rate Percentage collection of copays Cash receipts as a percentage of net revenues
Charge Capture	Accuracy of recording billable supplies

Coding	Percentage of correct procedure codes
	Percentage of correct diagnostic codes
	Discharged not final billed (DNFB)
	  Accounts awaiting coding
	  Accounts awaiting dictation
	Properly coding Present on Admission (POA) complications
	Case mix index based upon submitted MSDRGs

Electronic Billing	Percentage of claims submitted cleanly Lag days from date of service until posting date
Payment	Average days in accounts receivable Percentage accounts receivable over 90 days Percentage accounts receivable over 120 days Percentage accounts receivable over 6 months (probably uncollectible accounts) Percentage of unpaid accounts Bad debt expense as a percentage of total gross revenues

Source: Jonathan J Clark "Strengthening the revenue cycle: A 4-step method for optimizing payment."*Healthcare Financial Management*; Oct 2008; 62, 10; pg. 44–46

LAWS AND REGULATION FOR BILLING COMPLIANCE

Hospitals and other health care organizations must comply with numerous laws and regulation restrictions that include areas such as patient billing, cost reporting, physician transactions, and occupational health and safety. Given the rise in health care fraud and abuse, federal and state governments have a strong incentive to reduce any abusive practices in patient billing. Likely, the most stringent restrictions are those passed down by the Centers for Medicare and Medicaid Services (CMS) for the billing of Medicare patients. An example of a billing practice likely to be considered fraud by Medicare is unbundling, where a hospital charges for multiple laboratory tests when in reality a single battery of tests was performed. Another example of Medicare fraud is when a health care provider submits claims for medical supplies that were never provided to the patient.

To ensure compliance with laws and regulations, health care providers need to implement and maintain an effective corporate compliance plan. The plan should ensure that corporate policies, practices, and culture promote the understanding and adherence to appropriate legal requirements. This means that health care providers must develop effective programs to detect and prevent violations of the law. Listed below are questions that will help health care providers assess their billing compliance:

- Is there consistency in charging patients the same dollar amount for the same service, regardless of the patient's payor and where the service was rendered?

- Are controls implemented to ensure proper recording and billing of services and supplies?

- Do the medical records document that services billed were indeed provided, deemed medically necessary, and record the results of the tests?

- Is there a practice in place ensuring that adjustments to patient accounts (bad debt, discounts, etc.) are allowed and performed only by designated and responsible individuals?

- Are overpayments received by Medicare and other federal government programs refunded in a timely manner?

- Are policies and procedures developed to collect copayments and deductibles from patients?

- Are the changes in billing codes completed in a timely manner?

- Are charges listed and bundled properly?

Health Insurance Portability and Accountability Act

One of the major compliance regulations that hospitals face is the *Health Insurance Portability and Accountability Act (HIPAA)*. HIPAA provides reform in several areas ranging from portability of health insurance, preventing fraud and abuse, information security, and administrative simplification. HIPAA regulations covering fraudulent activities are enforced under codes of criminal conduct. For example, individuals who

knowingly defraud a health care benefit program by giving false statements or embezzling money can face personal fines, imprisonment, or
both. In addition, organizations must take important measures to ensure
that patient-specific information is kept confidential, especially in the
electronic age, and that organizations can be held accountable if reasonably appropriate measures have not been put into place.

> **Health Insurance Portability and Accountability Act (HIPAA)**
> A public law designed to improve efficiency in health care delivery by standardizing EDI and by protecting the confidentiality and security of health data by setting and enforcing recognized standards.

HIPAA also requires the adoption of industry standards for the electronic transmission of health information. According to the Department
of Health and Human Services (DHHS), at the start of the new millen-
nium there were about four hundred formats in use nationwide for electronic health care claims processing. As a result, health care providers
and health plans are unable to standardize claims processing, which increases the
expense of developing and maintaining software and reduces the overall efficiency
and savings in administrative transactions. Health care providers and health plans will
need to achieve this standardization in the following administrative and financial
health care transactions: health claims and equivalent encounter information, enroll-
ment and disenrollment in a health plan, eligibility for a health plan, health care
payment and remittance advice, health plan premium payments, health claim status,
referral certification and authorization, and coordination of benefits. By meeting the
HIPAA standards in the areas of content and format, health care providers and plans
could save over $3 to $5 billion annually. However, there is a significant investment
cost beforehand to become compliant.

To meet these standards, health care providers need to do the following:

- Train personnel on the standards
- Develop a management team that assesses the impact of these standards across the organization
- Identify and select vendors that support complying software
- Budget for the information system costs to adhere to these standards

Health care providers also face obstacles of state variation in billing codes for
government programs, health plans, and other commercial insurers, as well as local
variation in clinical codes.

SUMMARY

Working capital refers to the current assets
and current liabilities of a health care
organization. Working capital is important
because it turns the capacity of an organization (its long-term assets) into services
and revenues. All health care organizations must have sufficient working capital
available at appropriate times to meet
day-to-day needs.

The management of working capital involves managing the working capital
cycle: (1) obtaining cash, (2) purchasing
resources and paying bills, (3) delivering services, and (4) billing and collecting

for services rendered. There are two components to a working capital management strategy: determining asset mix and financing mix. Asset mix is the amount of working capital the organization keeps on hand relative to its potential working capital obligations, whereas financing mix refers to how the organization chooses to finance its working capital needs. To determine its level of working capital, a health care facility must evaluate the risk-return trade-off between overinvestment or underinvestment in working capital. A conservative approach with a higher investment in working capital increases an organization's liquidity but does so at the expense of lower returns. An aggressive approach with less investment in working capital decreases liquidity but frees funds to invest in higher returning fixed assets. The decision to select either option or some comfortable medium depends on the health care provider's environment, financial condition, and risk tolerance.

A major component of current assets is cash and cash equivalents. There are three reasons to hold cash: daily operations, precautionary reasons, and speculative purposes. The sources of temporary cash are bank loans, trade credit and billing, collections, and disbursement policies and procedures. Types of bank loans include normal and revolving lines of credit and transaction notes. Lines of credit are usually pre-established and allow a health care organization to borrow money in a reasonably expeditious manner. Transaction notes are short-term, unsecured loans made for specific purposes, such as the purchase of supplies. Both of these borrowing methods may involve either a commitment fee or compensating balance.

A second important source of temporary cash is trade credit, which does not actually bring in cash but instead slows its outflow. Although not commonly thought of in this way, it is a loan by a vendor to the health care organization, and vendors often provide discounts for early payment. It is normally beneficial for a health care organization to take the discount. To determine the approximate interest rate, see formula (1) below.

For another formula of the effective interest rate, see formula (2) below.

Because the approximate interest rate declines the longer the payment is delayed, a prudent policy is to make the payment as close to the last day of the discount period as is operationally feasible or, if the discount is not taken, on the last day of the "net" period. Although interest costs decrease as the number of days increases for which the bill is not paid, at a certain point new costs are encountered. These costs include late fees, loss of discounts in the future, loss

$$\text{Approximate Interest Rate} = \text{Discount \% / (1 - Discount \%)} \times (365 / \text{Net Period}) \tag{1}$$

$$\text{Effective Interest Rate} = \frac{(\text{Interest Expense on Amount Borrowed} + \text{Total Fees})}{(\text{Amount Borrowed} - \text{Compensating Balance})} \tag{2}$$

of priority status with this supplier, and so forth.

To enhance the timely and accurate collection of receivables, health care organizations implement sophisticated revenue cycle management techniques. The six key elements of this process are: scheduling or preregistration to gather as much information as possible in preparation for the patient's upcoming visit; registration of the patient on arrival to validate insurance information and review payment policies; systematic charge capture to ensure all services provided and supplies consumed have been recorded; coding audits to reconcile and maximize individual charges with services; electronic billing to submit invoice information in automated, standardized formats; and payment follow-up to track down and recover lost charges. The final step in the process undermines the need to use various methods to monitor revenue cycle management performance, including measurement of days in accounts receivable and calculating cost-to-collect ratios, among others.

There are several well-used techniques to reduce collection float (the time between the issuance of a bill and the monies are available for use) and transit float (the time it takes for a check to clear the banking system). These techniques include using decentralized collection centers, lockboxes, and electronic deposit of funds. The tools to reduce disbursement float include taking suppliers' discounts and using remote disbursement accounts.

A major function of cash management is to ensure that any excess cash is earning a reasonable return at an acceptable level of risk. There are four primary vehicles for short-term investment of cash: treasury bills, certificates of deposit, commercial paper, and money market mutual funds. These financial vehicles may differ in degrees of risk, return, and initial outlay.

A well-managed cash strategy is based on accurate forecasting of cash flow. The principal tool for this is the cash budget. A cash budget should forecast not only cash inflows and outflows, but also when excess cash will become available or when cash deficiencies that necessitate borrowing will occur.

In addition to managing cash, good working capital management involves managing accounts receivable. Most of the methods used to decrease accounts receivable are the same methods discussed under ways to speed up the inflows of cash. Managing receivables is based on good record keeping and periodic review. There are three main tools used to monitor receivables: creating an aging schedule, monitoring days in accounts receivable, and monitoring receivables as a percentage of revenues. Although days in accounts receivable is probably the most used ratio to monitor receivables, it may be overly sensitive to the timing of revenues. Therefore, receivables as a percentage of revenues is used to overcome this problem. Organizations can also improve their bottom line simply by keeping a well-trained staff, implementing good information systems, and maintaining good relations with payors. Finally, health care organizations need to develop a compliance program to ensure that its payroll, billing, and other financial transactions comply with governmental regulations.

KEY TERMS

a. Aging schedule	m. Lockbox
b. Approximate interest rate	n. Net working capital
c. Asset mix	o. Normal line of credit
d. Claims scrubbing	p. Required cash balance
e. Collateral	q. Revenue cycle management
f. Commitment fee	r. Revolving line of credit
g. Compensating balance	s. Trade credit
h. Effective interest rate	t. Trade payables
i. Factoring	u. Transaction note
j. Financing mix	v. Working capital
k. HIPAA	w. Working capital strategy
l. Liquidity	

KEY EQUATIONS

Approximate Interest Rate:

$$\text{Approximate Interest Rate} = \text{Discount \%} / (1 - \text{Discount \%}) \times (365 / \text{Net Period})$$

Effective Interest Rate:

$$\text{Effective Interest Rate} = (\text{Interest Expense on Amount Borrowed} + \text{Total Fees}) / (\text{Amount Borrowed} - \text{Compensating Balance})$$

QUESTIONS AND PROBLEMS

1. **Definitions.** Define the terms listed above.

2. **Working capital.** What is the function of working capital?

3. **Working capital cycle.** In terms of cash flow, what are the stages of the working capital cycle?

4. **Working capital management strategy.** Describe the two components of a working capital management strategy.

5. **Asset mix strategies.** Compare aggressive and conservative asset mix strategies. The comparison should address goals, liquidity, and risk.

6. **Borrowing.** What is the difference between temporary and permanent working capital needs? What is the general rule about when to borrow long term or short term?

7. **Borrowing.** In terms of risk and return (profit), compare the advantages and disadvantages of short- and long-term borrowing to meet working capital needs.

8. **Cash.** State the three reasons why a health care facility holds cash.

9. **Cash.** What are the main sources of temporary cash?

10. **Loans.** What is an unsecured loan?

11. **Loans.** What are the two types of unsecured bank loans? Describe each.

12. **Compensating balance.** Describe how compensating balances affect the "true" rate the borrower pays.

13. **Discounts.** What does "1.5/15 net 25" mean?

14. **Discounts.** What is the formula to determine the approximate annual interest cost for not taking a discount? When should discounts be taken?

15. **Revenue cycle management.** What are the objectives of billing, credit, and collections policies?

16. **Revenue cycle management.** Why is preregistration important within the revenue cycle management process?

17. **Revenue cycle management.** What is the major obstacle that health care providers face in receiving their payments electronically?

18. **Revenue cycle management.** Identify two problems that can delay the billing process.

19. **Billings.** In the hospital's billing process, why is medical records a critical department?

20. **Revenue cycle management.** As more health care costs are shifted to the patient through higher deductible health plans, what policy can a health care provider implement to ensure timely payment for elective surgery procedures?

21. **Lockboxes.** Describe the lockbox technique of collection float.

22. **Revenue cycle management.** What is the critical step toward capturing charges and identifying billing items?

23. **Investments.** Identify the alternatives for investing cash on a short-term basis, and discuss the general characteristics of each.

24. **Accounts receivable.** List three ways to measure accounts receivable performance.

25. **Accounts receivable.** Two methods to monitor accounts receivable are as a percentage of net patient revenues and as days in accounts receivable. What factor can cause the former to be a better measure than the latter with regard to collections activities?

26. **Accounts receivable.** Identify and define two methods to finance accounts receivable.

27. **Trade credit discount.** Compute the annual approximate interest cost of not taking a discount using the following scenarios. What conclusion can be drawn from the calculations?

    a. 1/10 net 20

    b. 1/10 net 30

c. 1/10 net 40

d. 1/10 net 50

e. 1/10 net 60

28. **Trade credit discount.** Compute the annual approximate interest cost of not taking a discount using the following scenarios. What conclusion can be drawn from the calculations?

a. 2/15 net 20

b. 2/15 net 30

c. 2/15 net 40

d. 2/15 net 50

e. 2/15 net 60

29. **Trade credit discount.** Compute the annual approximate interest cost of not taking a discount using the following scenarios. What conclusion can be drawn from the calculations?

a. 1/5 net 30

b. 1/10 net 30

c. 1/15 net 30

d. 1/20 net 30

30. **Trade credit discount.** Compute the annual approximate interest cost of not taking a discount using the following scenarios. What conclusion can be drawn from the calculations?

a. 2/5 net 30

b. 2/10 net 30

c. 2/15 net 30

d. 2/20 net 30

31. **Trade credit discount.** Compute the annual approximate interest cost of not taking a discount using the following scenarios. What conclusion can be drawn from the calculations?

a. 1/10 net 30

b. 2/10 net 30

c. 3/10 net 30

d. 4/10 net 30

32. **Trade credit discount.** Compute the annual approximate interest cost of not taking a discount using the following scenarios. What conclusion can be drawn from the calculations?

    a. 1/15 net 30

    b. 2/15 net 30

    c. 3/15 net 30

    d. 4/15 net 30

33. **Accounts receivable management.** There are two physician groups, Radnor Physician Group and Haverford Physician Group. Both groups have contracts with two major health plans. For Part A use the information below to compute Radnor Physician Group's days in accounts receivable, aging schedule, and accounts receivable as a percentage of net patient revenues for Health Plan A and Health Plan B for Quarter 1, 20X2. Compare the two health plans to determine which plan is a faster payer. (*Note*: For simplicity, assume that each month is thirty days. Dollar figures are expressed in thousands.)

Health Plan A, Quarter 1, 20X2	Quarter	Mar	Feb	Jan
Days outstanding	Total	1–30	31–60	61–90
Net accounts receivable	$2,500	$1,800	$500	$200
Net patient revenue	$7,500	$4,500	$2,500	$500

Health Plan B, Quarter 1, 20X2	Quarter	Mar	Feb	Jan
Days outstanding	Total	1–30	31–60	61–90
Net accounts receivable	$2,500	$1,200	$500	$800
Net patient revenue	$7,500	$3,000	$2,500	$2,000

For Part B use the information below to compute Haverford Physician Group's days in accounts receivable, aging schedule, and accounts receivable as a percentage of net patient revenues for Health Plan A and Health Plan B for Quarter 1, 20X2. Compare the two health plans to determine which plan is a faster payer. (*Note*: For simplicity, assume that each month is thirty days. Dollar figures are expressed in thousands.)

Health Plan A, Quarter 1, 20X2	Quarter	Mar	Feb	Jan
Days outstanding	Total	1–30	31–60	61–90
Net accounts receivable	$9,000	$5,000	$2,500	$1,500
Net patient revenue	$15,000	$9,000	$4,000	$2,000

Health Plan B, Quarter 1, 20X2	Quarter	Mar	Feb	Jan
Days outstanding	Total	1–30	31–60	61–90
Net accounts receivable	$9,000	$7,000	$1,500	$500
Net patient revenue	$15,000	$10,000	$3,000	$2,000

34. **Accounts receivable management.** Given the information below, compute the days in accounts receivable, aging schedule, and accounts receivable as a percentage of net patient revenues for Quarter 1 and Quarter 2, 20X1. Compare the two quarters to determine if the organization's collection procedure is improving. (*Note*: For simplicity, assume that each month is thirty days. Dollar figures are expressed in thousands.)

Quarter 1, 20X1				
Time	Quarter	Sep	Aug	Jul
Days outstanding	Total	1–30	31–60	61–90
Net accounts receivable	$20,000	$6,000	$2,000	$12,000
Net patient revenue	$38,000	$12,000	$6,000	$20,000
Quarter 2, 20X1				
Time	Quarter	Dec	Nov	Oct
Days outstanding	Total	1–30	31–60	61–90
Net accounts receivable	$20,000	$12,000	$2,000	$6,000
Net patient revenue	$38,000	$20,000	$6,000	$12,000

35. **Accounts receivable management.** Given the information below, compute the days in accounts receivable, aging schedule, and accounts receivable as a percentage of net patient revenues for Quarter 1 and Quarter 2, 20X1. Compare the two quarters to determine if the organization's collection procedure is improving. (*Note*: For simplicity, assume that each month is thirty days. Dollar figures are expressed in thousands.)

Quarter 1, 20X1				
Time	Quarter	Sep	Aug	Jul
Days outstanding	Total	1–30	31–60	61–90
Net accounts receivable	$5,000	$400	$1,000	$3,600
Net patient revenue	$15,000	$1,000	$5,000	$9,000
Quarter 2, 20X1				
Time	Quarter	Dec	Nov	Oct
Days outstanding	Total	1–30	31–60	61–90
Net accounts receivable	$5,000	$3,600	$1,000	$400
Net patient revenue	$15,000	$4,000	$5,000	$6,000

36. **Accounts receivable management.** Given the information below, compute the days in accounts receivable, aging schedule, and accounts receivable as a percentage of net patient revenues for Quarter 1 and Quarter 2 of FY 20X2, which runs from October 20X1 through September 20X2. Compare the two quarters to determine if the organization's collection procedure is improving. (*Note*: For simplicity, assume that each month is thirty days. Dollar figures are expressed in thousands.)

Quarter 1, 20X1				
Time	Quarter	Dec	Nov	Oct
Days outstanding	Total	1–30	31–60	61–90
Net accounts receivable	$19,600	$1,600	$4,000	$14,000
Net patient revenue	$60,000	$4,000	$20,000	$36,000

Quarter 2, 20X2

Time	Quarter	Mar	Feb	Jan
	Total	1–30	31–60	61–90
Days outstanding				
Net accounts receivable	$19,600	$14,000	$4,000	$1,600
Net patient revenue	$60,000	$36,000	$20,000	$4,000

37. **Compensating balance.** On January 2, 20X1, City Hospital established a line of credit with First Union National Bank. The terms of the line of credit called for a $400,000 maximum loan with an interest rate of 6 percent. The compensating balance requirement is 5 percent of the total line of credit (with no additional fees charged).

   a. What is the effective interest rate for City Hospital if 50 percent of the total amount were used during the year?

   b. What is the effective interest rate if only 25 percent of the total loan were used during the year?

   c. How would the answer to *a* change if the additional fees were $500?

   d. How would the answer to *b* change if the additional fees were $1,000?

38. **Compensating balance.** Lawrence Hospital wishes to establish a line of credit with a bank. The first bank's terms call for a $600,000 maximum loan with an interest rate of 5 percent and a $2,000 fee. The second bank for the same line of credit charges an interest rate of 6 percent but no fee. The compensating balance requirement is 5 percent of the total line of credit for either bank.

   a. What is the effective interest rate for Lawrence Hospital from the first bank if 50 percent of the total amount were used during the year?

   b. What is the effective interest rate for Lawrence Hospital from the first bank if 25 percent of the total amount were used during the year?

   c. What is the effective interest rate for Lawrence Hospital from the second bank if 50 percent of the total amount were used during the year?

   d. What is the effective interest rate for Lawrence Hospital from the second bank if 25 percent of the total amount were used during the year?

   e. Which bank would be the better choice for Lawrence Hospital?

39. **Cash budget.** Jay Zeeman Clinic provided the financial information in Exhibit 5–14. Prepare a cash budget for the quarter ending March 20X1.

40. **Cash budget.** Iowa Diagnostics Center provided the financial information in Exhibit 5–15. Prepare a cash budget for the quarter ending March 20X1.

41. **Cash budget.** Stacie Zeeman Clinic provided the financial information in Exhibit 5–16. Prepare a cash budget for the quarter ending March 20X1.

42. **Cash budget.** Happy Valley Rehab Facility provided the financial information in Exhibit 5–17. Prepare a cash budget for the quarter ending March 20X1.

Exhibit 5–14 Jay Zeeman Clinic

Givens

Revenues and Expenses

	Patient Revenues, 20X0			Estimated Patient Revenues, 20X1	
Given 1	October	$3,000,000	**Given 2**	January	$3,400,000
	November	$3,200,000		February	$3,600,000
	December	$3,400,000		March	$3,800,000

	Other Revenues, 20X1			Estimated Cash Outflows, 20X1[a]	
Given 3	January	$88,000	**Given 4**	January	$2,000,000
	February	$110,000		February	$2,200,000
	March	$100,000		March	$2,400,000
				April	$2,000,000

	Receipt of Payment for Patient Revenues and Services			Ending Cash Balances	
Given 5	Current month of service	60%	**Given 6**	December 20X0	$800,000
	1st month of prior service	30%		[b]	40%
	2nd month of prior service	10%			
	3rd+ months of prior services	0%			

[a] "Cash outflows" for the current month.

[b] The ending balance for each month as a percentage of the estimated cash outflows for the next month.

Exhibit 5–15   Iowa Diagnostics Center

Givens

Revenues and Expenses

	Patient Revenues, 20X0			Estimated Patient Revenues, 20X1	
Given 1	October	$2,000,000	**Given 2**	January	$2,300,000
	November	$2,200,000		February	$2,350,000
	December	$2,300,000		March	$2,400,000

	Other Revenues, 20X1			Estimated Cash Outflows, 20X1[a]	
Given 3	January	$80,000	**Given 4**	January	$2,250,000
	February	$100,000		February	$2,300,000
	March	$120,000		March	$2,350,000
				April	$2,400,000

	Receipt of Payment for Patient Revenues and Services			Ending Cash Balances	
Given 5	Current month of service	60%	**Given 6**	December 20X0	$700,000
	1st month of prior service	30%		[b]	40%
	2nd month of prior service	10%			
	3rd+ months of prior services	0%			

[a] "Cash outflows" for the current month.

[b] The ending balance for each month as a percentage of the estimated cash outflows for the next month.

Exhibit 5–16   Stacie Zeeman Clinic

Revenues:

Patient Revenues, 20X0	
July	$3,500,000
August	$3,350,000
September	$3,530,000

Patient Revenues, 20X0	
October	$3,420,000
November	$3,210,000
December	$3,800,000

Estimated Patient Revenues, 20X1	
January	$3,600,000
February	$3,350,000
March	$3,220,000

Receipt of Payment for Patient Services / Revenues

Current month of service	45%
1st month of prior service	25%
2nd month of prior service	10%
3–6 months of prior services	5%

Other Revenues, 20X1	
January	$88,000
February	$110,000
March	$115,000

Expenses:[a]

Supplies Purchases 20X0	
October	$800,000
November	$1,000,000
December	$1,600,000

Estimated Supplies Purchases, 20X1	
January	$1,000,000
February	$1,200,000
March	$1,400,000
April	$1,000,000

Other Estimated Expenses, 20X1

	Nursing	Admin.	Other
January	$1,700,000	$70,000	$245,000
February	$1,750,000	$70,000	$335,000
March	$1,700,000	$70,000	$275,000
April	$1,450,000	$70,000	$205,000

Timing of Cash Payment for Supplies Purchases

0%	Month purchased
60%	+1 Month
35%	+2 Months
5%	+3 Months

Ending Cash Balances

December, 20X0	$800,000
[b]	50%

a All estimated expenses are cash outflows for the given month.

b The ending balance for each month as a percentage of the estimated cash outflows for the next month.

Exhibit 5-17 Happy Valley Rehab Facility

Revenues:

Patient Revenues, 20X0		Patient Revenues, 20X0		Estimated Patient Revenues, 20X1	
July	$4,200,000	October	$4,500,000	January	$4,600,000
August	$4,400,000	November	$4,550,000	February	$4,500,000
September	$4,500,000	December	$4,600,000	March	$4,500,000

Receipt of Payment for Patient Services / Revenues

Current month of service	45%
1st month of prior service	25%
2nd month of prior service	10%
3–6 months of prior services	5%

Other Revenues, 20X1

January	$900,000
February	$910,000
March	$950,000

Other Estimated Expenses, 20X1

	Nursing	Admin.	Other
January	$2,000,000	$100,000	$700,000
February	$2,100,000	$100,000	$675,000
March	$2,200,000	$100,000	$650,000
April	$2,300,000	$100,000	$525,000

Expenses:[a]

Estimated Supplies Purchases, 20X1

January	$1,000,000
February	$1,025,000
March	$1,050,000
April	$1,075,000

Supplies Purchases 20X0

October	$900,000
November	$950,000
December	$1,000,000

Ending Cash Balances

December, 20X0	$700,000
[b]	50%

Timing of Cash Payment for Supplies Purchases

	Month purchased
0%	
60%	+1 Month
30%	+2 Months
10%	+3 Months

[a] All estimated expenses are cash outflows for the given month.
[b] The ending balance for each month as a percentage of the estimated cash outflows for the next month.

43. **Cash budget.** How would the cash budget in Problem 41 change if new credit and collection policies were implemented such that collections resulted as follows:

   a. 30%: current month of patient revenues

   b. 20% each: past 1–2 months of patient revenues

   c. 10% each: past 3–4 months of patient revenues

   d. 5% each: past 5–6 months of patient revenues

44. **Cash budget.** How would the cash budget in Problem 42 change if new credit and collection policies were implemented such that collections resulted as follows:

   a. 40%: current month of patient revenues

   b. 15% each: past 1–2 months of patient revenues

   c. 10% each: past 3–4 months of patient revenues

   d. 5% each: past 5–6 months of patient revenues

45. **Discounts.** Stacie Zeeman Clinic in Exhibit 5–16 is going to take better advantage of credit terms offered by suppliers. The clinic has negotiated a 3 percent discount for all supplies purchased beginning in 20X1, if paid in full during the month of service with the following credit terms for supplies listed below. How does this change the answer to Problem 43?

   Timing of payment for 20X0 supply purchases

   55 percent: month purchased

   30 percent: first prior month

   10 percent: second prior month

   5 percent: third prior month

46. **Discounts.** Happy Valley Clinic in Exhibit 5–17 is going to take better advantage of credit terms offered by suppliers. The clinic has negotiated a 3 percent discount for all supplies purchased beginning in 20X1, if paid in full during the month of service with the following credit terms for supplies listed below. How does this change the answer to Problem 44?

   Timing of payment for 20X0 supply purchases

   50 percent: month purchased

   30 percent: first prior month

   15 percent: second prior month

   5 percent: third prior month

47. **Revenue cycle management.** Ridley Hospital generated net patient revenues of $50 million for 20X1, and its cash collections were $35 million. The revenue cycle management costs to collect these revenues were $3 million.

    a. Compute Ridley's cost to collect for the year and provide an assessment of how it compares with the hospital industry benchmark of 3 percent.

    b. Compute Ridley's cost to collect for the year if 55 percent of the cash collections during the year required human intervention and its EDI costs were $200,000. Provide an assessment of how it compares with the hospital industry benchmark of 3 percent.

48. **Revenue cycle management.** Interboro Hospital generated net patient revenues of $125 million for 20X1, and its cash collections were $110 million. The revenue cycle management costs to collect these revenues were $4 million.

    a. Compute Interboro's cost to collect for the year and provide an assessment of how it compares with the hospital industry benchmark of 3 percent.

    b. Compute Interboro's cost to collect for the year if 35 percent of the cash collections during the year required human intervention and its EDI costs were $400,000. Provide an assessment of how it compares with the hospital industry benchmark of 4 percent.

6

THE TIME VALUE OF MONEY

Is it better to receive $10,000 today or at the end of the year? The clear answer is today, for a variety of reasons:

- *Certainty*. A dollar in hand today is certain, whereas a dollar to be received sometime in the future is not.

- *Inflation*. During inflationary periods, a dollar will purchase less in the future than it will today. Thus, because of inflation, the value of the dollar in the future is worth less than it is today.

- *Opportunity cost*. A dollar today can be used or invested elsewhere. The interest forgone by not having the dollar to invest now is an opportunity cost.

Opportunity Cost
Proceeds lost by forgoing other opportunities.

The concept of *interest* determines how much an amount of money invested today will be worth in the future (its *future value*). It can also be used to determine how much a dollar received at some point in the future would be worth today (its *present value*) (see Exhibit 6–1). This chapter focuses on both future and present value, the basics of the *time value of money,* which is essential to making long-term decisions (the focus of Chapter Seven).

FUTURE VALUE OF A DOLLAR INVESTED TODAY

What a dollar invested today will be worth in the future depends on the length of the investment period, the method used to calculate interest, and the interest rate.

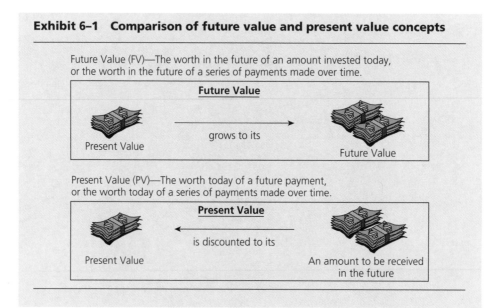

Exhibit 6–1   Comparison of future value and present value concepts

Future Value (FV)—The worth in the future of an amount invested today, or the worth in the future of a series of payments made over time.

Future Value

Present Value — grows to its → Future Value

Present Value (PV)—The worth today of a future payment, or the worth today of a series of payments made over time.

Present Value

Present Value ← is discounted to its — An amount to be received in the future

There are two types of methods to calculate interest: the simple method, and compounding. Under the *simple interest method*, interest is calculated only on the original principal each year. When the *compound interest method* is used, interest is calculated on both the original principal and on any accumulated interest earned up to that point.

Exhibit 6–2, part A uses the simple interest method to calculate how much $10,000 invested today at 10 percent interest would be worth in five years. Because the simple interest method calculates interest on the principal only, each year of investment would earn $1,000 interest (0.10 × $10,000). After five years, the net worth of the investment would be $15,000 ($10,000 plus $5,000 in interest).

Exhibit 6–2, part B uses the same scenario to illustrate the difference of compounded interest. In the first year, there is no difference between using the simple and compound interest methods because no interest has yet been earned. However, in the second and all subsequent years, more interest is earned using the compound interest method because 10 percent is earned on the original $10,000, plus 10 percent on the total amount of interest previously accumulated. Thus, the future value of $10,000 invested at 10 percent interest after five years is $16,105 using compound interest, as compared with $15,000 using simple interest.

Future Value (FV) What an amount invested today (or a series of payments made over time) will be worth at a given time in the future using the compound interest method, which accounts for the time value of money. See also *present value*.

Time Value of Money The concept that a dollar received today is worth more than a dollar received in the future.

Simple Interest Method A method in which interest is calculated only on the original principal. The principal is the amount invested.

Compound Interest Method A method in which interest is calculated on both the original principal and on all interest accumulated since the beginning of the investment time period.

Key point *Simple interest only calculates interest on the original principal, whereas compound interest calculates interest on both the principal and on any accumulated interest. Thus, the value in the future using compound interest will always be higher than that using simple interest, except in the first period.*

Key point *As commonly used, the term* future value *implies using the compound interest method. It is used in this way throughout this text unless noted otherwise.*

The difference between the two methods is considerable and increases with time. After ten years, $10,000 invested at 10 percent simple interest would grow to $20,000; after twenty years it would be worth $30,000; and after fifty years it would grow to $60,000. The comparable numbers for compound interest are $25,937, $67,275, and $1,173,909, respectively. These differences are illustrated in Exhibit 6–3, which compares the constant rate of growth using simple interest with the increasing growth rate using compound interest.

Exhibit 6–2   Investing $10,000 over five years at 10 percent using simple and compound interest

A. The future value of investing $10,000 over five years at 10 percent *simple* interest

A Year (Given)	B Total at Beginning of Year (D, Previous Year)	C Interest Earned ($10,000 × 10%)	D Amount at End of Year[a] (B + C)
1	$10,000	$1,000	$11,000
2	$11,000	$1,000	$12,000
3	$12,000	$1,000	$13,000
4	$13,000	$1,000	$14,000
5	$14,000	$1,000	$15,000
Summary			
Beginning balance	$10,000		
Interest earned		$5,000	
Ending balance			$15,000

B. The future value of investing $10,000 over five years at 10 percent *compound* interest

E Year (Given)	F Total at Beginning of Year (H, Previous Year)	G Interest Earned (F × 10%)	H Amount at End of Year[a] (F + G)
1	$10,000	$1,000	$11,000
2	$11,000	$1,100	$12,100
3	$12,100	$1,210	$13,310
4	$13,310	$1,331	$14,641
5	$14,641	$1,464	$16,105
Summary			
Beginning balance	$10,000		
Interest earned		$6,105	
Ending balance			$16,105

[a] Also called *future value*.

Exhibit 6–3   The future value of $10,000 earning 10 percent using simple and compound interest

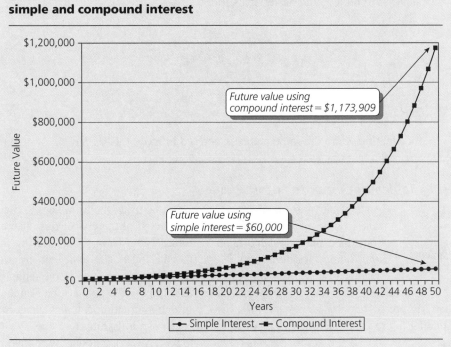

Using a Formula to Calculate Future Value

One approach to calculating future value is to use the formula:

$$FV = PV \times (1 + i)^n$$

where PV is the present value (initial investment amount), i is the interest rate, and n is the number of time periods of the investment. This formula says that an investment's worth in the future, FV, equals the investment's present worth today, PV, multiplied by a factor, $(1 + i)^n$, which takes into account the compounded growth in interest over the lifetime of the investment.

As an example, to calculate the future value of $10,000 in four years at 10 percent interest, the formula would be set up as follows:

$$FV = PV \times (1 + i)^n$$
$$FV = \$10,000 \times (1 + 0.10)^4$$
$$FV = \$10,000 \times (1.4641)$$
$$FV = \$14,641$$

Similarly, to calculate the future value of $10,000 earning 10 percent interest over five years, the formula would be set up as follows:

$$FV = PV \times (1 + i)^n$$
$$FV = \$10,000 \times (1 + 0.10)^5$$
$$FV = \$10,000 \times (1.6105)$$
$$FV = \$16,105$$

Notice that these are the same numbers derived in Exhibit 6–2, part B, for 4 and 5 years, respectively.

Using Tables to Compute Future Value

Future Value Table
Table of factors that shows the future value of a single investment at a given interest rate.

An alternative to calculating the future value using the formula is to use a *future value table*. Table B–1, in Appendix B at the end of this chapter, contains a pre-calculated range of future value factors (FVF) using the future value formula, $(1 + i)^n$. Across the top of the table, the column headings list various interest rates. The leftmost column in the table, or the row headings, provides the number of compounding periods (annual, semi-annual, quarterly, etc.). The intersecting cell for a row-column combination contains the corresponding future value factor (FVF). For example, as shown in Exhibit 6–4, the FVF to invest $10,000 at 10 percent for 5 years (abbreviated as $FVF_{10,5}$), is found by following the 10 percent column down to the fifth row (5 years), to the number 1.6105. This number is then inserted into the following formula to derive the future value:

$$FV = PV \times FVF_{i,n}$$

in a manner similar to the last two steps in the formula approach:

$$FV = \$10,000 \times (1.6105)$$
$$FV = \$16,105$$

 Key point *The future value factor (FVF): $(1 + i)^n$, where i is the interest rate and n is the number of periods.*

 Key point *The formula to find the future value: future value = present value × future value factor. It is abbreviated as*

$$FV = PV \times FVF_{i,n} \text{ or } FV = PV(1 + i)^n$$

Exhibit 6–4   Example of how to find the future value factor at 10 percent interest for 5 years using Table B–1

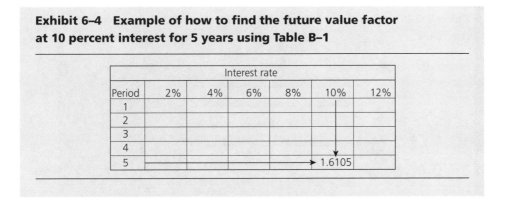

This is the same result calculated earlier by using the formula, $FV = PV \times (1 + i)^n$. Table B–1 can be used to find the FVF for numbers up to 50 percent interest and 50 periods.

Using a Spreadsheet to Calculate Future Value

Most spreadsheets have easy-to-use financial functions that can calculate future value. For example, to calculate the future value of $10,000 at 10 percent interest over five years in Excel, use the FV function in the Financial category. Enter the rate (10%), the number of periods (5), and the present value as a negative number (–10,000) to represent the cash outflow of the investment. The future value, $16,105, is automatically calculated at the bottom (see Exhibit 6–5). Note that the future value is a positive number because it represents a cash inflow of the principal and interest at a later point in time.

PRESENT VALUE OF AN AMOUNT TO BE RECEIVED IN THE FUTURE

The focus until now has been on the future value of money invested today. The example showed that $10,000 invested by a clinic today will be worth $16,105 in five years at 10 percent interest each year. In this section, the question is turned around to become: "How much is $16,105 to be received five years from now worth today?" The value today of a payment (or series of payments) to be received in the future taking into account the cost of capital is the *present value*. Taking future values back to the present is also called "discounting."

Present value = future value $\times$ present value factor

Present Value (PV)
The value today of a payment (or series of payments) to be received in the future, taking into account the cost of capital (sometimes called *discount rate*). It is calculated using the formula:

$$PV = FV \times PVF \text{ or } PV = FV \times [1 / (1 + i)^n]$$

Exhibit 6–5 Using Excel to calculate the future value for a single payment

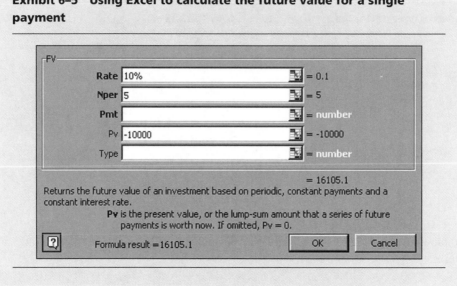

Rate	10%	= 0.1
Nper	5	= 5
Pmt		= number
Pv	-10000	= -10000
Type		= number

= 16105.1

Returns the future value of an investment based on periodic, constant payments and a constant interest rate.

Pv is the present value, or the lump-sum amount that a series of future payments is worth now. If omitted, Pv = 0.

Formula result = 16105.1   OK   Cancel

Using a Formula to Calculate Present Value

Just as the present value is multiplied by a future value factor (FVF) to determine the future value, the future value is multiplied by a present value factor to calculate present value. The present value factor, $1/(1 + i)^n$, is the inverse of the future value factor, $(1 + i)^n$.

Key point *The present value factor is the reciprocal of the future value factor and is calculated using the formula $1/(1 + i)^n$.*

Key point *The formula to find the present value: present value = future value × present value factor. It is abbreviated as: $PV = FV \times PVF_{i,n}$ or $PV = FV \times 1/(1 + i)^n$.*

Thus, using the formula, the present value of $16,105 at 10 percent interest for 5 years can be calculated as follows:

$$PV = FV \times 1/(1 + i)^n$$
$$PV = \$16,105 \times 1/(1 + 0.10)^5$$
$$PV = \$16,105 \times 1/(1.6105)$$
$$PV = \$16,105 \times (0.6209)$$
$$PV = \$10,000$$

The $1/(1.6105)$, which equals 0.6209, is the present value factor. It can be interpreted to mean that at 10 percent interest, a dollar received five years from now is

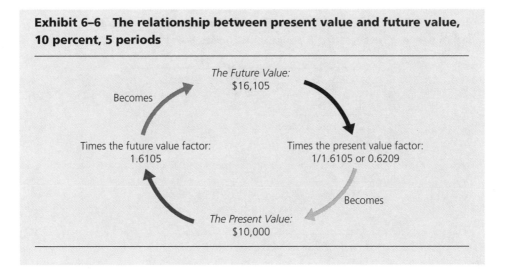

Exhibit 6–6   The relationship between present value and future value, 10 percent, 5 periods

worth only about 62 percent of its value in today's dollars. In the example, $16,105 received five years from now is only worth $10,000 in today's dollars.

Exhibit 6–6 illustrates the relationship between present value and future value. Just as $10,000 today grows to $16,105 over five years at 10 percent compound interest, $16,105 received five years from now is worth $10,000 today, assuming a 10 percent (discount) rate.

Compounding
Converting a present value into its future value taking into account the time value of money. See *compound interest method*. It is the opposite of discounting.

Key point *To find future value*, compound. *To find present value*, discount. *Discounting is the opposite of compounding.* Compound *toward the future*; discount *to the present.*

Discounting
Converting future cash flows into their present value taking into account the time value of money. It is the opposite of compounding.

Using Tables to Compute Present Value

Just as Table B–1 contains a list of pre-calculated future value factors (FVFs) based on the formula $(1 + i)^n$. Table B–3 contains a list of present value factors (PVF) based on the formula $1 / (1 + i)^n$, (Tables B–2 and B–4 will be discussed shortly.) Finding a present value factor (PVF) in Table B–3 is analogous to finding a future value factor (FVF) in Table B–1. The process to locate the present value factor (PVF) for 5 years at 10 percent interest is illustrated in Exhibit 6–7.

This present value factor (PVF) can be used in the formula $PV = FV \times PVF_{i,n}$ to derive the present value of $16,105 at 10 percent interest for five years:

$$PV = FV \times PVF_{10,5}$$
$$PV = \$16,105 \times 0.6209$$
$$PV = \$10,000$$

Exhibit 6–7   Example of how to find the present value factor at 10 percent interest for 5 years using Table B–3[a]

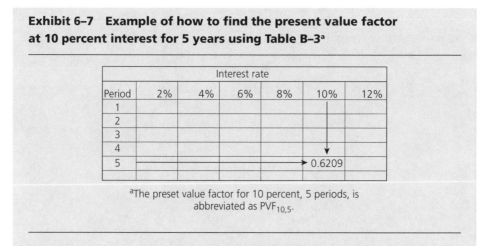

Period	2%	4%	6%	8%	10%	12%
1						
2						
3						
4						
5						0.6209	

[a]The preset value factor for 10 percent, 5 periods, is abbreviated as $PVF_{10,5}$.

Exhibit 6–8   Using Excel to calculate the present value for a single payment

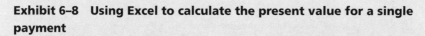

This is the same result derived by using the formula. Table B–3 can also be used to find the PVF for a wide range of numbers up to 50 percent interest and 50 periods.

Using a Spreadsheet to Calculate Present Value

As with future value, most spreadsheets have basic financial functions that can calculate present value. For example, to calculate the present value of $16,105 at 10 percent interest for 5 years in Excel, select the PV function in the Financial category. Enter the rate (10%), the number of periods (5), and the future value as a negative number: −16,105. The present value, 9999.937908 ($10,000), is automatically calculated at the bottom (see Exhibit 6–8).

ANNUITIES

The earlier discussion of present and future values shows how a single amount invested today grows over time and how a single amount to be received in the future is discounted to today's dollars. But sometimes, instead of a single amount, there is a series of payments. This section deals with a particular kind of series of payments called an annuity. An *annuity* is a series of equal payments made or received at equally spaced (regular) time intervals.

Annuity
A series of equal payments made or received at regular time intervals.

Future Value of an Ordinary Annuity

This section shows how to determine what an annuity to be received or invested will be worth at some future date. Suppose a donor were going to give $10,000 per year at the end of each year for the next three years. What would the donation be worth at the end of three years if it earned 10 percent interest each period? Based on the information previously discussed, at the end of three years there would be $33,100, computed as shown in Exhibit 6–9.

Future Value of an Annuity
What an equal series of payments will be worth at some future date using compound interest. See also *future value factor of an annuity* and *present value of an annuity.*

Using Tables to Calculate the Future Value of an Ordinary Annuity
Rather than making three separate calculations (one for each year, as shown), a shortcut is to add the future value factors, which total 3.3100 (1.2100 + 1.1000 + 1.000), then multiply the sum by $10,000. In this case, 3.3100 × $10,000 = $33,100, the same value as seen in Exhibit 6–9. Rather than adding the factors for each of the three years, an alternative approach is to use a *future value factor of an annuity* (FVFA) table, such as Table B–2. Such tables contain the same figures as achieved by adding together the separate future value factors for each year. For example,

Future Value Factor of an Annuity (FVFA)
A factor that when multiplied by a stream of equal payments equals the future value of that stream. See also *present value factor of an annuity.*

Exhibit 6–9   Calculating the future value of $10,000 to be received at the end of each of the next three years assuming 10 percent interest

Year (Given)	A Amount to Be Received at the End of the Year (Given)	B Future Value Formula (Given)	C Future Value Factor (Table B–1)	D Future Value at End of Year 3 (A × C)
1	$10,000	$(1 + i)^2$	1.2100	$12,100
2	$10,000	$(1 + i)^1$	1.1000	$11,000
3	$10,000	$(1 + i)^0$	1.0000	$10,000
Total			3.3100	$33,100

Future Value of an Annuity Table
Table of factors that shows the future value of equal flows at the end of each period, given a particular interest rate.

in Table B–2, the future value factor of an annuity at 10 percent interest for 3 years, $FVFA_{10,3}$, is 3.3100, the same number derived by adding the future value factors for each of the three years in Exhibit 6–9. Thus, whenever a series of equal payments is to be made or received at the end of each period, the *future value of an annuity table* can be used rather than computing the future value of each year's cash flow and adding the results.

Ordinary Annuity
A series of equal annuity payments made or received at the end of each period.

$$FV = \text{Annuity} \times FVFA_{10,3}$$
$$FV = \$10,000 \times 3.3100$$
$$FV = \$33,100$$

Incidentally, a series of payments made or received at the end of each period is called an *ordinary annuity*, whereas a series of payments made or received at the beginning of each period is called an *annuity due* (discussed shortly).

Key point *Whenever a series of payments is to be invested or received at the end of the year, an ordinary annuity table can be used to determine future value, rather than computing the future value of each year's cash flow.*

Using a Spreadsheet to Calculate the Future Value of an Ordinary Annuity Most spreadsheets can easily calculate the future value of an ordinary annuity. For example, in Excel, to calculate the future value of a series of $10,000 payments to be received at the end of each of three years, assuming a 10 percent interest rate, the financial FV function is again used. Enter the rate (10%), the number of periods (3), and the annuity or Pmt input value as a negative number: $-10,000$. The future value automatically appears at the bottom (see Exhibit 6–10).

Future Value of an Annuity Due

Annuity Due
A series of equal annuity payments made or received at the beginning of each period.

The future value of an annuity table, such as Table B–2, is developed for ordinary annuities: cash flows that occur at the end of each period. Sometimes however, a series of cash flows occurs at the beginning of each period, instead of at the end. Such an annuity is called an *annuity due*. The future value factor (FVF) for an annuity due is equal to the factor from the future value of an ordinary annuity table for n + 1 years, less 1.

Suppose a lessee has agreed to pay an organization $10,000 today and at the beginning of each of the next four years, for a total of five $10,000 payments over five years. The organization thinks it can invest this money at 10 percent. To determine the future value of the investment after five years, the organization (1) takes the future value factor for an ordinary annuity in Table B–2 at 10 percent interest for 5 + 1 = 6

Exhibit 6–10   Using Excel to calculate the future value for an ordinary annuity payment

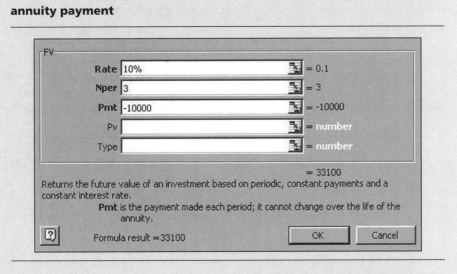

years (7.7156); (2) subtracts 1 from this future value factor (7.7156 − 1 = 6.7156); and (3) multiplies this value by $10,000.

$$\text{FV annuity due} = (\text{FVFA}_{i, n+1} - 1) \times \text{annuity}$$

$$\text{FV annuity due} = (\text{FVFA}_{10.5+1} - 1) \times \$10,000$$

$$\text{FV annuity due} = (7.7156 - 1) \times \$10,000$$

$$\text{FV annuity due} = 6.7156 \times \$10,000$$

$$\text{FV annuity due} = \$67,156$$

This procedure can also be performed on a spreadsheet using the future value function. In Excel, the same function to find an ordinary annuity is used, but a "1" is entered in the space for Type to indicate that this is an annuity due (see Exhibit 6–10).

Present Value of an Ordinary Annuity

As with future value, it is possible to calculate the *present value of an ordinary annuity* or annuity due. Suppose a donor wants to give $10,000 per year at the end of each of the next three years. What is it worth today if the donations can earn 10 percent interest each period? One way to approach this problem would be to calculate the present value of each year's cash flow and then add them, which equals $24,869 (see Exhibit 6–11).

Present Value of an Annuity
What a series of equal payments in the future is worth today taking into account the time value of money.

Exhibit 6–11   Calculating the present value of $10,000 to be received at the end of each year for the next three years assuming 10 percent interest

	A	B	C	D
Year (Given)	Amount to Be Received at the End of the Year (Given)	Present Value Formula (Given)	Present Value Factor (Table B–3)	Present Value at End of Year 0 (A × C)
1	$10,000	$1/(1 + i)^1$	0.9091	$9,091
2	$10,000	$1/(1 + i)^2$	0.8264	$8,264
3	$10,000	$1/(1 + i)^3$	0.7513	$7,513
Total			2.4869	$24,869

Using Tables to Calculate the Present Value of an Ordinary Annuity The same result can be derived by first adding the three present value factors (PVFs) (0.9091 + 0.8264 + 0.7513 = 2.4869) and then multiplying the result by $10,000 (2.4869 × $10,000 = $24,869), as shown in Exhibit 6–11. A shortcut is to use a *present value of an annuity table,* such as Table B–4. Such tables contain the same numbers as would be derived by adding the separate present value factors (PVFs) for each year (differences due to rounding). For example, in Table B–4, the present value factor (PVF) of an annuity (PVFA) for 10 percent interest for 3 years, $PVFA_{10,3}$, is 2.4869.

Present Value of an Ordinary Annuity Table Table of factors that shows the value today of equal flows at the end of each future period, given a particular interest rate.

$$PV = Annuity \times PVFA_{10,3}$$
$$PV = \$10,000 \times 2.4869$$
$$PV = \$24,869$$

 Key point *Whenever a series of payments is to be received at the end of the year, an ordinary annuity table can be used to determine its present value rather than computing the present value of each year's cash flow.*

Each factor in the present value of an annuity table is the sum of each of the present value factors for each year of the annuity. Present value annuity tables are set up as ordinary annuities.

Using a Spreadsheet to Calculate the Present Value of an Ordinary Annuity Most spreadsheets easily calculate the present value of an ordinary annuity (in Excel, the

Exhibit 6–12   Using Excel to calculate the present value for an ordinary annuity payment

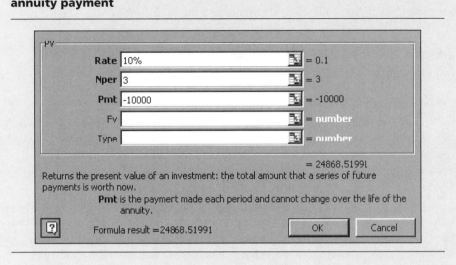

function is called PV). Exhibit 6–12 shows the result of entering the numbers in the appropriate category to calculate the present value of a $10,000 annuity to be received at the end of each of the next three years, assuming 10 percent interest.

Present Value of an Annuity Due

Table B–4, which shows the present value factors (PVFs) for an ordinary annuity (PVFA), can be used to calculate the present value factor for an annuity due (PVFA). This is done by finding the present value factor (PVF) for n–1 years and then adding 1 to this factor.

Suppose a lessee has agreed to pay an organization $10,000 today and at the beginning of each of the next four years, for a total of five $10,000 payments over five years. To find the present value of this series of payments, assuming an interest rate of 10 percent, the organization (1) determines the present value factor (PVF) for an ordinary annuity (PVFA) from Table B–4 at 10 percent interest and $5 - 1 = 4$ years (3.1699); (2) adds 1 to this factor to get the factor for an annuity due (3.1699 + 1 = 4.1699); and (3) multiplies this new factor by $10,000.

$$\text{PV annuity due} = (\text{PVFA}_{i,n-1} + 1) \times \text{annuity}$$
$$\text{PV annuity due} = (\text{PVFA}_{10,5-1} + 1) \times \$10{,}000$$
$$\text{PV annuity due} = (3.1699 + 1) \times \$10{,}000$$
$$\text{PV annuity due} = 4.1699 \times \$10{,}000$$
$$\text{PV annuity due} = \$41{,}699$$

This procedure can also be performed on a spreadsheet using the present value function. In Excel, the function to find an ordinary annuity is used, but a "1" is entered in the space for Type to indicate that this is an annuity due (see Exhibit 6–12).

SPECIAL SITUATIONS TO CALCULATE FUTURE OR PRESENT VALUE AND OTHER EXCEL FUNCTIONS

What if the Interest Rate Is Not Expressed as an Annual Rate?

In the examples presented thus far, the interest rate has been expressed as an annual interest rate, and periods have been expressed in years. However, periods can also refer to other periods of time, such as months or days. If periods of time other than a year are being used, then the interest rate must be expressed for an equivalent period of time. For example, 12 percent annually is 1 percent a month.

Suppose an investment of $10,000 is invested at an interest rate of 12 percent and compounded semi-annually for ten years. Because interest rates are always annual unless stated otherwise, the formula must be adjusted to account for periods other than annual. The future value formula to compound at intervals more frequent than annual is

$$FV = PV \times (1 + i/m)^{n \times m}$$

where i = annual interest rate, m = number of times per year that compounding occurs (e.g., $m = 4$ for quarterly, $m = 12$ for monthly), and n = number of years.
Using the figures in the example:

$$FV = PV \times (1 + i/m)^{n \times m}$$
$$FV = \$10,000 \times (1 + 0.12/2)^{10 \times 2}$$
$$FV = \$10,000 \times (1 + 0.06)^{20}$$
$$FV = \$10,000 \times 3.2071$$
$$FV = \$32,071$$

Note that the final value, $32,071, is higher than it would have been had the same amount been invested and compounded annually rather than semi-annually. For example, had it been compounded annually using the standard formula $FV = PV \times FVF_{12,10}$, the future value factor (FVF) would have been 3.1058, yielding a future value of $31,058 ($10,000 × 3.1058). This discrepancy is not a mistake (see Exhibit 6–13). It happens because compounding in the first instance is occurring twice per year rather than once per year, so interest is growing upon interest more frequently. With quarterly compounding over the same 10-year period (i.e., 3 percent per quarter for 40 quarters),

Exhibit 6–13   Effect of compounding using various compounding periods

Givens	
Initial amount	$10,000
Annualized interest rate	12%
Time horizon, years	10

Compounding Period	Future Value
Annually	$31,058
Semi-annually	$32,071
Quarterly	$32,620
Monthly	$33,004
Daily	$33,195
Continuously	$33,201

the answer would be still higher, and with monthly compounding (i.e., 1 percent per month for 120 months), still higher yet. Although the equation to calculate future value with continuous compounding is beyond the scope of this text, the key point here is that the more frequent the compounding for any given interest level and time period, the higher the future value.

 Key point *The more frequent the compounding for any given interest level and time period, the higher the future value.*

How to Compute Periodic Loan Payments Using Excel

Excel can also calculate periodic loan payments with the Pmt (payment) function. This function can only be used for loans that involve equal periodic payments over the length of the loan. Exhibit 6–14 provides an example of how to compute annual loan payments for a ten-year, $1,000,000 loan that has an interest rate of 10 percent. Note that the present value, $1,000,000 is entered as a negative number to make the final result positive. This final result, $162,745, is interpreted to mean that by paying this annual amount under these conditions, the loan will be completely paid off at the end. This type of analysis is also called a *loan amortization*, which will be discussed in more detail in Chapter Eight.

How to Calculate the Compounded Growth Rate

When examining data, researchers often like to present the compounded growth rate for numerical data, such as revenues, expenses, and earnings. Suppose Memorial

Exhibit 6–14 Using the Excel payment function to compute loan payments

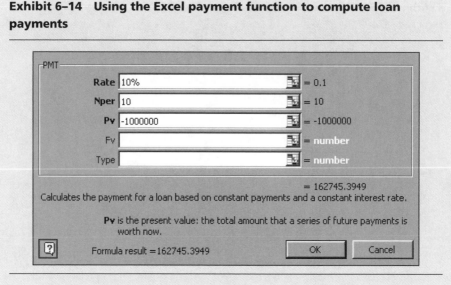

Exhibit 6–15 Patient revenues for Memorial Hospital

Year	Patient Revenues
20X0	$2,123,000
20X1	$2,245,000
20X2	$2,555,000
20X3	$2,700,000
20X4	$2,889,000
20X5	$3,145,000
20X6	$3,496,000
20X7	$3,650,000

Hospital would like to determine the compounded growth rate for patient revenues between 20X0 and 20X7, as shown in Exhibit 6–15.

Solving this problem requires finding the compound growth rate (which is similar to compound interest) that causes 20X0 revenues to have a future value equal to 20X7 revenues (seven time periods into the future). To do this analysis:

■ **Step 1.** Solve for FVF in the equation $FV = PV \times FVF_{i,n}$ where

FV = 20X7 amount ($3,650,000) and PV = 20X0 amount ($2,123,000)

$$FV = PV \times FVF_{i,n}$$

$$\$3,650,000 = \$2,123,000 \times FVF_{i,7}$$

$$\$3,650,000 / \$2,123,000 = FVF_{i,7}$$

$$1.7192 = FVF_{i,7}$$

■ **Step 2.** Using Table B–1, Memorial then compares the calculated FVF, 1.7192, against all FVF factors in the row for 7 time periods to find the factor closest to 1.7192. The appropriate interest rate is the rate given at the top of that column. In this case, 1.7138 comes closest to 1.7192. Therefore, the appropriate interest rate is approximately 8 percent, which also represents the average compound growth rate per year in revenues from 20X0 to 20X7; however, year-to-year changes may be more or less than 8 percent.

How to Calculate the Present Value of Perpetual Annuities

All the annuities in the earlier sections of this chapter were calculated using a finite number of time periods, such as ten years. In some instances, however, an organization needs to make an investment to generate an annuity (cash flow) for an infinite period. Such an annuity is called a *perpetual annuity*, or a *perpetuity*. For example, a donor may bequeath a large sum of money to a hospital under the condition that it generates a specified income every year for Alzheimer's research. Because there is no stipulation as to when this research funding should cease by allowing the funds to become depleted, the hospital would treat the donation as a perpetuity.

The concept of perpetuities and the calculations involved are actually simple. If $1,000,000 were reinvested each year forever at an annual 10 percent interest rate, $100,000 in interest income could be extracted every year ($1,000,000 × 10%) without ever depleting the principal. Every year after withdrawal of the interest income, the investment would still be worth $1,000,000 in real terms. Looked at another way, how much principal would need to be invested at 10 percent to earn $100,000 per year forever? The answer is obviously $1,000,000. This leads to the formula for a perpetuity:

Amount of perpetuity = initial investment × interest rate

Thus, using this formula, to generate a $100,000 perpetuity at a 10 percent interest rate, $100,000 / 0.10, or $1,000,000, would be needed.

Suppose that in her will, a wealthy donor leaves a $2,500,000 donation on her death to her alma mater's university hospital. The funds are to be used solely to buy gifts for pediatric cancer patients and to subsidize hotel costs for visiting parents. The donor's only son died at age eight from leukemia, and she wished to give other children hope and

Perpetuity
An annuity for an infinite period of time. Also called a *perpetual annuity*.

happiness. She stipulates in her will that no less than $150,000 in gift monies be available every year from the donation. It is at the hospital's discretion to decide how to invest the money prudently. What rate of return must the investment generate after the donor's death to ensure that her wishes be granted?

The formula for a perpetuity can be rearranged to solve for rate of return, given the other two factors:

Interest rate = amount of perpetuity / initial investment

Interest rate = $150,000 / $2,500,000

Interest rate = 0.06 = 6%

Therefore, as long as the hospital can invest the $2,500,000 at a minimum 6 percent rate of return, the donor's wishes will be granted indefinitely.

How to Solve for the Interest Rate of a Loan with Fixed Loan Payments

Assuming equal loan payments over the life of the loan, it is also possible to solve for the interest rate. If the present value of the loan, the annuity payments over time, and the length of the loan are given, the unknown interest rate of the loan, i, can be determined.

For example, suppose Mt. Moriah Hospital needs to borrow $10,000 for a new computer system. The annual loan payments are $3,019 per year at the end of each year for the next four years. What is the interest rate of this loan? Using the present value formula for an ordinary annuity, solve for the interest rate, i:

$$PV = \text{annuity} \times PVFA_{i,4}$$
$$\$10,000 = \$3,019 \times PVFA_{i,4}$$
$$\$10,000 / \$3,019 = PVFA_{i,4}$$
$$3.3124 = PVFA_{i,4}$$
$$3.3124 = PVFA_{8,4}$$
$$i = 8\%[1]$$

This could also be done in a spreadsheet, such as by using the Rate function in Excel, as shown in Exhibit 6–16. This is a 4-year, $10,000 loan with equal annual payments of $3,019. This Rate function can be used only for loan payments that are equal over the life of the loan. The loan payment value must be a negative value (cash outflow); otherwise, the rate function will give an incorrect value if both Pmt and PV values are positive.

Exhibit 6–16 Using the Excel rate function to compute a loan rate

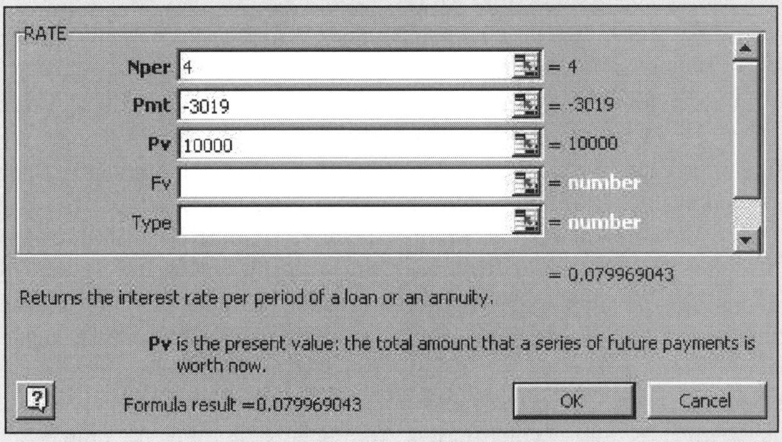

The prior example could also be used to solve for the time period *n*, given an interest rate *i* of 8 percent instead, by going down the 8 percent column in the present value annuity table to the $PVFA_{8\%, n}$ of 3.3124 and going across to the period row of *n* to identify 4 periods or 4 years. The time period could also be derived in a spreadsheet, such as by using the "Nper" function in Excel. This is a 4-year, $10,000 loan with equal annual payments of $3,019. This Nper function can be used only for loan payments that are equal over the life of the loan, and as before, the loan payment value must be a negative value (cash outflow).

Key point *In the Excel Rate and Nper functions, the Pmt box or loan payment box must be a negative value to represent cash outflows.*

SUMMARY

Future value is used to determine the value of dollar payments in the future, whereas present value indicates the current value of future dollars. Either simple interest, where interest is only calculated on the principal, or compound interest, where the interest is calculated on the principal *and* the interest, can be used to determine the future value of money. The compound interest method produces a larger sum of money in the future and is the standard method used.

The FVF, or $(1 + i)^n$, where *i* is the interest rate and *n* is the number of periods of the investment, is part of the formula to determine how much an

Present Value Table
Table of factors that
shows what a single
amount to be received in
the future is worth today
at a given interest rate.

investment will be worth in the future. This entire formula to find future value is: future value = present value × future value factor, abbreviated as FV = PV × FVF$_{i,n}$ *or* FV = PV(1 + i)^n. The opposite formula calculates the present value: present value = future value × present value factor, abbreviated as PV = FV × PVF$_{i,n}$ *or* PV = FV / (1 + i)^n. Similar formulas are used to calculate the present value or future value of an annuity; all that changes is the factor. All these factors can be found in pre-calculated tables, which are known as future value tables and *present value tables*.

If a series of payments is to be paid or received at the end of each period, it is called an *ordinary annuity*. If the series of payments is to be paid or received at the beginning of each period, it is called an *annuity due*. The steps used to calculate each of these two types of annuities are somewhat different. An understanding of present and future values and annuities can be used to answer a number of key questions, such as "How much will an investment today be worth in the future?" or "What is the rate of return for a loan?" Special situations and applications are described in the Appendices, and all calculations can be made either through the use of the accompanying tables or with the aid of a spreadsheet.

KEY TERMS

a. Annuity
b. Annuity due
c. Compound interest method
d. Compounding
e. Discounting
f. Future value
g. Future value factor
h. Future value factor of an annuity
i. Future value of an annuity
j. Future value of an annuity table
k. Future value table
l. Opportunity cost

m. Ordinary annuity
n. Perpetuity
o. Present value
p. Present value factor
q. Present value factor of an annuity
r. Present value of an annuity
s. Present value of an annuity table
t. Present value table
u. Simple interest method
v. Time value of money

KEY EQUATIONS

Future value equation: $FV = PV \times (1 + i)^n$
Future value formula: $FV = PV \times FVF_{i,n}$
Future value formula, annuity due: $FV = \text{annuity} \times (FVFA_{i,n+1} - 1)$
Future value formula, ordinary annuity: $FV = \text{annuity} \times FVFA_{i,n}$
Future value formula, period < 1 year: $FV = PV \times (1 + i/m)^{n \times m}$

Perpetuity formula: Amount of perpetuity $=$ initial investment $\times$ interest rate

Present value equation: $PV = FV \times 1 / (1 + i)^n$

Present value formula: $PV = FV \times PVF_{i,n}$

Present value formula, annuity due: $PV = \text{annuity} \times (PVFA_{i,n-1} + 1)$

Present value formula, ordinary annuity: $PV = \text{annuity} \times PVFA_{i,n}$

QUESTIONS AND PROBLEMS

1. **Definitions.** Define the terms listed on the previous page.

2. **Simple and compound interest.** What is the difference between simple interest and compound interest?

3. **Defining future value equation terms.** Write out the equation to find the future value of a single amount, and define each of the terms in it.

4. **Defining the exponent.** Does the n in the formula $(1 + i)^n$ always mean compounding on an annual basis?

5. **Multiple compounding periods in a year.** How should the future value equation be modified if compounding occurs more frequently than annually?

6. **Multiple compounding periods in a year (continued).** What is the future value of $10,000 with an interest rate of 16 percent and one annual period of compounding? With an annual interest rate of 16 percent and two semi-annual periods of compounding? With an annual interest rate of 16 percent and four quarterly periods of compounding?

7. **Multiple compounding periods in a year (continued).** Based on the answer to Question 6, explain why the investment increases in value when the number of compounding periods increases.

8. **Present and future value factors.** What is the relationship between the present value factor and the future value factor?

9. **Present value factor and discount rate.** What happens to the present value factor as the discount rate or interest rate increases for a given time period? If the discount rate or interest rate decreases?

10. **Relationship between ordinary annuity and annuity due.** Compare the results of the present value of a $6,000 ordinary annuity at 10 percent interest for ten years with the present value of a $6,000 annuity due at 10 percent interest for eleven years. Explain the difference.

11. **Perpetuities.** How many years in a typical perpetuity?

12. **Factors.** What is the relationship between the future value factor for five years at 5 percent and the present value factor for five years at 5 percent?

13. **Future value of an annuity table.** In the future value annuity table at any interest rate for one year, why is the future value interest factor of this annuity equal to 1.00?

14. **Present value of an amount and present value of an annuity.** What is the relationship between the present value of a single dollar payment formula and the present value of an ordinary annuity formula for the same number of years and the same discount rate? Assume a discount rate of 10 percent and an *n* value of five periods. Explain with an example.

15. If a nurse deposits $2,000 today in a bank account and the interest is compounded annually at 10 percent, what will be the value of this investment:

   a.   five years from now?

   b.   ten years from now?

   c.   fifteen years from now?

   d.   twenty years from now?

16. If a nurse deposits $12,000 today in a bank account and the interest is compounded annually at 11 percent, what will be the value of this investment:

   a.   three years from now?

   b.   six years from now?

   c.   nine years from now?

   d.   twelve years from now?

17. If a business manager deposits $30,000 in a savings account at the end of each year for twenty years, what will be the value of her investment:

   a.   at a compounded rate of 12 percent?

   b.   at a compounded rate of 18 percent?

   c.   What would the outcome be in both cases if the deposits were made at the beginning of each year?

18. If a business manager deposits $30,000 in a savings account at the end of each year for twenty years, what will be the value of her investment:

   a.   at a compounded rate of 13 percent?

   b.   at a compounded rate of 20 percent?

c. What would the outcome be in both cases if the deposits were made at the beginning of each year?

19. The chief financial officer of a home health agency needs to determine the present value of a $10,000 investment received at the end of year 10. What is the present value if the discount rate is:

   a. 6 percent?

   b. 9 percent?

   c. 12 percent?

   d. 15 percent?

20. The chief financial officer of a home health agency needs to determine the present value of a $40,000 investment received at the end of year 15. What is the present value if the discount rate is:

   a. 5 percent?

   b. 10 percent?

   c. 15 percent?

   d. 20 percent?

21. If a hospital received $5,000 in payments per year at the end of each year for the next twelve years from an uninsured patient who underwent an expensive operation, what would be the current value of these collection payments:

   a. at a 3 percent rate of return?

   b. at a 13 percent rate of return?

   c. If the funds were received at the beginning of the year, what would be the current value of these collection payments for each of the two rates of return?

22. If a hospital received $25,000 in payments per year at the end of each year for the next six years from an uninsured patient who underwent an expensive operation, what would be the current value of these collection payments:

   a. at a 5 percent rate of return?

   b. at a 15 percent rate of return?

   c. If the funds were received at the beginning of the year, what would be the current value of these collection payments for each of the two rates of return?

23. After completing her residency, an obstetrician plans to invest $12,000 per year at the end of each year into a low-risk retirement account. She expects to earn 6 percent for thirty-five years. What will her retirement account be worth at the end of those thirty-five years?

24. After completing her residency, an oncologist plans to invest $20,000 per year at the end of each year into a high-risk retirement account. She expects to earn 8 percent for thirty-five years. What will her retirement account be worth at the end of those thirty-five years?

25. Lincoln Memorial Hospital has just been informed that a private donor is willing to contribute $5 million per year at the beginning of each year for fifteen years. What is the current dollar value of this contribution if the discount rate is 9 percent?

26. Boulder City Hospital has just been informed that a private donor is willing to contribute $10 million per year at the beginning of each year for fifteen years. What is the current dollar value of this contribution if the discount rate is 14 percent?

27. If a community clinic invested $3,000 in excess cash today, what would be the value of its investment at the end of three years:

    a. at a 12 percent rate compounded semiannually?

    b. at a 12 percent rate compounded quarterly?

28. If a community hospital invested $10,000 in excess cash today, what would be the value of its investment at the end of three years:

    a. at a 28 percent rate compounded semiannually?

    b. at a 28 percent rate compounded quarterly?

29. Love Canal General Hospital wants to purchase a new blood analyzing device today. Its local bank is willing to lend it the money to buy the analyzer at a 3 percent monthly rate. The loan payments will start at the end of the month and will be $1,600 per month for the next eighteen months. What is the purchase price of the device?

30. General Hospital wants to purchase a new MRI today. Its local bank is willing to lend it the money to buy the MRI at a 4 percent monthly rate. The loan payments will start at the end of the month and will be $100,000 per month for the next thirty months. What is the purchase price of the MRI?

31. Midstate Medical Center is starting an endowment fund to pay for the expenses of a medical research program. The expenses are $1,000,000 per year, and the program is expected to last ten years. Assuming payments are made at the end of each year and the interest rate is 8 percent per year, what should be the initial size of the endowment?

32. Seaside Medical Center is starting an endowment fund to pay for the expenses of a community outreach pediatric program. The expenses are $600,000 per year, and the program is expected to last five years. Assuming payments are made at the end of each year and the interest rate is 5 percent per year, what should be the size of the initial endowment?

33. In 2010 Lilliputian County Hospital's total patient revenues were $15 million. In 2019 patient revenues are expected to be $30 million. What is the compound growth rate in patient revenues over this time period?

34. In 2011 Wythe County Hospital's total patient revenues were $5 million. In 2020 patient revenues are expected to be $27.75 million. What is the compound growth rate in patient revenues over this time period?

35. Shawnee Valley Family Practice Center plans to invest $30,000 in a money market account at the beginning of each year for the next five years. The investment pays 8 percent annual interest. How much would this investment be worth after five years of investing?

36. Starting today and every six months thereafter for the next ten years, St. Luke's Hospital plans to invest $750,000 at 6 percent annual interest in an account. How much would this investment be worth after ten years of investing?

37. Dr. Thomas plans to retire today and would like an income of $400,000 per year for the next fifteen years with the income payments starting one year from today. He will be able to earn interest of 8 percent per year compounded annually from his investment account. What must he deposit today in his investment account to achieve this income of $400,000 per year?

38. Today Williamson Hospital lends its Home Health Care Center $886,330. The center expects to repay the loan in quarterly installments of $100,000 for three years, with the first payment starting one quarter from now. What annual interest rate is the hospital charging for this loan?

39. Goldfarb Cancer Research Institute just received a $3 million gift to cover the salary for a permanent research scientist in perpetuity to study Hodgkin's disease. What would be the required rate of return on the investment if the position paid an annual salary of:

    a. $75,000 per year?

    b. $100,000 per year?

    c. $125,000 per year?

40. Upon the untimely and tragic death of their wealthy aunt, the heirs wanted to memorialize her with a named donation to the local hospital. They offered the hospital a choice of $40,000 annual payments forever or a lump sum payment of $500,000 today.

    a. What should be the decision if the hospital thinks it could earn an average of 5 percent annually on this donation?

    b. What should be the decision if the hospital thinks it could earn an average of 9 percent annually on this donation?

c. What should be the decision if the hospital thinks it could earn an average of 13 percent annually on this donation?

41. Stillwater Hospital is borrowing $1,000,000 for its medical office building. The annual interest rate is 5 percent. What will be the equal annual payments on the loan if the length of the loan is four years and payments occur at the end of each year?

42. Williamsburg Nursing Home is investing in a restricted fund for a new assisted-living home that will cost $6,000,000. How much do they need to invest each year to have $6,000,000 in fifteen years:

   a. If the expected rate of return on the investment is 12 percent, and the hospital invests at the end of each year?

   b. If the expected rate of return on the investment is 12 percent, and the hospital invests at the beginning of each year?

43. Carondelet Hospital is evaluating a lease arrangement for its ambulance fleet. The total value of the lease is $420,000. The hospital will be making equal monthly payments starting today.

   a. What is the monthly interest rate if the lease payments are $24,000 per month for twenty-four months?

   b. What is the monthly interest rate if the lease payments are $24,000 per month for thirty-six months?

   c. What is the monthly interest rate if the lease payments are $30,000 per month for thirty-six months?

44. A wealthy philanthropist has established the following endowment for a hospital. The details of the endowment include the following:

   a. A cash deposit of $9 million one year from now

   b. An annual cash deposit of $4 million per year for the next fifteen years. The first $4 million deposit will start today

   c. At the end of year 15, the hospital will also receive a lump sum payment of $16 million.

   Assuming the cost of money is 4 percent, what is the value of this endowment in today's dollars?

NOTES

1. From Table B–4, the PVFA equal or closest to 3.3124 is found in the row for 4 time periods. At this PVFA, the interest rate of this column heading is 8%.

APPENDIX B

FUTURE AND PRESENT VALUE TABLES

Appendix B presents pre-calculated tables to assist in determining future and present values (FV and PV). Future value is used to determine the future value of dollar payments made earlier; present value indicates the current value of future dollars. Although the formulas to compute these values appear in Chapter Six, pre-calculated tables provide a quick and flexible reference for this information.

Appendix B presents this information in four ways. Table B–1 presents the future value factor (FVF) of $1: what the future value of a single investment today will be worth at a future time at a given interest rate. Table B–2 reflects the future value factor of an annuity (FVFA): what the future value of an annuity received or invested over equal time periods will be worth at a future time, given a specified interest rate and number of periods involved. Table B–3 presents the present value factor (PVF) of $1: how much a single, one time amount to be received in the future at a specified interest rate is worth today. Table B–4 reflects the present value factor of an annuity (PVFA): the amount an annuity at a specified rate to be received at equal flows at the end of a specified number of periods, is worth today.

Table B–1 Future value factor of $1: $FVF_{i,n} = PV(1 + i)^n$; $FV = PV(FVF_{i,n})$

Period	1%	2%	3%	4%	5%	6%	7%	8%	9%	10%	11%	12%	13%	14%	15%
1	1.0100	1.0200	1.0300	1.0400	1.0500	1.0600	1.0700	1.0800	1.0900	1.1000	1.1100	1.1200	1.1300	1.1400	1.1500
2	1.0201	1.0404	1.0609	1.0816	1.1025	1.1236	1.1449	1.1664	1.1881	1.2100	1.2321	1.2544	1.2769	1.2996	1.3225
3	1.0303	1.0612	1.0927	1.1249	1.1576	1.1910	1.2250	1.2597	1.2950	1.3310	1.3676	1.4049	1.4429	1.4815	1.5209
4	1.0406	1.0824	1.1255	1.1699	1.2155	1.2625	1.3108	1.3605	1.4116	1.4641	1.5181	1.5735	1.6305	1.6890	1.7490
5	1.0510	1.1041	1.1593	1.2167	1.2763	1.3382	1.4026	1.4693	1.5386	1.6105	1.6851	1.7623	1.8424	1.9254	2.0114
6	1.0615	1.1262	1.1941	1.2653	1.3401	1.4185	1.5007	1.5869	1.6771	1.7716	1.8704	1.9738	2.0820	2.1950	2.3131
7	1.0721	1.1487	1.2299	1.3159	1.4071	1.5036	1.6058	1.7138	1.8280	1.9487	2.0762	2.2107	2.3526	2.5023	2.6600
8	1.0829	1.1717	1.2668	1.3686	1.4775	1.5938	1.7182	1.8509	1.9926	2.1436	2.3045	2.4760	2.6584	2.8526	3.0590
9	1.0937	1.1951	1.3048	1.4233	1.5513	1.6895	1.8385	1.9990	2.1719	2.3579	2.5580	2.7731	3.0040	3.2519	3.5179
10	1.1046	1.2190	1.3439	1.4802	1.6289	1.7908	1.9672	2.1589	2.3674	2.5937	2.8394	3.1058	3.3946	3.7072	4.0456
11	1.1157	1.2434	1.3842	1.5395	1.7103	1.8983	2.1049	2.3316	2.5804	2.8531	3.1518	3.4785	3.8359	4.2262	4.6524
12	1.1268	1.2682	1.4258	1.6010	1.7959	2.0122	2.2522	2.5182	2.8127	3.1384	3.4985	3.8960	4.3345	4.8179	5.3503
13	1.1381	1.2936	1.4685	1.6651	1.8856	2.1329	2.4098	2.7196	3.0658	3.4523	3.8833	4.3635	4.8980	5.4924	6.1528
14	1.1495	1.3195	1.5126	1.7317	1.9799	2.2609	2.5785	2.9372	3.3417	3.7975	4.3104	4.8871	5.5348	6.2613	7.0757
15	1.1610	1.3459	1.5580	1.8009	2.0789	2.3966	2.7590	3.1722	3.6425	4.1772	4.7846	5.4736	6.2543	7.1379	8.1371
16	1.1726	1.3728	1.6047	1.8730	2.1829	2.5404	2.9522	3.4259	3.9703	4.5950	5.3109	6.1304	7.0673	8.1372	9.3576
17	1.1843	1.4002	1.6528	1.9479	2.2920	2.6928	3.1588	3.7000	4.3276	5.0545	5.8951	6.8660	7.9861	9.2765	10.761
18	1.1961	1.4282	1.7024	2.0258	2.4066	2.8543	3.3799	3.9960	4.7171	5.5599	6.5436	7.6900	9.0243	10.575	12.375
19	1.2081	1.4568	1.7535	2.1068	2.5270	3.0256	3.6165	4.3157	5.1417	6.1159	7.2633	8.6128	10.197	12.056	14.232
20	1.2202	1.4859	1.8061	2.1911	2.6533	3.2071	3.8697	4.6610	5.6044	6.7275	8.0623	9.6463	11.523	13.743	16.367
21	1.2324	1.5157	1.8603	2.2788	2.7860	3.3996	4.1406	5.0338	6.1088	7.4002	8.9492	10.804	13.021	15.668	18.822
22	1.2447	1.5460	1.9161	2.3699	2.9253	3.6035	4.4304	5.4365	6.6586	8.1403	9.9336	12.100	14.714	17.861	21.645
23	1.2572	1.5769	1.9736	2.4647	3.0715	3.8197	4.7405	5.8715	7.2579	8.9543	11.026	13.552	16.627	20.362	24.891
24	1.2697	1.6084	2.0328	2.5633	3.2251	4.0489	5.0724	6.3412	7.9111	9.8497	12.239	15.179	18.788	23.212	28.625
25	1.2824	1.6406	2.0938	2.6658	3.3864	4.2919	5.4274	6.8485	8.6231	10.835	13.585	17.000	21.231	26.462	32.919
26	1.2953	1.6734	2.1566	2.7725	3.5557	4.5494	5.8074	7.3964	9.3992	11.918	15.080	19.040	23.991	30.167	37.857
27	1.3082	1.7069	2.2213	2.8834	3.7335	4.8223	6.2139	7.9881	10.245	13.110	16.739	21.325	27.109	34.390	43.535
28	1.3213	1.7410	2.2879	2.9987	3.9201	5.1117	6.6488	8.6271	11.167	14.421	18.580	23.884	30.633	39.204	50.066
29	1.3345	1.7758	2.3566	3.1187	4.1161	5.4184	7.1143	9.3173	12.172	15.863	20.624	26.750	34.616	44.693	57.575
30	1.3478	1.8114	2.4273	3.2434	4.3219	5.7435	7.6123	10.063	13.268	17.449	22.892	29.960	39.116	50.950	66.212
35	1.4166	1.9999	2.8139	3.9461	5.5160	7.6861	10.677	14.785	20.414	28.102	38.575	52.800	72.069	98.100	133.18
40	1.4889	2.2080	3.2620	4.8010	7.0400	10.286	14.974	21.725	31.409	45.259	65.001	93.051	132.78	188.88	267.86
45	1.5648	2.4379	3.7816	5.8412	8.9850	13.765	21.002	31.920	48.327	72.890	109.53	163.99	244.64	363.68	538.77
50	1.6446	2.6916	4.3839	7.1067	11.467	18.420	29.457	46.902	74.358	117.39	184.56	289.00	450.74	700.23	1,083.7

Period	16%	17%	18%	19%	20%	21%	22%	23%	24%	25%	30%	35%	40%	45%	50%
1	1.1600	1.1700	1.1800	1.1900	1.2000	1.2100	1.2200	1.2300	1.2400	1.2500	1.3000	1.3500	1.4000	1.4500	1.5000
2	1.3456	1.3689	1.3924	1.4161	1.4400	1.4641	1.4884	1.5129	1.5376	1.5625	1.6900	1.8225	1.9600	2.1025	2.2500
3	1.5609	1.6016	1.6430	1.6852	1.7280	1.7716	1.8158	1.8609	1.9066	1.9531	2.1970	2.4604	2.7440	3.0486	3.3750
4	1.8106	1.8739	1.9388	2.0053	2.0736	2.1436	2.2153	2.2889	2.3642	2.4414	2.8561	3.3215	3.8416	4.4205	5.0625
5	2.1003	2.1924	2.2878	2.3864	2.4883	2.5937	2.7027	2.8153	2.9316	3.0518	3.7129	4.4840	5.3782	6.4097	7.5938
6	2.4364	2.5652	2.6996	2.8398	2.9860	3.1384	3.2973	3.4628	3.6352	3.8147	4.8268	6.0534	7.5295	9.2941	11.391
7	2.8262	3.0012	3.1855	3.3793	3.5832	3.7975	4.0227	4.2593	4.5077	4.7684	6.2749	8.1722	10.541	13.476	17.086
8	3.2784	3.5115	3.7589	4.0214	4.2998	4.5950	4.9077	5.2389	5.5895	5.9605	8.1573	11.032	14.758	19.541	25.629
9	3.8030	4.1084	4.4355	4.7854	5.1598	5.5599	5.9874	6.4439	6.9310	7.4506	10.604	14.894	20.661	28.334	38.443
10	4.4114	4.8068	5.2338	5.6947	6.1917	6.7275	7.3046	7.9259	8.5944	9.3132	13.786	20.107	28.925	41.085	57.665
11	5.1173	5.6240	6.1759	6.7767	7.4301	8.1403	8.9117	9.7489	10.657	11.642	17.922	27.144	40.496	59.573	86.498
12	5.9360	6.5801	7.2876	8.0642	8.9161	9.8497	10.872	11.991	13.215	14.552	23.298	36.644	56.694	86.381	129.75
13	6.8858	7.6987	8.5994	9.5964	10.699	11.918	13.264	14.749	16.386	18.190	30.288	49.470	79.371	125.25	194.62
14	7.9875	9.0075	10.147	11.420	12.839	14.421	16.182	18.141	20.319	22.737	39.374	66.784	111.12	181.62	291.93
15	9.2655	10.539	11.974	13.590	15.407	17.449	19.742	22.314	25.196	28.422	51.186	90.158	155.57	263.34	437.89
16	10.748	12.330	14.129	16.172	18.488	21.114	24.086	27.446	31.243	35.527	66.542	121.71	217.80	381.85	656.84
17	12.468	14.426	16.672	19.244	22.186	25.548	29.384	33.759	38.741	44.409	86.504	164.31	304.91	553.68	985.26
18	14.463	16.879	19.673	22.901	26.623	30.913	35.849	41.523	48.039	55.511	112.46	221.82	426.88	802.83	1,477.9
19	16.777	19.748	23.214	27.252	31.948	37.404	43.736	51.074	59.568	69.389	146.19	299.46	597.63	1,164.1	2,216.8
20	19.461	23.106	27.393	32.429	38.338	45.259	53.358	62.821	73.864	86.736	190.05	404.27	836.68	1,688.0	3,325.3
21	22.574	27.034	32.324	38.591	46.005	54.764	65.096	77.269	91.592	108.42	247.06	545.77	1,171.4	2,447.5	4,987.9
22	26.186	31.629	38.142	45.923	55.206	66.264	79.418	95.041	113.57	135.53	321.18	736.79	1,639.9	3,548.9	7,481.8
23	30.376	37.006	45.008	54.649	66.247	80.180	96.889	116.90	140.83	169.41	417.54	994.66	2,295.9	5,145.9	11,223
24	35.236	43.297	53.109	65.032	79.497	97.017	118.21	143.79	174.63	211.76	542.80	1,342.8	3,214.2	7,461.6	16,834
25	40.874	50.658	62.669	77.388	95.396	117.39	144.21	176.86	216.54	264.70	705.64	1,812.8	4,499.9	10,819	25,251
26	47.414	59.270	73.949	92.092	114.48	142.04	175.94	217.54	268.51	330.87	917.33	2,447.2	6,299.8	15,688	37,877
27	55.000	69.345	87.260	109.59	137.37	171.87	214.64	267.57	332.95	413.59	1,192.5	3,303.8	8,819.8	22,748	56,815
28	63.800	81.134	102.97	130.41	164.84	207.97	261.86	329.11	412.86	516.99	1,550.3	4,460.1	12,348	32,984	85,223
29	74.009	94.927	121.50	155.19	197.81	251.64	319.47	404.81	511.95	646.23	2,015.4	6,021.1	17,287	47,827	127,834
30	85.850	111.06	143.37	184.68	237.38	304.48	389.76	497.91	634.82	807.79	2,620.0	8,128.5	24,201	69,349	191,751
35	180.31	243.50	328.00	440.70	590.67	789.75	1,053.4	1,401.8	1,861.1	2,465.2	9,727.9	36,449	130,161	444,509	1,456,110
40	378.72	533.87	750.38	1,051.7	1,469.8	2,048.4	2,847.0	3,946.4	5,455.9	7,523.2	36,119	163,437	700,038	2,849,181	11,057,332
45	795.44	1,170.5	1,716.7	2,509.7	3,657.3	5,313.0	7,694.7	11,110	15,995	22,959	134,107	732,858	3,764,971	18,262,495	83,966,617
50	1,670.7	2,566.2	3,927.4	5,988.9	9,100.4	13,781	20,797	31,279	46,890	70,065	497,929	3,286,158	20,248,916	117,057,734	637,621,500

Table B-2 Future value factor of an annuity (FVFA): Future value factor of an annuity of $1: $FVFA_{i,n} = [(1 + i)^n - 1] / i$

$FVA = PMT$ or annuity $\times (FVFA_{i,n})$

Period	1%	2%	3%	4%	5%	6%	7%	8%	9%	10%	11%	12%	13%	14%	15%
1	1.0000	1.0000	1.0000	1.0000	1.0000	1.0000	1.0000	1.0000	1.0000	1.0000	1.0000	1.0000	1.0000	1.0000	1.0000
2	2.0100	2.0200	2.0300	2.0400	2.0500	2.0600	2.0700	2.0800	2.0900	2.1000	2.1100	2.1200	2.1300	2.1400	2.1500
3	3.0301	3.0604	3.0909	3.1216	3.1525	3.1836	3.2149	3.2464	3.2781	3.3100	3.3421	3.3744	3.4069	3.4396	3.4725
4	4.0604	4.1216	4.1836	4.2465	4.3101	4.3746	4.4399	4.5061	4.5731	4.6410	4.7097	4.7793	4.8498	4.9211	4.9934
5	5.1010	5.2040	5.3091	5.4163	5.5256	5.6371	5.7507	5.8666	5.9847	6.1051	6.2278	6.3528	6.4803	6.6101	6.7424
6	6.1520	6.3081	6.4684	6.6330	6.8019	6.9753	7.1533	7.3359	7.5233	7.7156	7.9129	8.1152	8.3227	8.5355	8.7537
7	7.2135	7.4343	7.6625	7.8983	8.1420	8.3938	8.6540	8.9228	9.2004	9.4872	9.7833	10.089	10.405	10.730	11.067
8	8.2857	8.5830	8.8923	9.2142	9.5491	9.8975	10.260	10.637	11.028	11.436	11.859	12.300	12.757	13.233	13.727
9	9.3685	9.7546	10.159	10.583	11.027	11.491	11.978	12.488	13.021	13.579	14.164	14.776	15.416	16.085	16.786
10	10.462	10.950	11.464	12.006	12.578	13.181	13.816	14.487	15.193	15.937	16.722	17.549	18.420	19.337	20.304
11	11.567	12.169	12.808	13.486	14.207	14.972	15.784	16.645	17.560	18.531	19.561	20.655	21.814	23.045	24.349
12	12.683	13.412	14.192	15.026	15.917	16.870	17.888	18.977	20.141	21.384	22.713	24.133	25.650	27.271	29.002
13	13.809	14.680	15.618	16.627	17.713	18.882	20.141	21.495	22.953	24.523	26.212	28.029	29.985	32.089	34.352
14	14.947	15.974	17.086	18.292	19.599	21.015	22.550	24.215	26.019	27.975	30.095	32.393	34.883	37.581	40.505
15	16.097	17.293	18.599	20.024	21.579	23.276	25.129	27.152	29.361	31.772	34.405	37.280	40.417	43.842	47.580
16	17.258	18.639	20.157	21.825	23.657	25.673	27.888	30.324	33.003	35.950	39.190	42.753	46.672	50.980	55.717
17	18.430	20.012	21.762	23.698	25.840	28.213	30.840	33.750	36.974	40.545	44.501	48.884	53.739	59.118	65.075
18	19.615	21.412	23.414	25.645	28.132	30.906	33.999	37.450	41.301	45.599	50.396	55.750	61.725	68.394	75.836
19	20.811	22.841	25.117	27.671	30.539	33.760	37.379	41.446	46.018	51.159	56.939	63.440	70.749	78.969	88.212
20	22.019	24.297	26.870	29.778	33.066	36.786	40.995	45.762	51.160	57.275	64.203	72.052	80.947	91.025	102.44
21	23.239	25.783	28.676	31.969	35.719	39.993	44.865	50.423	56.765	64.002	72.265	81.699	92.470	104.77	118.81
22	24.472	27.299	30.537	34.248	38.505	43.392	49.006	55.457	62.873	71.403	81.214	92.503	105.49	120.44	137.63
23	25.716	28.845	32.453	36.618	41.430	46.996	53.436	60.893	69.532	79.543	91.148	104.60	120.20	138.30	159.28
24	26.973	30.422	34.426	39.083	44.502	50.816	58.177	66.765	76.790	88.497	102.17	118.16	136.83	158.66	184.17
25	28.243	32.030	36.459	41.646	47.727	54.865	63.249	73.106	84.701	98.347	114.41	133.33	155.62	181.87	212.79
26	29.526	33.671	38.553	44.312	51.113	59.156	68.676	79.954	93.324	109.18	128.00	150.33	176.85	208.33	245.71
27	30.821	35.344	40.710	47.084	54.669	63.706	74.484	87.351	102.72	121.10	143.08	169.37	200.84	238.50	283.57
28	32.129	37.051	42.931	49.968	58.403	68.528	80.698	95.339	112.97	134.21	159.82	190.70	227.95	272.89	327.10
29	33.450	38.792	45.219	52.966	62.323	73.640	87.347	103.97	124.14	148.63	178.40	214.58	258.58	312.09	377.17
30	34.785	40.568	47.575	56.085	66.439	79.058	94.461	113.28	136.31	164.49	199.02	241.33	293.20	356.79	434.75
35	41.660	49.994	60.462	73.652	90.320	111.43	138.24	172.32	215.71	271.02	341.59	431.66	546.68	693.57	881.17
40	48.886	60.402	75.401	95.026	120.80	154.76	199.64	259.06	337.88	442.59	581.83	767.09	1,013.7	1,342.0	1,779.1
45	56.481	71.893	92.720	121.03	159.70	212.74	285.75	386.51	525.86	718.90	986.64	1,358.2	1,874.2	2,590.6	3,585.1
50	64.463	84.579	112.80	152.67	209.35	290.34	406.53	573.77	815.08	1,163.9	1,668.8	2,400.0	3,459.5	4,994.5	7,217.7

Period	16%	17%	18%	19%	20%	21%	22%	23%	24%	25%	30%	35%	40%	45%	50%
1	1.0000	1.0000	1.0000	1.0000	1.0000	1.0000	1.0000	1.0000	1.0000	1.0000	1.0000	1.0000	1.0000	1.0000	1.0000
2	2.1600	2.1700	2.1800	2.1900	2.2000	2.2100	2.2200	2.2300	2.2400	2.2500	2.3000	2.3500	2.4000	2.4500	2.5000
3	3.5056	3.5389	3.5724	3.6061	3.6400	3.6741	3.7084	3.7429	3.7776	3.8125	3.9900	4.1725	4.3600	4.5525	4.7500
4	5.0665	5.1405	5.2154	5.2913	5.3680	5.4457	5.5242	5.6038	5.6842	5.7656	6.1870	6.6329	7.1040	7.6011	8.1250
5	6.8771	7.0144	7.1542	7.2966	7.4416	7.5892	7.7396	7.8926	8.0484	8.2070	9.0431	9.9544	10.946	12.022	13.188
6	8.9775	9.2068	9.4420	9.6830	9.9299	10.183	10.442	10.708	10.980	11.259	12.756	14.438	16.324	18.431	20.781
7	11.414	11.772	12.142	12.523	12.916	13.321	13.740	14.171	14.615	15.073	17.583	20.492	23.853	27.725	32.172
8	14.240	14.773	15.327	15.902	16.499	17.119	17.762	18.430	19.123	19.842	23.858	28.664	34.395	41.202	49.258
9	17.519	18.285	19.086	19.923	20.799	21.714	22.670	23.669	24.712	25.802	32.015	39.696	49.153	60.743	74.887
10	21.321	22.393	23.521	24.709	25.959	27.274	28.657	30.113	31.643	33.253	42.619	54.590	69.814	89.077	113.33
11	25.733	27.200	28.755	30.404	32.150	34.001	35.962	38.039	40.238	42.566	56.405	74.697	98.739	130.16	171.00
12	30.850	32.824	34.931	37.180	39.581	42.142	44.874	47.788	50.895	54.208	74.327	101.84	139.23	189.73	257.49
13	36.786	39.404	42.219	45.244	48.497	51.991	55.746	59.779	64.110	68.760	97.625	138.48	195.93	276.12	387.24
14	43.672	47.103	50.818	54.841	59.196	63.909	69.010	74.528	80.496	86.949	127.91	187.95	275.30	401.37	581.86
15	51.660	56.110	60.965	66.261	72.035	78.330	85.192	92.669	100.82	109.69	167.29	254.74	386.42	582.98	873.79
16	60.925	66.649	72.939	79.850	87.442	95.780	104.93	114.98	126.01	138.11	218.47	344.90	541.99	846.32	1,311.7
17	71.673	78.979	87.068	96.022	105.93	116.89	129.02	142.43	157.25	173.64	285.01	466.61	759.78	1,228.2	1,968.5
18	84.141	93.406	103.74	115.27	128.12	142.44	158.40	176.19	195.99	218.04	371.52	630.92	1,064.7	1,781.8	2,953.8
19	98.603	110.28	123.41	138.17	154.74	173.35	194.25	217.71	244.03	273.56	483.97	852.75	1,491.6	2,584.7	4,431.7
20	115.38	130.03	146.63	165.42	186.69	210.76	237.99	268.79	303.60	342.94	630.17	1,152.2	2,089.2	3,748.8	6,648.5
21	134.84	153.14	174.02	197.85	225.03	256.02	291.35	331.61	377.46	429.68	820.22	1,556.5	2,925.9	5,436.7	9,973.8
22	157.41	180.17	206.34	236.44	271.03	310.78	356.44	408.88	469.06	538.10	1,067.3	2,102.3	4,097.2	7,884.3	14,962
23	183.60	211.80	244.49	282.36	326.24	377.05	435.86	503.92	582.63	673.63	1,388.5	2,839.0	5,737.1	11,433	22,443
24	213.98	248.81	289.49	337.01	392.48	457.22	532.75	620.82	723.46	843.03	1,806.0	3,833.7	8,033.0	16,579	33,666
25	249.21	292.10	342.60	402.04	471.98	554.24	650.96	764.61	898.09	1,054.8	2,348.8	5,176.5	11,247	24,041	50,500
26	290.09	342.76	405.27	479.43	567.38	671.63	795.17	941.46	1,114.6	1,319.5	3,054.4	6,989.3	15,747	34,860	75,752
27	337.50	402.03	479.22	571.52	681.85	813.68	971.10	1,159.0	1,383.1	1,650.4	3,971.8	9,436.5	22,047	50,548	113,628
28	392.50	471.38	566.48	681.11	819.22	985.55	1,185.7	1,426.6	1,716.1	2,064.0	5,164.3	12,740	30,867	73,296	170,443
29	456.30	552.51	669.45	811.52	984.07	1,193.5	1,447.6	1,755.7	2,129.0	2,580.9	6,714.6	17,200	43,214	106,280	255,666
30	530.31	647.44	790.95	966.71	1,181.9	1,445.2	1,767.1	2,160.5	2,640.9	3,227.2	8,730.0	23,222	60,501	154,107	383,500
35	1,120.7	1,426.5	1,816.7	2,314.2	2,948.3	3,755.9	4,783.6	6,090.3	7,750.2	9,856.8	32,423	104,136	325,400	987,794	2,912,217
40	2,360.8	3,134.5	4,163.2	5,529.8	7,343.9	9,749.5	12,937	17,154	22,729	30,089	120,393	466,960	1,750,092	6,331,512	22,114,663
45	4,965.3	6,879.3	9,531.6	13,203	18,281	25,295	34,971	48,302	66,640	91,831	447,019	2,093,876	9,412,424	40,583,319	167,933,233
50	10,436	15,090	21,813	31,515	45,497	65,617	94,525	135,992	195,373	280,256	1,659,761	9,389,020	50,622,288	260,128,295	1,275,242,998

265

Table B–3 Present value factor of $1. $PVF(i,n) = 1/(1 + i)^n$; $PV = FV(PVF_{i,n})$

Period	1%	2%	3%	4%	5%	6%	7%	8%	9%	10%	11%	12%	13%	14%	15%
1	0.9901	0.9804	0.9709	0.9615	0.9524	0.9434	0.9346	0.9259	0.9174	0.9091	0.9009	0.8929	0.8850	0.8772	0.8696
2	0.9803	0.9612	0.9426	0.9246	0.9070	0.8900	0.8734	0.8573	0.8417	0.8264	0.8116	0.7972	0.7831	0.7695	0.7561
3	0.9706	0.9423	0.9151	0.8890	0.8638	0.8396	0.8163	0.7938	0.7722	0.7513	0.7312	0.7118	0.6931	0.6750	0.6575
4	0.9610	0.9238	0.8885	0.8548	0.8227	0.7921	0.7629	0.7350	0.7084	0.6830	0.6587	0.6355	0.6133	0.5921	0.5718
5	0.9515	0.9057	0.8626	0.8219	0.7835	0.7473	0.7130	0.6806	0.6499	0.6209	0.5935	0.5674	0.5428	0.5194	0.4972
6	0.9420	0.8880	0.8375	0.7903	0.7462	0.7050	0.6663	0.6302	0.5963	0.5645	0.5346	0.5066	0.4803	0.4556	0.4323
7	0.9327	0.8706	0.8131	0.7599	0.7107	0.6651	0.6227	0.5835	0.5470	0.5132	0.4817	0.4523	0.4251	0.3996	0.3759
8	0.9235	0.8535	0.7894	0.7307	0.6768	0.6274	0.5820	0.5403	0.5019	0.4665	0.4339	0.4039	0.3762	0.3506	0.3269
9	0.9143	0.8368	0.7664	0.7026	0.6446	0.5919	0.5439	0.5002	0.4604	0.4241	0.3909	0.3606	0.3329	0.3075	0.2843
10	0.9053	0.8203	0.7441	0.6756	0.6139	0.5584	0.5083	0.4632	0.4224	0.3855	0.3522	0.3220	0.2946	0.2697	0.2472
11	0.8963	0.8043	0.7224	0.6496	0.5847	0.5268	0.4751	0.4289	0.3875	0.3505	0.3173	0.2875	0.2607	0.2366	0.2149
12	0.8874	0.7885	0.7014	0.6246	0.5568	0.4970	0.4440	0.3971	0.3555	0.3186	0.2858	0.2567	0.2307	0.2076	0.1869
13	0.8787	0.7730	0.6810	0.6006	0.5303	0.4688	0.4150	0.3677	0.3262	0.2897	0.2575	0.2292	0.2042	0.1821	0.1625
14	0.8700	0.7579	0.6611	0.5775	0.5051	0.4423	0.3878	0.3405	0.2992	0.2633	0.2320	0.2046	0.1807	0.1597	0.1413
15	0.8613	0.7430	0.6419	0.5553	0.4810	0.4173	0.3624	0.3152	0.2745	0.2394	0.2090	0.1827	0.1599	0.1401	0.1229
16	0.8528	0.7284	0.6232	0.5339	0.4581	0.3936	0.3387	0.2919	0.2519	0.2176	0.1883	0.1631	0.1415	0.1229	0.1069
17	0.8444	0.7142	0.6050	0.5134	0.4363	0.3714	0.3166	0.2703	0.2311	0.1978	0.1696	0.1456	0.1252	0.1078	0.0929
18	0.8360	0.7002	0.5874	0.4936	0.4155	0.3503	0.2959	0.2502	0.2120	0.1799	0.1528	0.1300	0.1108	0.0946	0.0808
19	0.8277	0.6864	0.5703	0.4746	0.3957	0.3305	0.2765	0.2317	0.1945	0.1635	0.1377	0.1161	0.0981	0.0829	0.0703
20	0.8195	0.6730	0.5537	0.4564	0.3769	0.3118	0.2584	0.2145	0.1784	0.1486	0.1240	0.1037	0.0868	0.0728	0.0611
21	0.8114	0.6598	0.5375	0.4388	0.3589	0.2942	0.2415	0.1987	0.1637	0.1351	0.1117	0.0926	0.0768	0.0638	0.0531
22	0.8034	0.6468	0.5219	0.4220	0.3418	0.2775	0.2257	0.1839	0.1502	0.1228	0.1007	0.0826	0.0680	0.0560	0.0462
23	0.7954	0.6342	0.5067	0.4057	0.3256	0.2618	0.2109	0.1703	0.1378	0.1117	0.0907	0.0738	0.0601	0.0491	0.0402
24	0.7876	0.6217	0.4919	0.3901	0.3101	0.2470	0.1971	0.1577	0.1264	0.1015	0.0817	0.0659	0.0532	0.0431	0.0349
25	0.7798	0.6095	0.4776	0.3751	0.2953	0.2330	0.1842	0.1460	0.1160	0.0923	0.0736	0.0588	0.0471	0.0378	0.0304
26	0.7720	0.5976	0.4637	0.3607	0.2812	0.2198	0.1722	0.1352	0.1064	0.0839	0.0663	0.0525	0.0417	0.0331	0.0264
27	0.7644	0.5859	0.4502	0.3468	0.2678	0.2074	0.1609	0.1252	0.0976	0.0763	0.0597	0.0469	0.0369	0.0291	0.0230
28	0.7568	0.5744	0.4371	0.3335	0.2551	0.1956	0.1504	0.1159	0.0895	0.0693	0.0538	0.0419	0.0326	0.0255	0.0200
29	0.7493	0.5631	0.4243	0.3207	0.2429	0.1846	0.1406	0.1073	0.0822	0.0630	0.0485	0.0374	0.0289	0.0224	0.0174
30	0.7419	0.5521	0.4120	0.3083	0.2314	0.1741	0.1314	0.0994	0.0754	0.0573	0.0437	0.0334	0.0256	0.0196	0.0151
35	0.7059	0.5000	0.3554	0.2534	0.1813	0.1301	0.0937	0.0676	0.0490	0.0356	0.0259	0.0189	0.0139	0.0102	0.0075
40	0.6717	0.4529	0.3066	0.2083	0.1420	0.0972	0.0668	0.0460	0.0318	0.0221	0.0154	0.0107	0.0075	0.0053	0.0037
45	0.6391	0.4102	0.2644	0.1712	0.1113	0.0727	0.0476	0.0313	0.0207	0.0137	0.0091	0.0061	0.0041	0.0027	0.0019
50	0.6080	0.3715	0.2281	0.1407	0.0872	0.0543	0.0339	0.0213	0.0134	0.0085	0.0054	0.0035	0.0022	0.0014	0.0009

Period	16%	17%	18%	19%	20%	21%	22%	23%	24%	25%	30%	35%	40%	45%	50%
1	0.8621	0.8547	0.8475	0.8403	0.8333	0.8264	0.8197	0.8130	0.8065	0.8000	0.7692	0.7407	0.7143	0.6897	0.6667
2	0.7432	0.7305	0.7182	0.7062	0.6944	0.6830	0.6719	0.6610	0.6504	0.6400	0.5917	0.5487	0.5102	0.4756	0.4444
3	0.6407	0.6244	0.6086	0.5934	0.5787	0.5645	0.5507	0.5374	0.5245	0.5120	0.4552	0.4064	0.3644	0.3280	0.2963
4	0.5523	0.5337	0.5158	0.4987	0.4823	0.4665	0.4514	0.4369	0.4230	0.4096	0.3501	0.3011	0.2603	0.2262	0.1975
5	0.4761	0.4561	0.4371	0.4190	0.4019	0.3855	0.3700	0.3552	0.3411	0.3277	0.2693	0.2230	0.1859	0.1560	0.1317
6	0.4104	0.3898	0.3704	0.3521	0.3349	0.3186	0.3033	0.2888	0.2751	0.2621	0.2072	0.1652	0.1328	0.1076	0.0878
7	0.3538	0.3332	0.3139	0.2959	0.2791	0.2633	0.2486	0.2348	0.2218	0.2097	0.1594	0.1224	0.0949	0.0742	0.0585
8	0.3050	0.2848	0.2660	0.2487	0.2326	0.2176	0.2038	0.1909	0.1789	0.1678	0.1226	0.0906	0.0678	0.0512	0.0390
9	0.2630	0.2434	0.2255	0.2090	0.1938	0.1799	0.1670	0.1552	0.1443	0.1342	0.0943	0.0671	0.0484	0.0353	0.0260
10	0.2267	0.2080	0.1911	0.1756	0.1615	0.1486	0.1369	0.1262	0.1164	0.1074	0.0725	0.0497	0.0346	0.0243	0.0173
11	0.1954	0.1778	0.1619	0.1476	0.1346	0.1228	0.1122	0.1026	0.0938	0.0859	0.0558	0.0368	0.0247	0.0168	0.0116
12	0.1685	0.1520	0.1372	0.1240	0.1122	0.1015	0.0920	0.0834	0.0757	0.0687	0.0429	0.0273	0.0176	0.0116	0.0077
13	0.1452	0.1299	0.1163	0.1042	0.0935	0.0839	0.0754	0.0678	0.0610	0.0550	0.0330	0.0202	0.0126	0.0080	0.0051
14	0.1252	0.1110	0.0985	0.0876	0.0779	0.0693	0.0618	0.0551	0.0492	0.0440	0.0254	0.0150	0.0090	0.0055	0.0034
15	0.1079	0.0949	0.0835	0.0736	0.0649	0.0573	0.0507	0.0448	0.0397	0.0352	0.0195	0.0111	0.0064	0.0038	0.0023
16	0.0930	0.0811	0.0708	0.0618	0.0541	0.0474	0.0415	0.0364	0.0320	0.0281	0.0150	0.0082	0.0046	0.0026	0.0015
17	0.0802	0.0693	0.0600	0.0520	0.0451	0.0391	0.0340	0.0296	0.0258	0.0225	0.0116	0.0061	0.0033	0.0018	0.0010
18	0.0691	0.0592	0.0508	0.0437	0.0376	0.0323	0.0279	0.0241	0.0208	0.0180	0.0089	0.0045	0.0023	0.0012	0.0007
19	0.0596	0.0506	0.0431	0.0367	0.0313	0.0267	0.0229	0.0196	0.0168	0.0144	0.0068	0.0033	0.0017	0.0009	0.0005
20	0.0514	0.0433	0.0365	0.0308	0.0261	0.0221	0.0187	0.0159	0.0135	0.0115	0.0053	0.0025	0.0012	0.0006	0.0003
21	0.0443	0.0370	0.0309	0.0259	0.0217	0.0183	0.0154	0.0129	0.0109	0.0092	0.0040	0.0018	0.0009	0.0004	0.0002
22	0.0382	0.0316	0.0262	0.0218	0.0181	0.0151	0.0126	0.0105	0.0088	0.0074	0.0031	0.0014	0.0006	0.0003	0.0001
23	0.0329	0.0270	0.0222	0.0183	0.0151	0.0125	0.0103	0.0086	0.0071	0.0059	0.0024	0.0010	0.0004	0.0002	0.0001
24	0.0284	0.0231	0.0188	0.0154	0.0126	0.0103	0.0085	0.0070	0.0057	0.0047	0.0018	0.0007	0.0003	0.0001	0.0001
25	0.0245	0.0197	0.0160	0.0129	0.0105	0.0085	0.0069	0.0057	0.0046	0.0038	0.0014	0.0006	0.0002	0.0001	0.0001
26	0.0211	0.0169	0.0135	0.0109	0.0087	0.0070	0.0057	0.0046	0.0037	0.0030	0.0011	0.0004	0.0002	0.0001	0.0000
27	0.0182	0.0144	0.0115	0.0091	0.0073	0.0058	0.0047	0.0037	0.0030	0.0024	0.0008	0.0003	0.0001	0.0000	0.0000
28	0.0157	0.0123	0.0097	0.0077	0.0061	0.0048	0.0038	0.0030	0.0024	0.0019	0.0006	0.0002	0.0001	0.0000	0.0000
29	0.0135	0.0105	0.0082	0.0064	0.0051	0.0040	0.0031	0.0025	0.0020	0.0015	0.0005	0.0002	0.0001	0.0000	0.0000
30	0.0116	0.0090	0.0070	0.0054	0.0042	0.0033	0.0026	0.0020	0.0016	0.0012	0.0004	0.0001	0.0000	0.0000	0.0000
35	0.0055	0.0041	0.0030	0.0023	0.0017	0.0013	0.0009	0.0007	0.0005	0.0004	0.0001	0.0000	0.0000	0.0000	0.0000
40	0.0026	0.0019	0.0013	0.0010	0.0007	0.0005	0.0004	0.0003	0.0002	0.0001	0.0000	0.0000	0.0000	0.0000	0.0000
45	0.0013	0.0009	0.0006	0.0004	0.0003	0.0002	0.0001	0.0001	0.0001	0.0000	0.0000	0.0000	0.0000	0.0000	0.0000
50	0.0006	0.0004	0.0003	0.0002	0.0001	0.0001	0.0000	0.0000	0.0000	0.0000	0.0000	0.0000	0.0000	0.0000	0.0000

Table B–4 Present value factor of an annuity (PVFA): Present value factor of an annuity of $1: $PVFA_{i,n} = [1 - 1/(1+i)^n]/i$;
PVA = PMT or annuity $\times$ ($PVFA_{i,n}$)

Period	1%	2%	3%	4%	5%	6%	7%	8%	9%	10%	11%	12%	13%	14%	15%
1	0.9901	0.9804	0.9709	0.9615	0.9524	0.9434	0.9346	0.9259	0.9174	0.9091	0.9009	0.8929	0.8850	0.8772	0.8696
2	1.9704	1.9416	1.9135	1.8861	1.8594	1.8334	1.8080	1.7833	1.7591	1.7355	1.7125	1.6901	1.6681	1.6467	1.6257
3	2.9410	2.8839	2.8286	2.7751	2.7232	2.6730	2.6243	2.5771	2.5313	2.4869	2.4437	2.4018	2.3612	2.3216	2.2832
4	3.9020	3.8077	3.7171	3.6299	3.5460	3.4651	3.3872	3.3121	3.2397	3.1699	3.1024	3.0373	2.9745	2.9137	2.8550
5	4.8534	4.7135	4.5797	4.4518	4.3295	4.2124	4.1002	3.9927	3.8897	3.7908	3.6959	3.6048	3.5172	3.4331	3.3522
6	5.7955	5.6014	5.4172	5.2421	5.0757	4.9173	4.7665	4.6229	4.4859	4.3553	4.2305	4.1114	3.9975	3.8887	3.7845
7	6.7282	6.4720	6.2303	6.0021	5.7864	5.5824	5.3893	5.2064	5.0330	4.8684	4.7122	4.5638	4.4226	4.2883	4.1604
8	7.6517	7.3255	7.0197	6.7327	6.4632	6.2098	5.9713	5.7466	5.5348	5.3349	5.1461	4.9676	4.7988	4.6389	4.4873
9	8.5660	8.1622	7.7861	7.4353	7.1078	6.8017	6.5152	6.2469	5.9952	5.7590	5.5370	5.3282	5.1317	4.9464	4.7716
10	9.4713	8.9826	8.5302	8.1109	7.7217	7.3601	7.0236	6.7101	6.4177	6.1446	5.8892	5.6502	5.4262	5.2161	5.0188
11	10.368	9.7868	9.2526	8.7605	8.3064	7.8869	7.4987	7.1390	6.8052	6.4951	6.2065	5.9377	5.6869	5.4527	5.2337
12	11.255	10.575	9.9540	9.3851	8.8633	8.3838	7.9427	7.5361	7.1607	6.8137	6.4924	6.1944	5.9176	5.6603	5.4206
13	12.134	11.348	10.635	9.9856	9.3936	8.8527	8.3577	7.9038	7.4869	7.1034	6.7499	6.4235	6.1218	5.8424	5.5831
14	13.004	12.106	11.296	10.563	9.8986	9.2950	8.7455	8.2442	7.7862	7.3667	6.9819	6.6282	6.3025	6.0021	5.7245
15	13.865	12.849	11.938	11.118	10.380	9.7122	9.1079	8.5595	8.0607	7.6061	7.1909	6.8109	6.4624	6.1422	5.8474
16	14.718	13.578	12.561	11.652	10.838	10.106	9.4466	8.8514	8.3126	7.8237	7.3792	6.9740	6.6039	6.2651	5.9542
17	15.562	14.292	13.166	12.166	11.274	10.477	9.7632	9.1216	8.5436	8.0216	7.5488	7.1196	6.7291	6.3729	6.0472
18	16.398	14.992	13.754	12.659	11.690	10.828	10.059	9.3719	8.7556	8.2014	7.7016	7.2497	6.8399	6.4674	6.1280
19	17.226	15.678	14.324	13.134	12.085	11.158	10.336	9.6036	8.9501	8.3649	7.8393	7.3658	6.9380	6.5504	6.1982
20	18.046	16.351	14.877	13.590	12.462	11.470	10.594	9.8181	9.1285	8.5136	7.9633	7.4694	7.0248	6.6231	6.2593
21	18.857	17.011	15.415	14.029	12.821	11.764	10.836	10.017	9.2922	8.6487	8.0751	7.5620	7.1016	6.6870	6.3125
22	19.660	17.658	15.937	14.451	13.163	12.042	11.061	10.201	9.4424	8.7715	8.1757	7.6446	7.1695	6.7429	6.3587
23	20.456	18.292	16.444	14.857	13.489	12.303	11.272	10.371	9.5802	8.8832	8.2664	7.7184	7.2297	6.7921	6.3988
24	21.243	18.914	16.936	15.247	13.799	12.550	11.469	10.529	9.7066	8.9847	8.3481	7.7843	7.2829	6.8351	6.4338
25	22.023	19.523	17.413	15.622	14.094	12.783	11.654	10.675	9.8226	9.0770	8.4217	7.8431	7.3300	6.8729	6.4641
26	22.795	20.121	17.877	15.983	14.375	13.003	11.826	10.810	9.9290	9.1609	8.4881	7.8957	7.3717	6.9061	6.4906
27	23.560	20.707	18.327	16.330	14.643	13.211	11.987	10.935	10.027	9.2372	8.5478	7.9426	7.4086	6.9352	6.5135
28	24.316	21.281	18.764	16.663	14.898	13.406	12.137	11.051	10.116	9.3066	8.6016	7.9844	7.4412	6.9607	6.5335
29	25.066	21.844	19.188	16.984	15.141	13.591	12.278	11.158	10.198	9.3696	8.6501	8.0218	7.4701	6.9830	6.5509
30	25.808	22.396	19.600	17.292	15.372	13.765	12.409	11.258	10.274	9.4269	8.6938	8.0552	7.4957	7.0027	6.5660
35	29.409	24.999	21.487	18.665	16.374	14.498	12.948	11.655	10.567	9.6442	8.8552	8.1755	7.5856	7.0700	6.6166
40	32.835	27.355	23.115	19.793	17.159	15.046	13.332	11.925	10.757	9.7791	8.9511	8.2438	7.6344	7.1050	6.6418
45	36.095	29.490	24.519	20.720	17.774	15.456	13.606	12.108	10.881	9.8628	9.0079	8.2825	7.6609	7.1232	6.6543
50	39.196	31.424	25.730	21.482	18.256	15.762	13.801	12.233	10.962	9.9148	9.0417	8.3045	7.6752	7.1327	6.6605

Period	16%	17%	18%	19%	20%	21%	22%	23%	24%	25%	30%	35%	40%	45%	50%
1	0.8621	0.8547	0.8475	0.8403	0.8333	0.8264	0.8197	0.8130	0.8065	0.8000	0.7692	0.7407	0.7143	0.6897	0.6667
2	1.6052	1.5852	1.5656	1.5465	1.5278	1.5095	1.4915	1.4740	1.4568	1.4400	1.3609	1.2894	1.2245	1.1653	1.1111
3	2.2459	2.2096	2.1743	2.1399	2.1065	2.0739	2.0422	2.0114	1.9813	1.9520	1.8161	1.6959	1.5889	1.4933	1.4074
4	2.7982	2.7432	2.6901	2.6386	2.5887	2.5404	2.4936	2.4483	2.4043	2.3616	2.1662	1.9969	1.8492	1.7195	1.6049
5	3.2743	3.1993	3.1272	3.0576	2.9906	2.9260	2.8636	2.8035	2.7454	2.6893	2.4356	2.2200	2.0352	1.8755	1.7366
6	3.6847	3.5892	3.4976	3.4098	3.3255	3.2446	3.1669	3.0923	3.0205	2.9514	2.6427	2.3852	2.1680	1.9831	1.8244
7	4.0386	3.9224	3.8115	3.7057	3.6046	3.5079	3.4155	3.3270	3.2423	3.1611	2.8021	2.5075	2.2628	2.0573	1.8829
8	4.3436	4.2072	4.0776	3.9544	3.8372	3.7256	3.6193	3.5179	3.4212	3.3289	2.9247	2.5982	2.3306	2.1085	1.9220
9	4.6065	4.4506	4.3030	4.1633	4.0310	3.9054	3.7863	3.6731	3.5655	3.4631	3.0190	2.6653	2.3790	2.1438	1.9480
10	4.8332	4.6586	4.4941	4.3389	4.1925	4.0541	3.9232	3.7993	3.6819	3.5705	3.0915	2.7150	2.4136	2.1681	1.9653
11	5.0286	4.8364	4.6560	4.4865	4.3271	4.1769	4.0354	3.9018	3.7757	3.6564	3.1473	2.7519	2.4383	2.1849	1.9769
12	5.1971	4.9884	4.7932	4.6105	4.4392	4.2784	4.1274	3.9852	3.8514	3.7251	3.1903	2.7792	2.4559	2.1965	1.9846
13	5.3423	5.1183	4.9095	4.7147	4.5327	4.3624	4.2028	4.0530	3.9124	3.7801	3.2233	2.7994	2.4685	2.2045	1.9897
14	5.4675	5.2293	5.0081	4.8023	4.6106	4.4317	4.2646	4.1082	3.9616	3.8241	3.2487	2.8144	2.4775	2.2100	1.9931
15	5.5755	5.3242	5.0916	4.8759	4.6755	4.4890	4.3152	4.1530	4.0013	3.8593	3.2682	2.8255	2.4839	2.2138	1.9954
16	5.6685	5.4053	5.1624	4.9377	4.7296	4.5364	4.3567	4.1894	4.0333	3.8874	3.2832	2.8337	2.4885	2.2164	1.9970
17	5.7487	5.4746	5.2223	4.9897	4.7746	4.5755	4.3908	4.2190	4.0591	3.9099	3.2948	2.8398	2.4918	2.2182	1.9980
18	5.8178	5.5339	5.2732	5.0333	4.8122	4.6079	4.4187	4.2431	4.0799	3.9279	3.3037	2.8443	2.4941	2.2195	1.9986
19	5.8775	5.5845	5.3162	5.0700	4.8435	4.6346	4.4415	4.2627	4.0967	3.9424	3.3105	2.8476	2.4958	2.2203	1.9991
20	5.9288	5.6278	5.3527	5.1009	4.8696	4.6567	4.4603	4.2786	4.1103	3.9539	3.3158	2.8501	2.4970	2.2209	1.9994
21	5.9731	5.6648	5.3837	5.1268	4.8913	4.6750	4.4756	4.2916	4.1212	3.9631	3.3198	2.8519	2.4979	2.2213	1.9996
22	6.0113	5.6964	5.4099	5.1486	4.9094	4.6900	4.4882	4.3021	4.1300	3.9705	3.3230	2.8533	2.4985	2.2216	1.9997
23	6.0442	5.7234	5.4321	5.1668	4.9245	4.7025	4.4985	4.3106	4.1371	3.9764	3.3254	2.8543	2.4989	2.2218	1.9998
24	6.0726	5.7465	5.4509	5.1822	4.9371	4.7128	4.5070	4.3176	4.1428	3.9811	3.3272	2.8550	2.4992	2.2219	1.9999
25	6.0971	5.7662	5.4669	5.1951	4.9476	4.7213	4.5139	4.3232	4.1474	3.9849	3.3286	2.8556	2.4994	2.2220	1.9999
26	6.1182	5.7831	5.4804	5.2060	4.9563	4.7284	4.5196	4.3278	4.1511	3.9879	3.3297	2.8560	2.4996	2.2221	1.9999
27	6.1364	5.7975	5.4919	5.2151	4.9636	4.7342	4.5243	4.3316	4.1542	3.9903	3.3305	2.8563	2.4997	2.2221	2.0000
28	6.1520	5.8099	5.5016	5.2228	4.9697	4.7390	4.5281	4.3346	4.1566	3.9923	3.3312	2.8565	2.4998	2.2222	2.0000
29	6.1656	5.8204	5.5098	5.2292	4.9747	4.7430	4.5312	4.3371	4.1585	3.9938	3.3317	2.8567	2.4999	2.2222	2.0000
30	6.1772	5.8294	5.5168	5.2347	4.9789	4.7463	4.5338	4.3391	4.1601	3.9950	3.3321	2.8568	2.4999	2.2222	2.0000
35	6.2153	5.8582	5.5386	5.2512	4.9915	4.7559	4.5411	4.3447	4.1644	3.9984	3.3330	2.8571	2.5000	2.2222	2.0000
40	6.2335	5.8713	5.5482	5.2582	4.9966	4.7596	4.5439	4.3467	4.1659	3.9995	3.3332	2.8571	2.5000	2.2222	2.0000
45	6.2421	5.8773	5.5523	5.2611	4.9986	4.7610	4.5449	4.3474	4.1664	3.9998	3.3333	2.8571	2.5000	2.2222	2.0000
50	6.2463	5.8801	5.5541	5.2623	4.9995	4.7616	4.5452	4.3477	4.1666	3.9999	3.3333	2.8571	2.5000	2.2222	2.0000

7

THE INVESTMENT DECISION

LEARNING OBJECTIVES

- Explain the financial objectives of health care providers
- Evaluate various capital investment alternatives
- Calculate and interpret net present value (NPV)
- Calculate and interpret internal rate of return (IRR)

Capital Investment Decision
Decisions involving high-dollar investments expected to achieve long-term benefits for an organization.

Strategic Decision
Capital investment decision designed to increase a health care organization's strategic (long-term) position.

Expansion Decision
Capital investment decision designed to increase the operational capability of a health care organization.

Replacement Decision
Capital investment decision designed to replace older assets with newer, cost-saving ones.

Capital investment decisions involve large monetary investments expected to achieve long-term benefits for an organization. Such investments, common in health care, fall into three categories:

- **Strategic decisions:** Capital investment decisions designed to increase a health care organization's strategic (long-term) position (e.g., purchasing physician practices to increase horizontal integration)

- **Expansion decisions:** Capital investment decisions designed to increase the operational capability of a health care organization (e.g., increasing examination space in a group practice to accommodate increased volume)

- **Replacement decisions:** Capital investment decisions designed to replace older assets with newer, cost-saving ones (e.g., replacing a hospital's existing cost-accounting system with a newer, cost-saving one).

A capital investment decision has two components: determining if the investment is worthwhile, and determining how to finance the investment. Although these two decisions are interrelated, they should be separated. This chapter focuses on the first component: determining whether a capital investment should be undertaken. It is organized around three factors related to analyzing capital investment decisions: the objectives of capital investment analysis, three techniques to analyze capital investment decisions, and technical concerns related to capital budgeting. Chapter Eight focuses on capital financing alternatives. Perspectives 7–1 and 7–2 offer some examples of capital investments.

Caution: Although determining if an investment is worthwhile and how to finance the investment are interrelated, they should be considered separately.

OBJECTIVES OF CAPITAL INVESTMENT ANALYSIS

A capital investment is expected to achieve long-term benefits for the organization that generally fall into three categories: nonfinancial benefits, financial returns, and the ability to attract more funds in the future (see Exhibit 7–1). Clearly, these three objectives are highly interrelated. In the following discussion, it is important to keep in mind that "investors" are not just those external to an organization. When an organization purchases new assets or starts a new program, it is also an investor: it is investing in itself.

Perspective 7–1   Major Health Care System's Capital Spending

In 1999, the merger of two larger Catholic systems—Daughters of Charity National Health System and Sisters of St. Joseph of Nazareth system—created the St. Louis-based Ascension's health care system. The financial strength allowed the system to gain additional market share and expand its capital spending—to $1.2 billion per year through 2011. The health care system includes a range of urban, rural, and critical-access hospitals.

To support this capital spending, Ascension has more than $5.6 billion in unrestricted investments and operating revenues of over $11.2 billion, which ranks behind only two health systems: Nashville-based HCA and the federal Veterans Affairs Department. Its operating margin has increased fivefold. This sizeable revenue base has allowed Ascension to aggressively allocate over $1.6 billion of its investment portfolio into hedge funds, real estate, and private equity firms.

Its market share has enabled the system to achieve favorable rates with health plan contracts, which has raised its cash flow despite slowing patient volume. The system has also started a venture capital firm that helps fund medical devices and other health care-related companies. The criteria for allocating these funds include health care products that have the potential to improve Ascension's patient care, operations, or finances. The total amount allocated for the venture capital fund totaled $125 million, and over a five-year period, the return of the fund has been over $29 million.

Source: Evans, M. 2007 (May 14). Ascending in healthcare; Roman Catholic Ascension Health has made a Fortune 500 name for itself with business acumen, risk-taking and efficiency. *Modern Healthcare*, 37(20).

Exhibit 7–1   The objectives of the capital investment decision

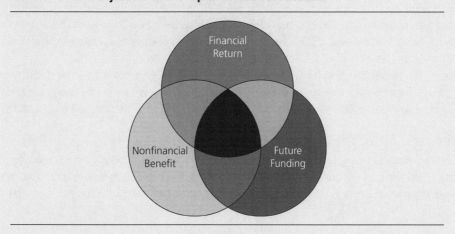

Perspective 7–2   HCA's Capital Investment after Leverage Buyout

In 2006, Hospital Corporation of America (HCA) recapitalized itself (issued debt to buy back its stock equity) by undertaking a $33 billion leveraged buyout that made it a private company again. Stock analysts expected HCA to make capital expenditures of around 6 percent of its operating revenues. Even with the high financial demands to pay off its debt payments, analysts expect that this greater level of capital spending is essential for this company to attract patients and physicians. Going forward, HCA was expected to invest on the outpatient services, especially surgery centers, as well as continue with its inpatient expansion to retain its existing levels of revenue and increase its incremental patient volume. On December 31, 2007, HCA owned 169 hospitals and operated 108 free-standing surgery centers.

In 2007, HCA sold off three of its hospitals for $661 million to help make its debt service repayment of $1.1 billion and reduce its debt load to $27 billion. In 2008, HCA was expected to sell additional hospitals in 2008 to lower its outstanding debt.

In the future, analysts expect HCA owners to generate their returns from higher multiples in stock price rather than by increasing equity through deleveraging and/or earnings growth. The owners were also projected to have a three- to five-year investment horizon before they sell the company and will more likely wait until multiples for health care stocks are higher.

Source: Galloro, V. 2008 (Feb. 11). Bad debt hits HCA; 4th quarter saw increase in uninsured. *Modern Healthcare*. p. 4.

Nonfinancial Benefits

How well an investment enhances the survival of the organization and supports its mission, patients, employees, and the community becomes a primary concern with many capital investment decisions. A particularly interesting movement in health care is the increasing number of governmental agencies with taxing authority asking for proof of community benefit. Community benefits include increased access to different types of care, higher quality of care, lower charges, the provision of charity care, and the employment of community members. Perspective 7–3 illustrates such an instance.

Financial Returns

Direct financial benefits are a primary concern not only to health care organizations, but also to many—if not all—investors who invest in health care organizations and their projects. Direct financial benefits to investors can take two forms. The first is

Perspective 7–3 Community Benefits in a Capital Investment Decision

The Palo Alto Medical Foundation (PAMF) will spend $300 million for a new medical center in San Carlos, California. However, this new capital expansion is expected to be delayed by the city's approval process. Besides traffic issues, the primary point of contention for the city relates to the inability of the new hospital to generate the tax revenues that a for-profit organization would provide. PAMF plans on guaranteeing some income to the city to offset the tax losses from property and sales tax revenue. To justify its tax-exempt status, PAMF would also support more than $25 million in community benefits over thirty years. The benefits range from a $9 million endowment for various charitable activities: $1 million investment to develop athletic fields and facilities, and $1.5 million to fund health care programs in local schools. More importantly, the new medical center is expected to fund a projected $3 million in annual medical benefits to city residents in the form of charity care, discounted care, and health education and philanthropic activities.

Source: Rauber, C. 2007 (Jan. 19). Plans for new hospital face delays. *San Francisco Business Times*. *http://sanfrancisco.bizjournals.com/sanfrancisco/stories/2007/01/22/story12.html*.

periodic payments in the form of dividends to stockholders, interest to bondholders, or both. (Bonds are discussed in Chapter Eight). *Dividends* represent the portion of profit that an organization distributes to equity investors, whereas *interest* is a payment to creditors, those who have loaned the organization funds or otherwise extended credit.

> **Retained Earnings**
> The portion of profits that an organization keeps for itself in-house to use in growth and support of its mission.

The second type of benefit to an investor is in the form of *retained earnings*, the portion of the profits the organization keeps in-house to use in growth and support of its mission. This describes the plowing back or investing of funds (including retained earnings) into capital projects that appreciate in value. *Capital appreciation* takes place whenever an investment is worth more when it is sold than when it was purchased. For investor-owned organizations, this appreciation in value increases the value of their stock.

> **Capital Appreciation**
> Occurs whenever an asset is worth more when sold than when purchased. Common examples would be land, property, or stocks.

Although almost all organizations can make periodic payments to their investors in the form of interest, by law, only investor-owned health care organizations can distribute dividends outside the organization.

Ability to Attract Funds in the Future

Without new capital funds, many health care organizations would be unable to offer new services, support medical research, or subsidize unprofitable services. Therefore, another objective of capital investment is to invest in profitable projects or services that will attract debt (borrowing) and equity financing in the future by external investors. (Capital financing is discussed at length in Chapter Eight. Capital financing includes funds from a variety of sources including government entities, foundations, and community-based organizations.)

ANALYTIC METHODS

An investment decision involves many factors (see Perspectives 7–4 and 7–5). Three commonly used financial techniques to analyze capital investment decisions for health care organizations are

- Payback
- Net present value
- Internal rate of return

Perspective 7–4 Demand for Cancer Services Creates Investment in Plant and Equipment

In Portland, Oregon, cancer care is a primary service for the area's major hospitals and medical centers. Over 20 years ago, a number of people in this city were exposed to hepatitis C through intravenous drug use or blood transfusions. As a result, area hospitals invested in cancer care including building new facilities to procuring high-tech equipment and implementing education programs. In the case of Providence Health System, it plans to open an eleven-story cancer center building at a cost of $130 million. Once the 500,000-square-foot Providence Cancer Center is built, it will support all of the cancer services, which include diagnosis, treatment, and support plus research, education, and prevention efforts. In addition, it offers an integrative medicine clinic that provides massage therapy, acupuncture, and a medical spa for cancer patients.

In the case of Kaiser Permanente health care system, its Northwest Interstate Radiation Oncology Center in North Portland has one of three linear accelerators to serve about eighty patients a day. The linear accelerators provide high doses of radiation in tightly focused beams to control and kill cancer cells. Kaiser Sunnyside Medical Center developed an inpatient palliative care program to serve cancer patients and patients suffering from other life-threatening diseases with the primary purpose to give patients increased control over their symptoms.

Source: Goldfield, R. 2007 (June 15). New cancer facilities, technology arrive at hospitals. *Portland Business Journal*. http://portland.bizjournals.com/portland/stories/2007/06/18/focus3.html

Perspective 7–5   Market Factors and Hospital Inefficiencies: A Case of Capital Investment in Rural Hospitals

Health care investors and systems invest in rural hospitals because they can achieve a greater rate of return on their investment than with hospitals located in urban markets. Rural hospitals are expected to achieve higher volume and profitability gains in excess of industry averages. Investors expect rural hospitals to generate a steady source of cash flow with significant upside returns if investors or the health care system can address inefficiencies. The upside returns are due to the vast number of nonprofit county- or city-owned facilities that are managed by administrative officials with limited hospital experience and who are not motivated to maximize cash flow. In addition, rural hospitals operate with higher staffing levels and are typically the largest employer in a county. Health care systems with an acquisition to invest in rural hospitals view them as an "add-on" to an existing platform of rural hospitals. As a platform investment, these health care systems will centralize duplicated support functions such as accounting, legal, and regulatory compliance to save costs and improve operational cash flow. The system network will also allow these hospitals to gain more leverage in negotiating reimbursement rates with various payers in any given market than would a stand-alone rural hospital.

The other benefits of a rural hospital are that they typically are located in smaller populations and are the only health care provider in their market. As a result, these facilities operate in a captive market with little pricing pressure. In addition, smaller-market rural facilities do not have to negotiate with large health plans, and therefore they are not confronted with the same pricing pressures of hospitals located in urban markets. However, rural facilities also face the out-migration of patients to urban hospitals. To combat this movement, health care systems that purchase rural hospitals invest in renovating the facility, adding new equipment, and implementing new technology.

Source: Fisk, H. 2006 (Dec. 15). Banker explains why investors are focusing on rural hospital sector. *Memphis Business Journal*. http://memphis.bizjournals.com/memphis/stories/2006/12/18/focus4.html.

Key Point *Until now, this book has stressed the accrual method of accounting. However, the techniques introduced in this chapter—payback, net present value (NPV), and the internal rate of return (IRR)—use only cash flows. Therefore, when only accrual information is available (such as information from financial statements), accrual items must be converted into cash flows. An example is shown in the discussion of net present value.*

Suppose Marquee Valley Hospital has $1,000,000 available to invest in a new business (Exhibit 7–2, Rows 1 and 3). After examining the marketplace, the hospital has narrowed its possibilities to two promising options, each of which would expend the full amount of money available: it could either buy an existing physician practice, or it could build its own small satellite clinic. If it buys the physician practice, it would expect to generate new net cash inflows of $333,333 each year for six years (Exhibit 7–2, Row 2). By investing in its own satellite clinic, Marquee Valley could expect to generate net cash flows of $200,000, $250,000, $300,000, $350,000, $450,000, and $650,000 over the next six years (Exhibit 7–2, Row 4).

Key Point *The term* cash flow *is used interchangeably with* net cash flow. Net cash flow *is the result of subtracting* cash outflows *from* cash inflows.

Payback Method
A method to evaluate the feasibility of an investment by determining how long it would take until the initial investment is recovered, disregarding the time value of money.

Payback Method

One way to analyze these investments is to calculate the time to recoup the investment. This is called the *payback method* and is illustrated in Exhibit 7–3, which builds on Exhibit 7–2.

Analysis Exhibit 7–3 shows four rows for each investment: the initial investment, the beginning balance for each year, the cash flow for each year, and the cumulative cash flow for each year, in rows A through D, respectively. Although the satellite clinic begins the fourth year with a $250,000 deficit (row B), it has a positive net cash flow of $350,000 during the year (row C), resulting in a cumulative cash flow by the end of the fourth year of $100,000. Thus, as shown in row D, during the fourth year, the hospital would have recouped its investment. By bringing in $333,333 each year, the physician practice recoups its

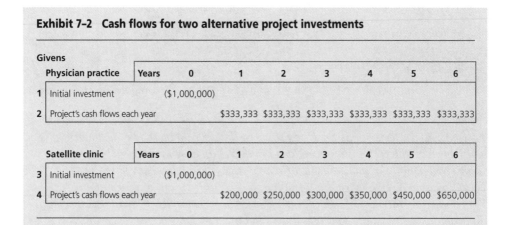

Exhibit 7–2 Cash flows for two alternative project investments

Givens								
Physician practice	**Years**	**0**	**1**	**2**	**3**	**4**	**5**	**6**
1 Initial investment		($1,000,000)						
2 Project's cash flows each year			$333,333	$333,333	$333,333	$333,333	$333,333	$333,333

Satellite clinic	**Years**	**0**	**1**	**2**	**3**	**4**	**5**	**6**
3 Initial investment		($1,000,000)						
4 Project's cash flows each year			$200,000	$250,000	$300,000	$350,000	$450,000	$650,000

Exhibit 7-3 Calculation of payback year for two alternative investments

Physician practice	Years	0	1	2	3	4	5	6
A	Initial investment	a	($1,000,000)						
B	Beginning of year balance	b		($1,000,000)	($666,667)	($333,333)	($0)	$333,333	$666,667
C	Project's cash flows each year	c		$333,333	$333,333	$333,333	$333,333	$333,333	$333,333
D	Cumulative cash flow	A + B + C	($1,000,000)	($666,667)	($333,333)	($0)	$333,333	$666,667	$1,000,000

a Exhibit 7–2, Row 1
b Balance from end of previous year, Row D
c Exhibit 7–2, Row 2
Break-even year = Year 3

Satellite clinic	Years	0	1	2	3	4	5	6
A	Initial investment	d	($1,000,000)						
B	Beginning of year balance	e		($1,000,000)	($800,000)	($550,000)	($250,000)	$100,000	$550,000
C	Project's cash flows each year	f		$200,000	$250,000	$300,000	$350,000	$450,000	$650,000
D	Cumulative cash flow	A + B + C	($1,000,000)	($800,000)	($550,000)	($250,000)	$100,000	$550,000	$1,200,000

d Exhibit 7–2, Row 3
e Balance from end of previous year, Row D
f Exhibit 7–2, Row 4
Break-even year = Year 4

$1,000,000 investment by the end of the third year. Under either scenario, the hospital would be tying up its money for at least three years.

The actual month that breakeven occurs can be obtained by dividing the deficit at the end of the year before breaking even by the average monthly inflow in the break-even year. For example, the deficit at the end of the third year for the satellite clinic is $250,000, with an average monthly inflow during the fourth year of $29,167 ($350,000 / 12). Thus, Marquee Valley would break even midway through September ($250,000 / $29,167 = 8.6 months) of the fourth year. If it bought the physician practice, it would break even at the end of the third year because it ends year 3 with no deficit.

If net cash inflows are equal each year (as with the physician practice), the number of years for an investment to break even simply equals the initial investment divided by the annual net cash flows resulting from the investment, and use of a more detailed analysis, such as in Exhibit 7–3 is unnecessary. Thus, the payback time for the physician practice would be $1,000,000 / $333,333, which equals 3 years, the same answer derived in Exhibit 7–3.

Key Point *Formula to calculate the break-even point in years if cash flows are equal each year:*

Initial Investment / Annual Cash Flows

Strengths and Weaknesses of the Payback Method The strengths of the payback method are that it is simple to calculate and easy to understand (see Exhibit 7–4). There are three major weaknesses to the payback method, however: it gives an answer in years, not dollars; it disregards cash flows after the payback time; and it does not account for the time value of money. Each of these is discussed briefly in the next section.

- *The payback is in years, not dollars.* Knowing that a project has a payback of three years does not provide key financial information such as the size of the dollar impact on the organization in future years.

- *The payback method disregards cash flows after the payback time.* For example, the physician practice has equal annual cash inflows and a payback of three

Exhibit 7–4 Strengths and weaknesses of the payback method

Strengths	Weaknesses
• Simple to calculate	• Answers in years, not dollars
• Easy to understand	• Disregards cash flows after payback
	• Does not account for the time value of money

years, whereas the satellite clinic has unequal annual cash inflows and does not reach payback until year 4. Thus, the physician practice with its shorter payback would appear to be the better investment. However, the satellite clinic has better cash flows in later years, and by the end of year 6, it brings in $200,000 more than does the physician practice. Hence, in addition to time until payback, it is important to consider the cash flows after the payback date when making an investment.

■ *The payback method does not account for the time value of money.* Chapter Six demonstrated that a dollar received sometime in the future is not worth the same as a dollar received today. The two evaluation methods discussed in the remainder of this chapter, net present value and internal rate of return, take the time value of money into account, whereas the payback method does not.

Net Present Value

Because of the deficiencies using the payback method to analyze capital investments, a preferred alternative is a net present value analysis. *Net present value* (NPV) is the difference between the initial amount paid for an investment and its associated future cash flows that have been adjusted (discounted) by the cost of capital. The cost of capital accounts for two costs: first, investors (bondholders and stockholders) are being asked to delay the consumption of their funds by investing in the project (time value of money); and second, these investors face a risk that the investment may not generate the revenues and net cash flows anticipated, leaving them with an inadequate rate of return, or the project may fail altogether, leaving the investors with perhaps nothing other than a tax loss.

Net Present Value The difference between the initial amount paid for an investment and the future cash inflows that the investment brings in, adjusted for the cost of capital.

Discounted Cash Flows Cash flows that have been adjusted to account for the cost of capital.

If the sum of the *discounted cash flows* resulting from the investment is greater than the initial investment itself, then the NPV is positive. Thus, from a purely financial standpoint, the project is acceptable, all else being equal. On the other hand, if the sum of the discounted cash flows resulting from the investment is less than the initial investment, then over time the investment brings in less than what was initially paid out, the NPV is negative, and the investment should be rejected.

Using the Satellite Clinic as an Example of a Net Present Value Analysis In the example used earlier (Exhibit 7–3), the annual cash flows were provided, but in real-world situations, organizations may not always have such information readily available. Therefore, in the following example (see Exhibit 7–5), the same annual cash flows are used as in the previous example ($200,000, $250,000, $300,000, $350,000, $450,000, and $650,000), but these numbers had to be derived using additional information commonly found in a budget forecast (revenues, expenses, depreciation, etc).

 Key Point *The following terms are used interchangeably:* cost of capital, discount rate, *and* hurdle rate.

Cost of Capital
The rate of return required to undertake a project; the cost of capital accounts for both the time value of money and risk; also called the *hurdle rate* or *discount rate*

The following steps are used to calculate the Net Present Value (NPV) of the satellite clinic alternative (Exhibit 7–5):

Step 1. Identify the initial cash outflow

Step 2. Determine revenues and expenses (net operating income):

    a. Identify annual net revenues

    b. Identify annual cash operating expenses and depreciation expense

    c. Compute annual net income

Step 3. Add back in depreciation expense to get net operating cash flows

Step 4. Add (subtract) any non-annual cash flows

Step 5. Adjust for working capital

Step 6. Determine the present value of each year's cash flow

Step 7. Sum the present values of all cash flows

Step 8. Determine the net present value of the project

1. Identify the initial cash outflow (row A).
   - The initial investment in the satellite clinic is $1,000,000
2. Determine net operating income (rows B, C, D, and E)
   - Identify annual cash inflows (revenues). Use net revenues rather than gross revenues to account for discounts and allowances that will not be collected.
   - Identify annual cash operating expenses and depreciation expense.
   - Compute annual net operating income.
3. Add back depreciation to compute net operating cash flows (rows F and G)

The annual expenses (Step 2b) include depreciation expenses, estimated at $145,000 annually. However, depreciation is an expense that does not require any cash outflow. Therefore, to calculate actual cash flows, an amount equal to depreciation expense is added back to net income, resulting in a higher cash flow.

4. Add (subtract) any non-annual cash flows (rows H and I)

Exhibit 7-5 Computation of NPV for the satellite clinic

Givens	Years	0	1	2	3	4	5	6
1 Initial investment		($1,000,000)						
2 Net revenue			$400,000	$550,000	$800,000	$900,000	$1,100,000	$1,370,000
3 Cash operating expense			$200,000	$300,000	$500,000	$550,000	$650,000	$850,000
4 Annual depreciation			$145,000	$145,000	$145,000	$145,000	$145,000	$145,000
5 Salvage value (end of year 6)								$130,000
6 Cost of capital	10%							

	Years	0	1	2	3	4	5	6
A Initial investment	Given 1	($1,000,000)						
B Net revenue	Given 2		$400,000	$550,000	$800,000	$900,000	$1,100,000	$1,370,000
C Less: cash operating expenses	Given 3		200,000	300,000	500,000	550,000	650,000	850,000
D Less: depreciation expense	Given 4		145,000	145,000	145,000	145,000	145,000	145,000
E Net operating income	B − C − D		55,000	105,000	155,000	205,000	305,000	375,000
F Add: depreciation expense	Given 4		145,000	145,000	145,000	145,000	145,000	145,000
G Net operating cash flows	E + F		200,000	250,000	300,000	350,000	450,000	520,000
H Add: sale of salvage value	Given 5							130,000
I Project cash flows	G + H		$200,000	$250,000	$300,000	$350,000	$450,000	$650,000
J Cost of capital	Given 6		10%	10%	10%	10%	10%	10%
K Present value interest factors[a]	$1/(1+i)^n$		0.9091	0.8264	0.7513	0.6830	0.6209	0.5645
L Annual PV of cash flows	I × K		$181,818	$206,612	$225,394	$239,055	$279,415	$366,908
M PV of cash flows	Sum L	$1,499,202						
N Net present value	A + M	$499,202						

[a] Present value interest factors in the table have been calculated by formula but are necessarily rounded for presentation. Therefore, there may be a difference between the number displayed and that calculated manually.

283

Some projects may have various non-annual cash flows that occur during the project. In this example, the only non-annual cash flow is a cash inflow in year 6 resulting from selling some assets of the investment project. The *salvage value* is estimated to be $130,000.

Key Point *In deriving the annual cash flows using pro forma operating statements that include depreciation expense, this or any other noncash expense (e.g., amortization of goodwill) is added back to the bottom line (operating income).*

Key Point *Interest expense should not be included as a cash flow because it is part of financing flows and is included in the discount rate. Therefore, if interest expense is included in the operating expenses, then for the non-taxpaying entity, it should be added back into revenue in excess of expenses or earnings.*

Salvage Value
The amount of cash to be received when an asset (e.g. equipment) is sold, usually at the end of its useful life; also called *terminal value, residual value,* and *scrap value*.

Goodwill
An amount paid above and beyond the book value of an asset (typically a business) when it is sold, representing the value of intangible factors such as brand reputation, customer or supplier relationships, employee competencies, and the like.

5. Adjust for working capital

Some projects affect working capital, and to the extent that this effect is material, it must be considered. This particular example assumes that there are no material working capital effects, but this concept is discussed in depth in Appendix D.

6. Determine the present value of each year's cash flow (rows I, J, K, and L)

Steps 1 through 5 estimate cash flows that will occur each year. Step 6 discounts these cash flows with an assumed discount rate of 10 percent using the methods discussed in Chapter Six. The $200,000 received at the end of year 1 (row I) is worth $181,818 in today's dollars (row L). The $250,000 received two years from now (row I) is worth only $206,612 today (row L). The cash flows received in years 3 through 6 are discounted similarly.

7. Sum the present values of all cash flows (row M)

8. Determine the net present value of the project (rows A, M, and N)

The net present value of the project is the difference between the discounted annual cash flows and the initial investment. The net present value (NPV), $499,202, is computed by adding the initial investment, $1,000,000, a cash outflow, to the present value of the annual cash flows, $1,499,202. If this were the only investment alternative, because the NPV is positive, this investment would be accepted based only on financial criteria.

Key Point *The terms* present value *and* net present value *should not be confused. Whereas present value is the sum of discounted future cash flows, net present value is equal to the present value net (less) the cost of the initial investment. Hence, in Exhibit 7–5, whereas the present value of the cash flows is $1,499,202 (the sum of the cash flows for years 1 through 6), the net present value is only $499,202 (the cash flows from years 1 through 6 less the cost of the initial $1,000,000 investment).*

It is also possible to calculate the NPV of the physician practice introduced in Exhibit 7–2. Because the cash flows from this investment are equal in both amount and timing, they can be treated as an ordinary annuity of $333,333 for six years at 10 percent. The present value factor for this ordinary annuity is 4.3553. Thus, the present value of the cash flows is $1,451,765 (4.3553 × $333,333), and the net present value of the physician practice would be $451,765 ($1,451,765 – $1,000,000).

Decision Rules Regarding NPV As noted in Exhibit 7–5, the net present value of the satellite clinic investment, after adjusting for depreciation and salvage value, is $499,202.

- The general decision rule regarding NPV is
  - If NPV > 0, accept the project.
  - If NPV < 0, reject the project.
  - If NPV = 0, then accept or reject.

Based on this rule, the satellite clinic should be purchased because it has a positive NPV of $499,202. This rule applies in most cases; however, the rule is modified for two other possible situations.

- If more than one mutually exclusive project is being considered, the one with the higher or highest positive NPV should be chosen. Thus, if a second project were being considered, such as the purchase of the physician practice, the satellite clinic project would be selected for having the higher NPV ($499,202 vs. $451,765). Only if the physician practice NPV were higher than the $499,202 would that project be selected instead.
- If more than one mutually exclusive project is being considered and one must be selected regardless of NPV, then the one with the higher or highest NPV should be chosen, even if its NPV is negative. Suppose the organization was considering developing either a burn unit or a school-based education program. An analysis determined that one project has an NPV of −$4,000,000, whereas the other has an NPV of −$1,500,000. If it had been decided in advance that one of the two projects will be undertaken, then the one with the higher NPV (lesser loss) should be chosen. In this case, –$1,500,000 would be the better choice.

Using Spreadsheets to Calculate NPV Any popular spreadsheet is an ideal platform to calculate net present value because most, if not all, have built-in functions that simplify the determination of NPV. Exhibit 7–6 shows how the NPV function in Excel can be used to compute the present value, $1,499,202, of the annual cash flows in Exhibit 7–5 (all six years' cash flows are entered, although only cash flows for the first four years are shown). Excel's NPV function is similar to its PV function, but allows for the use of unequal cash flows. Finally, the initial investment, –$1,000,000, must be added outside of the NPV function formula, which computes the present value of the annual project cash flows, $1,499,202, to obtain the NPV of $499,202. (A common mistake among users of the NPV function is to include the initial investment as a value in the NPV function formula. The initial investment must be added outside the function and needs to represent the negative outflow for the initial investment.)

Key Point *When using the Excel NPV function, the initial investment value must be added to the NPV function result and not entered as a value within the function itself.*

Strengths and Weakness of the NPV Method The NPV method has a number of strengths and weaknesses (see Exhibit 7–7). Its strengths are that it provides an answer in dollars, not years; it accounts for all cash flows in the project, including those beyond the payback period; and it discounts the cash flows at the cost of capital. Its main difficulties are developing estimates of cash flows and the discount rate.

Exhibit 7–6 Using Excel to calculate the net present value (NPV) of unequal annual cash flows, assuming a 10 percent discount rate

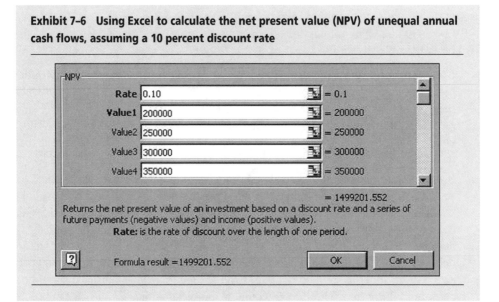

Exhibit 7-7 Strengths and weaknesses of an NPV analysis

Strengths

- Answers in dollars, not years
- Accounts for all the cash flows in the project
- Discounts at the cost of capital

Weaknesses

- Cash flow estimates may be difficult to develop
- Discount rate may be difficult to determine

Conceptually, NPV is strong because it accounts for all cash flows in a project and discounts at the cost of capital. However, the cost of capital can be difficult to determine, as discussed in Appendix C.

Internal Rate of Return (IRR)

The *internal rate of return* (IRR) on an investment can be defined and interpreted several ways. It is the discount rate at which the discounted cash flows over the life of the project exactly equal the initial investment; the discount rate that results in a net present value equal to zero; and the percentage return on the investment. In contrast, NPV is the dollar return on the investment. The method to use to solve for the IRR depends on whether the cash flows are equal or unequal.

Internal Rate of Return That rate of return on an investment that makes the net present value equal to $0, after all cash flows have been discounted at the same rate. It is also the discount rate at which the discounted cash flows over the life of the project exactly equal the initial investment.

Equal Cash Flows If the cash flows are equal each period, the IRR can be determined by first finding the present value factor for an annuity and then converting the answer to a discount rate depending on the number of years. Because the physician practice example used earlier has equal cash flows each period, its IRR can be found by:

- Computing the present value factor for an annuity (PVFA) (see Chapter Six):

$$PV = \text{Annuity} \times PVFA_{i, n}$$
$$\$1,000,000 = \$333,333 \times PVFA_{i, 6}$$
$$PVFA_{i, 6} = 3.0$$

- Finding the interest rate that yields this PVFA factor for 6 periods. In the present value of an annuity table (Appendix B, Table B–4), in the row for 6 time periods (because the investment is over 6 years), the column heading for the number closest to 3.0 (the PVFA factor) is the IRR. In this case, the

PVFA factor of 3.0 lies somewhere between the 24 percent and 25 percent columns; thus, the IRR is approximately 24.5 percent.

Unequal Cash Flows Business calculators and computer programs make finding the IRR for unequal cash flows relatively easy. Excel's function is called *IRR* (see Exhibit 7–8). All the operating cash flow values of the project, including the initial investment, either are entered individually, or else an array of cells is referenced (the initial investment must be a negative value in either case because it is a cash outflow). As shown in Exhibit 7–8, the IRR appears at the bottom of the box.

Key Point *In contrast to Excel's NPV function, the IRR function includes the initial investment as one of the entries in the function.*

Required Rate of Return An organization's minimally acceptable internal rate of return on any investment to justify an initial investment; also called *cost of capital* or *hurdle rate.*

Decision Rules with IRR When an organization chooses a project according to the IRR method, its financial decision depends on the value of the IRR relative to the *required rate of return* on the investment (which is also called the *cost of capital* or *hurdle rate*).

- If the IRR is greater than the required rate of return, the project should be accepted.

- If the IRR is less than the required rate of return, the project should be rejected.

- If the IRR is equal to the required rate of return, the facility should be indifferent about accepting or rejecting the project.

Exhibit 7–8   Using Excel to calculate the IRR of a $1,000,000 investment that yields unequal operating cash flows to be received at the end of each of six successive years

IRR

Values   A1:A7   = {-1000000;200000;2

Guess   = number

= 0.226362547

Returns the internal rate of return for a series of cash flows.

Values is an array or a reference to cells that contain numbers for which you want to calculate the internal rate of return.

Formula result =0.226362547   OK   Cancel

Note: The values in the array A1:A7 = −1000000; 200000; 250000; 300000; 350000; 450000; 650000

Strengths and Weaknesses of IRR Analysis There are three major strengths to using IRR as a decision criterion: it considers all the relevant cash flows related to the investment project; it is a time value of money-based approach; and managers are accustomed to evaluating projects by their respective rates of return. Similarly, there are three weaknesses to using internal rate of return (IRR) as a decision criterion: it assumes that proceeds are reinvested at the internal rate of return, which may or may not be equal to the cost of capital; developing estimates of cash flows is difficult; and the IRR sometimes generates multiple rates of return, if future cash flows are estimates. Still, this method is widely used in industry as the preferred way to make responsible investment decisions (see Exhibit 7–9).

USING AN NPV ANALYSIS FOR A REPLACEMENT DECISION

The previous analyses have focused on situations in which an organization was interested in either expanding its existing services or offering a new service altogether. However, a common and more complicated analysis is the replacement decision, which must be made by an organization when it contemplates replacing an older, existing asset with a newer, more cost-efficient one. There are two ways to undertake this problem, both using a net present value (NPV) approach and both yielding the same result. The first approach is to compare the NPVs of continuing as is with that of the replacement alternative, with the preferred investment alternative being the one yielding the higher NPV. The second approach is to perform a single NPV analysis using the *incremental differences* brought about by replacing an asset. If the single NPV is positive, then the replacement alternative is preferred.

Illustrative Example

Assume that a radiology department in a not-for-profit organization is considering renovating its x-ray processing area with new equipment that is faster and produces

---

Exhibit 7–9 Strengths and weaknesses of the IRR analysis

Strengths

- Considers all relevant cash flows of the investment project
- Time value of money-based approach
- Widely used by practitioners and easily understood

Weaknesses

- Assumes reinvestment of proceeds at the internal rate of return
- Estimates may be difficult to develop
- Can generate multiple rates of return if future cash flows are estimates

better, more reliable images. The existing equipment was purchased five years ago for $1,150,000 and is being depreciated on a *straight-line* basis over a ten-year life to a $150,000 salvage value. The old equipment can be sold now for its current book value of $650,000 ($1,150,000 original cost less $500,000 in accumulated depreciation).

The new equipment can be purchased for $1,500,000 and is estimated to have a five-year life. It would be depreciated on a straight-line basis to a $750,000 salvage value. The radiology department is a revenue-producing center. Presently, 45 patients per day, 260 days per year, can be screened by one radiology technologist at an average reimbursement of $75 per test, but a significant portion of these patients must be given a second test at no additional charge because the first image is inconclusive. The new equipment, because it is not only faster but produces images of better quality, can process 60 patients per day. (In this example, the hospital believes that sufficient demand exists to fully utilize the higher capacity of the new equipment.) An in-depth discussion of how to estimate future cash flows is found in Appendix C.

The old equipment costs $60,000 per year in utilities and maintenance. The new equipment would cost $30,000 per year in utilities and maintenance. The annual labor expenses will not change because one radiology technologist is needed to operate either piece of equipment. Cost of capital for this organization is 9 percent.

Solution

Exhibits 7–10a and 7–10b present the *comparative approach* to solve this problem. This approach employs the same eight steps outlined in Exhibit 7–5. An NPV is calculated for each alternative, and then the NPVs are compared to determine which is higher. As an alternative method, Exhibit 7–11 uses the *incremental approach* to solve the same problem, whereby instead of calculating two NPVs and comparing them, it calculates a single NPV based on marginal differences for each cash flow. The results are exactly the same.

Using the comparative approach, the net present value (NPV) over the next five years for the new equipment, $4,071,651 (Exhibit 7–10b, row N), is higher than that of the old equipment, $3,277,280 (Exhibit 7–10a, row N). Therefore, the decision in this case would be to renovate the area with the new equipment. Similarly, using the incremental approach, the NPV is $794,371 (Exhibit 7–11, row N). Thus, because the NPV is positive, the replacement decision should be made. Incidentally, note that the $794,371 NPV using the incremental method is exactly the difference between the two alternatives ($4,071,651 – $3,277,280) using the comparative approach. Thus, the results are the same using either method; just the method of calculation differs.

Before making a final decision, however, several issues must be considered:

■ The purchase of a new asset typically requires a large up-front expenditure, which may not always be feasible

■ Future cash flows are difficult to determine and may not always be accurate, especially the salvage value

Exhibit 7–10a NPV comparative analysis of a replacement decision: old equipment

Cash flows with the old equipment

Givens

1	Initial investment	$0
2	Annual revenues[a]	$877,500
3	Annual cash operating expenses	$60,000
4	Annual depreciation[b]	$100,000
5	Salvage value at 10 years (5 years hence)	$150,000
6	Cost of capital	9%

[a] $75 / exam × 45 exams / day × 260 operating days / year
[b] ($1,150,000 initial cost − $150,000 salvage value) / 10 years

		Years	0	1	2	3	4	5
A	Initial investment		$0					
B	Net revenues	Given 1		$877,500	$877,500	$877,500	$877,500	$877,500
C	Less: cash operating expenses	Given 2		60,000	60,000	60,000	60,000	60,000
D	Less: depreciation expense	Given 3		100,000	100,000	100,000	100,000	100,000
E	Operating income	B − C − D		717,500	717,500	717,500	717,500	717,500
F	Add: depreciation expense	Given 4		100,000	100,000	100,000	100,000	100,000
G	Net operating cash flows	E + F		817,500	817,500	817,500	817,500	817,500
H	Add: sale of salvage	Given 5						150,000
I	Project cash flows	G + H		$817,500	$817,500	$817,500	$817,500	$967,500
J	Cost of capital	Given 6		9%	9%	9%	9%	9%
K	Present value interest factors	$1/(1+i)^n$		0.9174	0.8417	0.7722	0.7084	0.6499
L	Annual PV of cash flows[c]	I × K		$750,000	$688,073	$631,260	$579,138	$628,809
M	PV of cash flows	Sum L	$3,277,280					
N	**Net present value**	A + M	**$3,277,280**					

[c] Present value interest factors in the exhibit have been calculated by formula, but are necessarily rounded for presentation. Therefore, there may be a difference between the number displayed and that calculated manually.

Exhibit 7–10b NPV comparative analysis of a replacement decision: new equipment

Cash flows with the new equipment

Givens

1	Initial investment amount[a]	($850,000)
2	Annual revenues[b]	$1,170,000
3	Annual cash operating expenses	$30,000
4	Annual depreciation[c]	$150,000
5	Salvage value (5 years hence)	$750,000
6	Cost of capital	9%

[a] −$1,500,000 initial cost + $650,000 sale of old equipment.
[b] $75 / exam × 60 exams / day × 260 operating days / year.
[c] ($1,500,000 initial cost − $750,000 salvage value) / 5 years.

	Years	0	1	2	3	4	5
A Initial investment	Given 1	($850,000)					
B Net revenues	Given 2		$1,170,000	$1,170,000	$1,170,000	$1,170,000	$1,170,000
C Less: cash operating expenses	Given 3		30,000	30,000	30,000	30,000	30,000
D Less: depreciation expense	Given 4		150,000	150,000	150,000	150,000	150,000
E Operating income	B − C − D		990,000	990,000	990,000	990,000	990,000
F Add: depreciation expense	Given 4		150,000	150,000	150,000	150,000	150,000
G Net operating cash flows	E + F		1,140,000	1,140,000	1,140,000	1,140,000	1,140,000
H Add: sale of salvage value	Given 5						750,000
I Project cash flows	G + H		$1,140,000	$1,140,000	$1,140,000	$1,140,000	$1,890,000
J Cost of capital	Given 6		9%	9%	9%	9%	9%
K Present value interest factors	1 / (1 + i)ⁿ		0.9174	0.8417	0.7722	0.7084	0.6499
L Annual PV of cash flows[d]	I × K		$1,045,872	$959,515	$880,289	$807,605	$1,228,370
M PV of cash flows	Sum L	$4,921,651					
N Net present value	A + M	**$4,071,651**					

[d] Present value interest factors in the exhibit have been calculated by formula, but are necessarily rounded for presentation. Therefore, there may be a difference between the number displayed and that calculated manually.

Exhibit 7-11 NPV analysis of a replacement decision: the incremental approach

Cash flows

Givens	Old Equipment	New Equipment	Incremental Difference (New − Old)	Incremental = New − Old
1 Initial investment		($850,000)	($850,000)	
2 Annual revenues[a]	$877,500	$1,170,000	$292,500	Incremental net revenues
3 Annual cash operating expenses	($60,000)	($30,000)	$30,000	Incremental operating cash savings
4 Annual depreciation[b]	$100,000	$150,000	$50,000	Incremental depreciation expenses
5 Salvage value	$150,000	$750,000	$600,000	Incremental salvage value
6 Cost of capital			9%	

[a] Old: $75 / exam × 45 exams / day × 260 operating days / year. New: $75 / exam × 60 exams / day × 260 operating days / year.
[b] Old: ($1,150,000 initial cost − $150,000 salvage value) / 10 years. New: ($1,500,000 initial cost − $750,000 salvage value) / 5 years.

	Years	0	1	2	3	4	5
A Initial investment	Given 1	($850,000)					
B Incremental net revenues	Given 2		$292,500	$292,500	$292,500	$292,500	$292,500
C Incremental operating cash savings	Given 3		30,000	30,000	30,000	30,000	30,000
D Incremental depreciation expenses	Given 4		50,000	50,000	50,000	50,000	50,000
E Incremental net operating income	(B + C) − D		272,500	272,500	272,500	272,500	272,500
F Add: incremental depreciation	Given 4		50,000	50,000	50,000	50,000	50,000
G Incremental net operating cash flow	E + F		322,500	322,500	322,500	322,500	322,500
H Add: incremental salvage value	Given 5						600,000
I Project incremental cash flows	G + H		$322,500	$322,500	$322,500	$322,500	$922,500
J Cost of capital	Given 6		9%	9%	9%	9%	9%
K Present value interest factors	$1/(1+i)^n$		0.9174	0.8417	0.7722	0.7084	0.6499
L Annual PV of incremental cash flows[c]	I × K		$295,872	$271,442	$249,029	$228,467	$599,562
M PV of incremental cash flows	Sum L	$1,644,371					
N Net present value	A + M	**$794,371**					

[c] Present value interest factors in the exhibit have been calculated by formula, but are necessarily rounded for presentation. Therefore, there may be a difference between the number displayed and that calculated manually.

- The exact cost of capital is difficult to determine

- Although not the case here, replacement of an old asset with a new asset may be more expensive (i.e., $NPV_{New} < NPV_{Old}$), but replacement may be necessary for other reasons, such as to remain competitive by being able to offer the latest technology to consumers.

SUMMARY

This chapter introduces three methods to evaluate large-dollar, multiyear investment decisions: payback, net present value, and internal rate of return. The payback method measures how long it takes to recover the initial investment. The strengths of the payback method are that it is simple to calculate and easy to understand. Its major weaknesses are that it does not account for the time value of money; it provides an answer in years, not dollars; and it disregards cash flows after the payback.

The NPV method overcomes the weaknesses of the payback method by accounting for cash flows after payback and discounting these cash flows by the project's cost of capital. The project's cost of capital is the rate of return that compensates investors for the time value of money and for the risk of the investment. The NPV measures the difference between the present value of the operating cash flows generated by the investment and the initial cost of that investment. The NPV technique measures the dollar return on the investment.

The general decision rule regarding NPV is: if NPV > 0, accept the project; if NPV < 0, reject the project; if NPV $= 0$, then accept or reject. If more than one mutually exclusive project is being considered, then the one with the higher or highest positive NPV should be chosen. If more than one mutually exclusive project is

being considered and one must be undertaken regardless of the NPV, then the one with the higher or highest NPV should be chosen, even if the NPV is negative.

The strengths of the NPV method of capital investment analysis are that it provides an answer in dollars, not years; it accounts for all cash flows from the project, including those beyond the payback period; and it discounts these cash flows at the cost of capital. The major weakness to the NPV method is that the discount rate is often difficult to determine and may be hard to justify. The calculation of an NPV can be accomplished in the eight steps presented in the chapter.

Step 1. Identify the initial cash outflow.

Step 2. Determine revenues and expenses (net income):

a. Identify annual net revenues.

b. Identify annual cash operating expenses and depreciation expense.

c. Compute annual net income.

Step 3. Add back in depreciation expense to get net operating cash flows.

Step 4. Add (subtract) any non-annual cash flows.

Step 5. Adjust for working capital.

Step 6. Determine the present value of each year's cash flow.

Step 7. Sum the present values of all cash flows.

Step 8. Determine the net present value of the project.

The IRR method determines the actual percentage return on the investment. When an organization chooses a project according to the IRR method, its decision depends on the value of the IRR relative to the required rate of return on the investment (also called the cost of capital or hurdle rate).

- If the IRR is greater than the required rate of return, the project should be accepted.

- If the IRR is less than the required rate of return, the project should be rejected.

- If the IRR is equal to the required rate of return, the facility should be indifferent about accepting or rejecting the project.

KEY TERMS

a. Cannibalization
b. Capital appreciation
c. Capital investment decisions
d. Capital investments
e. Cost of capital
f. Discount rate
g. Discounted cash flows
h. Dividends
i. Expansion decision
j. Goodwill
k. Hurdle rate
l. Incremental cash flows
m. Interest
n. Internal rate of return
o. Internal rate of return method
p. Net present value

q. Net present value method
r. Non-regular cash flows
s. Operating cash flows
t. Opportunity costs
u. Payback method
v. Regular cash flows
w. Replacement decision
x. Required rate of return
y. Residual value
z. Retained earnings
aa. Salvage value
bb. Scrap value
cc. Straight-line depreciation
dd. Strategic decision
ee. Sunk costs
ff. Terminal value

KEY EQUATION

Payback in years if cash flows are equal each year:

Initial Investment / Annual Cash Flows

QUESTIONS AND PROBLEMS

Note: Questions and problems include materials from the Appendices following this chapter.

1. Define the terms listed on the previous page.

2. Comment on the following statement: When a not-for-profit facility receives a contribution from a member of the community, the cost of capital is inconsequential when deciding how to use this contribution because it is, in effect, free money.

3. From a capital investment point of view, what are the goals of a health care facility?

4. What are the primary drawbacks of the payback method as a capital budgeting technique?

5. When using the IRR approach, when can the internal rate of return be determined simply by dividing the initial outlay by the cash flows?

6. Explain why pro forma income statements adjust for depreciation expense when developing projected cash flows for a project.

7. If a hospital were considering a new Women's Health Initiative, what spillover cash flows might result?

8. When performing a capital budgeting analysis, what costs should be included, and what costs should be excluded as part of the initial investment?

9. Why are financing flows such as interest expense and dividend payments excluded from the computation of cash flows?

10. Will a decision that is based on NPV ever change if it were based on IRR instead? Why or why not?

11. Marleboro Memorial Hospital is expecting its new cancer center to generate the following cash flows:

Givens	Years	0	1	2	3	4	5
Initial investment		($20,000,000)					
Net operating cash flows			$4,000,000	$6,000,000	$10,000,000	$12,000,000	$25,000,000

a. Determine the payback for the new cancer center.

b. Determine the net present value using a cost of capital of 12 percent.

c. Determine the net present value at a cost of capital of 16 percent, and compute the internal rate of return.

d. At a 12 percent cost of capital, should the project be accepted? At a16 percent cost of capital, should the project be accepted? Explain.

12. Buxton Community is expecting its new dialysis unit to generate the following cash flows:

Givens	Years	0	1	2	3	4	5
Initial investment		($10,000,000)					
Net operating cash flows			$1,500,000	$2,000,000	$4,000,000	$7,000,000	$14,000,000

a. Determine the payback for the new dialysis unit.

b. Determine the NPV using a cost of capital of 11 percent.

c. Determine the NPV at a cost of capital of 20 percent and compute the IRR.

d. At an 11 percent cost of capital, should the project be accepted? At a 20 percent cost of capital, should the project be accepted? Explain.

13. Letterman Hospital expects Projects A and B to generate the following cash flows:

Givens (in thousands)	Years	0	1	2	3	4	5
1 Initial investment		($2,500)					
2 Net operating cash flows for Project A			$1,800	$1,600	$900	$400	$200
3 Net operating cash flows for Project B			$200	$400	$900	$1,600	$1,800
4 Discount rate for Part a	15%						
5 Discount rate for Part b	5%						

a. Determine the NPV for both projects using a cost of capital of 15 percent.

b. Determine the NPV for both projects using a cost of capital of 5 percent.

c. At a 5 percent cost of capital, which project should be accepted? At a 15 percent cost of capital, which project should be accepted? Explain.

14. Castle Rock Medical Center expects Projects X and Y to generate the following cash flows:

Givens (in thousands)	Years	0	1	2	3	4	5
Initial investment		($6,500)					
Net operating cash flows for Project X			$5,000	$3,000	$2,000	$1,600	$1,000
Net operating cash flows for Project Y			$1,000	$1,600	$2,000	$3,000	$5,000
Discount rate for Part a	13%						
Discount rate for Part b	8%						

a. Determine the NPV for both projects using a cost of capital of 13 percent.

b. Determine the NPV for both projects using a cost of capital of 8 percent.

c. At an 8 percent discount rate, which project should be accepted? At a 13 percent discount rate, which project should be accepted? Explain.

15. Goodbar Practice expects projects 1 and 2 to generate the following cash flows:

Project 1 (in thousands)	Years	0	1	2	3	4	5
Givens							
Initial investment		($2,000)					
Net operating cash flows			$200	$300	$500	$1,000	$1,790

Project 2 (in thousands)	Years	0	1	2	3	4	5
Givens							
Initial investment		($3,800)					
Net operating cash flows			$1,000	$1,000	$1,000	$1,000	$1,000

a. Determine the payback for both projects.

b. Determine the IRR.

c. Determine the NPV at a cost of capital of 12 percent.

16. Martin Medical expects Alpha Project and Beta Project to generate the following:

Alpha Project 1 (in thousands)	Years	0	1	2	3	4	5
Givens							
Initial investment		($16,000)					
Net operating cash flows			($8,000)	$5,000	$10,000	$14,000	$24,000

Beta Project 2 (in thousands)	Years	0	1	2	3	4	5
Givens							
Initial investment		($24,000)					
Net operating cash flows			$6,000	$6,000	$6,000	$6,000	$6,000

a. Determine the payback for both projects.

b. Determine the IRR.

c. Determine the NPV at a cost of capital of 14 percent.

17. Tin Man Memorial Hospital, a non-taxpaying entity, is starting a new inpatient heart center on its third floor. The expected patient volume demands will generate $4,500,000 per year in revenues for the next five years. The new center will incur operating expenses, excluding depreciation, of $2,500,000 per year for the next five years. The initial cost of building and equipment is $6,500,000. Straight-line depreciation is used to estimate depreciation expense, and the building and equipment will be depreciated over a five-year life to their salvage value. The expected salvage value of the building and equipment at year five is $500,000. The cost of capital for this project is 8 percent.

a. Compute the NPV and IRR to determine the financial feasibility of this project.

b. Compute the NPV and IRR to determine the financial feasibility of this project if this were a taxpaying entity with a tax rate of 40 percent. (*Hint*: see Appendix E. Because the hospital is depreciating to the salvage value, there is no tax effect on the sale of the asset.)

18. Fall City Healthcare System, a non-taxpaying entity, is planning to purchase imaging equipment, including an MRI and ultrasonograms for its new imaging center. The equipment will generate $2,500,000 per year in revenues for the next five years. The expected operating expenses, excluding depreciation, will increase expenses by $950,000 per year for the next five years. The initial capital investment outlay for the imaging equipment is $4,500,000, which will be

depreciated on a straight-line basis to its salvage value. The salvage value at year five is $500,000. The cost of capital for this project is 9 percent.

a. Compute the NPV and IRR to determine the financial feasibility of this project.

b. Compute the NPV and IRR to determine the financial feasibility of this project if this were a taxpaying entity with a tax rate of 35 percent. (*Hint*: see Appendix E. Because the organization is depreciating to the salvage value, there is no tax effect on the sale of the asset.)

19. Due to rising utility costs, Eastern Community Hospital wants to replace its existing computer-controlled heating and cooling system (heating, ventilation, and air-conditioning [HVAC]) with a more efficient version. The existing system was purchased three years ago for $240,000 and is being depreciated on a straight-line basis over an eight-year life to zero salvage value. Although the current book value for the existing system is $150,000, this system could be sold for only $80,000 today. The new system would cost $500,000 and would be depreciated on a straight-line basis over a five-year life to a zero salvage value. The new heating and cooling system would reduce utility costs by $185,000 per year for five years and would not affect the level of net working capital. The economic life of the new system is five years, and the required rate of return on the project is 5 percent.

a. Should the existing HVAC system be replaced? Use the incremental NPV approach to evaluate the decision under a nonprofit assumption.

b. If the facility were a taxpaying entity with a tax rate of 40 percent, should the existing HVAC system be replaced? Use the incremental NPV approach to evaluate the decision. (*Hint*: see Appendix F.)

20. Because of its inability to control film and personnel costs in its radiology department, Carbone Valley Regional Hospital wants to replace its existing picture archive and communication (PAC) system with a newer version. The existing system, which has a current book value of $3,000,000, was purchased three years ago for $4,800,000 and is being depreciated on a straight-line basis over an eight-year life to zero salvage value. This system could be sold for $1,000,000 today. The new PAC system would reduce the need for staff by eight people per year for five years at a savings of $50,000 per person per year, and it would reduce film costs by $2,000,000 per year. The project would not affect the level of net working capital. The new PAC system would cost $10,000,000 and would be depreciated on a straight-line basis over a five-year life to a zero salvage value. The economic life of the new system is five years, and the required rate of return on the project is 6 percent.

a. Should the existing PAC system be replaced? Use the incremental NPV approach to evaluate the decision under a nonprofit assumption.

b. If the facility were a taxpaying entity with a tax rate of 40 percent, should the existing PAC system be replaced? Use the incremental NPV approach to evaluate the decision. (*Hint*: see Appendix F.)

21. Washington Federal Hospital plans to invest in a new MRI. The cost of the MRI is $1,500,000. The machine has an economic life of seven years, and it will be depreciated over a seven-year life to a $100,000 salvage value. Additional revenues attributed to the new machine will amount to $1,250,000 per year for seven years. Additional operating costs, excluding depreciation expense, will amount to $1,000,000 per year for seven years. Over the life of the machine, net working capital will increase by $25,000 per year for seven years.

a. Assuming that Washington Federal is a nontaxpaying entity, what is the project's NPV at a discount rate of 7 percent, and what is the project's IRR? Is the decision to accept or reject the same under either capital budgeting method, or does it differ?

b. Assuming that Washington Federal is a taxpaying entity and its tax rate is 40 percent, what is the project's NPV at a discount rate of 7 percent, and what is the project's IRR? Is the decision to accept or reject the same under either capital budgeting method, or does it differ? (*Hint*: see Appendices C, D, and E.)

22. Lima Oncology Center has seen a growth in patient volume since its primary competitor decided to relocate to a different area of the city. To accommodate this growth, a consultant has advised Lima to invest in a positron emission tomography (PET) scanner. The cost to implement the unit would be $3,700,000. The useful life of this equipment is typically about seven years, and it will be depreciated over a seven-year life to a $200,000 salvage value. Additional patient volume will yield $2,200,000 in new revenues the first year. These first-year total revenues will increase by $600,000 each year thereafter, but the unit is expensive to operate. Additional staff and variable costs, excluding depreciation expense, will come to $2,000,000 the first year, but these expenses are expected to rise by $400,000 each year thereafter. Over the life of the machine, net working capital will increase by $15,000 per year for seven years.

a. Assuming that Lima Oncology Center is a non-taxpaying entity, what is the project's NPV at a discount rate of 8 percent, and what is the project's IRR? Depending on the method used, what is the investment decision?

b. Assuming that Lima Oncology Center is a taxpaying entity and its tax rate is 35 percent, what is the project's NPV at a discount rate of 8 percent, and what is the project's IRR? Depending on the method used, what is the investment decision? (*Hint*: see Appendices C, D, and E.)

23. Rehab Center of Merion, Inc., owns an abandoned schoolhouse. The after-tax value of the land is $600,000. The furniture and fixtures of the school have been fully depreciated to an after-tax market value of $50,000. The two options the Rehab Center faces are either to sell the land and furniture and fixtures or to convert the building into a 40-bed free-standing rehabilitation hospital. To refurbish and renovate the facility would cost $4,000,000. The new building and equipment would be depreciated on a straight-line basis over a ten-year life to a $500,000 salvage value. At the end of ten years, the land could be sold for an after-tax value of $3,000,000. The new rehab facility lists its pro forma income statement below for the next ten years. Net working capital will increase at a rate of $15,000 per year over the life of the project. Rehab Center of Merion, Inc., has a 30 percent tax rate and a required rate of return of 7 percent. Use both the NPV technique and IRR method to evaluate this project. (*Hint*: see Appendices C, D, and E.)

Pro forma income statement	Years 1–5	Years 6–10
Net patient revenues / year	$7.5 million / year	$9.0 million / year
Operating expenses (excludes depreciation expense) / year	$7.0 million / year	$8.0 million / year

24. Ridgewood Healthcare Enterprises is in possession of a nonoperational 50-bed hospital. The after-tax value of the land is $2,000,000. The equipment and the building are fully depreciated and have an after-tax market value of $3,250,000. Ridgewood could either sell off its property or convert it into a new state-of-the-art acute care hospital. An analysis of the market reveals that the facility could attract 8,400 discharges per year, which is expected to increase at a rate of 3 percent per year. Projected net patient revenue per discharge is $9,000 for the first year and will increase annually by 4 percent thereafter. Projected operating expense per discharge is $7,500 for the first year and will increase annually by 6 percent thereafter. Renovation costs to create a plush facility would be $40,000,000. The new facility would be depreciated on a straight-line basis over a ten-year life to a $10 million salvage value. At the end of ten years, the land is expected to be sold for an after-tax value of $5 million. Net working capital will increase at a rate of $3,000,000 per year over the life of the project. Ridgewood has a 35 percent tax rate and a required rate of return of 9 percent. Use the NPV technique and IRR method to evaluate this project. (*Hint*: see Appendices C, D, and E.)

25. Faith Hospital, a taxpaying entity, wants to replace its current labor-intensive telemedicine system with a new automated version that would cost $3,000,000 to purchase. This new system has a five-year life and would be depreciated over a straight-line basis to a salvage value of $250,000. The current telemedicine system was purchased five years ago for $1,500,000,

has five years remaining on its useful life, and would be depreciated similarly to a salvage value of $200,000. This current system could be sold in the marketplace now for $300,000. The new telemedicine system has annual labor operating costs of $175,000, whereas the current system has annual labor operating costs of $900,000. Neither system will change patient revenues. The hospital has a 40 percent tax rate and required rate of return of 6 percent. The financial analysis will be projected over a five-year period. Use the NPV approach to determine if the new telemedicine system should be selected. (*Hint*: see Appendix F.)

26. Newtown Imaging Center, a for-profit institution, wants to replace its film-based mammography equipment with new digital models. The cost of the new digital models is $3,000,000. The current models were purchased three years ago for $1,300,000. The new digital models have a five-year life and will be depreciated over a straight-line basis to a salvage value of $500,000. The current models have five years remaining on their useful lives and will be depreciated over a straight-line basis to a salvage value of $300,000. The current models could be sold in the marketplace for $1,000,000. The new models are expected to generate annual cash cost savings on film of $400,000 per year relative to the current models. Neither system will change patient revenues. The imaging center has a 40 percent tax rate and required rate of return of 5 percent. The financial analysis will project over a five-year period. Use the NPV approach to determine if the new digital model should be selected. (*Hint*: see Appendix F.)

27. Alvin Hospital, a taxpaying entity, is considering a new ambulatory surgical center (ASC). The building and equipment for the new ASC will cost $5,000,000. The equipment and building will be depreciated on a straight-line basis over the project's five-year life to a $2,000,000 salvage value. The new ASC's projected net revenue and expenses are as follows. Net revenues are expected to be $4,800,000 the first year and will grow by 6 percent each year thereafter. The operating expenses, which exclude interest and depreciation expenses, will be $4,200,000 the first year and are expected to grow annually by 3 percent for every year after that. Interest expense will be $500,000 per year, and principal payments on the loan will be $1,000,000 a year. In the first year of operation, the new ASC is expected to generate additional after-tax cash flows of $500,000 from radiology and other ancillary services, which will grow at an annual rate of 5 percent per year for every year after that. Starting in year 1, net working capital will increase by $350,000 per year for the first four years, but during the last year of the project, net working capital will decrease by $250,000. The tax rate for the hospital is 40 percent, and its cost of capital is 15 percent. Use both the NPV and IRR approaches to determine if this project should be undertaken. (*Hint*: see Appendices C, D, and E.)

28. Blackmoore Health System, a taxpaying entity, is considering a new orthopedic center. The building and equipment for the new center will cost $7,000,000. The equipment and building will be depreciated on a straight-line basis over its five-year life to a $2,000,000 salvage value. The new orthopedic center's projected net revenue and expenses are listed below. The project will be financed partially by debt capital. Interest expense is expected to be $500,000 per year, and principal payments on the bank loan are expected to be $1,250,000 per year for the first five years of the loan. The new orthopedic center is expected to take away after-tax cash profits of $1,000,000 per year from inpatient orthopedic services. The tax rate for the institution is 40 percent, and its cost of capital is 10 percent. Two years ago, a $100,000 financial feasibility study was conducted and paid for. Pro forma working capital projections are listed below. These are the permanent account balances for inventory, accounts receivable, and accounts payable. Use the NPV and IRR approaches to determine if this project should be undertaken. (*Hint*: see Appendices C and E.)

Pro forma income statement before tax projections for the orthopedic center (in thousands)

Year	1	2	3	4	5
Net revenues	$6,000	$9,000	$11,000	$13,000	$15,000
Operating expenses	$5,500	$6,000	$6,500	$7,000	$8,000
Depreciation expense	$1,000	$1,000	$1,000	$1,000	$1,000
Interest expense	$500	$500	$500	$500	$500

Pro forma working capital for the orthopedic center (in thousands)

Year	1	2	3	4	5
Inventory / accounts receivable	$2,000	$3,000	$3,500	$2,500	$1,500
Accounts payable	$500	$1,000	$1,500	$2,000	$1,250

APPENDIX C

TECHNICAL CONCERNS REGARDING NET PRESENT VALUE

This appendix addresses three commonly asked questions about performing a net present value analysis:

- Determining the amount of the initial investment
- Determining the annual cash flows
- Determining a discount rate

DETERMINING THE AMOUNT OF THE INITIAL INVESTMENT

Included Costs

Expenditures for plant, property, and equipment usually comprise the primary initial investment items in a capital project. The amount recorded for these items is the purchase price plus all costs related to making the investment "ready to go," including labor, renovation of space, rewiring, transportation, and any investment in working capital (cash, inventory).

Along with these relatively tangible costs, the initial investment should include any additional planning costs incurred specifically for the project after it has been selected. General planning costs to decide which capital project to undertake would not be included because they are *sunk costs* (those costs incurred before a specific project has been selected).

Sunk Costs
Costs incurred in the past (they should not be included in NPV-type analyses).

Opportunity Costs
Lost proceeds by
forgoing or delaying
other opportunities.
The final category of costs to include in the initial cost estimate is the *opportunity cost*, which is proceeds lost by forgoing other opportunities. For example, suppose a health care facility has a plot of land it is holding for investment purposes on which it could build a long-term care facility. If it builds on the land, it will be earning a profit of $150,000 per year from the new facility; even though no cash is changing hands yet, losing the chance to collect $150,000 is a real cost to the organization. Thus, $150,000 would be included as part of the initial outlay as an opportunity cost or a cash outflow if the organization chose to delay building or not to build altogether.

Excluded Costs

In an NPV analysis, several categories of costs should explicitly not be included as part of the initial investment costs. For example, though the purchase price of assets should be included in the initial cost, interest paid from borrowing money to finance those assets should not be included because interest costs are financing flows and are reflected in the cost of capital.

Costs that have already occurred in the past are sunk costs and should not be included in the analysis. For example, $50,000 already spent by the health care organization to renovate a building should not be included as part of the cost for a new project. The initial investment should include only the cost of plant, property, and equipment; investment in working capital; additional planning costs; and opportunity costs (see Exhibit C–1).

DETERMINING THE ANNUAL CASH FLOWS

Incremental Cash Flows
Cash flows that occur
solely as a result of a
particular action, such as
undertaking a project.
An NPV analysis evaluates the relationship between an initial investment and the *incremental cash flows* in the future resulting from that investment. There are three types of incremental cash flows: operating, spillover, and non-regular.

Exhibit C-1 Initial costs of an investment

Included costs

- Plant, property, and equipment, and related preparation costs
- Additional planning costs
- Opportunity costs

Excluded costs

- Interest costs
- Sunk costs

Operating Cash Flows

Incremental operating cash flows are the new ongoing cash flows that occur solely as a result of undertaking a project. They include payments received for services rendered and expenditures for such things as labor, materials, marketing, utilities, and taxes. Excluded from NPV analyses are principal and interest payments made on loans to finance the project and any dividends that may result from the project. The purpose of maintaining this separation is to assess whether a project can generate enough positive cash flows from operations on its own merits to pay off its financing costs (interest, principal payments, and dividends).

Key Point *Operating flows are kept separate from financing flows. Operating cash flows include revenues, labor and supply expenses, etc. Financing cash flows include interest expenses, principal payments, and dividends.*

To realize these flows under the cash basis of accounting, the revenue and expense accounts are converted to a cash basis by changes in net working capital. These adjustments are discussed under the example for computing cash flows in Appendix D.

Key Point *If a facility is a for-profit organization, a project's positive net cash flows also entail tax payments according to the organization's tax rate. Therefore, operating cash flows are calculated* after tax. *Appendix E provides a detailed example of how to generate appropriate cash flows for taxable entities.*

Spillover Cash Flows

Spillover cash flows, which can be classified into two types, are increases or decreases in cash flows that occur elsewhere in an organization if a project is undertaken. The first type occurs when a new service produces additional cash flow to other departments. For example, if a facility were expanding its emergency department, additional revenues could be generated by ancillary support services, such as radiology or laboratory. The second type occurs when a new service diminishes cash flow elsewhere, sometimes called *cannibalization*. For example, if a facility were evaluating the development of an outpatient diagnostic center, it would have to consider the expected loss in cash flow for the existing inpatient diagnostic center. This loss in cash profits for inpatient services is a cash outflow.

Cannibalization
When a new service decreases the revenues from other services or service lines; these are considered cash outflows.

Operating Cash Flows
Cash flows that occur on a regular basis, often following implementation of a project; also called *regular cash* flows.

Non-Regular Cash Flows
Cash flows that occur sporadically or on an irregular basis. A common non-regular cash flow is salvage value, the receipt of funds following a one-time sale of an asset at the end of its useful life.

Non-regular Cash Flow and Terminal Value Cash Flow

As opposed to *operating cash flows*, which by definition occur on a regular basis, *non-regular cash flows* are incremental cash flows that typically occur on an irregular basis, typically at the end of the life of a project. One of the most common non-regular cash flows is salvage value, the money received from selling an asset at the termination of a project. Another typical cash flow at the end of a project's life is recovery of working capital, typically a cash inflow. Exhibit C–2 describes cash flows to be included or excluded, and Appendix D discusses the recovery of working capital.

Accuracy of Cash Flow Estimates

Because cash flows occur at some point in the future, they cannot be measured precisely. Expected revenues or projected cost savings can only be estimated based on a market analysis and the current operations of the organization. Unforeseeable events, such as new competition or an unexpected rise in energy prices, could significantly cut back on positive cash inflow. On the other hand, an investment such as a convenient new visitor parking deck may be so popular that it draws in unexpected patient volume, which would

---

Exhibit C–2   The components of incremental cash flows

Included items	Excluded items
Operating cash flows	***Existing cash flows not affected by the project being considered***
• Revenues in the form of payments (inflows)	
• Cash payments for labor, supplies, utilities, marketing, and taxes (outflows)	• Revenues already being generated by an existing service
Spillover cash flows	***Financing-related items***
• Effects of a new service on other departments, such as ancillary services (inflows)	• Interest
	• Principal payments
• Effects of a new service's cannibalizing similar existing services (outflows)	• Dividends
	Adjusted items
Non-regular cash flows (terminal value cash flows)	***Accrual-based items***
• Salvage value of equipment that will be sold at the end of a project (inflow)	• Revenues earned but not received in cash
	• Expenses recognized but no cash expended (i.e., depreciation, accrued expenses)
• Recovery of working capital (inflow)	
	Other
	• Changes in net working capital

increase revenues. Given that the future cash flows must be present to offset the cost of the initial investment, marked variation in these could alter the final NPV decision.

DETERMINING A DISCOUNT RATE

Although commonly thought of as an adjustment for the time value of money, the discount rate also accounts for project risk. The discount rate or cost of capital marks the required rate of return for investors who fund the project to compensate them for the risk of the investment opportunity and the temporary loss of funds to be used elsewhere. To estimate the required rate of return for investment projects with risk similar to the current risk of the health care organization, a facility can use its current cost of capital. This would be the rate an organization currently pays for its own financing. However, it should adjust the cost of capital to a higher (lower) value if the risk of the project is higher (lower) than the overall risk of the health care organization. The determination of precise models to estimate cost of capital is technical and beyond the scope of this text.

 Key Point *The discount rate is also called the opportunity cost of capital to the company undertaking the capital investment project. It is the cost of the next best alternative, those returns the company would be forgoing by making this investment as opposed to another. From the lenders' or investors' points of view, it is the returns they forgo by investing their money in this project rather than alternative projects of similar risk. For example, if an investor-owned hospital chain were issuing stock to purchase a health insurance business, investors considering buying this stock would expect at least the return on the stocks of other publicly held health insurance companies, such as Cigna or Aetna.*

APPENDIX D

ADJUSTMENTS FOR NET WORKING CAPITAL

To the extent that new projects affect working capital, adjustments in cash flows must be made. If working capital increases, then the organization has invested additional resources in working capital; that is, the project requires the organization to increase both its current asset accounts, which result in cash outflows, and current liability accounts, which are cash inflows, because they delay the use of cash (see example below). The difference between current assets and current liabilities is called *net working capital*, as discussed in Chapter Five. The effects of changes in net working capital must be accounted for each year. If there is an increase in net working capital, the amount is subtracted from net operating cash flows; likewise, for a decrease, the amount is added to net operating cash flows.

 Key Point *Increases in net working capital mean cash outlays. Decreases in net working capital mean cash inflows.*

An illustration of how to adjust for changes in net working capital is shown by continuing with the example of building a satellite hospital. Assume that the organization had balance sheet results as shown in rows 7 to 9 of Exhibit D–1. From row 9, its net working capital (current assets – current liabilities) is $1,000, $1,300, $1,800, $600, $400, and $300 in years 1 through 6, respectively.

The change in net working capital is the difference between the current year's net working capital and that from the previous year (row 10). For example, the change in net working capital the first year was $1,000 ($1,000 in year 1 – $0 in year 0). The second year's change in net working capital was $300 ($1,300 in year 2 – $1,000 in year 1). The same procedure is followed for years 3 through 6. As noted earlier, if net working capital increased, then cash decreased, which must be subtracted from the cash flows. If net working capital decreased, then cash increased, and that amount must be added to cash flows. Because net working capital increased by $1,000 in year 1 (row 10), $1,000 (row I) is subtracted from the net operating cash flows (row G). This process is continued for the remaining years.

Key Point *Increases in net working capital are cash* outflows. *Decreases in net working capital are cash* inflows.

In the first three years, cash outflows occurred, and net working capital for the project increased (row 10). But in year 4 and thereafter, the decreases in net working capital constituted cash inflows for the years. The facility is no longer investing cash in current assets and current liabilities. It is decreasing its investment in cash, collecting at a higher rate on its receivables, or reducing its outstanding payables (or all of these).

Once the changes in net working capital have been calculated, they are entered into the NPV calculation to adjust for changes in cash flows due to changes in net working capital (rows I and J).

Key Point *Interest-bearing, short-term debt (notes payable) should be excluded from calculations of changes in net working capital because it represents financing flows and is accounted for in the cost of capital.*

When a project ends, it is assumed that the total amount of net working capital investment is recaptured and accounted for as a cash inflow, and that plant and equipment will be sold or disposed of. In regard to the recapture of net working capital, typically all project receivables are collected, all project inventory gets sold, and all project payables are paid. The recapture of changes in net working capital is the sum of all the changes in net working capital during the life of the project, which is, in the case of the satellite hospital, –$300 [($1,000) + ($300) + ($500) + $1,200 + $200 + $100]. The negative $300 indicates an ending excess balance of $300 in net working capital to sell off; therefore, $300 in net working capital becomes a cash inflow that can be recaptured or recovered (see Exhibit D–1, row J).

Exhibit D-1 Computation of net present value for a satellite hospital, including working capital adjustments

Givens	Years	0	1	2	3	4	5	6
1 Initial investment		($1,000,000)						
2 Net revenues			$400,000	$550,000	$800,000	$900,000	$1,100,000	$1,370,000
3 Cash operating expenses			$200,000	$300,000	$500,000	$550,000	$650,000	$850,000
4 Depreciation expense			$145,000	$145,000	$145,000	$145,000	$145,000	$145,000
5 Sale of assets								$130,000
6 Cost of capital	10%							
7 Current assets			$2,200	$4,800	$7,400	$1,400	$1,300	$1,200
8 Current liabilities			$1,200	$3,500	$5,600	$800	$900	$900
9 Net working capital	(Given 7) – (Given 8)	$0	$1,000	$1,300	$1,800	$600	$400	$300
10 Change in net working capital [a]			$1,000	$300	$500	($1,200)	($200)	($100)

[a] Net working capital (current year) – Net working capital (previous year).

Exhibit D-1 (*Continued*)

Net present value for satellite hospital, adjusting for depreciation, working capital and salvage value

	Years	0	1	2	3	4	5	6
A	Initial investment	Given 1	($1,000,000)						
B	Net revenues	Given 2		$400,000	$550,000	$800,000	$900,000	$1,100,000	$1,370,000
C	Less: cash operating expenses before depreciation	Given 3		200,000	300,000	500,000	550,000	650,000	850,000
D	Less: depreciation expense	Given 4		145,000	145,000	145,000	145,000	145,000	145,000
E	Operating income	B – C – D		55,000	105,000	155,000	205,000	305,000	375,000
F	Add: depreciation expense	Given 4		145,000	145,000	145,000	145,000	145,000	145,000
G	Net operating cash flows	E + F		200,000	250,000	300,000	350,000	450,000	520,000
H	Add: sale of assets	Given 5							130,000
I	**Adjustments for changes in working capital**	**–Given 10**		**(1,000)**	**(300)**	**(500)**	**1,200**	**200**	**100**
J	**Recapture of net working capital**	**–Sum I**							**300**
K	Project cash flows	G + H + I + J		$199,000	$249,700	$299,500	$351,200	$450,200	$650,400
L	Cost of capital	Given 6		10%	10%	10%	10%	10%	10%
M	Present value interest factors	$1/(1+i)^n$		0.9091	0.8264	0.7513	0.6830	0.6209	0.5645
N	Annual PV of cash flows[b]	K × M		$180,909	$206,364	$225,019	$239,874	$279,539	$367,134
O	PV of cash flows	Sum N	$1,498,838						
P	**Net present value**	A + O	$498,838						

[b] Present value interest factors in the table have been calculated by formula, but are necessarily rounded for presentation. Therefore, there may be a difference between the number displayed and that calculated manually.

313

APPENDIX E

TAX IMPLICATIONS FOR FOR-PROFIT ENTITIES IN A CAPITAL BUDGETING DECISION AND THE ADJUSTMENT FOR INTEREST EXPENSE

This appendix introduces an NPV analysis for a for-profit entity. The total number of for-profit hospitals in the United States at the turn of the century represented less than 15 percent of the total number of short-term community hospitals. In contrast, there were more than 7,000 skilled and intermediate-care nursing homes nationwide, of which more than two-thirds were for-profit entities. Also, more than two-thirds of the managed care insurers were tax-paying entities. Therefore, it is imperative to consider the tax effects that can take place in a for-profit investment analysis. Appendix C discussed the separation of financing flows from the operating cash flow analysis for an NPV analysis. When computing a cash flow analysis from a projected income statement, interest expense needs to be taken out to be able to adjust for the tax effect if the entity is for-profit. The following analysis shows the calculations had the satellite hospital project been a for-profit endeavor.

The two most important tax adjustments that must be made for for-profit entities are accounting for the effect of taxes on operating income, and accounting for the tax effect from the gains or losses resulting from the sale of assets at the expected end of the project's life. This example focuses only on the first adjustment because gains and losses, like most other tax effects, are complicated and therefore only introduced in this text.

As shown in Exhibit E–1, the analysis looks nearly identical to that for not-for-profit entities (Exhibit D–1), except for the tax expense and interest expense accounts, and the inclusion of a new line for payment of taxes (Exhibit E–1, row G, which assumes that the organization has a 40 percent tax rate on its net income). In year 1, the organization had earnings before taxes of $30,000 (row F). Because the tax rate is 40 percent, it must pay an additional $12,000 in taxes ($30,000 $\times$ 0.40). In year 2, it pays $32,000 in taxes on earnings before tax of $80,000 (rows F and G). A similar analysis is conducted for years 3 through 6.

At this point, an adjustment must be made for interest because interest expense affected net income (and thus the amount of taxes paid), but interest expense is not itself an operating cash flow. Thus, interest expense must be added back at the amount of (1 – tax rate) to determine true cash outflows. This is done in row J, where $15,000 is added back [$25,000 $\times$ (1 − 0.40)]. In effect, the interest expense provided a tax deduction of $10,000 ($25,000 $\times$ 0.40 saved), which represents a cash inflow. Thus, the true cash outflow is only $15,000 ($25,000 – $10,000), which matches the value in row J. For nonprofit entities with interest expense in the projected income statement, the full amount of the interest expense is added back in because the tax rate is zero. The remainder of the analysis remains the same. Overall, the NPV for the hospital as a taxpaying entity equals $181,116 (row T) versus $498,838 as a not-for-profit hospital (Exhibit D–1, row P), which is much less.

Exhibit E-1 NPV decision assuming satellite hospital is for-profit

Givens		Years	0	1	2	3	4	5	6
1	Initial Investment		($1,000,000)						
2	Net revenues			$400,000	$550,000	$800,000	$900,000	$1,100,000	$1,370,000
3	Cash operating expenses			$200,000	$300,000	$500,000	$550,000	$650,000	$850,000
4	Depreciation expense			$145,000	$145,000	$145,000	$145,000	$145,000	$145,000
5	Interest expense			$25,000	$25,000	$25,000	$25,000	$25,000	$25,000
6	Sale of assets								$130,000
7	Cost of capital	10%							
8	Tax rate	40%							
9	Current assets			$2,200	$4,800	$7,400	$1,400	$1,300	$1,200
10	Current liabilities			$1,200	$3,500	$5,600	$800	$900	$900
11	Net working capital	(Given 9) − (Given 10)	$0	$1,000	$1,300	$1,800	$600	$400	$300
12	**Change in net working capital**	a		**$1,000**	**$300**	**$500**	**($1,200)**	**($200)**	**($100)**

a Net working capital (current year) − net working capital (previous year).

316

Exhibit E-1 (Continued)

Net present value for satellite hospital, adjusting for depreciation, interest, working capital and salvage value

		Years	0	1	2	3	4	5	6
A	Initial investment	Given 1	($1,000,000)						
B	Net revenues	Given 2		$400,000	$550,000	$800,000	$900,000	$1,100,000	$1,370,000
C	Less: cash operating expenses before dep. & int.	Given 3		200,000	300,000	500,000	550,000	650,000	850,000
D	Less: depreciation expense	Given 4		145,000	145,000	145,000	145,000	145,000	145,000
E	Less: interest expense	Given 5		25,000	25,000	25,000	25,000	25,000	25,000
F	Earnings before taxes	B − C − D − E		30,000	80,000	130,000	180,000	280,000	350,000
G	Less: tax expense (40% tax rate)	Given 8 × F		12,000	32,000	52,000	72,000	112,000	140,000
H	Earnings after tax	F − G		18,000	48,000	78,000	108,000	168,000	210,000
I	Add depreciation expense	Given 4		145,000	145,000	145,000	145,000	145,000	145,000
J	Add back interest expense at (1 − tax rate)	(1 − Given 8) × E		15,000	15,000	15,000	15,000	15,000	15,000
K	Net operating cash flow	H + I + J		178,000	208,000	238,000	268,000	328,000	370,000
L	Add: sale of assets[b]	Given 6							130,000
M	**Adjustments for changes in working capital**	−Given 12		(1,000)	(300)	(500)	1,200	200	**100**
N	**Recapture of net working capital**	−Sum M							**300**
O	Project cash flows	K + L + M + N		$177,000	$207,700	$237,500	$269,200	$328,200	$500,400
P	Cost of capital	Given 7		10%	10%	10%	10%	10%	10%
Q	Present value interest factors	$1/(1+i)^n$		0.9091	0.8264	0.7513	0.6830	0.6209	0.5645
R	Annual PV of cash flows[c]	O × Q		$160,909	$171,653	$178,437	$183,867	$203,786	$282,463
S	PV of cash flows	Sum R	$1,181,116						
T	Net present value	A + S	**$181,116**						

[b] There is no tax effect from selling the asset because it was depreciated to the salvage value; therefore, salvage value equals book value.

[c] Present value interest factors in the table have been calculated by formula but are necessarily rounded for presentation. Therefore, there may be a difference between the number displayed and that calculated manually.

APPENDIX F

COMPREHENSIVE CAPITAL BUDGETING REPLACEMENT COST EXAMPLE

Assume that a cardiology laboratory is considering replacing its manual electrocardiography (EKG) management information system (MIS) with a new, more efficient product. The new system automatically stores EKG and stress records online. The existing system was purchased five years ago for $70,000 and is being depreciated over a ten-year life to a salvage value of $10,000. The old system can be sold now at a market price of $20,000 and has a book value of $40,000 ($70,000 original cost − $30,000 accumulated depreciation). The new system can be purchased for $100,000 and is estimated to have a five-year life. It can be depreciated to a salvage value of $20,000. Because the organization is paid on a per-procedure basis, there are no new revenues directly associated with the improved EKG system. Thus, the focus becomes the cash savings in operational expenses. Annual labor expenses will drop from $50,000 for the old system to $15,000 with the new system, resulting in a labor cash savings of $35,000. Purchasing the new system will increase net working capital by $1,000 each year compared with a $300 annual increase for the old system, starting in year 1. The remainder of this chapter provides comparative and incremental NPV analyses of this situation, first assuming that the lab is not-for-profit and then assuming that it is investor-owned. In both cases, the cost of capital is 5 percent.

COMPARATIVE APPROACH: NOT-FOR-PROFIT ANALYSIS

As its name implies, the comparative approach compares the cash flows resulting from continuing with the existing alternative to those that would result were the equipment being replaced. The comparative approach does this by separately calculating each of these cash flows and then comparing the end results (Exhibit F–1).

Were the organization to continue with the existing system, there would be no investment at year 0 (it has already been made), and the operating loss would be $56,000 a year (row D), which includes operating expenses (row B) and depreciation expense (row C). However, because operating loss contains depreciation, and depreciation is an expense that does not require a cash outlay, depreciation must be added back in order to derive cash flows from operations. This is done in row F by adding back $6,000 (row E) to the $56,000 operating loss (row D). Although the same result, $50,000 (row F), can be derived without first subtracting out and then adding back in depreciation expense, this approach makes it easier to compare the not-for-profit and for-profit analyses. Because the change in net working capital increases by $300 each year, the resultant cash outflow must be accounted for (row G). However, as explained in Appendix D, assume that this will be recovered at the end of the project (row I). The only other cash flow to account for would be the $10,000 salvage value that results in a cash inflow in year 5 (row H). Finally, the cash flows are computed for each of the five years (row J), and then discounted using the cost of capital (rows K and L). This information forms the basis to calculate NPV of the cash flows attributable to the existing machine: −$208,762 (row O).

The initial outlay, expenses, depreciation, salvage value, and working capital effects differ for the purchase of the replacement system (Exhibit F–1, lower half). The initial outlay is computed in row A. Although the new equipment costs $100,000, the organization has to pay only $80,000 from its existing funds because it can allocate $20,000 from the sale of the existing equipment.

Because net working capital increases by $1,000 each year, the resulting cash outflow must be accounted for (rows G and I). The remaining steps in the replacement analysis are the same as those in the previous analysis, and only the amounts differ. Using the comparative approach, the NPV of the replacement alternative is −$129,683 (row O). Thus, because the replacement alternative has the higher NPV (−$129,683 vs. −$208,762), the replacement alternative should be undertaken.

COMPARATIVE APPROACH: FOR-PROFIT ANALYSIS

The for-profit analysis is exactly the same as that for the not-for-profit analysis with two exceptions shown in Exhibit F–2, rows E and F, which arise as a result of the effects of taxes on cash flows and ultimately, which affects NPV. As in the not-for-profit analysis, earnings (or loss) before tax is calculated in row D. Because earnings get taxed at 40 percent, the resulting tax savings would be $22,400 for the existing alternative as compared with $12,400 for the replacement alternative, respectively (row E, both sections). Because earnings before tax is negative, the organization is losing

Exhibit F-1   Comparative approach to analyzing a capital budgeting decision: not-for-profit entity

Existing equipment

Givens	Years	0	1	2	3	4	5
1 Initial outlay		$0					
2 Operating expenses			($50,000)	($50,000)	($50,000)	($50,000)	($50,000)
3 Depreciation expense			($6,000)	($6,000)	($6,000)	($6,000)	($6,000)
4 Change in net working capital			$300	$300	$300	$300	$300
5 Salvage value							$10,000
6 Cost of capital	5%						

	Years	0	1	2	3	4	5
A Initial outlay	Given 1	$0					
B Operating expenses before depreciation	Given 2		($50,000)	($50,000)	($50,000)	($50,000)	($50,000)
C Depreciation expense	Given 3		(6,000)	(6,000)	(6,000)	(6,000)	(6,000)
D Operating income (loss)	B + C		(56,000)	(56,000)	(56,000)	(56,000)	(56,000)
E Add: depreciation expense	−Given 3		6,000	6,000	6,000	6,000	6,000
F Net operating cash flow	D + E		(50,000)	(50,000)	(50,000)	(50,000)	(50,000)
G Change in net working capital	−Given 4		(300)	(300)	(300)	(300)	(300)
Terminal value changes:							
H Salvage value	Given 5						10,000
I Recovery of net working capital	−Sum G						1,500
J Change in net cash flow	F + G + H + I		($50,300)	($50,300)	($50,300)	($50,300)	($38,800)
K Cost of capital	Given 6		5%	5%	5%	5%	5%
L Present value interest factor	$1/(1+i)^n$		0.9524	0.9070	0.8638	0.8227	0.7835
M Annual PV of cash flows[a]	J × L		($47,905)	($45,624)	($43,451)	($41,382)	($30,401)
N Sum of PV of cash flows	Sum M	($208,762)					
O Net present value	A + N	($208,762)					

[a] Present value interest factors in the table have been calculated by formula but are necessarily rounded for presentation. Therefore, there may be a difference between the number displayed and that calculated manually.

Exhibit F-1 (Continued)

Replacement Equipment

Givens	Years	0	1	2	3	4	5
1 Initial outlay	b	($80,000)					
2 Operating expenses			($15,000)	($15,000)	($15,000)	($15,000)	($15,000)
3 Depreciation expense			($16,000)	($16,000)	($16,000)	($16,000)	($16,000)
4 Change in net working capital			$1,000	$1,000	$1,000	$1,000	
5 Salvage value							$20,000
6 Cost of capital	5%						

	Years	0	1	2	3	4	5
A Initial outlay	Given 1	($80,000)					
B Operating expenses before depreciation	Given 2		($15,000)	($15,000)	($15,000)	($15,000)	($15,000)
C Depreciation expense	Given 3		(16,000)	(16,000)	(16,000)	(16,000)	(16,000)
D Operating income (loss)	B + C		(31,000)	(31,000)	(31,000)	(31,000)	(31,000)
E Add: depreciation expense	−Given 3		16,000	16,000	16,000	16,000	16,000
F Net operating cash flow	D + E		(15,000)	(15,000)	(15,000)	(15,000)	(15,000)
G Change in net working capital	−Given 4		(1,000)	(1,000)	(1,000)	(1,000)	(1,000)
Terminal value changes:							
H Salvage value	Given 5						20,000
I Recovery of net working capital	−Sum G						5,000
J Change in net cash flow	F + G + H + I		($16,000)	($16,000)	($16,000)	($16,000)	$9,000
K Cost of capital	Given 6		5%	5%	5%	5%	5%
L Present value interest factor	$1/(1+i)^n$		0.9524	0.9070	0.8638	0.8227	0.7835
M Annual PV of cash flows[a]	J × L		($15,238)	($14,512)	($13,821)	($13,163)	$7,052
N Sum of PV of cash flows	Sum M	($49,683)					
O Net present value	A + N	**($129,683)**					
P **NPV difference**	c	**$79,079**					

[b] — $100,000 purchase of new equipment + $20,000 sale of old equipment.
[c] — (−$129,683 replacement system) − (−$208,762 existing system) = $79,079.

money but will not be incurring negative taxes. However, the tax expense becomes a positive value because this tax loss can be either carried forward to offset future income or carried back to offset prior income to result in a tax refund. This has the same effect as a cash inflow: for each additional $1.00 in expenses, the organization pays $0.40 less in taxes. Therefore, these tax savings get added back to the loss in row D. Taking into account the tax effects, the NPV of the existing alternative is –$111,782, and the NPV of the replacement alternative is –$67,998. Again, showing a smaller loss, or a savings of $43,784 (row R, bottom table), the replacement alternative should be undertaken, all else being equal.

INCREMENTAL APPROACH—NOT-FOR-PROFIT ANALYSIS

Exhibit F–3 analyzes the same replacement decision using the incremental approach. It looks at the savings for each item (or lack thereof) that would result if the decision were made to replace the old EKG system with a new product. To make this decision, several aspects of cash flows must be taken into account.

To compute the initial outlay, though the new MIS system costs $100,000, the facility receives $20,000 from the sale of the old system. Thus, the initial outlay is $80,000 (row A). The change in operating cash flows produces a net operating cash flow savings of $35,000 per year (row B: $15,000 replacement equipment labor expense vs. $50,000 in labor expenses for the existing equipment).

As with the comparative analysis, in this non-taxpaying example, depreciation expense could be disregarded altogether because it has no effect on cash flow. However, to compare the not-for-profit and for-profit examples, operating income is first computed (which is needed to compute taxes in the for-profit example) by subtracting the $10,000 in depreciation expense (row C) and then adding it back in, to show that net operating cash flows do not change as a result of depreciation (rows E and F).

The effects of changes in working capital and the salvage value must be added to the analysis as well. Because net working capital increases by $700 annually ($300 existing system vs. $1,000 replacement system), cash flows decrease by $700 each year (rows 5 and G). In year 5, the year in which the investment is assumed to end, salvage value increases by $10,000 (row H, sale of assets), which equals the incremental difference between the salvage value of the new system, $20,000, and the salvage value of the old system, $10,000. Because the project presumably ends at this time, it is also necessary to recapture $3,500 in net working capital (row I: 5 years × $700 per year).

To determine the NPV, the cash flows each year are discounted at 5 percent and summed (rows J through O), and then the initial outlay (row A) is added. Because the NPV equals $79,079, which represents a positive return due to replacement, from a financial perspective, the new EKG system should be purchased. Note that this NPV equals the same number as that derived in Exhibit F–1, row P in the bottom section, as it should.

Exhibit F-2 Comparative approach to analyzing a capital budgeting decision: for-profit entity

Existing equipment

Givens	Years	0	1	2	3	4	5
1 Initial outlay		$0					
2 Operating expenses			($50,000)	($50,000)	($50,000)	($50,000)	($50,000)
3 Depreciation expense			($6,000)	($6,000)	($6,000)	($6,000)	($6,000)
4 Change in net working capital			$300	$300	$300	$300	$300
5 Salvage value							$10,000
6 Cost of capital	5%						
7 Tax rate	40%						

	Years	0	1	2	3	4	5
A Initial outlay	Given 1	$0					
B Operating expenses before depreciation	Given 2		($50,000)	($50,000)	($50,000)	($50,000)	($50,000)
C Depreciation expense	Given 3		(6,000)	(6,000)	(6,000)	(6,000)	(6,000)
D Earnings (loss) before tax	B + C		(56,000)	(56,000)	(56,000)	(56,000)	(56,000)
E Taxes at 40%	Given 7 × D		22,400	22,400	22,400	22,400	22,400
F Earnings after tax	D + E		(33,600)	(33,600)	(33,600)	(33,600)	(33,600)
G Add: depreciation expense	−Given 3		6,000	6,000	6,000	6,000	6,000
H Net operating cash flow	F + G		(27,600)	(27,600)	(27,600)	(27,600)	(27,600)
I Change in net working capital	−Given 4		(300)	(300)	(300)	(300)	(300)
Terminal value changes:							
J Salvage value	Given 5						10,000
K Recovery of net working capital	−Sum I						1,500
L Change in net cash flow	H + I + J + K		($27,900)	($27,900)	($27,900)	($27,900)	($16,400)
M Cost of capital	Given 6		5%	5%	5%	5%	5%
N Present value interest factor	$1/(1+i)^n$		0.9524	0.9070	0.8638	0.8227	0.7835
O Annual PV of cash flows[a]	L × N		($26,571)	($25,306)	($24,101)	($22,953)	($12,850)
P Sum of PV of cash flows	Sum O	($111,782)					
Q Net present value	A + P	**($111,782)**					

(Continued)

Exhibit F-2 Comparative approach to analyzing a capital budgeting decision: for-profit entity (Continued)

Replacement equipment

Givens	Years	0	1	2	3	4	5
1 Initial outlay	[b]	($72,000)					
2 Operating expenses			($15,000)	($15,000)	($15,000)	($15,000)	($15,000)
3 Depreciation expense			($16,000)	($16,000)	($16,000)	($16,000)	($16,000)
4 Change in net working capital			$1,000	$1,000	$1,000	$1,000	
5 Salvage value							$20,000
6 Cost of capital	5%						
7 Tax rate	40%						

Replacement equipment

		Years	0	1	2	3	4	5
A	Initial outlay	Given 1	($72,000)					
B	Operating expenses before depreciation	Given 2		($15,000)	($15,000)	($15,000)	($15,000)	($15,000)
C	Depreciation expense	Given 3		(16,000)	(16,000)	(16,000)	(16,000)	(16,000)
D	Earnings before tax (loss before tax)	B + C		(31,000)	(31,000)	(31,000)	(31,000)	(31,000)
E	Taxes at 40%	Given 7 × D		12,400	12,400	12,400	12,400	12,400
F	Net Income or earnings after tax	D + E		(18,600)	(18,600)	(18,600)	(18,600)	(18,600)
G	Add: depreciation expense	−Given 3		16,000	16,000	16,000	16,000	16,000
H	Net operating cash flow	F + G		(2,600)	(2,600)	(2,600)	(2,600)	(2,600)
I	Change in net working capital	−Given 4		(1,000)	(1,000)	(1,000)	(1,000)	
	Terminal value changes:							
J	Salvage value	Given 5						20,000
K	Recovery of net working capital	−Sum I						5,000
L	Change in net cash flow	H + I + J + K		($3,600)	($3,600)	($3,600)	($3,600)	$21,400
M	Cost of capital	Given 6		5%	5%	5%	5%	5%
N	Present value interest factor	$1/(1+i)^n$		0.9524	0.9070	0.8638	0.8227	0.7835
O	Annual PV of cash flows[a]	L × N		($3,429)	($3,265)	($3,110)	($2,962)	$16,767
P	Sum of PV of cash flows	Sum O	$4,002					
Q	Net present value	A + P	($67,998)					
R	**NPV difference**	[c]	**$43,784**					

[a] Present value interest factors in the exhibit have been calculated by formula, but are necessarily rounded for presentation. Therefore, there may be a difference between the number displayed and that calculated manually.

[b] —$100,000 purchase of new equipment + $20,000 sale of old equipment + $8,000 in tax savings from loss on sale of existing equipment (0.40 Tax Rate × $20,000 loss).

[c] ($67,998) − ($111,782) = $43,784.

Exhibit F-3 Incremental approach to analyzing a capital budgeting decision: not-for-profit entity

Givens

1	Initial outlay[a]	($80,000)	
2	Cost of capital	5%	
3	Change in annual operating expenses and depreciation expense:		

		Old MIS	New MIS	Change (New – Old)
3	Operating expense (labor)	($50,000)	($15,000)	$35,000
4	Depreciation expense[b]	($6,000)	($16,000)	($10,000)
5	Net working capital	($300)	($1,000)	($700)
6	Salvage value	$10,000	$20,000	$10,000

[a] ($100,000) Purchase of new equipment + $20,000 Sale of old equipment

[b] Old MIS: ($70,000 – $10,000) / 10 years = $6,000 / year. New MIS: ($100,000 – $20,000) / 5 years = $16,000 / year

		Years	0	1	2	3	4	5
A	Initial outlay	Given 1	($80,000)					
B	Cash savings due to decreased operating expenses	Given 3		$35,000	$35,000	$35,000	$35,000	$35,000
C	Increase in depreciation expense	Given 4		(10,000)	(10,000)	(10,000)	(10,000)	(10,000)
D	Change in operating income	B + C		25,000	25,000	25,000	25,000	25,000
E	Add: increase in depreciation expense	–Given 4		10,000	10,000	10,000	10,000	10,000
F	Change in net operating cash flow	D + E		35,000	35,000	35,000	35,000	35,000
G	Change in net working capital	Given 5		(700)	(700)	(700)	(700)	(700)
	Terminal value changes:							
H	Salvage value	Given 6						10,000
I	Recovery of net working capital	–Sum G						3,500
J	Change in net cash flow	F + G + H + I		$34,300	$34,300	$34,300	$34,300	$47,800
K	Cost of capital			5%	5%	5%	5%	5%
L	Present value interest factor	$1/(1+i)^n$		0.9524	0.9070	0.8638	0.8227	0.7835
M	Annual PV of cash flows[c]	J × L		$32,667	$31,111	$29,630	$28,219	$37,453
N	Sum of PV cash flows	Sum M	$159,079					
O	Net present value	A + N	**$79,079**					

MIS – Management Information System

[c] Present value interest factors in the table have been calculated by formula but are necessarily rounded for presentation. Therefore, there may be a difference between the number displayed and that calculated manually.

INCREMENTAL APPROACH: FOR-PROFIT ANALYSIS

Exhibit F–4 presents a similar incremental analysis, but for a for-profit, taxpaying organization. In this case, the new initial outlay is still reduced from $100,000 to $80,000 by the additional $20,000 from the sale of the old system, but it is also reduced another $8,000 (to $72,000) by the tax effect of that sale (row 1). This tax benefit arises because the organization sells a system with a $40,000 book value for $20,000, incurring a $20,000 loss. Assuming a 40 percent tax rate, it will pay $8,000 less in taxes (0.40 × $20,000) than had it not sold the machine.

Taxes also affect operating income and represent a real cash outflow. Because the change in earnings before tax is $25,000 (row D), assuming a 40 percent tax rate, taxes will increase by $10,000 (row E), thereby reducing the change in net income to $15,000 (row F). However, reflected in this $15,000 net income is the $10,000 in depreciation expense that does not require a cash outflow. Therefore, this $10,000 must be added back in, and cash flow becomes $25,000 (rows G and H). The remainder of the analysis remains the same as for the not-for-profit analysis, adjusting for the change in net working capital and the terminal value.

After accounting for the sale of the new system at its termination date and discounting at the cost of capital, the decision to make this investment results in a positive NPV of $43,784 (row Q). Because the NPV is positive, the investment should be made. Again, this value expectedly equals that shown in row R in the bottom section of Exhibit F–2.

Exhibit F–4 Incremental approach to analyzing a capital budgeting decision: for-profit entity

Givens

1	Initial outlay[a]	($72,000)	
2	Cost of capital	5%	
3	Tax rate	40%	
4	Change in annual operating expenses and depreciation expense		

		Old MIS	New MIS	Change (new – old)
4	Operating expense (labor)	($50,000)	($15,000)	$35,000
5	Depreciation expense[b]	($6,000)	($16,000)	($10,000)
6	Net working capital	($300)	($1,000)	($700)
7	Salvage value	$10,000	$20,000	$10,000

[a]($100,000) purchase of new equipment + $20,000 sale of old equipment + $8,000 (0.40 × $20,000) tax savings due to sale at a loss
[b]Old MIS: ($70,000 – $10,000) / 10 years = $6,000 / year
New MIS: ($100,000 – $20,000) / 5 years = $16,000 / year

		Years	0	1	2	3	4	5
A	Initial outlay	Given 1	($72,000)					
B	Cash savings due to decreased operating expenses	Given 4		$35,000	$35,000	$35,000	$35,000	$35,000
C	Increase in depreciation expense[c]	Given 5		(10,000)	(10,000)	(10,000)	(10,000)	(10,000)
D	Change in earnings before tax	B + C		25,000	25,000	25,000	25,000	25,000
E	Less: increased tax expense	Given 3 × D		10,000	10,000	10,000	10,000	10,000
F	Increase in net income or earnings after tax	D – E		15,000	15,000	15,000	15,000	15,000
G	Add: increase in depreciation expense	–Given 5		10,000	10,000	10,000	10,000	10,000
H	Change in net operating cash flow	F + G		25,000	25,000	25,000	25,000	25,000
I	Change in net working capital	Given 6		(700)	(700)	(700)	(700)	(700)
	Terminal value changes:							
J	Change in salvage value	Given 7						10,000
K	Recovery of net working capital	–Sum I						3,500
L	Change in net cash flow	H + I + J + K		$24,300	$24,300	$24,300	$24,300	$37,800
M	Cost of capital	Given 2		5%	5%	5%	5%	5%
N	Present value interest factor	1 / (1 + i)^n		0.9524	0.9070	0.8638	0.8227	0.7835
O	Annual PV of cash flows[d]	L × N		$23,143	$22,041	$20,991	$19,992	$29,617
P	Sum of PV cash flows	Sum O	$115,784					
Q	Net present value	A + P	**$43,784**					

[c]For row C, depreciation expense increased. However, it is an expense and must be deducted from cash savings.
[d]Present value interest factors in the table have been calculated by formula but are necessarily rounded for presentation. Therefore there may be a difference between the number displayed and that calculated manually.

APPENDIX SUMMARY

This appendix provided both a comparative and an incremental NPV analysis of purchasing a new EKG MIS system. The analysis was conducted for both a not-for-profit and a for-profit entity. The summary results are presented in Exhibit F–5, which show that the comparative and incremental approaches provide exactly the same answer. Thus, the method used depends only on preference but has no effect on the final result. In this case, though tax effects are considerable, they do not change the decision.

Exhibit F–5   Results of the comparative and incremental NPV analyses of replacing an existing EKG system

	Not-for-profit institution	For-profit institution
Replace equipment	($129,683)[a]	($67,998)[b]
Keep existing equipment	($208,762)[a]	($111,782)[b]
Difference (replace-keep)	$79,079	$43,784
Incremental approach	$79,079[c]	$43,784[d]

[a] Exhibit F–1, Comparative approach
[b] Exhibit F–2, Comparative approach
[c] Exhibit F–3, Incremental approach
[d] Exhibit F–4, Incremental approach

CAPITAL FINANCING FOR HEALTH CARE PROVIDERS

LEARNING OBJECTIVES

- Describe the types of equity and debt financing
- Define various bond terminology
- Compare tax-exempt with taxable financing
- Explain lease financing

In Chapters Two and Three, the basic accounting equation was defined as Assets = Liabilities + Net Assets. Because liabilities are debts and net assets represent the community's equity in a not-for-profit health care organization, in terms of the sources of financing, the basic accounting equation can also be thought of as

$$\text{Assets} = \text{Debt} + \text{Equity}$$

The equation shows that any increase in assets must be balanced by a similar increase in debt, equity or both. The structuring of debt relative to equity is called the *capital structure decision* and is becoming increasingly important to both for-profit and not-for-profit providers. This was not always the case: in the 1970s and early 1980s, the cost of capital was never a major concern for health care providers. As with other operational costs, health care organizations simply passed on the costs of debt and equity financing to third-party payors. Hospitals had no trouble accessing capital markets because they were virtually guaranteed any income needed to cover debts. In today's environment, however, health policymakers need to recognize that governmental policy cutbacks in Medicare and Medicaid reimbursement, the implementation of at-risk prospective payment systems, industry changes stemming from the increased usage of outpatient services, and the rise in competition among physician and freestanding surgical centers all can limit the access to debt and equity financing among hospital industry entities. For example, a hospital system with a poor bond credit rating due to an increase in Medicaid volume and lower Medicaid payments may experience a downgrade in its credit rating, which in turn may increase its cost of capital, thereby restricting its ability to purchase or replace its plant and equipment. A hospital system unable to maintain and update its facilities could impact its ability to attract and retain physicians and patients, which in turn may reduce patient volume and result in further financial distress. Perspective 8–1 provides an example of how higher debt and greater dependence on one commercial payer can affect the credit rating of a hospital. Finally, the recent change sweeping financial markets in the use of debt financing (leveraged buyouts, or LBOs) by private equity firms to buy back the stock and privatize a company has affected the health care industry as well. Several companies in health care have made this transformation, specifically HCA in 2006 and Manor Care in 2007. Perspective 8–2 offers insight into HCA's LBO.

The first section of this chapter briefly examines equity financing. The remaining sections focus on the issuance of bonds, which is the main source of debt financing for many health care organizations, and lease financing, which is similar to debt financing.

Perspective 8–1   Market, Strategic, and Financial Factors Improve a Hospital's Credit Rating

Moody's Investor Services raised the credit rating of Evanston Northwestern Healthcare System tax-exempt bonds to Aa2 from Aa3. There are several underlying reasons for this improved credit rating, which relate to market, financial, and strategic factors. Evanston has expanded its commercial patient base by aligning itself with a large multi-specialty medical group. Financially, Evanston is earning operating cash flow that is 4.3 times its maximum debt service payment. In 2007, the hospital raised its cash flow margin to 10 percent compared with 9.4 percent in 2006. The higher cash flow stems from expanding its medical group, increasing outpatient revenue, and achieving efficiencies from the system's advanced information technology. The hospital also maintains a strong liquidity position with its unrestricted cash and unrestricted investments totaling over $1.6 billion, which equates to 509 days of cash on hand. Evanston is expected over the next three years to have capital outlays of over $100 million annually, which will be used for the replacement and/or expansion of intensive care units, operating rooms, and cancer centers. A concern that Moody's has relates to the increasing competition from hospitals that are merging in their service area, and Evanston's dependency on one commercial payer, which generates 25 percent of its patient revenue.

Source: Moody's Investor Service. 2008 (May). Moody's upgrades Evanston Northwestern Healthcare's bond rating to Aa2 and Aa2/Vmig1 from Aa3 and Aa3/Vmig1, respectively; outlook is stable. *Moody's Investors Service Press Release.*

Perspective 8–2   HCA's Leveraged Buyout by Private Equity Firm

In July 2006, HCA Inc., the nation's largest hospital chain, agreed to be acquired by private equity firms including Bain Capital; Kohlberg, Kravis, Roberts & Co.; and Merrill Lynch Global Private Equity, as well as HCA founder Thomas F. Frist, Jr., MD. The private equity group will pay approximately $33 billion, which includes the assumption of approximately $11.7 billion of debt and the issuance of new bonds and loans (leverage), $10 billion to $15 billion, to buy out HCA stockholders. Analysts expected the privately held HCA to produce annual returns of greater than 20 percent and to go public again in five years. Analysts believe the key to the deal's success will be cash flow. The private buyout group was attracted to HCA because of the consistency and reliability of its cash flows.

Source: Berman, D. K., Naik, G., and Winslow, R. 2006 (July 25). Behind $21 billion buyout of HCA lies a high-stakes bet on growth. *Wall Street Journal,* A1.

EQUITY FINANCING

The primary sources of equity financing for not-for-profit health care organizations are internally generated funds, philanthropy, government grants, and sale of real estate or other medical office buildings, whereas the primary sources of equity financing for for-profit organizations are internally generated funds and stock issuances. Unfortunately, internally generated funds—those funds retained from operations (retained earnings)—are shrinking. As discussed in Chapter One, financial pressures have lowered revenues and eroded earnings for health care organizations, especially hospitals. However, these organizations still must be able to generate new sources of capital to be able to survive.

Because the equity account on the balance sheet represents the claim on assets, as earnings increase an organization builds its asset base. Typically, health care organizations use their most liquid assets on a balance sheet (i.e., cash, marketable securities, long-term investments) to finance small capital purchases. But by doing so, an organization incurs an opportunity cost, which represents the lost financial returns from not putting these funds into short- and long-term investments. Assuming these funds are not invested in tax-exempt debt funds, the financial returns from these short- and long-term investments are higher than the interest cost on tax-exempt debt. Because tax-exempt debt financing is a cheaper source of capital than equity financing, nonprofit health care organizations try to minimize their cost of capital by utilizing more debt than equity in their financing decision. As a result, nonprofit hospitals are motivated to enhance the liquidity of their organization, so bond rating agencies will assign them a higher credit rating, which in turn will lower their cost of debt. The opposite is true for for-profit hospitals because they are driven to enhance shareholder wealth; they seek to maximize cash flow and use the cash they retain to invest in capital projects, return the capital to shareholders in the form of dividends or stock buybacks, or both.

 Key point *Equity financing for not-for-profits is derived from retained earnings, government grants, sale of assets, and contributions. Equity financing for for-profits comes from issuing stock as well as retained earnings.*

The Tax Reform Act of 1986 was seen as a major setback for health care providers because it lowered the tax deduction available to private individuals who wanted to make philanthropic donations. Nevertheless, charitable giving remains a major source of capital for certain health care providers. Although individuals who make contributions do not receive a direct monetary return, they expect nonmonetary benefits for the community in terms of greater access to or increased quality of care. As health care providers reach their debt limits, equity financing becomes their only source of new funds. Besides externally generated equity, such as grants and appropriations, which are available to all health care organizations, for-profit organizations (commonly referred to as investor-owned) can also issue stock. Exhibit 8–1 lists selected advantages and disadvantages of issuing stock versus debt financing.

Exhibit 8–1 Comparison of stock and debt financing

	Stock	Debt Financing
Ownership	Gives up ownership to investors	No ownership rights given up
Tax implications	Dividends are not tax deductible	Interest on debt is deductible
Set payments	Dividends are not required to be paid	Debt service payments are legally required to be made
Amount of payments	Dividend payment at the organization's discretion	Debt service payments are legally specified as to amount
Time limit of payments	No limit	Time limit is part of borrowing agreement
Restrictions on other actions	Indirect through giving up of ownership	May place restrictions on operations and capital acquisition

The stock markets generally require a higher rate of return on equity financing (issuing stock) relative to debt financing (issuing bonds). This is because of the greater uncertainty associated with equity relative to debt: organizations are legally required to pay back debt, but there is no legal obligation on an issuer's part to pay back equity.

DEBT FINANCING

The major alternative to equity financing is debt financing: borrowing money from others at a cost. The remainder of this chapter describes several types of debt financing and then the process to issue bonds. Hospitals continue to depend on tax-exempt debt as their primary source of capital, which is attributable to low interest rates since the year 2000. Perspective 8–3 provides insight on how one health system issued tax-exempt debt to refinance taxable debt. Certainly, system-affiliated hospitals are able to achieve greater access to capital given the diversity of services, range of market areas, and overall financial strength.

Sources of Debt Financing by Maturity

The general rule of thumb is to borrow short term for short-term needs and long term for long-term needs. Short-term borrowing was discussed in Chapter Five, working capital. There are two important types of long-term financing: *term loans*, which typically must be paid off within ten years, and *bonds*, which typically can have a maturity of twenty to

Term Loan
A loan typically issued by a bank that has a maturity of one to ten years.

Bond
A form of long-term financing whereby an issuer receives cash from a lender (an investor), and in return issues a promissory note (a "bond") agreeing to make principal or interest payments on specific dates.

Perspective 8–3   Use of Tax-Exempt Debt to Refinance Taxable Debt

In July 2007, Wheaton Franciscan Health System issued $70 million in tax-exempt debt, of which $50 million will be used to retire taxable debt that was used to finance a heart center in 2003. The health system had to use taxable debt back in 2003 because the heart center did not qualify for tax-exempt debt owing to a joint-venture partnership arrangement it had with a for-profit physician group. However, in 2006 the system purchased the physician ownership interest, which allowed it to issue tax-exempt debt, resulting in annual interest savings of $1 million. This increased debt load, however, coupled with rising competition from other hospitals and physicians in its health care markets, specifically Milwaukee, Wisconsin, resulted in Moody's downgrading Wheaton's bond rating to Baa1 from A3.

Source: Sanders, E. 2007 (July 13). Wheaton sets $70M bond issue. *Business Journal of Milwaukee.* http://milwaukee.bizjournals.com/milwaukee/stories/2007/07/16/story9.html

thirty-five years. Bonds are the primary source of long-term financing for many tax-exempt health care entities. Term loans, such as bank loans, conventional mortgages, and Federal Housing Administration (FHA)-issued mortgages, require the borrower to pay off or amortize the principal value of the loan over its life. The amortization of a loan requires equal periodic payments for principal and interest obligations. (Appendix G provides a detailed analysis on the computation and development of a loan amortization schedule.) In contrast, the payment of a bond can require the payment of the principal at maturity, at which time the bondholder receives the face value of the bond, and interest payments either can be paid periodically or else all at once at maturity, along with the principal.

Sinking Fund
A fund into which monies are set aside each year to ensure that a bond can be liquidated at maturity.

As opposed to a bank, which lends funds, the issuer of a bond receives funds from the purchasers of the bond, typically the public. However, bond payments may be structured so that the issuer can make early repayments of the principal or equal payments over the life of the bond through a *sinking fund*. In the latter case, the issuer makes payments to the bond trustee, who then uses the funds to retire a portion of the debt.

 Key point Short-term financing *typically refers to a wide range of financing, from debt that must be paid back almost immediately to debt that may not have to be paid off for a year.* Long-term financing *typically refers to debt that will be paid off in a period longer than one year.*

Sources of Debt Financing by Type of Interest Rate

Fixed and Variable Interest Fixed interest rate debt is a security whose rate does not change during the lifetime of the bond; conversely, variable interest rate debt is a security whose rate changes based on market conditions and can fluctuate on a daily, weekly, or monthly basis. Health care providers are attracted to fixed-rate debt because of the predictability of future payments, but the generally higher cost of fixed-rate debt may encourage a health care provider to borrow on a lower-cost, variable basis. Types of variable rate bonds include *variable rate demand bonds* and *auction rate securities*. Variable rate demand bonds allow the investor to "put," which means "to sell" the bonds back to the trustee within a short time, typically thirty days, and which are then resold by the investment bank. Hospitals usually have a letter of credit from a bank to repurchase the bonds in case all the bonds are not resold by the investment bank. In contrast to fixed-rate debt, these bonds can also be paid off by the hospital within thirty days at par value without prepayment penalty.

Unlike demand variable rate bonds, auction variable rate bonds allow the bondholders to resell the bonds through an auction process rather than the put feature of the variable rate debt. As a result, the hospital does not need to establish and pay for a letter of credit from a bank. In 2008 the downgrading of bond insurers from insuring subprime mortgage securities resulted in no buyers for auction rate securities and essentially forced health care systems and hospitals from this market.

The primary concern about variable interest rates is that interest rates may increase, which could cause an unanticipated demand for cash flow. However, throughout the 1990s and up to 2005, the average interest difference or spread between fixed and variable rates was 2.88 percent, significantly mitigating the upward variable rate risk, In 2004 average variable rates fell as low as 1.74 percent, making variable rate debt appealing and allowing hospitals to lower their overall cost of capital. However, variable rates can also rise. Perspective 8–4 provides a detailed example of rising rates during the credit crisis of 2008 and 2009.

Perspective 8–4 Bank Credit Crisis Causes Rates for Variable Rate Debt to Rise

In September of 2008, during a two-week span, the Index for variable rate municipal bonds increased to 7.96 percent from 1.79 percent. This spike in variable rates was related to the pull out of money market funds from the municipal market. The reason these funds cashed out was the credit fear that banks, which act as a buyer in markets when the notes cannot be sold, did not have the available credit to purchase these bonds. As a result, the return rates on the thirty-year variable rate municipal bonds, which typically trade at rates below the taxable treasury bonds, were trading more than 1 percent higher than thirty-year treasury bonds.

Source: Gullapalli, D. 2008 (Sept. 27–28). Muni money-fund yields surge. *Wall Street Journal*, B2.

Hedging
The art of offsetting high variable rate debt payments with returns from high-rate investments.

Interest Rate Swaps
Hospital borrower exchanges or swaps interest rates (fixed to variable rate or variable to fixed rate) between another party, typically a bank or investment banking firm, with the intent of securing a more favorable rate.

Health care providers may use variable rate debt if they have sufficient cash flows and cash investment accounts to hedge against changes in interest rates, which is called *interest rate risk*. The concept of *hedging* is that as variable interest rates and debt payments increase, so, too, will the returns on the facility's investments, thereby offsetting increased debt payments. As result, hospital issuers with strong liquidity and cash flow may opt to use a mix of fixed and variable rate debt, such as 40 percent and 60 percent, respectively.

Interest Rate Swap Hospitals continually look for financial mechanisms to lower their cost of debt, especially when interest rates decline. One approach is to refinance the bond by issuing new debt to retire the old debt, which was typically utilized in the past. To avoid the issuance costs of new debt or refunding its existing debt, a hospital can utilize an *interest rate swap*, whereby the hospital borrower exchanges or "swaps" interest rates with another party, typically a bank or investment banking firm. One type of swap involves switching fixed-rate debt to floating or variable rate debt and is called a *fixed to floating rate swap.* Under this type of swap, the hospital pays a fixed interest rate to its bondholders and decides to exchange or swap to a variable interest rate. To carry out this swap, the hospital will pay a variable interest rate to the bank over the life of the swap, and the bank will pay a fixed interest rate to the hospital, which the hospital will use to pay the current bondholders their fixed interest rate. A hospital would consider using this type of swap or exchange in interest rates if the variable or "floating" rate tax-exempt debt is below the fixed rate the hospital is paying to its current bondholders, which in turn allows the facility to achieve a lower cost of debt. However, it is important for hospitals to have the cash and investment hedge to offset any unexpected rise in interest rates. From the bondholders' perspective, it is important to remember that they are not affected by the interest rate swap. The hospital is still obligated to pay them their fixed-rate interest rate. The hospital borrower could also exchange or swap from a floating or variable rate to a fixed rate. This type of swap is called a "floating to fixed rate swap," and its use can be considered when the hospital wants to avoid the risk of rising variable rates and to lock into a fixed rate without issuing new debt. Again, it is important to remember that the current bondholders are not affected by this exchange and will still receive their variable or floating rate.

For a further understanding how a swap works, Exhibit 8–2 presents an example of a hospital, in this case St. Mary's hospital, that is currently paying a 3 percent variable rate to its existing bondholders, which is based on the market rate index for tax-exempt bonds (see row A). St. Mary's wants to avoid the risk of rising variable interest rates, and it locks into a fixed rate by entering into a floating to fixed rate swap agreement. The hospital contracts with a local bank or counterparty to pay St. Mary's a variable rate of 3 percent based on the market rate index for tax-exempt bonds (see row B). The hospital uses this variable rate payment to pay the 3 percent for its existing variable rate bondholders. The net difference (see row C) is zero because the variable rate it

Exhibit 8–2   Selected advantages and disadvantages of fixed and variable rate debt and explanation of interest rate swap

	Advantages	Disadvantages
Fixed rate debt	1. Fixed debt service payments	1. Higher up-front or issuance expenses
	2. Fixed interest rate, no risk related to interest rate changes, which is called "interest rate risk"	2. Market conditions may result in low variable rate debt over the life of the fixed-rate loan; therefore, may result in paying higher interest cost over life of loan
	3. No risk that investor sell bond back, which is called "put risk"	3. Typically for first 10 years of bond, issuer cannot "call" or refund bonds back, unless issuer uses advance refunding, which can only be done once
	4. No letter of credit required from bank	4. Can result in negative arbitrage situation whereby income earned from investments is less than the interest cost of fixed debt
Variable rate debt	1. Lower up-front issuance costs	1. Higher interest costs if interest rates increase (interest rate risk)
	2. Lower initial interest rate	2. Unstable debt service payments
	3. Greater call or refund flexibility for issuer	3. Decline in cash flow if interest rates increase
	4. Greater matching or hedging between interest income from investments and interest expense from variable debt	4. Bondholders can sell or put the bonds back (put risk)
		5. Requires liquidity to pay off bondholders if unable to fund buyers. Hospitals typically pay for a bank letter of credit rather than use own liquidity
		6. Banks require renewed letter of credit every 3 to 5 years (renewal risk). High-credit-risk hospitals may have trouble renewing letter of credit

(Continued)

Exhibit 8–2   Selected advantages and disadvantages of fixed and variable rate debt and explanation of interest rate swap (Continued)

St. Mary's Hospital enters into an interest rate swap agreement with a bank, which is called a "counterparty"

Givens

1	Interest rate on hospital's existing variable rate debt		3%
2	Counterparty or bank contracts to pay hospital a variable interest rate		3%
3	Hospital contracts with counterparty to pay a fixed interest rate		5%
4	Maturity of bond and swap		10 years

Total interest cost to St. Mary's Hospital when entering into a floating to fixed rate swap agreement

A	Hospital pays variable rate debt for existing debt	Given 1	3%
B	Counterparty or bank pays hospital variable rate for existing bondholders	Given 2	3%
C	Net difference between hospital variable rate and bank variable rate	A - B	0%
D	Hospital pays fixed coupon rate to counterparty	Given 3	5%
E	Total interest rate cost to St. Mary's Hospital	C + D	5%

receives from the bank is equivalent to the variable rate it needs to pay its existing bondholders. Because St. Mary's is exchanging or swapping to a fixed rate, it needs to pay the bank or counterparty a fixed rate of 5 percent (see row D). The total interest rate cost to St. Mary's is 5 percent (row E), which is the sum of the fixed rate (row D) and the net difference 0 percent (row C), which is the difference between what St. Mary's needs to pay the existing variable rate bondholders and what it receives from the bank. In short, St. Mary's is able to lock into a fixed rate of 5 percent without issuing new debt and while its existing bondholders continue to receive their variable rate.

For some floating to fixed rate swap agreements, the hospital's interest rate to existing bondholders (row A) may be higher than the interest rate it receives from the counterparty because the hospital has a higher credit risk or the maturity of the swap is less than the maturity of the bond. Using the above example, the hospital may be paying one percentage point above the tax-exempt bond index (4% = 3% + 1%) to its current bondholders. Under this scenario, St. Mary's total interest rate cost is 6 percent, which is the sum of the fixed rate it pays the bank, 5 percent, and the net difference (1% + 4% − 3%) between what the hospital needs to pay the existing bondholders and what St. Mary's receives from the bank. It is beyond the scope of this textbook to address the other facets of interest rate swaps and the types of risk hospitals face when entering an interest rate swap contract.[1]

Selected Types of Health Care Debt Financing

This section discusses further several specific types of debt financing: bank loans, conventional mortgages, FHA program loans, and bonds.

Bank Term Loans Loans traditionally issued by banks with maturities of one to ten years are defined as term loans. These loans are usually paid off in equal or "level" amounts over the life of the loan.

Conventional Mortgages Under a conventional mortgage, the health care facility pledges its land or building(s) as *collateral* for a loan. Typical lenders include commercial banks, insurance companies, and savings and loan institutions. The term of a loan is normally twenty years. Unfortunately, the lender may allow the borrower to finance only a portion of the purchase, requiring a down payment on the rest.

> **Collateral**
> An asset with clear value (such as land or buildings) that is pledged against a loan to reduce risk to the lender. If the loan is not paid off satisfactorily, the lender has a legal claim to seize the pledged asset.

Pooled Equipment Financing To create greater access to tax-exempt debt financing for less expensive loans, a program of pooled equipment financing was developed. Given the high fixed issuance costs of borrowing, pooled financing spreads these costs over a number of health care borrowers, who each receive a portion of the loan. State or regional hospital associations typically sponsor pooled equipment financing programs.

FHA Program Loans To improve marketability and encourage lower interest rates, the government-sponsored FHA provides mortgage insurance for health care facilities' loans. The insurance guarantees the principal and interest on a loan, which reduces risk to the bondholders. The disadvantages are the fees charged and the time it takes to have a loan approved. Many FHA-insured loans can take a year or more to implement.

Bonds A *bond* is a long-term contract whereby on specific dates a borrower agrees to make principal or interest payments (or both) to the holder of the bond who lent the funds. The section below describes key terms used in the rest of this chapter as they relate to bonds and the bond issuance process.

- *Indenture and covenant:* A legal document that states the conditions and terms of a bond is called an *indenture.* It usually is a lengthy document—often one hundred pages or more—and discusses interest mode (daily, weekly, or long-term rates), payment provisions, call features, and repayment years of the debt. It also

---

[1]To learn more about these issues, refer to David L. Taub's "Understanding Municipal Derivatives" (*Government Finance Review*, August 2005: http://www.sifma.org/capital_markets/docs/Understanding MuniDerivatives.pdf)

lists the numerous covenants of the bond. A loan covenant is a legal provision stated in the bond that the issuer must follow, such as the security backing the bond, the amount of future debt that can be offered, and acceptable ranges for liquidity and debt service coverage ratios. Covenants protect the claims of bondholders on the facility's assets in case of default.

- *Debenture:* A *debenture* is an unsecured bond; that is, it is not backed by specific assets of the organization.

- *Subordinated debenture:* A *subordinated debenture* is an unsecured bond that is junior to debenture bonds. In the case of default, debenture bondholders are paid first. A subordinated debenture is more risky to the investor and thus pays a higher interest rate.

- *Par value:* The *par value* of a bond is the security's face value, such as $1,000 or $5,000. This is the amount that a bondholder is paid at the time of the bond's maturity.

- *Coupon rate and coupon payment:* The *coupon rate* is the stated interest rate on the bond, as promised by the issuer. The *coupon payment* is the amount the holder of the coupon receives periodically, usually semi-annually. It equals the coupon rate times the face value of the bond payment. For example, if the coupon rate is 10 percent for a bond with a $1,000 par value, the coupon payment is $100 annually or $50 semi-annually.

- *Callable bonds: Callable bonds* may be redeemed by the issuer before they mature. An issuer may call a bond if its coupon rate is higher than the presently prevailing interest rates for bonds, or if the issuer wants to eliminate restrictions caused by having the bond outstanding. To attract investors, most callable bonds guarantee a certain coupon payment for ten years (the *call protection period*) and contain a call price feature that equals par value plus a call premium, usually equal to 1 to 2 percent of the outstanding balance.

- *Zero coupon bonds:* The term *coupon* refers to the amount of interest that will be paid by the issuer to the bondholders. Bonds issued with no coupon at all are called *zero coupon bonds*. The trade-off to the issuer for not making any coupon payments over the lifetime of a bond is that the bond must be issued at a deep discount, that is, less than face value, which means that the issuer receives less initially in bond proceeds. Investors are attracted to these bonds not only because of their bigger discount rates, but also because they need not concern themselves with managing and reinvesting coupon payments (although they still must pay annual taxes on portions of taxable bonds).

- *Serial bonds:* A smaller portion of a fixed rate bond issue that matures during the early due dates of the issue, typically during the first ten to fifteen years with their own interest rate are called *serial bonds*. Bonds of this nature allow the investor to purchase bonds with shorter maturities in addition to investing in bonds with longer maturities. In contrast, term bonds represent the remaining larger portion and have longer maturities (between twenty and thirty years).

■ *Basis points:* Security traders discuss the changes in a bond's interest rate by basis points. A basis point is 1/100th of 1 percent. Thus, 100 basis points is equal to 1 percent; one bond yielding 5.75 percent and one bond yielding 5.65 percent have a spread of 10 basis points. Traders also consider the basis point spread between different types of bonds. For example, the spread between taxable and tax-exempt bonds may be 300 basis points, or there may be a spread of 30 basis points between AAA and A-rated bonds (bond ratings are discussed more later).

■ *Sinking fund:* As part of the bond contract, a covenant may establish that part of the principal be paid back each year, earmarked for the orderly retirement or the redemption of bonds before maturity. These funds, called sinking funds, are paid periodically to the trustee who maintains the fund for the health care provider. They are analogous to the principal repayment of a mortgage.

■ *Secondary market: Secondary markets* deal in the buying and selling of bonds that have already been issued.

■ *Debt service reserve fund: Debt service reserve funds*, typically equivalent to one year of principal and interest payments, are set aside with the trustee to act as a safeguard against default during the life of the loan period.

Tax-Exempt Bonds *Tax-exempt bonds* are bonds in which the interest payments to the investor have exempt status from federal income taxes, and possibly state and local income taxes as well; thus, the interest payments are typically lower than those from other bonds that do not have tax-exempt status (either taxable municipal or corporate bonds). The lower interest payments of tax-exempt financing have made it the primary choice of debt financing for not-for-profit health care organizations. These bonds can be issued only by an organization that has received tax exemption as designated by the Internal Revenue Service, such as a state, city, or local government, and their respective agencies and the funds must be used for projects that qualify as "exempt uses." Rather than having assets as collateral, these bonds are backed by either the issuer's general obligations or specific revenues; the latter are called *tax-exempt revenue bonds*.

For most health care organizations, the issuance of a tax-exempt revenue bond will require the security of a *mortgage*, meaning the health care provider will pledge its real property and equipment as security or collateral in the case of default. In today's market, health care providers with an A or higher bond rating normally are not required to pledge their fixed assets as collateral; in the unlikely case of default, creditors are secured by the pledge of the health care provider's revenues. However, creditors can enhance their security indirectly by requiring a negative pledge on a health care provider's real estate. A *negative pledge* prohibits the health care provider from giving a lien (claim) on its real estate to any other creditor.

Another advantage to the issuer of tax-exempt bonds other than the lower interest rates is their long maturity to term, often thirty to thirty-five years, as compared with seven to twenty years typical of taxable bonds. One disadvantage is the higher issuance cost due to documentation fees for the issuing authority, bond counsel fees, and other documentation required to achieve tax-exempt status on the issue. Slower issuance is another drawback. Because the facility must act through a governmental authority, the bureaucratic approval and issuance process increases the time it takes to bring the security to market.[2]

Key point *Tax-exempt bonds have lower interest rates than do taxable bonds because investors in tax-exempt bonds do not have to pay taxes on the interest income they receive*

Taxable Bonds Taxable bonds differ from tax-exempt bonds primarily in that the coupon payments must be reported as taxable income by the investor, resulting in a higher interest rate for the health care issuer. Taxable bonds typically have shorter maturity (twenty years) and do not have restrictions on the use of proceeds. The proceeds of tax-exempt debt can benefit only the tax-exempt entity; therefore, projects partnering with another taxpaying entity, such as a physician practice or specific medical office buildings or parking garages used by physician offices can be financed only with taxable debt and do not qualify for tax-exempt debt.

BOND ISSUANCE PROCESS

Before a bond can be issued, it must be sold by either public or private placement. Health care providers, whether they are issuing a taxable or a tax-exempt bond, must select between public or private placement. In a *public offering*, a bond is sold to the investing public through an *underwriter*, sometimes called an *investment banker*. *Private placements* are sold to a particular institution or group of institutions (banks, pension funds, or insurance companies), also with the assistance of an underwriter. Exhibit 8–3 introduces the key parties involved in the bond issuance process, which is discussed in more detail below.

Public versus Private Placement

The advantage of private over public placement is that the issuer primarily avoids public disclosure in the form of a bond rating, credit enhancement, and official statement (OS) at the time of issuance as well as after the issuance. Removing these parts from the issuance process also lowers the costs and shortens the time to issue the bonds. Although there is no OS, there is a private placement memorandum, which is limited in scope to "OS" and is circulated to all buyers of the private placement. The primary disadvantage of private placement is that because of the bond's reduced liquidity in a narrower market, buyers demand higher interest rates. If the buyer desires to resell the bonds, there is no public secondary market, only other qualified institutional buyers.

---

[2]To learn more about tax-exempt bonds and the issuance process, go to the Electronic Municipal Market Access Educational Web site (http://www.emma.msrb.org/EducationCenter/EducationCenter.aspx).

Exhibit 8–3   Parties involved in a tax-exempt bond issuance process

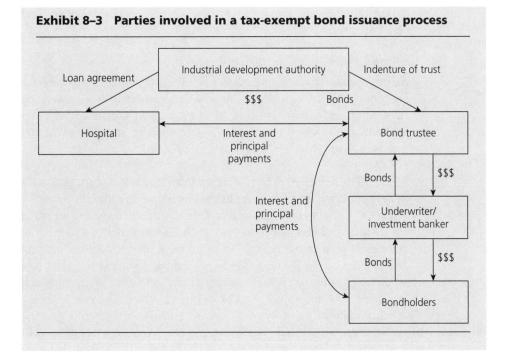

In the past, most health care facilities selected public placement because the lower interest cost differential over the lifetime of the bond offsets the front-end savings of a private placement. However, in today's market, hospitals are finding private placement attractive because they can match the length of the project with the length of the financing, particularly when it comes to projects related to medical and information technology equipment.

Public offering of a bond by a tax-exempt health care institution requires an offering prospectus to investors (OS). These tax-exempt bond issuers do not have to file a registration statement with the Securities and Exchange Commission (SEC). If required by the bond covenants, underwriters of these bonds may have to comply with Nationally Recognized Municipal Securities Information Repositories (NRMSIRs) and submit the OS as well as annual updates of financial information (audited financials and key ratios related to bond covenants) to these repositories. In contrast, stock or bond issues by for-profit corporations require stiffer disclosure requirements for investors, registration with the SEC, and annual and quarterly reports to stockholders. The OS must fully disclose information about the obligated organization (i.e., the one that promises to pay) and the project for which the bonds are issued. This allows investors to assess the risk of the issue, which includes the financial state of the facility (audited financial statements), operational background (medical and management staff, service area, services offered, sources of revenues),

Feasibility Study
A preliminary study undertaken by an organization and compiled by a third party to determine and document a project's financial viability. Depending on the results of this study, a decision will be made whether or not to proceed with said project.

Debt Capacity
The amount of total debt that an organization can be reasonably expected to take on and pay off in a timely manner.

the terms of the issue, and in some cases, a *feasibility study* of the project being financed.[3]

Steps in the Bond Issuance Process

An organization considering issuing bonds as its source of capital must go through a long and arduous process before it actually receives any cash. The bond-issuing process for not-for-profit organizations using public markets, which can take twelve to eighteen months before any cash is received, is described below.

1. The health care borrower updates its capital plan, measures its *debt capacity*, and attempts to "get its house in order."

Over a year before actually starting the bond issuance process, a health care provider needs to "get its house in order" to receive an investment grade bond rating. For example, it may attempt to build up cash reserves, decrease receivables, or liquidate some existing debt—or all three. In addition, it may update its strategic and capital plan and improve its information system or other parts of its infrastructure. The provider may also conduct a financial feasibility study of the project (see Chapter Seven regarding NPV and IRR), as well as assess its debt borrowing capacity. Appendix G, and specifically Exhibit G–4 (discussed later), presents an example of how debt capacity is measured. A hospital may spend $750,000 on plans for a $55 million project, only to find out later its cash flow and liquidity limit its debt capacity to $35 million.

2. The health care borrower identifies and selects the key parties involved in the bond issuance process.

The bond issuance process involves a host of parties involved in the issuance of tax-exempt financing. The primary members include an underwriter or investment banker, issuing authority, and bond *trustee*. Other members include lawyers, accountants, financial advisors, and feasibility consultants, if needed. The underwriters, sometimes referred to as investment bankers, are the main coordinators of the bond issuance process, though in some cases an independent financial advisor is hired instead. They provide advice during the capital planning stage, assist in identifying the debt structure (for example, the use of fixed vs. variable rate debt), oversee the purchase of credit insurance, select rating agencies and bond insurers, participate in the writing of the bond documents, organize the key party members, and plan the timetable of the bond deal. At the time of the bond issuance, the primary role of the underwriter is to purchase the bonds from the hospital via the governmental authority and then market and sell the bonds to investors.

Trustee
An agent for bondholders who ensures that the health care facility is making timely principal and interest payments to the bondholders and complies with legal covenants of the bond.

---

[3]The Web site http://www.munios.com provides electronic access to official statements of tax-exempt health care provider bond issues.

To spread the risk, the leading investment banker may invite other investment bankers to help sell the bonds. The co-managers, selling group, or both, may consist of local investment banking firms (to enhance marketability and lower the interest rate through state tax deductions as well) or national investment banking firms such as JP Morgan Chase, Goldman Sachs, or Merrill Lynch.

The trustee, typically a bank, acts as an agent for the bondholders and performs two important functions. First, the trustee collects the principal and interest payments from the health care providers and makes these payments to the bondholders. Second, the trustee ensures that the health care provider complies with the legal covenants of the bond. For example, if the health care provider were required to maintain a debt service coverage ratio above 2.5 and debt to total capital less than 50 percent, the trustee would monitor its performance with respect to these ratios. If the health care provider did not comply, it would be in default on the bond.

3. The health care borrower is evaluated by a credit rating agency.

When issuing either tax-exempt or taxable bonds to the public, health care providers turn to bond rating agencies to objectively evaluate their creditworthiness. They normally seek a credit rating from two out of the three rating agencies: Fitch, Moody's, or Standard & Poor's (S&P). Creditworthiness measures the borrower's ability to make interest and principal payments at the contracted times over the life of the bond. Rating agencies consider a range of factors to evaluate a borrower's credit risk, including financial, market, physician, utilization, and management data. They also assess any capital budgeting or financial feasibility studies related to the financed project. However, if the health care borrower does not expect its facility to receive a quality rating, it may forgo disclosure of the rating and issue a nonrated bond. (For conventional mortgage loans, a commercial bank performs the evaluation.)

Financial Evaluation From a financial standpoint, the lender or rating agency is primarily interested in evaluating a health care provider's ability to pay. This can be measured by the debt service coverage ratio as discussed in Chapter Four:

Debt service coverage = (net income + interest + depreciation + amortization) / maximum annual debt service payments

The numerator represents the health care provider's operating cash flow before its interest payments, depreciation, and amortization expenses and is divided by the *maximum* annual loan payments of principal and interest required over the life of the bond. Lenders or rating agencies expect a minimum debt service coverage ratio of 1.2. They also measure ability to pay using several other financial ratios, such as days cash on hand, operating margin, cash and investments to long-term debt, and long-term debt to total capital.

Key point *Debt service coverage ratio is one of the primary financial ratios used to evaluate a health care provider's ability to meet debt service payments.*

Market Evaluation In this step, the lender or rating agency evaluates the demand for the investment project. A wide range of factors are considered in this step, including local demographics (population growth, income levels, unemployment rate in the market area), competition from other health care providers, penetration of managed care, the industrial base of the local economy, and last, the borrower's market share for key service lines, such as cardiology, orthopedics, and oncology.

Physician and Management Evaluation Because physicians are responsible for admissions, lenders pay particular attention to the characteristics of the staff, including the number of medical staff members by specialties, their ages, the percentage of admissions by staff members, the number of board-certified physicians, and the recruitment and retention of staff.

The lender or credit rating agency also examines the health care provider's management staff for such things as background and experience, how they are organized, and how they relate to the medical staff. Any recent turnover of management staff and its effect on the organization would be scrutinized closely.

4. The bond is rated by a credit rating agency.

Rating agencies visit the facility to gain further insight into operation of the hospital and the relationship among management, board members, and medical staff. After reviewing quantitative data and performing an on-site assessment, the rating analysts recommend a final rating, which can be appealed by the borrower. The ratings assess the organization's creditworthiness or the likelihood of default of a bond. The higher the rating, the lower the interest rate the organization has to pay (a higher rating implies less risk of default to investors but means a lower coupon). The three primary rating agencies are Fitch, Moody's, and Standard & Poor's (S&P). The rating assigned to an issue affects the interest rate and marketability of the bond. Depending on the size and complexity of the issue, simply getting a rating can cost the issuer from $1,000 to $50,000. The assigned ratings for all agencies are listed in Exhibit 8–4. *Investment grade* ratings range from AAA to BBB (S&P and Fitch), or Aaa to Baa (Moody's), of which the highest are called *quality* ratings. *Junk bonds* are rated BB and below by S&P and Ba and below by Moody's. Within the junk bond category are *substandard* and *speculative* bonds, both of which are considered risky investments. Some providers may choose not to have their bonds rated because they are relatively small or they will receive a "below investment grade" rating.

Key point *Investment grade bonds are at or above S&P's BBB rating or Moody's Baa rating. Bonds below this rating in either category may be considered junk bonds.*

Exhibit 8–4   Comparison of Moody's, Fitch, and S&P's bond ratings

Moody's Rating	Fitch & S&P's Rating	Interpretation	Grade of the Bond
Aaa	AAA	Judged to be the best quality	Quality
Aa	AA	High quality, smaller amount of protection than AAA	Quality
A	A	Many favorable investment attributes	Investment grade
Baa	BBB	Medium grade; neither highly protected nor poorly secured	Investment grade
Ba	BB	Speculative elements; future cannot be considered as well assured	Substandard junk bonds
B	B	Generally lack characteristics of desirable investment	Substandard junk bonds
Caa	CCC	Poor standing; may be in default or have elements of danger	Speculative junk bonds
Ca, C	CC, C	Very speculative; often in default; very poor prospects	Speculative junk bonds
DDD	D	Bond in default	Speculative junk bonds

Typically a health care provider is unable to achieve the top AAA or Aaa rating unless it purchases a credit enhancement via bond insurance. Health care providers in the AA/Aa rating category not only have excellent financial strength but are more likely to be health care systems with strong management, large bed size, and a superior medical staff. These hospitals tend to rely less on Medicare and Medicaid revenues, exhibit low debt ratios, generate strong profits, and possess large cash reserves. Health care providers in the BBB/Baa and substandard categories are normally smaller facilities located in competitive or rural markets and serve a high proportion of Medicare and Medicaid patients. Furthermore, their cash reserves tend to be low, and they possess a high amount of debt. Exhibit 8–5 lists three Fitch bond ratings for not-for-profit hospitals and offers a sample of their respective financial ratios. Perspective 8–5 discusses the process that the Fitch rating agency follows in rating a health care provider's bond.

A health care provider can strengthen its credit rating, and thereby lower its interest rate and increase its marketability, through either bond insurance or a letter of credit. For a fee of 0.07 to 2 percent of the bond's total value, a facility can obtain bond insurance that guarantees the timely payments of principal and interest to bondholders in the unlikely event of default by the health care provider. The rating then

Exhibit 8–5   Selected median ratio values for not-for-profit hospitals and health systems: 2005

Measure	Bond Rating		
	AA	A	BBB
Bad debt expense to operating revenues	4.7%	5.7%	5.8%
Debt service coverage ratio	5.6	4.0	3.0
Operating margin	4.1%	3.2%	2.2%
Total profit margin	7.8%	5.2%	3.8%
Investment income to net income	45.0%	43.0%	41.0%
Age of plant, years	9.5	9.7	9.5
Days cash on hand	237	185	120
Days in accounts receivable	51	51	48
Average payment period, days	61	62	61
Long-term debt to total capital	32.8%	38.9%	47.0%
Cash and investment to total debt	153%	111%	74%

Source: 2007 Median Ratios for Nonprofit Hospitals and Health Systems, Aug. 8, 2007, Fitch Rating Agency.

Perspective 8–5   Health Care Rating Process

Fitch Credit Rating Agency considers an array of quantitative and qualitative factors in rating a health care provider. After the agency conducts an initial review of this information, the rating agency will send its credit analysts to visit the health care provider. The agency believes that the time spent visiting the hospital allows their analysts to hear directly from management about their philosophy, operation, mission, and strategic plans, as well as seeing the actual physical layout of the hospital and its surrounding market area. During the visit, the analysts expect the hospital to focus on such issues as the role of the board and medical staff, retention policy for employees, market trends, strengths and weaknesses of the hospital, future capital outlays and financing needs, and current financial condition. Another important aspect of the visit includes educating the credit analysts on the economic climate of the hospital's service area as well as driving distances among competing hospitals and other competing providers. After the visit, the rating analysts more than likely have follow-up questions to the hospital. Finally, the analysts will correspond to the hospital their recommended rating to Fitch's credit committee. The committee votes on the recommended rating, with the rating determined by a majority vote. The hospital executives can appeal if they contend that certain issues were left out of the analysis.

Source: Rating process for nonprofit health care credits, *Fitch Rating Agency,* July 11, 2005.

assigned to the bond is a function of the credit strength of the bond insurance company. In 2008, major bond insurers such as AMBAC and MBIA lost their "AAA" credit ratings due to insuring high-risk, mortgage-backed securities. To raise their credit rating to "AA and higher," so that they could sell bond insurance for health care providers, in 2009, these companies were trying to form separate subsidiaries that insured only tax-exempt bonds.

A *letter of credit* through a bank is another option to enhance the rating of an issuer's bond. The cost is an initial fee plus an ongoing percentage of the outstanding amount remaining on the issue each year. Again, the bond's rating is dependent on the strength of the bank.

The rating of a bond traded in the marketplace, called an *outstanding bond issue*, is reviewed on a periodic basis and could be either upgraded or downgraded, depending on the issuer's present financial or operational conditions. For example, S&P lowered the rating of a hospital in North Carolina from BBB to BB after it had issued debt to pay for a replacement hospital. The agency cited decreased patient volume, loss of key physicians, and poor economic conditions in the market area that contributed to a lower debt service coverage ratio of 1.0, an operating margin of –1.6%, and declines in other key financial ratios. Conversely, during the late 2000s, hospital and health system bonds rated above investment grade demonstrated improved financial and utilization indicators. As a result, S&P upgraded more of its hospital bonds than it downgraded because of improved financial and operating performance. These improvements ranged from higher profitability and cash flow, higher returns from investments, and stronger liquidity position coupled with operational changes related to the return of hospitals to their core business of patient care and an overall gain in hospital efficiency. Perspective 8–6 lists specific factors affecting the change in the credit rating of tax-exempt hospital bonds.

Bond Insurance
By purchasing bond insurance, which protects against default, a hospital borrower can lower its cost of debt and improve the bond's marketability.

Outstanding Bond Issue
A bond that trades in the marketplace.

5. The health care borrower enters into a loan agreement with the governmental authority, the issuer of the bonds.

The hospital borrower issues its bonds through a governmental authority, which is either a city, county, or state entity. A loan agreement that is equivalent to the bond payments establishes this relationship and specifies that the hospital borrower, not the issuer, is responsible for the debt payments.

Net Proceeds from a Bond Issuance
Gross proceeds less the underwriter's and others' issuance fees.

6. The underwriters sell the bonds to bondholders at the public offering price, and the trustee provides the health care provider with the *net proceeds from a bond issuance*.

The issuance process actually begins several weeks before the official pricing date of the bonds, when the underwriter(s) issue a preliminary official statement *(POS)* to prospective buyers approximately two weeks before pricing. This document allows investors to assess the

POS
A preliminary official statement offered to prospective buyers of a bond by the underwriters to help determine a fair market price for the bond.

Perspective 8–6　Factors Affecting Credit Ratings of Hospital Bonds

Over the next ten years, Moody's has listed several key rating issues that will challenge the credit ratings of hospital bonds. These factors include

1. Declining payments for Medicare and Medicaid due to rising federal deficits and shortfalls in state budgets as well
2. Increasing competition from ambulatory surgical and imaging centers, which may impact their most profitable services
3. Rising capital spending to improve quality of care and patient amenities (such as private rooms), to replace aging facilities, and to increase technology and medical equipment in order to remain competitive may increase costs, deplete cash reserves, and raise level of debt capital
4. Changing to high deductible health plans will increase patients' copayments and deductibles and result in higher bad debt for hospitals
5. Increasing government scrutiny with respect to hospital's policies in the areas of charity care, pricing, and billing and collection practices, which may force hospitals to provide more charity care and community benefits

If these factors contribute to declining liquidity in terms of lower days cash on hand and operating financials, specifically debt service coverage, cash flow margin, and falling volume because of competition, one would expect a downgrade in a hospital's bond rating.

Source: Moody's Public Finance. 2008 (Jan). Moody's rating methodology: not-for-profit hospitals and health systems. *Moody's Investor Service.*

borrower's creditworthiness. After assessing the market for current interest rates, the underwriters construct a pre-pricing scale of interest rates for various maturities. The underwriter's primary objective is to achieve the lowest interest rate for the borrower that will still attract investors to purchase the bond. Thus, the objective of the underwriter is to achieve an equilibrium interest rate that ensures marketability, yet avoids oversubscription of the issue. If on the pricing date oversubscription occurs, this indicates that the interest rate is set too high and, thus, unfavorable to the borrower (health care provider). In this case, the underwriter will lower the interest rate, which will decrease the number of bond orders and make the interest rate fairer to the borrower (health care provider).

Once the final interest rates for given maturities have been set, an agreement is signed by the issuer and the leading underwriter. Shortly thereafter, the underwriter purchases the bonds and sells them to investors at the predetermined price. The bond issuance process closes approximately two weeks later when the underwriter transfers the proceeds to the health care provider via the trustee. In short, the pricing period allows the underwriter to obtain indications of market interest rates from institutional buyers to reduce its own risk before buying the bonds.

The cost of the issuance process includes service payments for legal, accounting, feasibility, underwriting or investment banking, financial advisors, trustee, and any credit enhancement (bond insurance or letter of credit). The fees may vary from 1 to 2 percent of the total amount issued.

After the issuance process has been completed, the health care provider makes monthly interest and principal payments to the trustee, who in turn pays the investors or bondholders on a semi-annual basis for interest payments and on an annual basis (or so directed by the maturity schedule) for the principal payments.

LEASE FINANCING

As health care facilities find it more difficult to acquire capital to finance equipment, many consider lease arrangements as a necessary and viable alternative. Leasing now accounts for 20 to 25 percent of all health care provider equipment spending. A lease involves two parties: the *lessor*, who owns the asset, and the *lessee*, who pays the lessor for the use of the asset but does not own it. A health care provider may decide to enter into a lease arrangement for several reasons:

Lessor
An entity who owns an asset that is then leased out.

1. *To avoid the bureaucratic delays of capital budget requests.* Because of the longer, closer scrutiny given capital budgeting requests by top management and the board, an administrator may find it more convenient to lease a piece of medical equipment rather than to request it in the capital budget. This is especially true for state- or city-owned facilities whose capital purchases require governmental approval.

Lessee
An entity who negotiates the use of another's asset via a lease.

Key point *The lessor owns the asset, and the lessee makes lease payments to the lessor for the use of the asset.*

---

2. *To avoid technological obsolescence.* Given the rapid changes in health care technology, lessees can avoid paying for high-tech equipment that may become outdated shortly. By leasing, a facility can continually upgrade its equipment; the risk of technological obsolescence then shifts to the lessor.

3. *To receive better maintenance services.* Most full-service leases include maintenance for the equipment. Some believe that because the lessor owns the equipment, maintenance is better.

4. *To allow for convenience.* If an asset is to be used for only a short time, leasing is less time-consuming and costly than buying and selling shortly thereafter. Because leasing constitutes 100 percent financing, leasing companies advertise that it

frees cash for other purposes. A facility could also avoid a cash down-payment by borrowing enough to cover the full cost of the lease, which is less than buying the asset outright. Thus, from a financial perspective, lease financing appears equivalent to debt financing, with the only major difference being that a facility never actually owns a leased asset.

Operating Lease
A lease that lasts shorter than the useful life of the leased asset, typically one year or less. This type of leasing arrangement can be canceled at any time without penalty, but there is no option to purchase the asset once the lease has expired.

Capital Lease
A lease that lasts for an extended period, up to the life of the leased asset. This type of lease cannot be canceled without penalty, and at the end of the lease period, the lessee may have the option to purchase the asset. Also called a *financial lease*.

Financial Lease
See capital lease.

Sale and Leaseback Arrangement
A type of capital lease whereby an institution sells an owned asset and then simultaneously leases it back from the purchaser. The selling institution retains rights to use the asset but benefits from the immediate acquisition of cash from the sale.

The two major types of leases are operating leases and capital leases.

Operating Lease

An *operating lease* is for service equipment leased for periods shorter than the equipment's economic life, usually between a few days and a year. The lessor's aim is to lease for less than the equipment's full cost but to recover the cost by leasing the same asset many times over its economic life. The usual types of assets covered by operating leases are computers, copier machines, and vehicles. The lessor incurs all the ownership costs of maintenance, service, and insurance on the leased equipment.

A second characteristic of operating leases is a cancellation clause, which gives the lessee the option to return the leased asset to the lessor with little or no penalty at any time during the life of the lease. Finally, if the operating lease complies with specific accounting standards (e.g., no automatic transfer of title), it can be treated as "*off balance sheet financing.*" This means that the lease is not reported on the balance sheet under long-term debt but instead is reflected on the income statement as an operating expense. The Financial Accounting Standards Board (FASB) has specific conditions that define an operating versus a capital lease.[4]

Capital Lease

In a *capital lease*, also called a *financial lease*, the lessor aims to lease the asset for virtually all of its economic life. In return, the lessee is committed to lease payments for the entire lease period. The lessee does not have the option to cancel a capital lease immediately without a substantial penalty but does have an option to buy the leased asset at the end of the lease agreement. The latter option tends to be more expensive than if the facility had initially bought the equipment outright because the lessor always operates with a margin for profit; however, the lessee may not be in a financial position initially to be able to afford the full cost of the asset.

One type of capital lease used by the health care industry is the *sale and leaseback arrangement*, whereby a health care provider sells an

---

[4]A discussion of this issue is beyond the scope of this textbook, but a detailed explanation of these conditions can be found under FASB statement number 13, specifically http://www.fasb.org/pdf/fas13.pdf

owned asset (such as a clinic) to a third party and simultaneously leases it back from the purchaser. By selling the owned asset, the facility is able to obtain immediate capital, though it still retains use of the asset.

From a financial management perspective, a capital lease has implications similar to buying an asset and financing it with debt. Buying through borrowing and negotiating a capital lease are similar in that both require contractual payments (debt or lease payments) over the life of the asset, and both options incur the costs of operating the asset. In addition, the capital lease, just like a debt obligation, is reported in the balance sheet under long-term debt obligations. The primary difference occurs at the end of the asset's life, when the lease provisions require the asset to be returned to the lessor (the owner), unless the contract stipulates an option to buy or renew. In contrast, under the buy-borrow option, the owner may either sell or continue to use an asset at any point.

Key point *In contrast to an operating lease, a capital lease has attributes similar to owning an asset. The latter type of leasing arrangement also provides the option to buy the asset.*

Analysis of the Lease versus Purchase Decision

One of the most common financial decisions made by a health care organization is whether to buy or lease a needed asset. The usual approach is to compare the present value cost of a buy decision with the present value cost of a lease decision over a specified time. From a purely financial standpoint, the option with the lower present value cost is preferable. In making this assessment, several factors must be considered. Taxpaying entities realize either an effective lower net lease payment from the tax deduction of the lease payment, or an interest and depreciation tax shield from buying the asset. The cost of ownership includes the outflow of cash to maintain the asset offset by the inflow of cash from its salvage value. Interest and depreciation expenses act as *tax shields* because they are tax-deductible expenses, which reduce the taxes paid to the government. Last, the cash flows under the lease option are discounted back at the after-tax cost of debt rather than at the cost of capital.

Tax Shield
An investment for a for-profit entity that reduces the amount of income tax to be paid, often because interest and depreciation expenses are tax deductible.

Suppose Five-Star General Hospital is undecided about purchasing a $10 million piece of equipment or leasing it. If it decides to buy the asset, it can borrow the full amount from its local bank at a rate of 10 percent; the equipment would be depreciated at a rate of $2 million per year over its five-year life to a zero salvage value. Under the lease arrangement, the gross lease payments would be $3 million per year, starting one year from now. Assuming the organization is a taxpaying entity with a 30 percent tax rate, which is the better alternative from an economic standpoint?

Exhibit 8–6 presents the analysis of this purchasing versus leasing decision. Because the present value sum of the financing flows for purchasing is the higher of the two options (less of a loss), –$7,540,000 versus –$8,610,000, purchasing the asset is the desired alternative to leasing.

Exhibit 8-6 Comparison of purchasing arrangement with leasing arrangement for Five-Star General Hospital

Givens (in thousands)

1	Annual annuity payment[a]	$2,638
2	Interest rate	10%
3	Annual depreciation expense[b]	$2,000
4	Tax rate	30%
5	Depreciation expense tax shield[c]	$600
6	After-tax cost of debt[d]	7%
7	Before-tax lease payments	$3,000

[a] PVFA, 10%, 5 yrs = 3.7908. $10,000 initial investment / 3.7908
[b] $10,000 purchase price / 5 years useful life = $2,000 depreciation expense per year
[c] $2,000 depreciation expense per year x 30% tax rate = $600 tax shield per year
[d] (Interest Rate) x (1 – Tax Rate) = 10% x (1 – 30%) = 7%

Purchasing Arrangement

	A	B	C	D	E	F	G	H	I
	Annuity Payment	Interest Expense (D* ×	Principal Payment	Remaining Balance	Interest Expense Tax Shield (B ×	Depreciation Expense Tax Shield	Net Cash Outflow (if Owned)	PV Factor from	PV of Net Cash Outflows (if Owned)
Year	(Given 1)	Given 2)	(A – B)	(D* – C)	Given 4)	(Given 5)	[A – (E + F)]	(Given 6)	(G × H)
0				$10,000 – (₣3)					
1	$2,638	$1,000	= $1,638	8,362	$300	$600	$1,738	0.9346	$1,624
2	2,638	836	1,802	6,560	251	600	1,787	0.8734	1,561
3	2,638	656	1,982	4,578	197	600	1,841	0.8163	1,503
4	2,638	458	2,180	2,398	137	600	1,901	0.7629	1,450
5	2,638	240	2,398	0	72	600	1,966	0.7130	1,402
Total									$7,540

Note: D* is the previous year's Column D value.

Exhibit 8-6 *(Continued)*

Leasing Arrangement

Year	J Before-Tax Lease Payments (Given 7)	K Lease Tax Shield (J × Given 4)	L Net after Lease Payments (J – K)	M PV Factor from (Given 6)	N PV of Net Cash Outflows (if Leased) (L × M)
0					
1	$3,000	$900	$2,100	0.9346	$1,963
2	3,000	900	2,100	0.8734	1,834
3	3,000	900	2,100	0.8163	1,714
4	3,000	900	2,100	0.7629	1,602
5	3,000	900	2,100	0.7130	1,497
Total					$8,610

Note: All dollar figures are expressed in thousands.

- A loan amortization schedule similar to the one in Exhibit G–3 is presented in columns A through D in the top section for the purchasing arrangement. The loan amortization amount ($2,638,000, Given 1) is calculated by dividing the initial investment amount ($10 million) by the present value factor for an annuity at 10 percent interest for five years (3.7908). Column A represents the only cash outflows, which are the loan payments.

- Columns E and F present cash inflows from interest and depreciation expense tax shields. The interest expense tax shield was computed by multiplying the interest expense in column B by the same tax rate of 30 percent (Given 4). The depreciation tax shield inflow ($600,000) was computed by multiplying the annual depreciation expense, $2 million, by the tax rate, 30 percent (Givens 3 and 4).

- The net cash outflow, column G, equals the annual loan payment from column A less the tax shield amounts in columns E and F. Finally, the net cash outflow is discounted back at the net after-tax cost of debt: $10\% \times (1 - 0.30) = 7\%$. Because the cash flows are net of taxes, the calculations should be based on the net after-tax cost of debt as well. Column H gives the present value factors at 7 percent, and column I shows the net present value of the decision to purchase the asset, –$7,540,000.

- The lower section shows the calculations for the leasing alternative. Cash outflows, column L, are also examined net of taxes; thus, the net payment equals only $2.1 million per year [$3 million $\times$ (1 – 0.30)]. These payments are also discounted back at the same net after-tax cost of debt rate of 7 percent. Column N shows the present value of the leasing decision, –$8,610,000.

If Five-Star General were a non-taxpaying entity, there would be no tax shield benefits. In this case, the analysis would be simplified by comparing only the present value of the loan payments with the present value of the lease payments, but the cost of debt would be 10 percent, not 7 percent. Although normally it would be necessary to go through these calculations if the payments differed each year, it can easily be seen here that with flat payments every year under both options ($2.638 million borrowing vs. $3.0 million leasing), purchasing would be less costly than leasing. Therefore, the present value of the loan of $10 million would be less than the present value of the lease, and the decision would be to borrow the funds and buy the asset.

Caution: Salvage or residual value of an asset should also be considered in the buy-or-borrow evaluation. Residual values are a cash inflow. Because the cash flow of the residual value is less certain than the debt and lease cash flows, some financial analysts may use a higher rate than the after-tax cost of debt to discount this cash flow.

SUMMARY

There are three ways to finance assets: using debt (liabilities), equity, or a combination of the two.

$$\text{Assets} = \text{Debt} + \text{Equity}$$

Any increase in assets must be balanced by a similar increase in debt, equity, or both. The structuring of debt relative to equity is called the capital structure decision and is increasingly important to both for-profit and not-for-profit providers. In today's environment characterized by prospective and capitated payments, the increased use of managed care and outpatient services, and increasing cutbacks caused by competition, obtaining debt and equity financing is a much more complicated undertaking. Both types of financing have advantages and disadvantages.

The primary sources of equity financing for not-for-profit health care organizations are internally generated funds, philanthropy, and government grants, whereas for-profit facilities primarily rely on internally generated funds and stock issuances. Unfortunately, internally generated funds—funds retained from operations (retained earnings)—are shrinking.

A rule of thumb is to borrow short term for short-term needs and long term for long-term needs. Short-term financing typically refers to a wide range of financing, from debt that must be paid back almost immediately to debt that may not have to be paid off for up to a year. Long-term financing typically refers to debt that must be paid off in a period longer than a year. The two major types of long-term

financing are term loans, which must be paid off in one to ten years, and bonds, which may have a final maturity of up to twenty to thirty-five years. Bonds are the primary source of long-term financing for tax-exempt health care entities.

Types of debt financing available to not-for-profit health care organizations include bank term loans, conventional mortgages, FHA-insured mortgages, tax-exempt financing (available only to not-for-profit organizations), and taxable bonds.

Organizations that decide to issue bonds generally go through a series of six steps:

Step 1. The health care borrower updates its capital plan, measures its debt capacity, and attempts to "get its house in order."

Step 2. The health care borrower selects the key parties involved in the bond issuance.

Step 3. The health care borrower is evaluated by a credit rating agency.

Step 4. Bond is rated by the credit rating agency.

Step 5. The health care borrower enters into a loan agreement with the governmental authority, the issuer of the bonds.

Step 6. The underwriters sell the bonds to bondholders at the public offering price, and the trustee provides the health care provider with the net proceeds.

Bonds can be issued with either fixed-rate or variable-rate interest, each of which has advantages and disadvantages.

An alternative to traditional equity and debt financing is leasing. Leasing is undertaken for four reasons: to avoid the bureaucratic delays of capital budget requests, to avoid technological obsolescence, to receive better maintenance services, and to allow for convenience.

There are two types of leases: operating and capital. An operating lease is for service equipment leased for periods shorter than the equipment's economic life, usually between a few days and a year. Under a capital lease, also called a financial lease, the lessor aims to lease the asset for virtually all of its economic life. In return, the lessee is committed to lease payments for the entire lease period.

KEY TERMS

a. Amortization
b. Bond
c. Bond issuance
d. Capital lease
e. Collateral
f. Debt capacity
g. Discount
h. Feasibility study
i. Financial lease
j. Fixed income security
k. Hedging
l. Interest rate swap
m. Lessee
n. Lessor
o. Letter of credit
p. Market value

q. Net proceeds from a bond issuance
r. Off balance sheet financing
s. Operating lease
t. Outstanding bond issue
u. Par value
v. POS
w. Premium
x. Rating of bond
y. Required market rate
z. Sale-leaseback arrangement
aa. Sinking fund
bb. Tax shield
cc. Term loan
dd. Trustee
ee. Yield to maturity

KEY EQUATIONS

Bond valuation (annual coupon payments):

$$\text{Market value} = (\text{coupon payment}) \times \text{PVFA}(k, n) + (\text{par value}) \times \text{PVF}(k, n)$$

Bond valuation (semi-annual periods for coupon payments):

Market value = (coupon payment / 2) × PVFA(k / 2, n × 2) + (par value) × PVF(k / 2, n × 2)

QUESTIONS AND PROBLEMS

1. **Definitions.** Define the terms listed on the previous page.

2. **Equity position.** What avenues are available for for-profit and not-for-profit health care providers to increase their equity position?

3. **Debt versus equity financing.** What are the advantages and disadvantages to a taxpaying entity in issuing debt as opposed to equity?

4. **Debt financing.** Does adding debt increase or decrease the flexibility of a health care provider? Why?

5. **Basis points.** How much is a basis point? How many basis points between 6⅝ percent and 6¾ percent?

6. **Debentures.** Explain the difference between subordinated debentures and debentures.

7. **Bonds.** Name at least two factors that might cause a facility to call in its bond.

8. **Bonds.** What are the advantages and disadvantages of a taxable bond relative to a tax-exempt bond? Who is the issuer of tax-exempt bonds?

9. **Bonds.** What party acts on behalf of bondholders to ensure that the issuing facility not only is complying with the covenants of the bond but also is making timely principal and interest payments to the bondholders?

10. **Investment bankers.** Why would an investment banker syndicate a bond issue with other investment bankers?

11. **Bonds.** Compare private placement bond issues with public placement bond issues.

12. **Credit ratings.** Identify two ways that a health care provider can strengthen its credit rating. What are some of the ramifications of these options?

13. **Credit ratings.** What can cause a health care provider's credit rating to be downgraded?

14. **Market rates.** What impact do required market rate changes have on bonds of longer maturities?

15. **Leasing.** What are the two types of leasing arrangements and their primary differences?

16. **Leasing.** Why might an organization enter into a leasing arrangement?

17. **Bond valuation.** If a $1,000 zero coupon bond with a twenty-year maturity has a market price of $376.90, what is its rate of return? (*Hint:* see Appendix G.)

18. **Bond valuation.** If a $1,000 zero coupon bond with a fifteen-year maturity has a market price of $315.20, what is its rate of return? (*Hint:* see Appendix G.)

19. **Bond valuation.** A tax-exempt bond was recently issued at an annual 12 percent coupon rate and matures twenty years from today. The par value of the bond is $1,000. (*Hint:* see Appendix G)

   a. If required market rates are 12 percent, what is the market price of the bond?

   b. If required market rates fall to 6 percent, what is the market price of the bond?

   c. If required market rates rise to 18 percent, what is the market price of the bond?

   d. At what required market rate (6 percent, 12 percent, or 18 percent) does the above bond sell at a discount? At a premium?

20. **Bond valuation.** A tax-exempt bond was recently issued at an annual 10 percent coupon rate and matures thirty years from today. The par value of the bond is $5,000. (*Hint:* see Appendix G.)

   a. If required market rates are 10 percent, what is the market price of the bond?

   b. If required market rates fall to 5 percent, what is the market price of the bond?

   c. If required market rates rise to 20 percent, what is the market price of the bond?

   d. At what required market rate (5 percent, 10 percent, or 20 percent) does the above bond sell at a discount? At a premium?

21. **Bond valuation.** Assuming that the bond in problem 19 matures in five years, what would be the market prices under the various required market interest rate changes? (See Appendix G.)

22. **Bond valuation.** Assuming that the bond in problem 20 matures in ten years, what would be the market prices under the various required market interest rate changes? (See Appendix G.)

23. **Bond valuation.** Charles City Hospital plans on issuing a tax-exempt bond at an annual coupon rate of 8 percent with a maturity of thirty years. The par value of the bond is $1,000. (See Appendix G.)

   a. If required market rates are 8 percent, what is the value of the bond?

   b. If required market rates fall to 4 percent, what is the value of the bond?

   c.   If required market rates fall to 12 percent, what is the value of the bond?

   d.   At what required market rate (4 percent, 8 percent, or 12 percent) does the above bond sell at a discount? At a premium?

24. **Bond valuation.** Assuming that the bond in problem 23 matures in ten years, what would be the market prices under the various required interest rate changes? (See Appendix G.)

25. **Bond valuation.** A $1,000 par value bond with an annual 6 percent coupon rate will mature in twelve years. Coupon payments are made semi-annually. What is its market price if the required market rate is 4 percent? (See Appendix G.)

26. **Bond valuation.** A $1,000 par value bond with an annual 10 percent coupon rate will mature in twenty years. Coupon payments are made semi-annually. What is the market price if the required market rate is 8 percent? (See Appendix G.)

27. **Bond valuation.** Currently, Boston Common Community Hospital's tax-exempt bond is selling for $626.53 per bond and has a remaining maturity of twenty years. If the par value is $1,000 and the coupon rate is 7 percent, what is the yield to maturity? (See Appendix G.)

28. **Bond valuation.** Haven Hospital's tax-exempt bond is currently selling for $818.46 and has a remaining maturity of twenty-five years. If the par value is $1,000 and the coupon rate is 8 percent, what is the yield to maturity? (See Appendix G.)

29. **Loan amortization.** Land Hope Hospital needs to borrow $1,000,000 to purchase an MRI. The interest rate for the loan is 8 percent. Principal and interest payments are equal debt service payments, made on an annual basis. The length of the loan is five years. The CEO of Land Hope wants to develop a loan amortization schedule for this debt borrowing for tomorrow morning's meeting. Prepare such a schedule. (See Appendix G.)

30. **Loan amortization.** Petersville Hospital needs to borrow $60 million to finance its new facility. The interest rate is 6 percent for the loan. Principal and interest payments are equal debt service payments, made on an annual basis. The length of the loan is ten years. The CFO would like to develop a loan amortization schedule for this debt issuance. (See Appendix G.)

31. **Purchase versus lease.** Mercy Medical Mega Center, a taxpaying entity, has made the decision to purchase a new laser surgical device. The device costs $500,000 and will be depreciated on a straight-line basis over five years to a zero salvage value. Mercy Medical could borrow the full amount at a 12 percent rate for five years. The after-tax cost of debt equals 8 percent. Alternatively, it could lease the device for five years. The before-tax lease payments per year would be $90,000. The tax rate for this Mega Center is 40 percent. From a financial perspective, should Mercy lease the surgical device or borrow the money to purchase it?

32. **Purchase versus lease.** New Health Hospital Systems wants to either borrow money to purchase a hospital or else enter into a lease agreement with the city of Chesterville. The purchase price of the hospital is $35 million. Assuming 100 percent financing, the interest rate is 8 percent for the loan with an after-tax cost of debt of 5 percent. The length of the loan is five years. The before-tax lease payments are expected to be $8 million per year. The tax rate is 40 percent for New Health System. Should New Health System lease or borrow the money to purchase the hospital?

33. **Purchase versus lease.** Carolina Ancillary Services for Hospitals (CASH), a tax-paying entity, is considering the purchase of a 64-slice computed tomographic scanner. The cost of the scanner is $2,000,000. The scanner would be depreciated over ten years on a straight-line basis to a zero salvage value. At the end of five years, the scanner could be sold for its book value, $1,000,000. The tax rate is 40 percent. The financing options include either borrowing for the full cost of the scanner and selling it at the end of year 5 or leasing one. The lease option is a five-year lease with equal before-tax lease payments of $550,000 per year. The borrowing alternative is a five-year loan covering the entire cost of the scanner at an interest rate of 6 percent. The after-tax cost of debt is 4 percent. Should CASH lease the scanner or borrow the full amount to purchase it?

34. **Purchase versus lease.** Tidewater Hospital, a taxpaying entity, is considering a leasing arrangement for its ambulance fleet. The fleet of ambulances costs $250,000 and will be depreciated over a ten-year life to a salvage value of $50,000. Tidewater could finance the entire fleet with equal annual debt and principal payments at a before-tax cost of debt of 9 percent and an after-tax cost of debt at 6 percent for ten years. Alternatively, it could lease the fleet for ten years. The before-tax lease payments are $45,000 per year for ten years. Tidewater's tax rate is 40 percent. From a financial perspective, should Tidewater lease or borrow the money to buy the ambulances?

35. **Debt capacity.** Exton Hospital is considering a new replacement hospital and plans to issue long-term bonds to finance the project. Before it meets with its investment bankers, the hospital wants to estimate how much additional debt it can take on. Currently, the hospital has annual debt service payments of $2 million, and its cash flow available to meet debt service payment is $10 million per year. For its new debt issuance, the hospital plans to issue fixed-rate debt for thirty years. It also assumes that Fitch Rating Agency will assign it a BBB rating. Fitch's median debt service coverage ratio for BBB bonds is 3.0×. The expected fixed interest rate for a thirty-year BBB rate tax-exempt bond is 5 percent. Using Fitch's median debt service coverage ratio for a BBB-rated bond along with the prior information, how much additional debt could Exton Hospital take on? (See Appendix G.)

36. **Debt capacity.** Springfield Health System is considering developing full-service imaging centers across its service area and plans to issue long-term debt to finance these centers. Before it meets with its investment bankers, it wants to estimate how much additional debt it can take on. Currently, Springfield Health System has annual debt service payments of $5 million, and its cash flow available to meet debt service payment is $25 million per year. For its new debt issuance, it plans to issue fixed-rate debt for thirty years. It also assumes Fitch Rating Agency will assign it a BBB rating. Fitch's median debt service coverage ratio for BBB-rated large health care systems is 2.75×. The expected fixed rate for a thirty-year BBB-rate long-term bond is 5 percent. Using Fitch's median debt service coverage ratio for a BBB-rated bond along with the prior information, how much additional debt could Springfield take on? (See Appendix G.)

APPENDIX G

BOND VALUATION, LOAN AMORTIZATION, AND DEBT BORROWING CAPACITY

A facility plans to market bonds at the lowest possible interest rate, but to do so, it first must carefully scrutinize the current market's relationship between bond prices and yield to maturity. Because many bonds have a call feature as well, the facility must also examine how this will affect interest rates. The facility must understand the process of paying off its debt.

BOND VALUATION FOR YIELD TO MATURITY

Most bonds are *fixed income securities*, which mean the investor receives a fixed amount of interest periodically, usually semi-annually, over the lifetime of the bond. With fixed interest rate securities, the coupon payment does not change from year to year, even though the market interest rate may change. A bond's *market value* is the price at which a bond can be bought or sold today in the open market. Although market value should not be confused with *par value*, a bond's face value, a bond may be issued with an equal market value and par value.

The *yield to maturity* (YTM), or *required market rate* of a bond, is used by analysts to determine the return on the bond. The YTM is the rate at which the market value of a bond is equal to the bond's present value of future coupon payments plus par value. The *bond valuation formula* is defined as:

Fixed Income Security
A bond that pays fixed amounts of interest at regular periodic intervals, usually semi-annually.

Market Value
What a bond would sell for in today's open market.

Par Value
The face value amount of a bond, the amount the bondholder is paid at maturity; it does not include any coupon payments.

$$MV = \left[\sum_{t=1}^{n} CP_t / (1 + k)^t\right] + PV / (1 + k)^n$$

where MV is the market value (price) of the bond, CP represents the coupon payment on the bond, PV is the bond's par value, n is the number of periods to maturity, t represents 1, 2, 3 . . . n periods, and k indicates the yield to maturity (required market rate).

Fortunately, it is not necessary to use this formula in its present form, which can get lengthy and complicated. In fact, the first part of the formula after the summation sign is simply the calculation for the present value of an annuity; the latter part of the formula reduces to a basic present value term. In line with the terms discussed in Chapter Six, the formula can be simplified to:

Yield to Maturity
The rate at which the market value of a bond is equal to the bond's present value of future coupon payments plus par value.

Required Market Rate
The market interest rate on similar risk bonds.

Market value = (coupon payment) × PVFA(k,n) + (par value) × PVF(k,n)

Exhibit G–1a and Exhibit G–1b show how to use the formula by proving that when the coupon rate equals the required market rate, market value equals par value. Suppose a hospital wants to issue $100,000 worth of bonds with a twenty-year maturity date.

Exhibit G–1a   Example of how to use the bond valuation formula where coupon rate equals required market rate

	Givens	
1	Par value	$5,000
2	Market rate (k)	8%
3	Time horizon in years (n)	20
4	Coupon rate	8%
5	Coupon payment[a]	$400

[a] Coupon Payment = (Coupon Rate) × (Par Value)

Market value = (coupon payment) × PVFA(k,n) + (par value) × PVF(k,n)
Market value = $400 × PVFA(0.08, 20) + $5,000 × PVF(0.08, 20)
Market value = $400 × 9.8181 + $5,000 × 0.2145
Market value = $3,927 + $1,073 = $5,000

Exhibit G–1b   Using IRR formula to solve for yield to maturity or market rate, k

Using Excel IRR formula to compute the Market Rate, k, of the bond.
    The values in the array D11:X11 include −1211, 90, 90, 90,....1090), and the function calculates a value of 7%.

Function Arguments ☒

IRR

Values D11:X11 ▦ = {-1211,90,90,90,90

Guess ▦ = number

= 0.070071953

Returns the internal rate of return for a series of cash flows.

Guess is a number that you guess is close to the result of IRR; 0.1 (10 percent) if omitted.

Formula result =   7%

Help on this function   [OK] [Cancel]

The present market interest rate is 8 percent, and the hospital sets its coupon rate at 8 percent to equal the required market rate. Bonds are sold in denominations of $1,000 or $5,000 each, which is the par value.

As with the techniques to find the internal rate of return (IRR), trial and error is used to find the yield to maturity, k. For example, if the coupon rate is 9 percent, par value is $1,000, market price is $1,200, and the time to maturity is twenty years, what is the yield to maturity? Solving for k through trial and error yields a value of about 7 percent:

$$\$1,200 = \$90 \times PVFA(k,20) + \$1,000 \times PVF(k,20)$$

$$\$1,211 = \$90 \times 10.594 + \$1,000 \times 0.258 \text{ when } k = \text{exactly } 0.07$$

BOND VALUATION FOR MARKET PRICE

The formula also can be used to solve for the market value of a bond. It shows that market value equals the present value of the cash flows in the form of principal and interest payments, discounted back at the required market rate. The required market rate is estimated by examining market rates from publicly traded bonds of similar risk and maturity. This market rate is also how the market perceives the issuer's financial condition, the loan covenants, and a bond's collateral. (A more complete discussion of how market rates change is in the next section.)

There is an inverse relationship between market value and required market rate: when the required market rate is higher than a bond's coupon rate, the market value is less than par value; when the required market rate is lower, the required market value is higher. And, as stated before, when the coupon rate and the required market rate are equal, the market value will be equal to the par value.

When the required market rate is higher than the coupon rate, a bond is said to be selling at a *discount* from its par value. The reason lies with the action of the market: no one will pay par value for a bond with 9 percent coupon payments if the market rate is 10 percent. Consequently, the price of the outstanding bond must fall to a point that produces an effective market rate of 10 percent with the same coupon payment.

Conversely, when the required market rate is lower than the coupon rate, a bond is said to be selling at a *premium*. Market factors again are the reason for this: if the present market rate is only 8 percent, but the coupon payments are at 9 percent, investors will be willing to pay more for the bonds than their par value, which pushes the market price up.

Discount
When the market rate is higher than the coupon rate, a bond is said to be selling at a discount from its par value. See also *Premium*.

Premium
When the market rate is lower than the coupon rate, a bond is said to be selling at a premium. See also *discount*.

Although the focus to this point has been on the effect of changing interest rates in the marketplace, the time to maturity can have a significant impact as well. If the required market rate equals the coupon rate, then regardless of maturity date, market value will always be equal to par value. However, when these two rates differ, maturity date has an effect. If a bond is selling at a discount (determined by interest rates), longer maturity bonds sell at a lesser price than do bonds of shorter maturities. Conversely, if a bond is selling at a premium, the longer maturity bonds sell for more than those of shorter maturity. Exhibit G–2a shows the impact of both required market rates and maturity on the market value for a $1,000 bond with 9 percent annual coupon payments, and Exhibit G–2b shows how the NPV function in Excel can be used to compute the

Exhibit G–2a   Effect of market rates and maturity on a bond's market value

Par Value:	$1,000			
Coupon rate:	9%			
		k = 0.08	k = 0.09	k = 0.10
Maturity = 10 years		$1,067	$1,000	$939
Maturity = 20 years		$1,099	$1,000	$915
Maturity = 30 years		$1,112	$1,000	$905
k = market interest rate				

Exhibit G–2b   Using NPV function to solve for market value of bond

Function Arguments	☒

NPV

Rate	0.1	= 0.1
Value1	E11:X11	= {90,90,90,90,90,90
Value2		= number

= 914.8643628

Returns the net present value of an investment based on a discount rate and a series of future payments (negative values) and income (positive values).

   Rate: is the rate of discount over the length of one period.

Formula result = $914.86

Help on this function   OK   Cancel

Note: With coupon payments of $90 per year for twenty years plus an additional $1,000 at year 20 for the par value, which are discounted back to the present value at 10 percent, this results in a market price of $915.

market price of the bond for a 9 percent coupon rate bond, required market rate of 10 percent, par value of $1,000, and maturity of twenty years.

Longer maturity makes bond prices more sensitive to changes in required market interest rates. Thus, in response to interest rate changes, the prices of longer maturity bonds change more than do those of shorter maturity bonds. When the coupon rate and the market rate are equal, the market price of a bond equals its face value, regardless of maturity.

BOND VALUATION FOR OTHER PAYMENT PERIODS

Many bonds pay interest semi-annually—in some cases, quarterly. If so, the bond valuation formula can be adjusted to account for any number of payment periods within a year, q, using the following formula:

$$MV = \left[\sum_{t=1}^{n} (CP_t/q) \times (1 + k/q)^t \right] + PV / (1 + k/q)^{nq}$$

where MV is the market value (price) of the bond, CP is the coupon payment on the bond, PV represents the bond's par value of the bond, n indicates the number of periods to maturity, t represents $1, 2, 3, \ldots n$ periods, k is the yield to maturity (required market rate), and q is the number of payment periods per year. For example, suppose the previously described bond, which had an annual coupon rate of 9 percent, required payments semi-annually instead of annually. If the term or maturity of the bond were fifteen years, required market rate 8 percent, and the par value $1,000, the market value of the bond would be computed as follows:

$$\text{Market value} = (\text{coupon payment} / 2) \times \text{PVFA}(k/2, n \times 2) + (\text{par value}) \times \text{PVF}(k/2, n \times 2)$$

$$MV = (\$90/2) \times \text{PVFA}(0.08/2, 15 \times 2) + \$1,000 \times \text{PVF}(0.08/2, 15 \times 2)$$

$$MV = \$45 \times \text{PVFA}(0.04, 30) + \$1,000 \times \text{PVF}(0.04, 30)$$

$$MV = \$45 \times 17.292 + \$1,000 \times 0.308 = \$1,086.14$$

AMORTIZATION OF A TERM LOAN

The *amortization* of a term loan is the gradual process of paying off debt through a series of equal periodic payments. Each payment covers a portion of the principal plus current interest. The periodic payments are equal over the lifetime of the loan, but the proportion going toward the principal gradually increases. For most long-term debt, health care providers opt for this form of level debt service. This option usually is not

Amortization
The gradual process of paying off debt through a series of equal periodic payments. Each payment covers a portion of the principal plus current interest. The periodic payments are equal over the lifetime of the loan, but the proportion going toward the principal gradually increases. The amount of a payment can be determined by using the formula to calculate the present value of an annuity.

available for short-term financing. Some short-term debt loans require equal interest payments over the life of the loan and a total principal payment at the end of the loan.

To illustrate how an issuer computes its level debt service requirement, assume a health care provider borrows $1,000,000 at an interest rate of 10 percent for 10 years. The first step is to determine the periodic debt service requirements, which equate to the present value of an annuity:

$$\$1,000,000 = (\text{annuity payment}) \times \text{PVFA}(0.10, 10)$$

The present value interest factor for an annuity at 10 percent for 10 years is 6.1446.

$$\$1,000,000 = \text{annuity payment} \times 6.1446$$
$$\$1,000,000 / 6.1446 = \text{annual payment}$$
$$\$162,745 = \text{annual payment}$$

Thus, the annual loan payment amount from the health care provider is $162,745 for 10 years. Also, one could use the Excel PMT function to arrive at annual payments, which was discussed in Chapter Six. As noted earlier, each payment is composed of both principal and interest. The loan amortization schedule for this example is given in Exhibit G–3.

DEBT BORROWING CAPACITY

A hospital or health system can estimate its debt borrowing capacity, specifically how much additional debt it can take on, by selecting a capital structure ratio value for a given bond rating. Hospitals can reference either of the three credit rating agencies' annual reports (Fitch, Moody's, or Standard & Poor's) that publish the median ratio values for their rated bonds. Within the report, the agencies list key capital structure ratio values by each bond rating category. The key ratios include debt service coverage ratio, cash to total debt, long-term debt to total capital, and so forth.

For example, a hospital expecting to issue more debt to fund a renovation assumes that its bond rating would be BBB by Fitch. Exhibit G–4 shows that with a BBB rating, the median ratio value for debt service coverage ratio is 2.50. Currently, the hospital has $30 million in cash flow available to fund the debt service payments. To estimate its new projected debt service payments, the facility first divides the $30 million of

Exhibit G–3   Loan amortization schedule for a $1,000,000 loan at 10 percent interest over 10 years

	Givens			
1	Annuity payment	$162,745		
2	Interest rate	10%		

Year	A Annuity Payment (Given 1)	B Interest Expense (Given 2 × D*)	C Principal Payments (A − B)	D Remaining Balance[a,b] (D* − C)
0				$1,000,000
1	$162,745	$100,000	$62,745	937,255
2	162,745	93,725	69,020	868,235
3	162,745	86,823	75,922	792,313
4	162,745	79,231	83,514	708,799
5	162,745	70,880	91,866	616,933
6	162,745	61,693	101,052	515,881
7	162,745	51,588	111,157	404,724
8	162,745	40,472	122,273	282,451
9	162,745	28,245	134,500	147,950
10	$162,745	$14,795	$147,950	$0

[a] D* is the previous year's value of D.
[b] Columns may not total due to rounding.

cash available for debt service payments by the debt service coverage ratio value of 2.50, arriving at $12,000,000:

Debt service payments = cash available for debt service payments / debt service coverage

Debt service payments = $30,000,000 / 2.50

Debt service payments = $12,000,000

This $12,000,000 is the total amount that the hospital could afford to pay per year toward its overall debt obligations However, assume that the hospital already has current debt service payments of $4,000,000. In this scenario, the hospital would be able to afford additional annual debt service payments of $8,000,000 ($12,000,000 – $4,000,000). See Exhibit G–4, rows A through E.

Exhibit G–4   Steps to compute added debt capacity based on debt service coverage (DSC) ratio

	Givens		
1	Cash flow available for debt service payments[a]		$30,000,000
2	Debt service coverage at given rating of BBB		2.50
3	Current debt service payments		$4,000,000
4	Maturity of new bond, years		30
5	Fixed interest rate for new bond		6%
6	Assumed bond rating		BBB

[a] Cash flow available for debt service = Net Income + Interest Expense + Depreciation Expense

A	Cash flow available for debt service payments	Given 1	$30,000,000
B	Debt service coverage at given rating of BBB	Given 2	2.50
C	Projected debt service payments	A/B	$12,000,000
D	Current debt service payments	Given 3	$4,000,000
E	Additional debt service payments	C – D	$8,000,000
F	Maturity of new bond, years	Given 4	30
G	Fixed Interest rate for new bond	Given 5	6%
H	Present value annuity factor	PVFA(0.06, 30)	13.76
I	Additional debt borrowings	E × H	$110,118,649

Alternative option is to use present value function to compute value of the loan

Function Arguments ☒

PV

Rate	.06		= 0.06
Nper	30		= 30
Pmt	-8000000		= -8000000
Fv			= number
Type			= number

= 110118649.2

Returns the present value of an investment: the total amount that a series of future payments is worth now.

Pmt is the payment made each period and cannot change over the life of the investment.

Formula result =   110118649.2

Help on this function   [OK]   [Cancel]

Assuming a 6 percent fixed rate for tax-exempt debt for a 30-year bond with additional annual debt service payments of $8,000,000, the hospital can compute its additional debt borrowing capacity. The additional total debt can be computed by identifying the present value factor for an annuity at 6 percent interest for 30 years (13.76) and then multiplying this value by $8,000,000:

Present value of loan = annuity payment × PVFA(0.06, 30)

Present value of loan = $8,000,000 × 13.76

Present value of loan = $110,118,649

One could also use the present value function to solve for the value of the loan as well (see Exhibit G–4). Based on these assumptions, the hospital could borrow an additional $110 million over thirty years, assuming its financial status remained intact during the loan period. The hospital could also estimate its additional debt borrowing capacity based on other key financial ratios, such as long-term debt to total capital and cash to total debt ratios, from the credit rating agencies' median ratio values for a given rating.

9

USING COST INFORMATION TO MAKE SPECIAL DECISIONS

LEARNING OBJECTIVES

- ■ Define fixed and variable costs
- ■ Compute price, fixed cost, variable cost per unit, or quantity, given the others
- ■ Construct and interpret a break-even chart
- ■ Apply the concepts of contribution margin and product margin to the following types of decisions: make or buy, adding or dropping a service, and expanding or reducing a service

From time to time, administrators face such decisions as:

- Should we offer a particular service or group of services?
- What volume of services do we need to provide to break even?
- How much must we charge or be reimbursed for a service to be financially viable?
- Should we offer a service in-house or should we contract with another organization?
- Should we replace equipment?

Questions such as these are called *special decisions* because they are made on an as-needed basis as opposed to a standard schedule. This chapter provides tools to help answer these and similar questions. It begins with a discussion of break-even analysis and the role of fixed and variable costs in decision making. It then turns to the related topics of the break-even chart, contribution margin, and product margin.

Key Point *When the special decisions discussed in this chapter involve multiyear periods, the time value of money must be considered, as discussed in Chapters Six and Seven.*

Although this chapter focuses primarily on financial concerns, nonfinancial criteria must also be considered when making special decisions. In certain cases, nonfinancial criteria may even outweigh the results of a financial analysis. For instance, though a financial analysis shows that a project meets the financial criteria, such as breaking even, management may decide not to undertake the project because it does not sufficiently meet its community service goals. As shown in Exhibit 9–1, the course of action is clear only when it meets or fails to meet both financial and nonfinancial criteria.

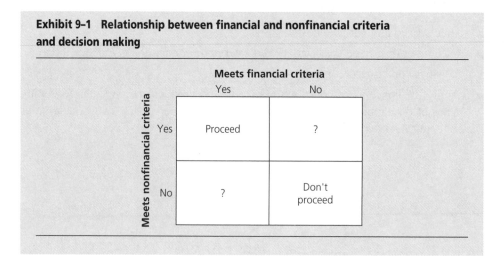

Exhibit 9–1 Relationship between financial and nonfinancial criteria and decision making

BREAK-EVEN ANALYSIS

One of the most fundamental financial criteria used to make special decisions is whether or not, in the future, a service's revenues will be sufficient to cover its costs. In attempting to answer such a question, management must understand the relationship of revenues, costs, and volume. *Break-even analysis*, also called *cost-volume-profit* (CVP) analysis, provides tools to study these relationships. The remainder of this section explores break-even analysis and how it can be used to help answer numerous questions facing health care organizations.

Break-Even Analysis
A technique to analyze the relationship among revenues, costs, and volume. It is also called *cost-volume-profit* or CVP analysis.

Using the Break-Even Approach to Determine Prices, Charges, and Reimbursement

Suppose a home health director wants to know how much her agency must be reimbursed per visit for her commercial home health service line to break even. Assuming for the moment that the only costs for this service line are $200,000 for staffing (2 RNs and 3 nursing assistants), then to break even, revenues must also equal $200,000.

> Revenues =   Costs
> $200,000 = $200,000

Although knowing that $200,000 is necessary to cover costs is useful information, the director still does not know how much she must be reimbursed *for each visit* to reach her $200,000 target. The fewer the number of visits, the higher the reimbursement needs to be; conversely, the higher the number of visits, the lower that reimbursement needs to be to earn the $200,000. Thus, to determine the necessary per visit reimbursement to break even, she must know the number of visits.

Key Point *Formula to determine total revenue when price and quantity are known: Total Revenue = Price × Quantity*

Key Point *The terms quantity, volume, and activity are often used interchangeably when referring to the number of visits, number of patients, number of services, or the activities of providers and patients related to the delivery or receipt of health care goods and services.*

As shown in Exhibit 9–2, if only 1,000 visits were made, she would have to receive $200 (column D, $200,000/1,000) for each visit. However, if there were

Exhibit 9-2 Illustration of how price and fixed cost per visit vary with volume, holding total revenue and total fixed costs constant

A	B	C	D	E
Number of Visits (Given)	Total Revenues (Given)	Total Fixed Costs (Given)	Price/Visit (B/A)	Fixed Cost/Visit (C/A)
1,000	$200,000	$200,000	$200	$200
2,000	$200,000	$200,000	$100	$100
3,000	$200,000	$200,000	$67	$67
4,000	$200,000	$200,000	$50	$50
5,000	$200,000	$200,000	$40	$40

5,000 visits, she would have to receive only $40 per visit ($200,000/5,000). This inverse relationship between price and volume to obtain a specified amount of revenue (i.e., $200,000) is summarized in the equation:

$$\text{Total Revenue} = \text{Price} \times \text{Quantity}$$

where quantity is used generically to stand for such things as number of visits, number of patients, number of services, and so forth. Because price times quantity equals total revenue, and total revenues equal total costs, the basic break-even formula can be restated as:

$$(\text{Price} \times \text{Quantity}) = \text{Total Costs}$$

This is shown in row II in Exhibit 9–3.

Caution: For simplification purposes, the terms *price* and *reimbursement* are used interchangeably in the following discussion. To the extent they differ in any particular situation, an adjustment should be made.

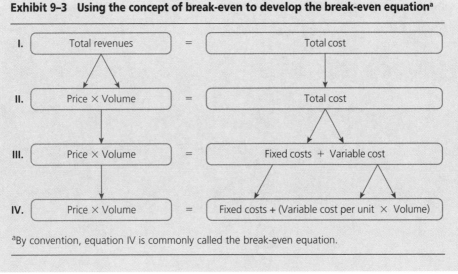

Exhibit 9–3   Using the concept of break-even to develop the break-even equation[a]

I.	Total revenues	=	Total cost
II.	Price × Volume	=	Total cost
III.	Price × Volume	=	Fixed costs + Variable cost
IV.	Price × Volume	=	Fixed costs + (Variable cost per unit × Volume)

[a]By convention, equation IV is commonly called the break-even equation.

Break-Even Analysis: The Role of Fixed Costs

Just as price per visit varies inversely with volume, if total revenue remains constant, the average fixed cost per visit is also inversely related to volume as long as total fixed cost remains constant (Exhibit 9–2, column E). If the fixed costs remain at $200,000 and only 1,000 visits are delivered, the average fixed cost per visit is $200 ($200,000 / 1,000 visits). But at 5,000 visits, the average fixed cost per visit drops to $40 ($200,000 / 5,000 visits).

This example illustrates the two major attributes of fixed costs:

- Fixed costs stay the same in total as volume increases (in Exhibit 9–2 they remained at $200,000).
- Fixed costs per unit change inversely with volume (in Exhibit 9–2 they decreased from an average of $200 per visit to $40 per visit as volume increased from 1,000 to 5,000 visits).

Key Point   *The term* cost per unit *is shorthand for* average cost per unit. *Thus, the terms* average fixed cost per unit *and* fixed cost per unit *are used interchangeably. Similarly, the terms* average variable cost per unit *and* variable cost per unit *are used interchangeably.* Note: *variable costs will be discussed shortly.*

Although fixed cost per unit decreases as volume increases, it does so at a decreasing rate. Exhibit 9–4 shows that cost per visit drops quickly at first, but as the number

Exhibit 9–4 Illustration of how fixed cost per unit decreases at a decreasing rate

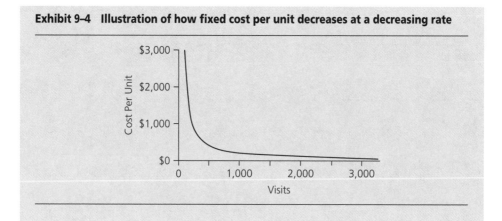

Perspective 9–1 Cardinal, Sage Announce Layoffs

Medical products and services supplier Cardinal Health, Dublin, Ohio, will cut 600 jobs, while health care information technology developer Sage Software Healthcare, Tampa, Florida, will lay off 235 employees, the companies announced.

According to a Cardinal Health news release, the company will reorganize into two business units. It will combine its network of pharmaceutical and medical product distribution centers and nuclear pharmacies into a new health care supply-chain services unit under the direction of vice chairman George Barrett. The company will sell infusion, medication-dispensing, respiratory care, and infection-prevention products under a clinical and medical products segment led by vice chairman David Schlotterbeck. The job cuts include about 160 positions currently open within the company that won't be filled. The company will take a restructuring charge of about $63 million, the "substantial majority of which" will be posted during the current fiscal year that began July 1.

Sage Software Healthcare will lay off 235 people from its workforce of about 1,700. "Every area of the company was touched; however, we did everything we could to minimize the impact on customer-facing jobs, sales, customer service, and account management," said company spokeswoman Lynne Durham.

Source: Conn, J. 2009 (July 8). Modern Healthcare.com.
© 2008 Crain Communications, Inc., 360 N Michigan Avenue, Chicago, IL 60601.

of visits increases toward capacity, each additional visit decreases the per unit cost at a gradually decreasing rate. In other words, fixed assets provide the capacity to provide service, and if these assets are being used inefficiently (low volume relative to capacity), considerable gains can be made in per unit cost by increasing volume. However, if these assets are already being used efficiently (high volume relative to capacity), the less per unit cost decreases for each additional unit of service provided. Perspective 9–1 illustrates how organizations supplying services to the health care industry have been forced to cut their fixed costs.

Of course, at some point the capacity of the assets is reached, and there is a need to expand (for instance, by buying new equipment or hiring new staff). In such a case, fixed costs would no longer remain fixed at $200,000 but would step up to a new level. When the lower or upper limits of capacity are reached, and it becomes necessary to add or drop capacity (e.g., full-time staff), the organization is said to be going beyond the *relevant range* of its *fixed costs*. However, within the relevant range, fixed costs remain fixed.

Relevant Range
The range of activity over which *total fixed costs* or *per unit variable cost* (or both) do not vary.

Fixed Costs
Costs that stay the same in total over the relevant range but change inversely on a per unit basis as activity changes.

Exhibit 9–5 shows that the fixed costs of $200,000 in labor are considered fixed up to 5,000 visits (relevant range 1). Then, assuming an additional full-time RN is needed if volume exceeds 5,000 visits, the fixed costs would take a step up to $285,000 (assuming that each new RN costs $85,000). The fixed costs then remain at this level (relevant range 2) until visits reach 7,500, at which point they step up to $370,000 (relevant range 3), when another full-time RN again has to be hired. To the extent that there are *step-fixed costs*, the break-even formula can become complicated. Thus, it is strongly suggested that break-even analyses with step-fixed costs be done on electronic spreadsheets.

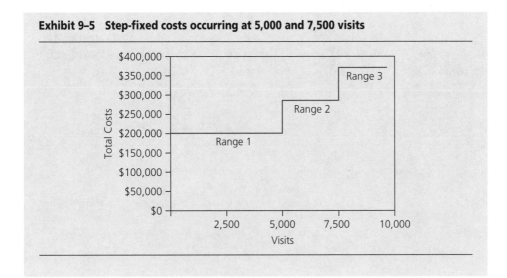

Exhibit 9–5 Step-fixed costs occurring at 5,000 and 7,500 visits

Caution There are two major errors that must be avoided when using fixed cost information to make decisions: assuming that cost per unit does not change when volume changes and using fixed cost per unit derived at one level to forecast total fixed costs at another level.

Step-Fixed Costs
Costs that increase in total over wide, discrete steps.

Relative to the above caution, how fixed cost per unit changes with a change in volume was just illustrated. In regard to the second type of error: suppose that the home health agency, which has $200,000 in fixed costs, made 4,000 visits this year (Exhibit 9–6, second row). Using this information, the administrator correctly calculates the average fixed cost per visit to be $50 ($200,000/4,000 visits). The next year the agency plans to make 5,000 visits (third row). The administrator would be making an error if she assumed that the average fixed cost per visit would remain at $50. Because volume increases from 4,000 visits to 5,000, and total fixed cost remains at $200,000 (it's fixed!), the average fixed cost per visit decreases from $50 per visit ($200,000/4,000 visits) to $40 per visit ($200,000/5,000 visits). Thus, if the administrator were trying to set her price to cover her fixed cost, she may set it too high ($50) instead of recognizing that cost has decreased (to $40) because of increased volume. Conversely, as shown in Exhibit 9–6, if the administrator were using the $50 per visit derived at 4,000 visits to estimate her fixed cost at 3,000 visits, her estimate would be too low.

Exhibit 9–6   Illustration of the error of using fixed cost per unit derived at one level of activity to calculate total fixed cost at another level

A	B	C	D	E
	Assumed Per	Estimated Total	Actual	Overestimate
Volume	Unit Fixed Cost[a]	Fixed Cost	Fixed Cost	(Underestimate)
(Estimated)	(Given)	(A × B)	(Given)	(C − D)
3,000	$50	$150,000	$200,000	($50,000)[b]
4,000	$50	$200,000	$200,000	$0[c]
5,000	$50	$250,000	$200,000	$50,000[d]

[a] All three examples use the unit cost derived at 4,000 visits to estimate total fixed cost.
[b] If the unit fixed cost is originally derived at a higher volume, the total fixed cost estimate will be too low.
[c] If the unit fixed cost is originally derived at the same volume, the total fixed cost estimate will be correct.
[d] If the unit fixed cost is originally derived at a lower volume, the total fixed cost estimate will be too high.

Break-Even Analysis: The Role of Variable Costs

Thus far, it has been assumed that all costs are fixed or step-fixed. In this example, assume that a home health agency pays employees an average of $25 a visit, rather than a salary. Thus, 100 visits would cost $2,500 (100 × $25). For 1,000 or 10,000 visits, costs would increase to $25,000 (1,000 × $25) and $250,000 (10,000 × $25), respectively. Because total cost varies *directly* with activity (in this case visits), these costs are called *variable costs*, though the cost per unit remains the same, $25.

Variable Costs
Costs that stay the same per unit but change directly in total with a change in activity over the relevant range. Total Variable Cost = Variable Cost Per Unit × Number of Units of Activity.

Thus, the two major characteristics of variable costs have been identified, and they are just the opposite of those for fixed costs:

- Total variable cost changes directly with a change in activity.
- Variable cost per unit stays the same with a change in activity.

The formula that describes the relationship between variable cost and activity is:

> Total Variable Cost = Variable Cost Per Unit × Number of Units of Activity

As discussed earlier, when total fixed costs go beyond the relevant range, they often take the form of step-fixed costs, though it is possible to substitute variable costs for fixed costs (e.g., paying a home health nurse by the visit rather than hiring another full-time nurse). When variable costs per unit go beyond the relevant range, it is possible to have either an increase or decrease in cost per unit. For instance, if volume increases significantly, an organization may be able to obtain a volume discount on supplies. Of course, if volume dropped, the opposite effect may occur: the loss of discounts and an increase in variable cost per unit. As with fixed costs, as volume goes beyond the relevant range, it becomes difficult to use the break-even formula to solve break-even problems with variable costs, and using a spreadsheet model is recommended.

Key Point *By convention, when the terms* fixed costs *and* variable costs *are used, it is understood that they remain constant in total (fixed costs) or on a per unit basis (variable costs), respectively, only within a relevant range*

Exhibit 9–7 summarizes and compares the major characteristics of fixed and variable costs in relation to volume within a relevant range. Fixed costs stay the same in total but change per unit as volume changes, whereas variable costs change in total but remain constant per unit with changes in volume. That some costs are necessary to meet regulations is shown in Perspective 9–2, and Perspective 9–3 illustrates the complex interaction between cost and inpatient care.

Exhibit 9–7   Illustration of how fixed and variable costs are affected by changes in volume

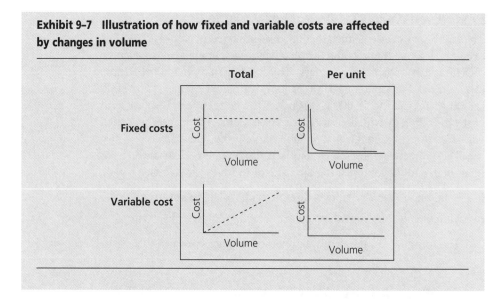

Perspective 9–2   Study Estimates Cost of ICD-10 Implementation

Implementing the new ICD-10 [International Classification of Diseases, 10th revision] codes will cost the typical small medical practice (3 doctors and 2 administrative staffers) $83,200, the typical medium-sized practice (ten providers, six staffers, one full-time coder) $285,195, and the typical large practice (one hundred providers, fifty-four medical records staffers, ten full-time coders) almost $2.73 million, according to a new study conducted by Reisterstown, Maryland-based Nachimson Advisors, a health care information technology consultant.

The study was funded by eleven medical organizations, including the American Medical Association and the Medical Group Management Association, and it researched the costs associated with replacing the current ICD-9 codes with the new, more detailed ICD-10 system by 2011 as proposed by HHS [Department of Health and Human Services].

Some of the costs would be one-time only, such as staff training, changing superbills to include ten times as many codes, upgrading IT systems and insurance plan review, the study concluded. Cash flow disruption during the transition was listed as the second-largest cost, and would equal $19,500 for the typical small practice, $65,000 for the medium-sized practice, and $650,000 for large practices.

Source: Robeznieks, A. 2008 (Oct. 15). Modern Healthcare.com.
© 2008 Crain Communications, Inc.

Perspective 9–3   Study Finds Cost-Savings with Palliative Care

Palliative care reduced unnecessary care and costs in a study of eight U.S. hospitals that was published in the *Archives of Internal Medicine*. Researchers estimated that hospitals saved roughly $280 to $370 per day, per palliative-care patient when compared with patients who did not receive such services. For palliative-care patients who died, researchers reported an estimated savings of $4,908 per admission. For those who did not die, savings were estimated at $1,696 per admission.

Palliative care aids patients and families with symptom management, communication, support for medical decisions in line with treatment goals, and safe movement from one location to another. Researchers analyzed costs for patients at eight hospitals between 2002 and 2004 who were aged eighteen or older and hospitalized for seven to thirty days.

Findings suggest that palliative services prevent the use of unnecessary care, which is no small task, the authors wrote. "While it may appear self-evident that discontinuing costly nonbeneficial interventions among seriously ill patients reduces hospital costs, such a fundamental shift in the usual hospital-care pathway is neither a simple nor straightforward process, given the highly patterned treatment culture of the U.S. hospitals, which is structured to prolong life and avert death at all costs," the authors wrote. The Center to Advance Palliative Care, the National Palliative Care Research Center, and the National Institute on Aging supported the study.

Source: Evans, M. 2008 (Sept. 9). Modern Healthcare.com.
© 2008 Crain Communications, Inc.

Using the Break-Even Equation

The break-even formula can now be expanded and modified to include variable costs (see Exhibit 9–3, row III):

$$\text{Price} \times \text{Volume} = \text{Fixed Cost} + \text{Variable Cost}$$

Expanding this equation based on the above discussion yields the basic break-even equation:

$$\text{Price} \times \text{Volume} = \text{Fixed Cost} + (\text{Variable Cost Per Unit} \times \text{Volume})$$

as shown in row IV in Exhibit 9–3.

Exhibit 9–8 illustrates how the break-even formula can be used to find the price, quantity (volume), fixed cost, or variable cost per unit needed to break even, if each of

Exhibit 9-8   Applying the break-even formula

Givens	A	B	C	D	E
				Total	Variable
	Situation	Price	Quantity[a]	Fixed Cost	Cost Per Unit[b]
	Situation 1	?	4,000	$200,000	$25
	Situation 2	$100	?	$200,000	$25
	Situation 3	$100	4,000	?	$25
	Situation 4	$100	4,000	$200,000	?

[a] For example, number of visits
[b] For example, cost of supplies per visit

Situation 1.   Finding the break-even *price*, given quantity, total fixed cost, and variable cost per unit

						Total		Variable Cost		
Setup:	Price	×	Quantity	=	Fixed Cost	+	Per Unit	×	Quantity
	Price	×	4,000	=	$200,000	+	$25	×	4,000
Solution:	Price	×	4,000	=	$200,000	+		$100,000	
	Price	×	4,000	=	$300,000				
	Price			=	$75				

Situation 2.   Finding the break-even *quantity*, given price, total fixed cost, and variable cost per unit

					Total		Variable Cost		
Setup:	Price	×	Quantity	=	Fixed Cost	+	Per Unit	×	Quantity
	$100	×	Quantity	=	$200,000	+	$25	×	Quantity
Solution:	$75	×	Quantity	=	$200,000				
			Quantity	=	$2,667				

Situation 3.   Finding the break-even *total fixed* cost, given price, quantity, and variable cost per unit

					Total		Variable Cost		
Setup:	Price	×	Quantity	=	Fixed Cost	+	Per Unit	×	Quantity
	$100	×	4,000	=	TFC	+	$25	×	4,000
Solution:	$400,000			=	TFC	+		$100,000	
	$300,000			=	TFC				

Situation 4.   Finding the break-even *variable cost per unit*, given price, quantity, and total fixed cost

					Total		Variable Cost		
Setup:	Price	×	Quantity	=	Fixed Cost	+	Per Unit	×	Quantity
	$100	×	4,000	=	$200,000	+	VCu	×	4,000
Solution:	$400,000			=	$200,000	+	VCu	×	4,000
	$200,000			=			VCu	×	4,000
	$50			=			VCu		

the other factors is known. In situation 1 of Exhibit 9–8, price is unknown; in situation 2, quantity (volume) is unknown; in situation 3, total fixed cost is unknown; and in situation 4, variable cost per unit is unknown.

Expanding the Break-Even Equation to Include Indirect Costs and Required Profit

Up to this point, the example has looked at situations where revenues exactly match those costs that the organization can directly associate with a service, such as those of the 2 RNs and 3 nursing assistants, and miscellaneous variable costs such as supplies and transportation. However, it is often desirable that revenues cover other costs, such as overhead, and perhaps provide a margin (profit). As discussed in more detail in Chapter Twelve, *direct costs* are those that an organization can measure or trace to a particular patient or service (e.g., the time a nurse or nursing assistant spends with a client), whereas *indirect costs* are those that the organization is not able to associate with a particular patient or service (e.g., the cost of the billing clerk or computer system). Exhibit 9–9 extends the break-even equation in Exhibit 9–3 to account for indirect costs and profit, and Exhibit 9–10 expands the example from Exhibit 9–8 to illustrate how to use the extended equation. Because it is usually the case, these examples assume that both indirect costs and profits are fixed amounts, though the equation can be modified to account for other instances.

In situations 1 to 3 of Exhibit 9–10, price is unknown, and various combinations of indirect costs and desired profit are added to the information originally provided in Exhibit 9–8. Such analyses would be used when an organization is trying to determine if the reimbursement it will receive is sufficient to cover its costs and desired profit for a particular service. For example, in situation 3, if the organization were not reimbursed at least $111 per visit, management could conclude that the reimbursement would be insufficient to cover its direct and indirect costs and desired margin and perhaps decide not to provide the service at this rate or try to renegotiate a higher rate.

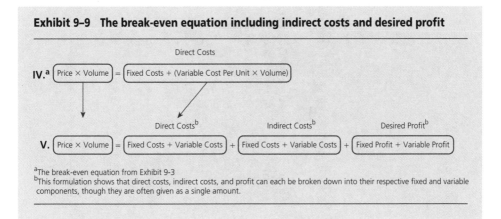

Exhibit 9–9 The break-even equation including indirect costs and desired profit

Direct Costs

IV.[a] Price × Volume = Fixed Costs + (Variable Cost Per Unit × Volume)

Direct Costs[b]   Indirect Costs[b]   Desired Profit[b]

V. Price × Volume = Fixed Costs + Variable Costs + Fixed Costs + Variable Costs + Fixed Profit + Variable Profit

[a]The break-even equation from Exhibit 9-3
[b]This formulation shows that direct costs, indirect costs, and profit can each be broken down into their respective fixed and variable components, though they are often given as a single amount.

Exhibit 9-10 Applying the break-even equation to situations with indirect costs or desired profit (or both)

Situation	Price	Quantity[a]	Total Fixed Cost	Variable Cost Per Unit[b]	Indirect Costs	Desired Profit
1	?	4,000	$200,000	$50	$24,000	$0
2	?	4,000	$200,000	$50	$0	$20,000
3	?	4,000	$200,000	$50	$24,000	$20,000
4	$100	4,000	?	$50	$24,000	$20,000

[a] For example, number of visits.
[b] For example, cost of supplies per visit.

Situation 1. Finding the break-even *price*, given quantity, total fixed cost, variable cost per unit, and indirect costs

				Total Fixed		Variable Cost					Indirect		Desired	
Setup:	Price	×	Quantity	=	Cost	+	Per Unit	×	Quantity	+	Costs	+	Profit	
Solution:	Price	×	4,000	=	$200,000	+	$50	×	4,000	+	$24,000	+	$0	
	Price	×	4,000	=	$200,000	+	$200,000			+	$24,000			
	Price	×	4,000	=	$424,000									
	Price			=	**$106**									

Situation 2. Finding the break-even *price*, given quantity, total fixed cost, variable cost per unit, and desired profit

				Total Fixed		Variable Cost					Indirect		Desired	
Setup:	Price	×	Quantity	=	Cost	+	Per Unit	×	Quantity	+	Costs	+	Profit	
Solution:	Price	×	4,000	=	$200,000	+	$50	×	4,000	+	$0	+	$20,000	
	Price	×	4,000	=	$200,000	+	$200,000			+	$0	+	$20,000	
	Price	×	4,000	=	$420,000									
	Price			=	**$105**									

Exhibit 9-10 *(Continued)*

Situation 3. **Finding the break-even *price*,** given quantity, total fixed cost, variable cost per unit, indirect costs, and desired profit

			Total Fixed Cost	+	Variable Cost Per Unit	×	Quantity	+	Indirect Costs	+	Desired Profit
Setup:	Price	× Quantity =									
Solution:	Price	× 4,000 =	$200,000	+	$50	×	4,000	+	$24,000	+	$20,000
	Price	× 4,000 =	$200,000	+	$200,000			+	$44,000		
	Price	× 4,000 =	$444,000								
	Price	=	**$111**								

Situation 4. **Finding the break-even *total fixed cost*,** given price, quantity, variable cost per unit, indirect costs, and desired profit

			Total Fixed Cost	+	Variable Cost Per Unit	×	Quantity	+	Indirect Costs	+	Desired Profit
Setup:	Price	× Quantity =									
Solution:	Price	× 4,000 =	TFC	+	$50	×	4,000	+	$24,000	+	$20,000
	Price	× 4,000 =	TFC	+	$200,000			+	$44,000		
	Price	× 4,000 =	TFC	+	$244,000						
	Price	=	Total Fixed Cost								

Target Costing
Controlling costs, decreasing profit margins, or both to meet or beat a predetermined price or reimbursement rate.

In situation 4 of Exhibit 9–10, all the factors are given except for total fixed costs. A situation such as this occurs when an organization is given a set price (reimbursement) and must control its costs to ensure that its costs do not exceed that reimbursement. In this case, given the indirect costs and desired profit, the organization must ensure that its direct fixed costs do not exceed $156,000. Such an approach, called *target costing*, is common in health care, where the government is the price setter and the provider is the price taker. Perspective 9–4 shows how, rather than cutting back, others are growing as part of their strategic positioning. Perspective 9–5 illustrates that it is possible for cost savings and quality to go hand in hand. Finally, Perspective 9–6 discusses the importance of a strategic approach to controlling supply costs.

The Break-Even Chart

A break-even chart graphically displays the relationships in the break-even equation. For instance, Exhibits 9–11a, 9–11b, and 9–11c present different ways to graph the data in Exhibit 9–8, where the revenue per visit is $100, fixed costs are $200,000, and variable cost is $25 per visit. Exhibit 9–11a presents this information in the traditional break-even chart format but with considerable annotation. The three lines represent

Perspective 9–4   Planned Growth

Atlanta—Children's Healthcare of Atlanta expects to spend $2.5 billion over the next ten years as it lays out a strategy for capital and program expansions. The three-hospital system plans to break ground August 13 at its Hughes Spalding facility as part of that strategy. The $43 million expansion and renovation will help the hospital focus on primary care, sickle cell disease, asthma, and child protection, a spokeswoman said. The system recently completed the purchase of twenty-eight acres of land for a potential fourth hospital in the north suburbs of Atlanta and is developing a $17.6 million, 90,000-square-foot facility for its subsidiary, the Marcus Autism Center. In addition to the physical expansion, Children's will bolster its clinical, education, research, and wellness programs through the decade-long strategic plan, dubbed "Vision 2018." The system is building on its partnerships with nearby Emory University, the Georgia Institute of Technology, and Morehouse School of Medicine to conduct more pediatrics research and increase pediatrics education, the spokeswoman said. Wellness activities will focus on combating obesity in the community and increasing healthy lifestyles.

Source: 2008 (Aug. 4). Regionals, South. Modern Healthcare.com.
© 2008 Crain Communications, Inc.

Perspective 9–5   Premier Cites Gains Under CMS Pay-for-Performance Initiative

Hospital costs and mortality rates are declining under a CMS pay-for-performance project, according to an analysis released by the Premier healthcare alliance. The hospital quality incentive demonstration project was launched by the alliance and the CMS in 2003 to find out if economic incentives improve inpatient care at hospitals.

Apparently they do: In an analysis of more than a million patient records from participating hospitals, the median hospital cost per patient declined by more than $1,000 across the first three years of the project. Meanwhile, the median mortality rate decreased by 1.87 percent.

The more than 250 participating hospitals report process and outcome measures in five clinical areas, including acute myocardial infarction, congestive heart failure, coronary artery bypass graft, pneumonia, and hip and knee replacement. According to the analysis, hospitals nationally could save an estimated seventy thousand lives per year and reduce costs by more than $4.5 billion annually if they all achieved the cost and mortality improvements found among the project participants in each of the five clinical areas over a three-year period.

Source: Lubell, J. 2008 (Jan. 31). Modern Healthcare.com.
© 2008 Crain Communications, Inc.

---

fixed cost, total cost, and total revenues. The total revenue line begins at $0 (the amount of revenue earned if no services are offered) and increases by $100 for each home health visit made. Because by definition fixed costs do not change with volume, the fixed cost line begins at $200,000 and remains at that level. Because total cost is made up of fixed cost plus variable cost, the total cost line begins at $200,000 (the level of fixed cost at zero units of service) and grows by $25 (the variable cost per unit) for each unit of service provided.

At 2,667 visits, the total revenue and total cost lines cross. Before 2,667 visits, the net income is negative, whereas after 2,667 visits, it is positive. Thus, the *break-even point*, the point at which total revenues equal total costs, is 2,667 visits. Before the break-even point, the size of the space between the *total revenue* line and the *total cost* line equals the amount of loss. After the break-even point, the size of the space between the total revenue line and the total cost line equals the amount of profit.

Because it is so difficult to visually determine how much the actual loss or profit is by using the traditional version, increasingly a newer version is being used (see Exhibit 9–11c). In addition to the information typically presented in Exhibit 9–11b, the newer version presents net

Break-Even Point
The point where total revenues equal total costs.

Exhibit 9–11a   A traditional break-even chart with annotation

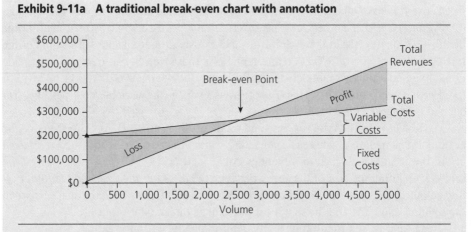

Note: This example is a fully labeled chart for learning purposes. Usually some of the information given is omitted and assumed to be understood, as in Exhibit 9–11b.

Exhibit 9–11b   A traditional break-even chart

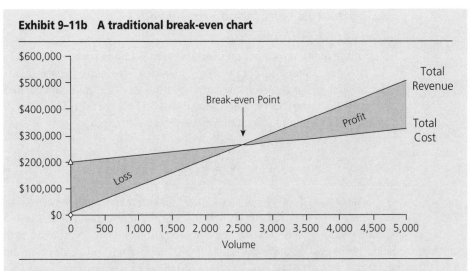

Note: Some presenters will include the fixed cost line. However, it is not absolutely necessary because it is equal to the amount where the total cost line crosses the Y axis: $200,000.

Exhibit 9–11c   A break-even chart emphasizing net income

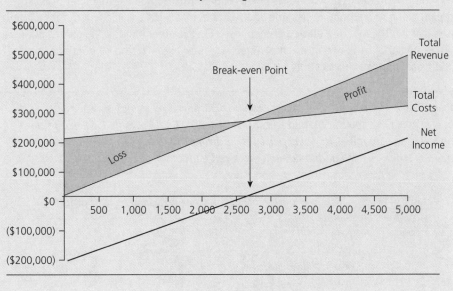

income, total revenues less total costs. Note that in all three charts, break-even is achieved at 2,667 visits. In general, the old version should be used where detailed cost information is important, and the new version should be used in cases where the amount of profit is the essential concern.

Contribution Margin Per Unit
Per unit revenue minus per unit variable costs.

Incremental Costs
Additional costs incurred solely as a result of an action or activity or a particular set of actions or activities.

Total Contribution Margin
Total revenues minus total variable costs.

A Shortcut to Calculating Break-Even: The Contribution Margin

Per unit revenue minus per unit variable cost is called *contribution margin per unit* because after covering *incremental (variable) costs*, this is the amount left to contribute toward covering all other costs and desired profit. If the contribution margin is known and all other costs are fixed, a shortcut formula to calculate break-even can be used:

> Break-Even Volume = Fixed Costs / Contribution Margin Per Unit

Assume that total fixed costs are $200,000, revenue per visit is $100, and variable cost is $25 per visit. Thus, contribution margin per unit is $75 ($100 - $25), which means that the organization makes $75 more on each visit than the incremental cost of that visit. Thus, using the above formula, to cover the $200,000 in fixed costs, there must be 2,667 visits ($200,000/$75; see Exhibit 9–12). This is the same answer that was derived using the longer formula in Exhibit 9–8, situation 2.

Finally, notice that even if the organization does not reach break-even, each unit of service it delivers contributes $75 toward covering its fixed costs and overhead. This leads to the *contribution margin rule*: *ceteris paribus* ("with all else being the same"), if the contribution margin per unit is positive, then it is in the best financial interest of the organization to continue to provide additional units of that service, even if the organization is not fully covering all of its other costs. On the other hand, if the contribution margin is negative, it is not in the best interest of the organization to continue to provide additional units of service.

 Key Point *The contribution margin can be determined on a total or a per unit basis.* Total Contribution Margin = *Total Revenue − Total Variable Cost.* Contribution Margin per Unit = *Revenue per Unit − Variable Cost per Unit. It is the amount of profit made on each additional unit produced if all other costs remain the same.*

Exhibit 9–12   Break-even equation using the contribution margin approach

Given:		
Revenue per visit	$100	
Variable cost per visit	$25	
Contribution margin per visit	$75	
Fixed cost	$200,000	

To determine the break-even quantity using the contribution margin approach:

$$\frac{\text{Fixed cost}}{\text{Contribution margin per unit}} = \frac{\$200,000}{\$75} = 2{,}667 \text{ Visits}$$

Effects of Capitation on Break-Even Analysis

With an increasing emphasis on cost control, various managed care companies have turned to capitation as their preferred method of payment. Because capitated payment systems are discussed in detail in Chapter Thirteen, the focus here is on how break-even analysis can be used with capitation. Briefly, under full capitation, the insurer prepays a health care provider an agreed-on amount per member that covers a designated set of services for the insured population over a defined time period. Typically, these payments are made on a per member per month (PMPM) basis. If there are no terms to the contrary, in return for the capitated payments, the provider agrees to bear all the risk for the costs of services provided. If the provider's costs are below the global capitation amount, the provider can keep the difference. If the provider's costs are more than the capitation, the provider is at risk for the difference. Obviously, negotiations on both the capitated amount and any particulars of the contract (e.g., services not covered and arrangements that limit the financial risk of the provider) are critical to the provider, who must estimate the volume and type of services that may have to be performed and the amount of money needed to cover them. The following example shows a break-even analysis for a health care provider under a capitated system.

Contribution Margin Rule If the contribution margin per unit is positive and no other additional costs will be incurred, then it is in the best financial interest of the organization to continue to provide additional units of that service, even if the organization is not fully covering all of its other costs. On the other hand, if the contribution margin is negative, it is not in the best interest of the organization to continue to provide additional units of service, ceteris parabis.

Hospital A, which has a capitation arrangement with a managed care organization, wants to negotiate a capitated contract with a multispecialty group practice to provide a major portion of the medical services that hospital A is obligated to provide. This type of arrangement is commonly called a *subcapitation arrangement*. The population covered under this subcapitation arrangement consists of 1,400 covered lives with no Medicare or Medicaid beneficiaries.

The director of managed care contracts for the clinic is under pressure to bring in new business. In weighing this opportunity, he must balance many factors, some of which will not be known until the contract is actually in effect, including the PMPM rate, the expected proportion of members needing services, and the average cost of the services that the members will actually receive. Exhibit 9–13 offers three separate scenarios, each varying one of these three factors while holding the other two constant.

In keeping with the same example used throughout the chapter, assume that fixed costs equal $200,000 and that the variable cost per unit equals $25. However, the fixed cost figure represents the *annual* amount, whereas capitation is being paid here on a *monthly* basis (PMPM). Thus, annual fixed costs must be converted into equivalent monthly amounts, or $16,667 ($200,000/12 months). Variable costs remain the same and do not need to be converted.

In the first scenario (Exhibit 9–13), only the capitation rate is unknown. The clinic either gains or loses depending on whether the capitation amount is above or below $14.40 PMPM. Note that in this scenario, total costs remain constant (columns H, I, and J), regardless of the capitation amount, but total revenues vary based on the

Exhibit 9–13 An example of how to perform a break-even analysis under a capitated arrangement

Givens	Number of Members	Total Fixed Cost	PMPM	Utilizaton Rate	Variable Cost/Unit
Scenario 1	1,400	$16,667	?	10%	$25
Scenario 2	1,400	$16,667	$15	?	$25
Scenario 3	1,400	$16,667	$15	10%	?

Scenario 1. Using the break-even equation to determine break-even *PMPM subcapitation rate*, given service cost and utilization rates

A. Monthly capitation amount (PMPM)	?
B. Fixed costs per month	$16,667
C. Variable costs of services per member receiving	$25
D. Percentage of members receiving services each month	10%
E. Total number of HMO capitated members	1,400

A Monthly Capitation (Estimate)	F Revenues (A × E)	G Members w/Services (D × E)	H Fixed Costs (B)	I Variable Costs (C × G)	J Total Costs (H + I)	K Net Income (F − J)
$5.00	$7,000	140	$16,667	$3,500	$20,167	($13,167)
$10.00	$14,000	140	$16,667	$3,500	$20,167	($6,167)
$14.40	**$20,167**	**140**	**$16,667**	**$3,500**	**$20,167**	**$0**
$15.00	$21,000	140	$16,667	$3,500	$20,167	$833
$20.00	$28,000	140	$16,667	$3,500	$20,167	$7,833
$25.00	$35,000	140	$16,667	$3,500	$20,167	$14,833

Exhibit 9–13 *(Continued)*

Scenario 2. Using the break-even equation to determine break-even *utilization rates*, given service cost and PMPM subcapitation rates.

A. Monthly capitation amount	**$15**
B. Fixed costs per month	**$16,667**
C. Variable costs of services per member receiving	**$25**
D. Percentage of members receiving services each month	**?**
E. Total number of HMO capitated members	**1,400**

D Average Util Rate (Estimate)	F Revenues (A × E)	G Members w/Services (D × E)	H Fixed Costs (B)	I Variable Costs (C × G)	J Total Costs (H + I)	K Net Income (F − J)
5.00%	$21,000	70	$16,667	$1,750	$18,417	$2,583
10.00%	$21,000	140	$16,667	$3,500	$20,167	$833
12.38%	**$21,000**	**173**	**$16,667**	**$4,333**	**$21,000**	**$0**
15.00%	$21,000	210	$16,667	$5,250	$21,917	($917)
20.00%	$21,000	280	$16,667	$7,000	$23,667	($2,667)
25.00%	$21,000	350	$16,667	$8,750	$25,417	($4,417)

Scenario 3. Using the break-even equation to determine break-even *service cost*, given PMPM subcapitation rates and utilization rate

A. Monthly capitation amount	**$15**
B. Fixed costs per month	**$16,667**
C. Variable costs of services per member receiving	**?**
D. Percentage of members receiving services each month	**10%**
E. Total number of HMO capitated members	**1,400**

C Variable Costs[a] (Estimate)	F Revenues (A × E)	G Members w/Services (D × E)	H Fixed Costs (B)	I Variable Costs[b] (C × G)	J Total Costs (H + I)	K Net Income (F − J)
$15.00	$21,000	140	$16,667	$2,100	$18,767	$2,233
$20.00	$21,000	140	$16,667	$2,800	$19,467	$1,533
$25.00	$21,000	140	$16,667	$3,500	$20,167	$833
$30.00	$21,000	140	$16,667	$4,200	$20,867	$133
$30.95	**$21,000**	**140**	**$16,667**	**$4,333**	**$21,000**	**$0**
$35.00	$21,000	140	$16,667	$4,900	$21,567	($567)

[a] Per Visit
[b] Total

capitation rate to be paid (column A). Although Exhibit 9–13 uses a spreadsheet approach to solving scenario 1, another way to solve this problem is to set it up as an equation:

$$\text{PMPM} \times \text{Enrollees} = (\text{Enrollees} \times \text{Utilization Rate} \times \text{Variable Cost/Unit}) + \text{Fixed Cost}$$

$$\text{PMPM} \times 1,400 = (1,400 \times 0.10 \times 25) + 16,667$$

$$1,400\ \text{PMPM} = 20,167$$

$$\text{PMPM} = \sim \$14.40$$

In the second scenario, the percentage of members each month receiving services is unknown, but capitation is held to $15 PMPM. As expected, the lower the percentage of members receiving services, the greater the net income for the clinic. Note that in this scenario, total revenues remain constant (column F), but total costs vary (columns I and J). As with the previous scenario, scenario 2 can also be set up as an equation:

$$\text{PMPM} \times \text{Enrollees} = (\text{Enrollees} \times \text{Utilization Rate} \times \text{Variable Cost/Unit}) + \text{Fixed Cost}$$

$$15 \times 1,400 = (1,400 \times \text{Utilization Rate} \times 25) + 16,667$$

$$4,333 = 35,000 \times \text{Utilization Rate}$$

$$\text{Utilization Rate} = 0.1238$$

In the final scenario, capitation and percentage of members receiving services are held constant, but the variable cost per member receiving services is unknown. As the variable cost per member receiving services rises (column C), net income falls for the clinic (column K), as would be expected. Note that in this third scenario, like the one before it, total revenues remain constant, but total costs vary. As with the previous scenarios, scenario 3 can also be set up as an equation:

$$\text{PMPM} \times \text{Enrollees} = (\text{Enrollees} \times \text{Utilization Rate} \times \text{Variable Cost/Unit}) + \text{Fixed Cost}$$

$$\$15 \times 1,400 = (1,400 \times 0.10 \times \text{Variable Cost/Unit}) + 16,667$$

$$\$4,333 = 140 \times \text{Variable Cost/Unit}$$

$$\text{Variable Cost/Unit} = \$30.95$$

As with noncapitated payments, a break-even chart can also be constructed under a capitated payment environment. Exhibit 9–14 provides an illustration of this using the same cost structure as in Exhibits 9–11a, 9–11b, and 9–11c (fixed cost = $16,667 and variable cost = $25 per visit), but revenue remains constant at $21,000 (PMPM = $15 × 1,400 patients). As opposed to the noncapitated situation where net income

Exhibit 9–14 Break-even chart with capitated payments

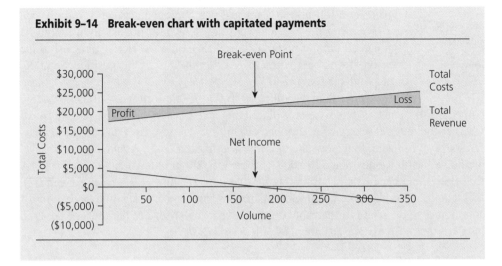

increases as volume increases, the more services provided here, the lower the net income. This is because revenues remain constant, but costs increase at $25 per visit.

The examples given in this chapter illustrate how a cost-volume-profit analysis can be used in both noncapitated and capitated environments. However, as the factors being considered increase, a more thorough analysis is suggested. Such an approach is presented in Chapter Ten, where such things as acuity level, payor mix, productivity, and labor force distribution are taken into account.

PRODUCT MARGIN

Whereas the above discussion dealt with breaking even regarding a single service, health care delivery is often quite complex. The next section of this chapter introduces tools and concepts applicable to situations involving multiple services. For instance, a home health agency might offer the following services: nursing assistant services, infusion therapy, physical therapy, registered dietitian services, and occupational therapy. Later the situation is expanded to cases where there are multiple payors.

Multiple Services

Where multiple services are being offered, both organizational fixed costs and service-specific fixed costs must be considered. Fixed costs incurred only because a service is being provided, and not otherwise, are called *avoidable fixed costs*. For instance, continuing with the home health example, assume that of the $200,000 in fixed costs, $85,000 is to

Avoidable Fixed Cost
A fixed cost that is avoided if a service is not provided. *Example:* full-time nursing costs saved if a service were closed.

Nonavoidable Fixed Costs
A fixed cost that will remain even if a particular service is discontinued. *Example:* full-time nursing costs in an organization that will continue, even though one of several services is dropped.

Common Costs
Costs that benefit a number of services shared by all. *Example:* rent, utilities, and billing. Also called *joint costs*.

be paid for a full-time RN for just one particular service (Exhibit 9–15, row D), and if the service were not delivered, this position would be eliminated (and not just transferred to another service). In regard to the decision of whether to drop the service, the cost of this position, $85,000, is an avoidable fixed cost.

Assume that the other $115,000 of the original $200,000 of the home health agency's fixed costs will remain and must be covered regardless of whether the particular service is dropped (Exhibit 9–15, row E). Because these costs cannot be eliminated, they are called *nonavoidable fixed costs*. Assume in the case of the home health agency that $100,000 of the $115,000 in nonavoidable fixed costs is for salaries and benefits and $15,000 is for overhead (Exhibit 9–15, rows E1 and E2). Incidentally, overhead (i.e., rent, administration, insurance, etc.) often is a type of common cost: one that is not attributable to any particular service but must be covered by all of them. *Common costs* are also called *joint costs*.

 Caution Note that even if an organization drops a service, if the employees are transferred within the organization, their costs are considered nonavoidable.

Product Margin
Total Contribution Margin – Avoidable Fixed Costs. It represents the amount that a service contributes toward covering all other costs after it has covered the costs that are there solely because the service is offered (its total variable cost and avoidable fixed costs) and would not be there if the service were dropped.

Product Margin Decision Rule
If a service's product margin is positive, the organization will be better off financially if it continues with the service, ceteris paribus. Conversely, if a service's product margin is negative, the organization will be better off financially if it discontinues the service, ceteris paribus.

Just as subtracting total variable cost from total revenue yields the total contribution margin, subtracting avoidable fixed cost from the total contribution margin yields the *product margin*. The *product margin decision rule* is the following: If a service's product margin is positive, the organization will be better off financially if it continues with the service than if it drops the service, ceteris paribus. Conversely, if a service's product margin is negative, the organization will be better off financially if it discontinues the service, ceteris paribus. It represents the amount that a service contributes toward covering all other costs after it has covered costs that are there solely because the service is offered (its total variable cost and avoidable fixed cost) and would not be there if the service were dropped. As shown in Exhibit 9–15, if an organization violates this rule and closes a service with a positive product margin (column K), the organization increases its loss by the amount of the product margin that it forgoes. Note that this rule holds for any particular service but does not work for all services taken together because common costs would not be covered.

Presume that the home health agency is trying to decide whether to continue this service next year, and it forecasts it will make 2,000 visits (Exhibit 9–15, column F). If the home health agency made its decision on the basis of net income, it would conclude that it should drop the service because it would conclude that it is losing $50,000 (column N). However, if it drops the service, it will be $65,000 worse off (the amount of the product margin, column K) than if it provided the 2,000 visits.

Exhibit 9–15 An illustration of the product margin rule

Given		
A	Net revenue per visit	$100
B	Variable cost per visit	$25
C	Contribution margin per visit (A − B)	$75
D	Avoidable fixed costs	$85,000
E	Other fixed costs	$115,000
	E1. Salaries and benefits	$100,000
	E2. Overhead costs	$15,000

F	G	H	I	J	K	L	M	N
Volume (Estimate)	Total Revenues (A × F)	Total Variable Costs (B × F)	Total Contribution Margin (G − H)	Avoidable Fixed Costs (D)	Product Margin (I − J)	Salaries and Benefits (E1)	Overhead Costs (E2)	Net Income (K − L − M)
2,000	$200,000	$50,000	$150,000	$85,000	$65,000	$100,000	$15,000	($50,000)
2,500	$250,000	$62,500	$187,500	$85,000	$102,500	$100,000	$15,000	($12,500)
2,667	**$266,700**	**$66,675**	**$200,025**	**$85,000**	**$115,025**	**$100,000**	**$15,000**	**$25**
3,000	$300,000	$75,000	$225,000	$85,000	$140,000	$100,000	$15,000	$25,000
3,500	$350,000	$87,500	$262,500	$85,000	$177,500	$100,000	$15,000	$62,500

Because the product margin is the amount left over after the service has covered all of its own costs, if the service were dropped, the home health agency would lose the $65,000 to help defray its other costs (rows E1 and E2). Note also that if they dropped the service, net income would drop from –$50,000 to –$115,000.

Multiple Payors

It is possible to extend the analysis presented in Exhibit 9–15 from one payor to multiple payors. The previous example assumed that revenues were $100 per visit, but in fact, this is really an average of $100. Three scenarios are shown in Exhibit 9–16. Scenario 1 presents the basic conditions of 4 payors paying different rates, with a weighted average revenue of $100 ("Total" row, columns F/E). Scenario 2 explores the effect on the product margin of increasing the rate for payor 1 by 10 percent (from $110 to $121) with a corresponding drop in volume of 10 percent (from 300 visits to 270 visits). The result is that the product margin increases from $0 to $1,170 (column J). Scenario 3 shows the effect on the original conditions if all patients in payor category 1 are on a flat-fee contract fixed at $33,000, and volume increases by 10 percent. Because there are no additional revenues for these patients, the variable cost increases, but there is no change in revenue. Therefore, the product margin decreases

---

Exhibit 9–16 Expansion of the product margin concept to multiple payors

Scenario 1. Original conditions

Payor	A. Payment/Unit	B. Variable cost/unit	$50
1	$110	C. Avoidable fixed costs	$50,000
2	$105		
3	$101		
4	$85		

D	E	F	G	H	I	J
			Total	Total	Avoidable	
Payor		Total	Variable	Contribution	Fixed	Product
Category	Volume	Revenues	Costs	Margin	Costs	Margin
(Given)	(Given)	(A × E)	(B × E)	(F − G)	(C)	(H − I)
1	300	$33,000	$15,000	$18,000		
2	175	$18,375	$8,750	$9,625		
3	250	$25,250	$12,500	$12,750		
4	275	$23,375	$13,750	$9,625		
Total	1,000	$100,000	$50,000	$50,000	$50,000	$0

Exhibit 9–16 *(Continued)*

Scenario 2. Original conditions with rate for payor 1 patients increased by 10%, but payor 1 volume is decreased by 10%

Payor	A. Payment/Unit	B. Variable cost/unit	$50
1	*$121*	C. Avoidable fixed costs	$50,000
2	$105		
3	$101		
4	$85		

D	E	F	G	H	I	J
			Total	Total	Avoidable	
Payor		Total	Variable	Contribution	Fixed	Product
Category	Volume	Revenues	Costs	Margin	Costs	Margin
(Given)	(Given)	(A × E)	(B × E)	(F − G)	(C)	(H − I)
1	*270*	*$32,670*	*$13,500*	*$19,170*		
2	175	$18,375	$8,750	$9,625		
3	250	$25,250	$12,500	$12,750		
4	275	$23,375	$13,750	$9,625		
Total	970	$99,670	$48,500	$51,170	$50,000	$1,170

Scenario 3. Original conditions with payor 1 patients being covered under a flat-fee contract in which the total payment remains $33,000, but payor 1 volume is increased by 10%.

Payor	A. Payment/Unit	B. Variable cost/unit	$50
1	*$33,000*[a]	C. Avoidable fixed costs	$50,000
2	$105		
3	$101		
4	$85		

D	E	F	G	H	I	J
			Total	Total	Avoidable	
Payor		Total	Variable	Contribution	Fixed	Product
Category	Volume	Revenues[a]	Costs	Margin	Costs	Margin
(Given)	(Given)	(A × E)	(B × E)	(F − G)	(C)	(H − I)
1	*330*	*$33,000*	*$16,500*	*$16,500*		
2	175	$18,375	$8,750	$9,625		
3	250	$25,250	$12,500	$12,750		
4	275	$23,375	$13,750	$9,625		
Total	1,030	$100,000	$51,500	$48,500	$50,000	($1,500)

[a]For payor 1, this formula is not used, and Total Revenues equals the fixed $33,000.

from $0 to −$1,500. This same paradigm can be used to judge the effects of similar changes occurring with any of the four payors.

APPLYING THE PRODUCT MARGIN PARADIGM TO MAKING SPECIAL DECISIONS

The product margin paradigm presented in Exhibits 9–15 and 9–16 can be used to address a number of special decisions, commonly categorized as make or buy, add or drop, and expand or reduce.

Make-or-Buy Decisions

Decision Rule After comparing the product margins between the make-and-buy alternatives, the alternative with the higher product margin should be chosen.

Example: Zacharias Community Clinic (ZCC) is deciding whether to produce a portion of its laboratory tests in-house or to purchase them from a reference lab. ZCC has $200,000 in fixed costs for the lab (primarily for facilities, equipment, and staffing), all of which would remain even if ZCC purchased the tests from a reference lab. Variable cost (primarily for reagents and other supplies) is $10 per test. The reference lab has offered to do the tests for a price of $17 each. ZCC currently receives $30 per test. If 10,000 tests are performed, is ZCC better off producing them in-house or contracting with the outside lab?

The solution is shown in Exhibit 9–17, solution 1. The product margin of the buy alternative is $70,000 less than that of the make alternative (line K). Therefore the *make* alternative is preferred. Notice that fixed costs do not have to be included in the analysis because they are the same for either alternative. However, if fixed costs do change between the two alternatives, then they have to be considered. For instance, if $80,000 of the fixed costs were avoidable, the analysis would be as shown in solution 2 of Exhibit 9–17, line J. As a result, the buy alternative becomes the preferred choice. Although it has a $70,000 lower total contribution margin (line I), it saves $80,000 in avoidable fixed costs, resulting in a positive product margin of $10,000 (line K).

Adding or Dropping a Service

Decision Rules If a proposed new service is expected to have a positive product margin, it should be added; and if an existing service has a negative product margin, it should be dropped.

Example: Geiser HMO asked Nathaniel Clinic, a pediatric group practice, to provide 3,000 well-baby visits. Nathaniel has excess capacity to see more patients but would have to hire additional staff for $85,000. It estimates additional variable costs (such as disposable thermometers, linens, etc.) of $10 per visit. Geiser is willing to pay $65 per visit. Should Nathaniel contract with Geiser and provide the well-baby clinic?

Exhibit 9–17 Example of a make-or-buy decision

		Alternative		Difference if Choose Buy Option (Buy - Make)
		Make[a]	Buy[b]	
Givens:				
A	Volume of tests (Given)	10,000	10,000	No change in volume
B	Revenue per test (Given)	$30	$30	No change in charge
C	Variable cost per test (Given)	$10	$17	Increase in VC/test
D	Contribution margin per test (Given)	$20	$13	Decrease in CM
E1	Avoidable fixed cost original (Given)	$0	$0	No change in AFC
E2	Avoidable fixed cost modified (Given)	$80,000	$0	Decrease in AFC
Solution 1. No avoidable fixed costs				
F	Volume (A)	10,000	10,000	0[c]
G	Revenues (A × B)	$300,000	$300,000	$0[d]
H	Variable costs (A × C)	$100,000	$170,000	$70,000[e]
I	Total contribution margin (G – H)	$200,000	$130,000	($70,000)[f]
J	Avoidable fixed cost (E1)	$0	$0	$0[g]
K	Product margin (I – J)	$200,000	$130,000	($70,000)[h]
Solution 2. Avoidable fixed costs				
F	Volume (A)	10,000	10,000	0[c]
G	Revenues (A × B)	$300,000	$300,000	$0[d]
H	Variable costs (A × C)	$100,000	$170,000	$70,000[e]
I	Total contribution margin (G – H)	$200,000	$130,000	($70,000)[f]
J	Avoidable fixed cost (E2)	$80,000	$0	($80,000)[g]
K	Product margin (I – J)	$120,000	$130,000	$10,000[h]

[a] Do test in-house.
[b] Purchase tests from outside lab.
[c] Increase (decrease) in volume from choosing buy option.
[d] Increase (decrease) in revenue from choosing buy option.
[e] Increase (decrease) in variable costs by choosing buy option.
[f] Increase (decrease) in total contribution margin by choosing buy option.
[g] Increase (decrease) in avoidable fixed costs by choosing buy option.
[h] Increase (decrease) in product margin from choosing buy option.

The solution is shown in Exhibit 9–18a. Because the project has a positive product margin of $80,000, Nathaniel should agree to offer the service. But what happens now if Geiser changes the terms of the contract and will only pay $35 per visit? In this case, as shown in Exhibit 9–18b, Nathaniel would have a positive total contribution margin, $75,000 (line I) but a negative product margin, -$10,000 (line K). Nathaniel should not agree to offer the service at this price.

Expanding or Reducing a Service

Decision Rule If only one alternative *will* or *must* be chosen, then the anticipated product margin of both alternatives should be compared. The alternative with the higher anticipated product margin should be chosen.

Example: Physicians Healthcare Group (PHG) is located in the greater Barnsboro metropolitan area. One of its major revenue centers, a radiology service, receives its revenues on a capitated basis: $55 per member per year to take care of all of their routine radiology needs. Assume that 20 percent of the 10,000 members will receive some routine radiological service each year at an average cost of $50 per service.

PHG operates 6 satellite clinics that offer general and specialty medicine services to their customers. X-ray service is also available at every clinic so that patients can be examined on site immediately. This has been a successful marketing feature, as shown by the annual patient satisfaction survey, but it has been costly. Stacy Helman, the new clinic manager, has suggested centralizing the radiology operations to two locations that have the capacity to serve all 6 clinics. She feels this would help reduce the current fixed costs of the organization by $200,000. However, if the services were relocated, Helman predicts a 10 percent reduction in members because they would probably change HMOs. The solution is shown in Exhibit 9–19.

Given the product margin results (row K), it appears that PHG should centralize its radiology service. Even though 10 percent of the patient volume would be lost, there would be significant equipment cost savings with this option. PHG would be better off by $155,000 per year by centralizing.

Although these examples illustrate the application of the product margin paradigm, other financial analysis tools should also be employed when making these decisions. For instance, the impact of these decisions on the financial ratios of the organization should be considered (see Chapter Four). Similarly, to the extent that these decisions have multiyear implications, a more thorough analysis would discount future cash flows and assess the net present value of these decisions (see Chapters Six and Seven). Finally, these financial concerns must be weighed against nonfinancial concerns when making these decisions.

Exhibit 9-18a Example of an add-or-drop decision

		Alternative		Difference if Choose to Add Service (Do - Don't)
		Don't Add[a]	Add[b]	
Givens:				
A	Volume	0	3,000	Increase in volume
B	Revenue per visit	$0	$65	Increase in charge
C	Cost per visit	$0	$10	Increase in VC/test
D	Contribution margin per visit	$0	$55	Increase in CM
E	Avoidable fixed cost	$0	$85,000	Increase in AFC
Solution				
F	Volume	(A)	0	3,000	3,000[c]
G	Revenues	(A × B)	$0	$195,000	$195,000[d]
H	Variable costs	(A × C)	$0	$30,000	$30,000[e]
I	Total contribution margin	(G – H)	$0	$165,000	$165,000[f]
J	Avoidable fixed costs	(E)	$0	$85,000	$85,000[g]
K	Product margin	(I – J)	$0	$80,000	$80,000[h]

[a] Do not open a new clinic.
[b] Open new clinic.
[c] Increase (decrease) in volume from choosing add option.
[d] Increase (decrease) in revenue from choosing add option.
[e] Increase (decrease) in variable costs by choosing add option.
[f] Increase (decrease) in avoidable fixed costs by choosing add option.
[g] Increase (decrease) in total contribution margin by choosing add option.
[h] Increase (decrease) in product margin from choosing add option.

407

Exhibit 9–18b Example of an add-or-drop decision

Givens:		Alternative		Difference if Choose to Add Service (Do - Don't)
		Don't Add[a]	Add[b]	
A	Volume	0	3,000	Increase in volume
B	Revenue per visit	$0	$35	Increase in charge
C	Cost per visit	$0	$10	Increase in VC/test
D	Contribution margin per visit	$0	$25	Increase in CM
E	Avoidable fixed cost	$0	$85,000	Increase in AFC
Solution				
F	Volume (A)	0	3,000	3,000[c]
G	Revenues (A × B)	$0	$105,000	$105,000[d]
H	Variable costs (A × C)	$0	$30,000	$30,000[e]
I	Total contribution margin (G – H)	$0	$75,000	$75,000[f]
J	Avoidable fixed costs (E)	$0	$85,000	$85,000[g]
K	Product margin (I – J)	$0	($10,000)	($10,000)[h]

[a] Do not open a new clinic.
[b] Open new clinic.
[c] Increase (decrease) in volume from choosing add option.
[d] Increase (decrease) in revenue from choosing add option.
[e] Increase (decrease) in variable costs by choosing add option.
[f] Increase (decrease) in avoidable fixed costs by choosing add option.
[g] Increase (decrease) in total contribution margin by choosing add option.
[h] Increase (decrease) in product margin from choosing add option.

Exhibit 9-19 Example of an add-or-drop decision

		Alternative		Difference if Choose to Reduce Service (Do - Don't)
		Don't Reduce[a]	Reduce[b]	
Givens:				
A	Members	10,000	9,000	Decrease in volume
B	Utilization rate	20%	20%	No change in utilization rate
C	PMPY	$55	$55	No change in PMPY
D	Cost per test	$50	$50	No change in cost per test
E	Avoidable fixed cost	$200,000	$0	Decrease in AFC
Solution				
F	Members (A)	10,000	9,000	(1,000)[c]
G	Revenues (A × C)	$550,000	$495,000	($55,000)[d]
H	Variable costs (A × B × D)	$100,000	$90,000	($10,000)[e]
I	Total contribution margin (G – H)	$450,000	$405,000	($45,000)[f]
J	Avoidable fixed costs (E)	$200,000	$0	($200,000)[g]
K	Product margin (I – J)	$250,000	$405,000	$155,000[h]

[a] Do not reduce number of locations.
[b] Reduce number of locations.
[c] Increase (decrease) in volume from reducing locations.
[d] Increase (decrease) in revenue from reducing locations.
[e] Increase (decrease) in variable costs by reducing locations.
[f] Increase (decrease) in avoidable fixed costs by reducing locations.
[g] Increase (decrease) in total contribution margin by reducing locations.
[h] Increase (decrease) in product margin from reducing locations.

409

SUMMARY

An understanding of fixed and variable costs provides a valuable tool to help make decisions of what price to charge, whether to add or drop a service, or whether to make or buy a service. Fixed costs are costs that do not vary in total but vary per unit over the relevant range. Variable costs vary in total but do not vary per unit over the relevant range. The relevant range is the range over which total fixed costs and/or per unit variable cost do not vary.

The break-even equation can be used to determine price, volume, fixed costs, or variable cost per unit, if each of the other factors is known. The break-even equation is (1) below.

The break-even point is that volume where total revenues equal total costs. The results of a break-even analysis are often presented on a break-even chart, which illustrates fixed costs, total costs, total revenues, and volume. The distance between the total cost and total revenue lines represents the amount of profit or loss the service is experiencing at any particular volume of service. An alternative form of this chart shows the difference between the total cost and total revenue lines: net income.

The break-even equation can be applied to capitated situations to determine capitation rates, utilization rates, or fixed or variable costs, given the others. The break-even equation can also be extended to multipayor and multiservice situations, though the latter is beyond the scope of this text. In conducting multipayor analyses that include capitated and fixed-fee patients, it is important not to adjust revenues for changes in volume, though variable costs may change. This caveat also holds for fixed-fee patients, such as those who pay on the basis of DRGs.

Per unit contribution margin is calculated by subtracting per unit variable cost from per unit revenues. It is the amount of profit made on each additional unit provided all other costs (fixed costs and overhead) remain the same. It is also the amount of incremental income from an average unit of service that is available to cover all other costs. If the contribution margin is known, a shortcut formula to calculate break-even can be used, (2) below.

If (1) the decision has been made not to close down a service, (2) no other additional costs will be incurred, and (3) the contribution margin is positive, then it is in the best financial interest of the organization to continue to provide additional units of that service, even if it is not fully covering all of its other costs.

$$(\text{Price} \times \text{Volume}) = \text{Fixed Costs} + (\text{Variable Cost per Unit} \times \text{Volume}) \qquad (1)$$

$$\text{Break-Even Volume} = \text{Total Fixed Costs} / \text{Contribution Margin per Unit} \qquad (2)$$

In instances where multiple services are offered, it is likely that there are both organizational fixed costs and service-specific fixed costs. Fixed costs that are present just because the service is being provided and would not be there if the service were not offered are called avoidable fixed costs. Product margin is computed as follows in equation (3) below:

The product margin decision rule states: if a service is covering its own variable and avoidable fixed costs, even if it does not fully cover its full share of other costs (nonavoidable fixed costs and common costs), the organization is better off delivering the service than not, all other things being equal (there are no better alternatives). If the organization violates this rule and closes a service with a positive product margin, the organization increases its loss by the amount of the product margin that it forgoes. The product margin concept is useful to help answer questions related to providing a service in-house or going outside (make-or-buy decision), adding or dropping a service, and expanding or reducing services. In all of these analyses, sunk costs should not be considered.

Other financial analysis tools should also be employed when making these decisions. For instance, the impact on the financial ratios of the organization should be considered. Also, decisions that have multiyear implications should include a more thorough analysis of future cash flows and net present value. Finally, as noted earlier, the financial concerns must be balanced with nonfinancial concerns to make these decisions.

$$\text{Total Revenues} - \text{Total Variable Costs} - \text{Avoidable Fixed Costs} \qquad (3)$$

KEY TERMS

a. Avoidable fixed cost
b. Break-even analysis
c. Break-even point
d. Capitation
e. Common costs
f. Contribution margin
g. Contribution margin per unit
h. Contribution margin rule
i. Fixed costs
j. Incremental costs

k. Joint costs
l. Nonavoidable fixed costs
m. Product margin
n. Product margin decision rule
o. Relevant range
p. Step-fixed costs
q. Target costing
r. Total Contribution Margin
s. Variable costs

KEY EQUATIONS

■ Basic break-even equation

$$\text{Price} \times \text{Volume} = \text{Fixed Cost} + (\text{Variable Cost per Unit} \times \text{Volume})$$

■ Contribution margin per unit

$$\text{Revenue per Unit} - \text{Variable Cost per Unit}$$

■ Total contribution margin

$$\text{Total Revenue} - \text{Total Variable Cost}$$

■ Short-cut to determine break-even volume

$$\text{Fixed Costs} / \text{Contribution Margin per Unit}$$

■ Break-even equation modified to include desired profit

$$\text{Price} \times \text{Volume} = \text{Fixed Costs} + (\text{Variable Cost per Unit} \times \text{Volume}) + \text{Desired Profit}$$

■ Break-even equation modified to include indirect cost and desired profit

$$\text{Price} \times \text{Volume} = \text{Direct Cost} + \text{Indirect Costs} + \text{Desired Profit}$$
$$\text{where Direct Costs} = \text{Direct Fixed Costs} + (\text{Direct Variable Cost per Unit} \times \text{Volume})$$

■ Break-even for capitation

$$\text{PMPM} \times \text{Enrollees} = (\text{Enrollees} \times \text{Utilization Rate} \times \text{Variable Cost/Unit}) + \text{Monthly Fixed Cost}$$

■ Product margin

$$\text{Total Contribution Margin} - \text{Avoidable Fixed Costs}$$

QUESTIONS AND PROBLEMS

1. **Definitions:** Define the previously listed key terms.

2. **Break-even formulas.** What are the formulas for:

   a. The basic break-even equation

   b. The basic break-even equation expanded to include indirect costs and desired profit?

3. **Understanding fixed and variable cost.** Briefly describe what happens to each of the following as volume increases. Assume all values stay within their relevant range.

   a. Total fixed cost

   b. Total variable cost

   c. Fixed cost per unit

   d. Variable cost per unit

4. **Step-fixed cost and the relevant range.** Explain the relationship between step-fixed costs and the relevant range.

5. **Product margin.** Based on the product margin, when is it in the best interests of an organization to continue or drop a service?

6. **Make-or-buy decision and related analyses.**

   a. What is a make-or-buy decision?

   b. What other analyses are relevant to the types of decisions discussed in this chapter?

7. **Break-even equation. Fill in the blank.** The following table contains selected data concerning several outpatient clinics in the new Ambulatory Care Center at Hope University Hospital. Fill in the missing information.

A Price per Visit	B Variable Cost/Visit	C Number of Visits	D Contribution Margin	E Fixed Costs	F Net Income
$85		3,000	$180,000		$80,000
$70	$20		$130,000	$90,000	
	$35	3,250		$78,000	$117,000
$65	$40	2,000		$60,000	

8. **Break-even equation. Fill in the blank.** Instead of the information in problem 7, assume Ambulatory Care Center's data looked like this:

A Price per Visit	B Variable Cost/Visit	C Number of Visits	D Contribution Margin	E Fixed Costs	F Net Income
$90		4,000	$200,000		$90,000
$85	$35		$150,000	$75,000	
	$55	4,500		$78,000	$120,000
$50	$60	2,000		$60,000	

9. **Expand-or-reduce decision.** Laurie Vaden is a physician with her own practice. She has developed contracts with several large employers to perform routine exams, fitness-for-duty exams, and initial screening of on-the-job injuries. She provides 100 exams per month, charging $100 per exam. Under this contract, she estimates her avoidable fixed costs attributable to the exams is $1,000 per month, and she pays a lab an average of $15 per exam. She has decided she needs to increase profit, so she is considering raising her fee to $125, even though there may be a 10 percent loss in the number of exams she does per month. Determine the current and predicted: revenues, variable costs, and total contribution margin. What do you recommend she do? Why?

10. **Expand-or-reduce decision.** Janet Gilbert is director of labs. She has some extra capacity and has contracted with some small neighboring hospitals to run some of their lab tests. She has recently had a study conducted and has determined that her costs for these contracts are $50,000, of which $7,000 is the variable cost of supplies. The rest is nonavoidable fixed cost. She currently charges an average of $20 per test. She is thinking of lowering her price by 20 percent in hopes of raising her current volume of 10,000 tests by 15 percent. If she does so, she expects her variable cost per test will go up by 4 percent. Determine the current and predicted: revenues, variable costs, and total contribution margin and product margin. What do you recommend she do? Why?

11. **Calculating break-even.** Jasmine Gonzales, administrative director of Small Imaging Center, has been asked by the practice members to see if it is feasible to add more staff to support the practice's mammography service, which currently has 2 analogue film or screen units and 2 technologists. She has compiled the following information:

a. What is the monthly patient volume needed per month to cover fixed and variable costs?

Reimbursement per screen:	$66.05
Equipment costs per month	$1,450.00
Technologist cost per mammography	$15.60
Technologist aide per mammography	$3.10
Variable cost per mammography	$15.00
Equipment maintenance per month per machine	$916.66

b. What is the patient volume needed per month if Small Imaging Center desires to cover its fixed and variable costs and make a $5,000 profit on this equipment to cover other costs associated with the organization?

c. If reimbursement decreases to $60 per screen, what is the patient volume needed per month to cover fixed and variable costs but not profit?

d. If a new technologist aide is hired, what is the patient volume needed per month at the original reimbursement rate to variable costs, but not profit?

(Problem developed by Michael Bohl)

12. **Break-even volume.** Monica Lee, administrative director of Digital Imaging Center, has been asked by the practice members to see if it is feasible to add more staff to support the practice's mammography service, which currently has 2 digital units and 2 technologists. She has compiled the following information:

Reimbursement per mammography	$126.30
Equipment lease per month per machine	$10,450.00
Equipment maintenance per month per machine	$12,500.00
Technologist cost per mammography	$31.92
Technologist aide per mammography	$18.20
Variable cost per mammography	$15.00

a. What is the patient volume needed per month to cover fixed and variable costs?

b. What is the patient volume needed per month if Digital Imaging Center desires to cover its fixed and variable costs and make a $5,000 profit on this equipment to cover other costs associated with the organization?

c. If reimbursement decreases to $120 per screen, what is the patient volume needed per month to cover fixed and variable costs but not profit?

d. If a new technologist aide is hired, what is the patient volume needed per month at the original reimbursement rate to cover costs, but not profit?

(Problem developed by Michael Bohl)

13. **Calculating break-even and graphing.** San Juan Health Department's dental clinic projects the following costs and rates for the year 20XX.

Total fixed costs	$175,000
Variable costs	$48 per patient
Charges	$150 per patient

a. Using this information, determine the break-even point in patients.

b. Using this information, determine the break-even point in dollars.

c. Graph this scenario in a break-even chart using a range of 0 to 3,500 patients in 500-patient increments.

d. If the clinic decides it would like to make a profit of $5,500, what is the new break-even point in patients?

e. If the clinic decides it would like to make a profit of $5,500 at 1,770 patients, what is the new break-even point in dollars?

14. **Calculating break-even and graphing.** The North Kingstown Cancer infusion therapy division expects tremendous growth over the next year and is projecting the following cost and rate structure for the service.

Revenue	$750	per patient
Costs:		
Rent	$3,600	per month
Staff	$195,000	per month
Leases	$10,000	per month
Other fixed costs	$20,000	per month
Pharmaceuticals	$500	per patient
Intravenous supplies	$25	per patient
Other patient supplies	$25	per patient

a. What volume of patients per month will it take for the center to break even?

b. What is the break-even point in dollars?

c. Graph the above scenario using a range of 0 to 2,500 patients in 500-patient increments.

d. If the clinic needs to make a profit of $75,000 per month, what is the new break-even point in volume per month?

e. If the clinic needs to make a profit of $75,000 per month, what is the new break-even point in revenue?

15. **Determining break-even price in a reduce-or-expand decision.** QuickCare is a health care franchise that functions as a primary family health clinic, seeing unscheduled patients twenty-four hours a day. Several months after the grand opening, a corporate office management engineering study showed that the clinic was experiencing some dips in volume in the midafternoon hours. To increase volume, efficiency, and revenues, the clinic administrator contracted with the area high schools to provide after-school physicals for the sports teams. The initial agreement was that QuickCare would charge $100 per exam, the market average. Fixed costs were $30,000 and variable costs are $25 per physical. Although this strategy proved somewhat successful, gross profit margin lagged behind the corporate expectations. To improve margin, the clinic is considering increasing the exam price to $125. QuickCare's administrator projects that this price increase will cause the high schools to send their athletes to other providers and that volume could drop by 33 percent. Last year, QuickCare performed 1,026 examinations. The administrator feels that if the program closes down, all $30,000 in fixed costs would be saved.

a. What should QuickCare's decision be, assuming that this price increase will decrease the number of patients seen by one-third?

b. What price would QuickCare have to charge to make up for the loss of patients?

c. Using the information from part a, should QuickCare make the same decision if 40 percent of the fixed costs are avoidable? Would it be better or worse off? Why?

16. **Expand-or-reduce.** The administrator of ABC Hospital, Mr. Stevens, has just received the latest financial report, and the news is not good. The hospital has been losing money for over a year, and if things don't improve, it may lose its AA bond rating. Stevens has met with his vice president of finance, Mr. Sanger, and has asked him to identify areas for cutting costs, beginning with services that are operating at a loss. The following information is for services provided at ABC Hospital's ambulatory care clinic:

Annual volume (in patient visits)	5,000
Charge per visit	$125
Variable cost per visit	$30
Fixed costs	$500,000

a. Suppose that all fixed costs are avoidable. What should Sanger recommend to Stevens regarding dropping the clinic?

b. What if only $150,000 of the fixed costs were avoidable? Would this change his recommendation?

c. Are there any other considerations that should be taken into account when making this decision?

17. **Add-or-drop decision.** The Ancome County Health Department is considering using 300 square feet of excess office space to provide a clinic for Healthchek visits. These visits are reimbursed at $67.30 under a Medicaid program. Variable costs per visit are $53.30, and providing the service requires an additional physician assistant and nurse with prorated salaries of $90,000 and $50,000, respectively. The state has mandated efforts to increase the utilization of Medicaid eligibility, so the Department of Social Services is conducting interventions to increase eligibility awareness in the community. As a result, the health department expects 10,000 Healthchek visits in the coming year. Unavoidable overhead costs for the health department are $300,000 per year and will be allocated to each program based on its proportional share of the health department's total office space of 2,700 square feet.

    a.   What are the total contribution margin and total product margin for a Healthchek visit?

    b.   Considering the total product margin, should the health department provide the service?

    c.   Are there any other considerations that should be taken into account when making this decision?

18. **Add-or-drop decision.** The Midtown Women's Center offers bone densitometry scans in the office as a convenience to its patients. The clinic volume is expanding, and Sam Loch, the center's administrator, is considering dropping the bone densitometry service and converting the space to an exam room to allow for more outpatient visits. The following information has been gathered to help with the decision.

Number of scans per year	425
Reimbursement for bone densitometry scan	$65
Bone densitometry supply cost per scan	$15
Part-time bone densitometry scan technician	$15,000
Reimbursement per office visit	$80
Supply cost per office visit	$20
Expected increase in outpatient volume if additional exam space is available	500

    a.   What is the contribution margin for the bone densitometry service per year?

    b.   Should this service continue as opposed to converting it to exam room space? Why or why not?

    c.   How many office visits would it take to replace the income from the bone densitometry service?

19. **Break-even.** Sure Care Health Maintenance Organization is seeking a managed care contract with a local manufacturing plant. Sure Care estimates that the cost of providing preventative and curative care for the 300 employees and their families will be $36,000 per month. The manufacturing company offered Sure Care a premium bid of $200 per employee per month.

    a. If Sure Care accepts this bid and contracts with the manufacturing firm, will Sure Care earn a profit or loss for the year? How much?

    b. What premium per employee per month does Sure Care need to break even?

    c. If Sure Care wants to earn $100,000 in profit for the year, what is the required premium per employee per month?

    d. What concerns do you have about this analysis?

20. **Break-even.** Zack Millman Clinic is seeking to provide sports-related health care services to high schools in the area. Zack Millman estimates that the cost to provide care would be $1,000 plus $12 per athlete per month on a 9-month basis. The high schools jointly offered to pay the clinic $10,000 for a 9-month contract to cover 75 athletes.

    a. If the clinic accepts this bid and contracts with the high schools, will it earn a profit or loss for the year? How much?

    b. What would the contract price have to be for Millman to break even?

    c. If Zack Millman Clinic wants to earn $5,000 in profit for the year, and the school system preferred to pay on a per athlete per month basis, what would the price have to be?

21. **Profit, charges, and break-even without and with overhead.** A number of years ago, at the request of its employees, Jake Winslow and Company converted one of its small rooms to house a small pharmacy for its employees in which they can buy a few popular prepackaged drugs. JWC only wants to break even on this service. Total cost of operating the pharmacy per year is $24,000: $1,000 a month for the contractor who operates the pharmacy and the remainder in drug costs. JWC charged $25 a month to each of 500 employees who participated last year.

    a. How much did the company make or lose during the year?

    b. In setting its rate for the coming year, how much would JWC have to charge per participating employee if it expects to break even? It estimates 500 employees per year will use this service.

    c. What if JWC also wants these employees to cover the estimated $100 overhead per month the pharmacy space costs?

    d. What would JWC have to charge if it expects drug costs to increase 10 percent per employee?

22. **Determining charges for private pay residents.** Shady Rest Nursing Home has 100 residents. The administrator is concerned about balancing the ratio of its private pay to non-private pay patients. Non-private pay sources reimburse an average of $150 per day whereas private pay residents pay on average 100 percent of full daily charges. The administrator estimates that variable cost per resident per day is $50 for supplies, food, and contracted services, and annual fixed costs are $4,562,500.

   a. What is the daily contribution margin of each non-private pay resident?

   b. If 25 percent of the residents are non-private pay, what will Shady Rest charge the private pay patients to break even?

   c. What if non-private pay payors cover 50 percent of the residents?

   d. The owner of Shady Rest Nursing Home insists that the facility earn $80,000 in annual profits. How much must the administrator raise the per day charge for the privately insured residents if 25 percent of the residents are covered by non-private pay payors?

23. **Determining charges for private pay residents.** Shady Grove Nursing Home has 220 private pay residents. The administrator is concerned about balancing the ratio of its private pay to non-private pay patients. Non-private pay sources reimburse an average of $125 per day whereas private pay residents pay on average 90 percent of full daily charges. The administrator estimates that variable cost per resident per day is $45 for supplies, food, and contracted services, and annual fixed costs are $6,000,000.

   a. What is the daily contribution margin of each non-private pay resident?

   b. If 25 percent of the residents are non-private pay, what will Shady Rest charge the private pay patients to break even?

   c. What if non-private pay payors cover 50 percent of the residents?

   d. The owner of Shady Rest Nursing Home insists that the facility earn $80,000 in annual profits. How much must the administrator raise the per day charge for the privately insured residents if 25 percent of the residents are covered by non-private pay payors?

24. **Add or drop with net present value analysis (builds on material in Chapters Six and Seven).** Franklin County Hospital, a nonprofit hospital, bought and installed a new computer system last year for $65,000. The system is designed to relay information between labs and medical units. Charlene Walker, the hospital's new computer specialist, had a meeting with Lou Campbell, vice president of finance. She began: "Lou, today I read in a journal that a new computer system has just been introduced. It costs $42,000, but I believe that by replacing our old system, we could

reduce operating and maintenance costs that are now being incurred." The following are Walker's estimates:

	Present System	**New System**
Purchase and installment price	$65,000	$42,000
Useful life when purchased	6 years	5 years
Computer operating costs per year	$30,000	$20,000
Computer operating and maintenance costs per year	$20,000	$18,000
Depreciation expenses per year	$10,833	$8,400
Cost of capital	10%	10%

a. Based on an analysis, what advice do you recommend that Walker give Campbell?

b. At what price for the new computer system would Campbell be indifferent?

c. Is this a typical make-or-buy decision? Why?

25. **Add or drop with net present value analysis (builds on material in Chapters Six and Seven).** Franklin County Hospital, a nonprofit hospital, bought and installed a new computer system last year for $150,000. The system is designed to relay information between labs and medical units. Charlene Walker, the hospital's new computer specialist, had a meeting with Lou Campbell, vice president of finance. She began: "Lou, today I read in a journal that a new computer system has just been introduced. It costs $100,000, but I believe that by replacing our old system, we could reduce operating and maintenance costs that are now being incurred." The following are Walker's estimates:

	Present System	**New System**
Purchase and installment price	$150,000	$100,000
Useful life when purchased	6 years	5 years
Computer operating costs per year	$45,000	$30,000
Computer operating and maintenance costs per year	$25,000	$12,000
Depreciation expenses per year	$10,833	$20,000
Cost of capital	10%	10%

a. Based on an analysis, what advice do you recommend that Walker give Campbell?

b. At what price for the new computer system would Campbell be indifferent?

c. Is this a typical make-or-buy decision? Why?

26. **Income statement and add or drop.** Lakespring Retirement Village is home to senior citizens who are fairly independent but need assistance with basic health care and occasional meals. Jill Thompson, a licensed beautician, works on salary 16 hours a week at Lakespring. Funds at the retirement village have been getting tight due to an increase in the number of Medicaid and other low-income residents. Carl Jones, Lakespring's administrator, told Thompson that the hair salon might have to be closed. Jones is sympathetic because he knows that it will be inconvenient for many residents to get this service elsewhere, and Thompson's charges are about all the residents can afford, but he wonders how he can keep any unit open that does not break even. Jones is looking for a way to save the hair salon and has provided the following information:

	Hair Cuts	Permanents	Brief Visits
Charge per resident	$10.00	$20.00	$5.00
Variable costs per service performed	$1.00	$4.00	$3.50
Cleaning/styling/setting products			
Variable water expense	$0.15	$0.25	$0.25
Laundry expenses for towels, smocks, etc.	$0.10	$0.30	$0.30

Jill is currently doing an average weekly business of 16 hair cuts, 7 permanents, and 4 brief visits, which take half an hour, an hour, and fifteen minutes, respectively. The hair salon is currently allocated rent of $250 per month and other upkeep expenses of $50 a month. Thompson is paid $12 per hour, and she earned $768 last month.

a. Prepare a monthly income statement and determine the total contribution margin and total product margin for each service line. Determine net income for the service taken as a whole.

b. How would you advise Jones: Should he close the hair salon? Why or why not?

c. Should Jones try to persuade Thompson to drop any service she now offers?

10

BUDGETING

LEARNING OBJECTIVES

- State the purposes of budgeting
- Describe the planning-and-control cycle and the five key dimensions of budgeting
- List the major budgets and explain their relationship to each other and to the income statement and balance sheet
- Construct each of the major budgets

The budget is one of the most important documents of a health care organization and is the central document of the planning-and-control cycle. The budget serves not only as a *planning* document that identifies the revenues and resources needed for an organization to achieve its goals and objectives but also as a *control* document that allows an organization to monitor the actual revenues generated and its use of resources against what was planned.

The Planning-and-Control Cycle

As illustrated in Exhibit 10–1, the planning-and-control cycle has four major components: strategic planning, planning, implementing, and controlling. Budgeting is the central element that affects all these areas.

Strategic Planning and Planning Strategic planning and planning activities provide the basis to develop the budget. The purpose of *strategic planning* is to identify the organization's vision, mission, goals, and strategy in order to position itself for the future. The purpose of *planning* is to identify the goals, objectives, tasks, activities, and resources necessary to carry out the strategic plan over a defined time period, commonly one year. The organization's mission is usually set forth in a mission statement, which is a broad, enduring statement of its vision and purpose. The *mission statement* guides the organization into the future by identifying the unique attributes of the organization, why it exists, and what it hopes to achieve (see Perspective 10–1).

Strategic Planning
Identifying an organization's mission, goals, and strategy to best position itself for the future.

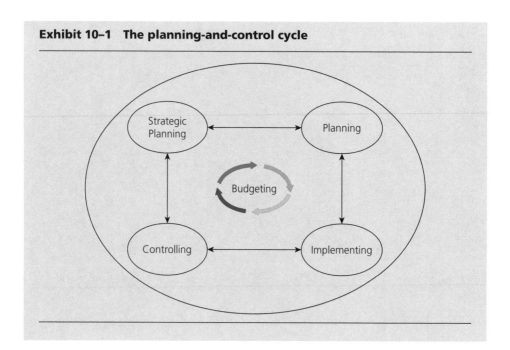

Exhibit 10–1   The planning-and-control cycle

Strategic Planning

Planning

Budgeting

Controlling

Implementing

Perspective 10–1 Mission Statement and Objectives of Shriners Hospitals

The mission of Shriners Hospitals for Children is to:

- Provide the highest quality care to children with neuro-musculoskeletal conditions, burn injuries and certain other special health care needs within a compassionate, family-centered and collaborative care environment
- Provide the education of physicians and other health care professionals
- Conduct research to discover new knowledge that improves the quality of care and quality of life of children and their families

The mission is carried out without cost to the patient or family, and without regard to race, color, creed, sex and sect.

Source: Shriners Hospitals for Children; available at: www.shrinershq.org/files/careeer_center/pdf/Mission_and_Vision.pdf Last accessed April 26, 2009.

A major activity of the strategic planning process is to assess the organization's external and internal environments. The external environment of most health care organizations is complex, and an environmental analysis must include surveying the local, regional, national, and international environments for changes that may occur in a variety of areas, including the economy, regulation, technology, and health status of populations. Other areas of the external environment that must be examined are listed in the top part of Exhibit 10–2. Failing to thoroughly and correctly assess even one of these domains could lead to major problems for, or even the demise of, the organization. In addition to its external environment, a health care organization has to examine its internal environment, which includes both *tangible factors*, such as financing, staff, services, and structure, and *intangible factors*, such as its history, reputation, and the strength of its board of directors.

An important outcome of the strategic planning process is to identify goals and objectives. In the past, goals and objectives for many health care organizations were fairly narrowly restricted to the nature and scope of services the organization hoped to provide. More recently, however, they have included population impacts (e.g., to reduce low-weight births in the covered population by 15 percent over the next five years), market penetration (e.g., to capture 25 percent of the HMO market within the next five years), and financial position (e.g., to increase return on assets by 10 percent over the next three years). The goals and

Planning
The process of identifying goals, objectives, tasks, activities, and resources necessary to carry out the strategic plan of the organization over the next time period, typically one year.

Mission Statement
A statement that guides the organization by identifying the unique attributes of the organization, why it exists, and what it hopes to achieve. Some organizations divide these attributes between a vision and a mission statement.

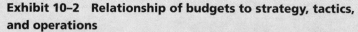

Exhibit 10–2 Relationship of budgets to strategy, tactics, and operations

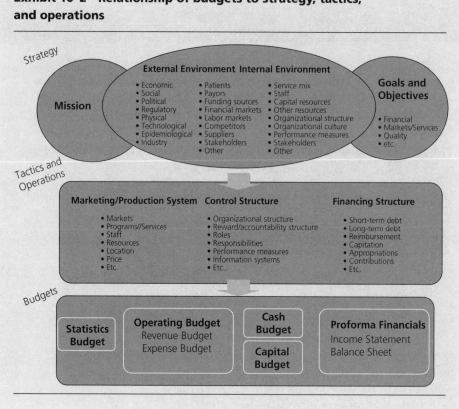

objectives the organization chooses to pursue impact the revenues and resources the organization will need, and these in turn must be reflected in the budgets.

Whereas the organization's strategic planning process focuses on the long term, the organization also develops shorter-term plans to help it achieve its short-term objectives. Whereas the strategic plan is fairly general, *short-term plans* are more specific and identify short-term goals and objectives in more detail, primarily in regard to marketing, production, control, and financing the organization.

Controlling Activities Planning activities provide input to develop a budget. Once the budget has been approved and implementation begins, *controlling activities* provide guidance and feedback to keep the organization within its budget (see Exhibit 10–1). Control tools vary from organizational structure and information systems to financially related controlling activities such as monthly reports to department managers

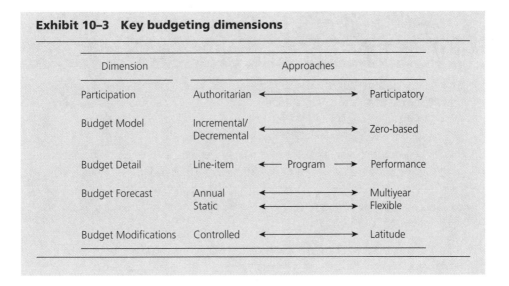

Exhibit 10–3   Key budgeting dimensions

Dimension	Approaches		
Participation	Authoritarian ←————→ Participatory		
Budget Model	Incremental/ Decremental ←————→ Zero-based		
Budget Detail	Line-item ←— Program —→ Performance		
Budget Forecast	Annual ←————→ Multiyear Static ←————→ Flexible		
Budget Modifications	Controlled ←————→ Latitude		

regarding their expenditures against budget and midyear bonuses based on financial performance.

Organizational Approaches to Budgeting

Exhibit 10–3 lists five key dimensions over which organizations vary in regard to budgeting: participation, budget model, budget detail, budget forecast, and budget modifications.

Participation The budgeting process can vary considerably from one organization to the next in terms of the roles and responsibilities of various positions in the organization. Under an authoritarian approach, the environmental assessment and planning of future activities are largely concentrated in a few hands at the top of the organization, and the budget is essentially dictated downward. The *authoritarian approach* is often called *top-down budgeting*. Perspective 10–2 illustrates a case where an outside authority's actions dictate budget cuts. Perspective 10–3 illustrates a case where an inside, overriding authority dictates program cuts.

The opposite of the authoritarian approach is the *participatory approach*, in which the roles and responsibilities of the budgeting process are diffused throughout the organization. The participatory approach often begins with some general guidelines from the top, based on top management's knowledge of the environment. Within the restrictions of these general guidelines, department heads and service-line managers (e.g., women's services, emergency services, outreach services) have great latitude to develop their own budgets to submit to upper management for approval. This approach is often called a *top-down-bottom-up approach*.

Authoritarian Approach
Budgeting and decision making that are done by relatively few people concentrated in the highest level of the organizational structure. Opposite of the *participatory approach.*

Top-down Budgeting
See *Authoritarian approach.*

Perspective 10–2   New Jersey Association Leader Rips Charity-Care Cuts

Calling the state Legislature's budgetary cuts to charity-care reimbursement "draconian," New Jersey Hospital Association president and chief executive officer designee Betsy Ryan said that patient care and the financial health of the state's hospitals will suffer as a result of the reduction, set to go into effect next year.

"Lost jobs, reduced services and longer drives and longer waits for needed healthcare services are becoming a real-life worry for a growing list of New Jersey communities," Ryan said. She added that financially strapped hospitals will have great difficultly keeping their doors open in light of the rising number of uninsured patients seeking care. . . .

Source: Rhea, S. 2008 (July 1)., N.J. association leader rips charity-care cuts. Modern Healthcare.com. © 2007 Crain Communications, Inc., 360 N Michigan Avenue, Chicago, IL 60601.

Perspective 10–3   Board OKs Plans to Close Inpatient Services at East St. Louis Facility

The Illinois Health Facilities Planning Board has approved the closing of inpatient services at 119-bed Kenneth Hall Regional Hospital, East St. Louis, according to the Southern Illinois Healthcare Foundation. Kenneth Hall will continue to operate an emergency department and behavioral health services, but other services will be shut down by July, as they duplicate services at 105-bed Touchette Regional Hospital, also in East St. Louis and about four miles from Kenneth Hall, said Ronda Sauget, a spokeswoman for the foundation and the hospitals. Both hospitals serve the same service area, which is declining in population, and are affiliates of the foundation.

The foundation, a network of twenty-seven federally qualified health centers, agreed to take over Kenneth Hall in 2004 as the hospital, then known as St. Mary's Hospital of East St. Louis, was on the brink of closing because of financial troubles, Sauget said. The foundation did so with the understanding that services would have to be consolidated eventually with Touchette Regional.

Source: Galloro, V. 2008 (April 9). Board OKs plans to close inpatient services at East St. Louis facility. Modern Healthcare.com. © 2008 Crain Communications, Inc.

Exhibit 10–4 The participatory approach to budgeting

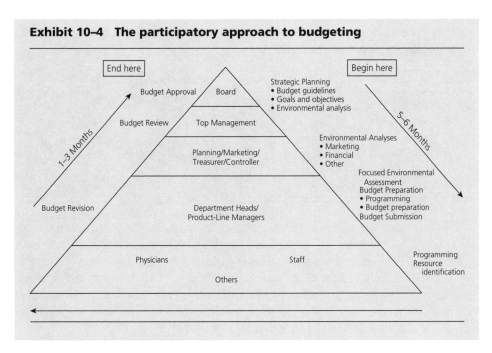

The roles and responsibilities of various positions in the organization in the participatory approach are summarized in Exhibit 10–4.

The participatory approach to budgeting has a number of advantages beyond just forcing management to plan (see Exhibit 10–5). These advantages include:

■ Developing a shared understanding of the goals and objectives of the organization by those who have participated in the budgeting process

■ Developing cooperation and coordination among the various departments

■ Clarifying roles and responsibilities throughout the organization (thus preventing overlap)

■ Motivating staff (by allowing them input into their roles, responsibilities, and accountability)

■ Bringing about cost awareness as a result of being involved in resource allocation decisions.

Although the participatory approach has many advantages, it has three important disadvantages:

■ Participation may result in loss of control

■ Participation is time-consuming and uses resources (mainly staff time) that could be devoted to other purposes

■ Participation may result in disappointment.

Participatory Approach
A method of budgeting in which the roles and responsibilities of putting together a budget are diffused throughout the organization, typically originating at the department level. There are guidelines to follow, and approval must be secured by top management. Opposite to the *Authoritarian approach*.

Top-down-bottom-up Approach
See *Participatory approach*.

Exhibit 10–5   Some key advantages and disadvantages of the participatory approach to budgeting

Advantages	Disadvantages
Shared understanding	Loss of control
Cooperation and competition	Time-consuming
Clarified roles and responsibilities	High resource use
Motivation	Disappointment
Cost awareness	

Incremental-Decremental Approach
A method of budgeting that starts with an existing budget to plan future budgets.

Zero-based Budgeting
An approach to budgeting that continually questions both the need for existing programs and their level of funding, as well as the need for new programs. Zero-based budgeting is often referred to as ZBB.

Budget Models There are two basic budget models: incremental-decremental budgeting and zero-based budgeting (see Exhibit 10–3). The *incremental-decremental approach* begins with what exists and usually gives a slight increase, no change, or slight decrease to various line items, programs, or departments. In some cases, all programs may receive an equal increase or decrease. In other instances, management may differentially give increases or decreases.

Where incremental-decremental budgeting begins by asking the question, "How much of an increase or decrease should each program receive?" *zero-based budgeting,* commonly called ZBB, continually questions both the need for each program and its level of funding. It asks: "Why does this program or department exist in the first place?" and "What will happen by changing (increasing or decreasing) its level of funding?"

In preparation for the zero-based budgeting process, each budgeting unit (department, program, or service line) prepares a budget package that provides an overall justification for the program and a series of requests to show what the program would look like at various levels of funding. After receiving all budget packages from all budgeting units, management chooses from among them to find the best combination of programs and levels of programs to meet the goals of the organization within existing resource constraints.

The following scenario illustrates what a zero-based budgeting package might look like at the general level for a small rural hospital that feels it must establish better relationships with physician practices. In this example, the zero state is no change. The alternatives are providing practice privileges to primary care physicians at one, two, or three physician practices. In addition to the information used in this example, many organizations would also require further detail of various line items. Such information can be found in the next section, Budget Detail.

The Situation San Valens Hospital continuously wants to attract more referring primary care physicians (PCPs) into sending their patients to San Valens, using the lure of the hospitalist service as a way to bypass twenty-four-hour, seven-days-a-week PCP inpatient coverage obligations. Currently there are three PCP groups in the local market area who have been referring their patients to a competing facility, but all practices have expressed interest in joining the medical staff at San Valens and referring their patients there instead. Crown Colony and Westover Family Practice, with six and eight PCPs, respectively, have a similar mix of adult patients across all insurance and age levels; Parkland Affiliates, on the other hand, is the largest practice with eleven PCPs but, being located adjacent to a growing retirement community, tends to have a much higher proportion of elderly patients. Parkland patients also predominantly have Medicare and steady retiree incomes, so their reimbursement is more favorable, but because of their age, they tend to utilize services at a disproportionately higher rate than is seen at the other two practices.

San Valens wants to establish itself as a regional referral center for patients and cannot discriminate based on ability to pay. However, at the same time, it wants to make financially prudent decisions and budget adequately for any changes in service capacity. As such, the hospital needs to explore the economic ramifications of gaining patients from any or all of these PCP groups as it strives to strategically position itself as the dominant area hospital. San Valens is not operating close to its full capacity.

Three alternatives are being proposed, each with considerably different costs and potential revenue, as well as impact on growth, image, and political concerns (Exhibits 10–6 and 10–7a). Although the costs are fairly predictable (mainly new staff), if volume projections are off, the revenues are not as predictable. Thus, San Valens must decide how much it wants to invest, if any, in the three alternatives. See Exhibits 10–7a, 10–7b, 10–7c, 10–7d, and 10–7e.

Exhibit 10–6 Summary zero-based budget[a]

Practice-Related Revenues	Crown Colony	Westover Family Practice	Parkland Affiliates
Initial services	$28,350	$36,800	$58,625
Follow-up services	$91,350	$115,200	$201,000
Total	$119,700	$152,000	$259,625
Practice-Related Expenses			
Labor expenses	$162,082	$202,603	$330,563
Total	$162,082	$202,603	$330,563
Hospitalist practice net income (loss)	($42,382)	($50,603)	($70,938)
Hospital Income			
Net inpatient revenues (loss)	$189,000	$235,750	$385,000
Incremental financial impact of proposal	$146,618	$185,147	$314,062
Performance measure: new admissions	900	1,150	1,750

[a] *Note:* The budgets for each practice separately are considered line item budgets. The three budgets presented together constitute a program budget and together or in combinations, could be chosen. Finally, when performance targets are added to a line item budget, it becomes a performance budget.

Exhibit 10–7a   Incremental revenue and cost summary for three additional PCP practices[a]

	Assumptions:	Formula	Crown Colony	Westover Family Practice	Parkland Affiliates
	Practice Profile				
A	Number of primary care physicians	(Given)	6	8	11
B	Proportion Medicare patients	(Given)	46%	51%	79%
C	Proportion Medicaid/Self-Pay patients	(Given)	10%	6%	4%
	Volume Projections				
D	Annual initial service RVUs	(Given)	900	1,150	1,750
E	Annual follow-up service RVUs	(Given)	2,900	3,600	6,000
F	Average LOS per admission, days	(Given)	4.2	4.1	4.4
	Financials				
G	Incremental practice costs per year[b]		$162,082	$202,603	$330,563
H	Average reimbursement per RVU	(Given)	$31.50	$32.00	$33.50
I	Average facility profit per inpatient day	(Given)	$200	$200	$200
	Calculations:				
J	Annual initial service revenues	(D × H)	$28,350	$36,800	$58,625
K	Annual follow-up service revenues	(E × H)	$91,350	$115,200	$201,000
L	Incremental practice costs per year	(G)	$162,082	$202,603	$330,563
M	*Incremental hospitalist group income (loss)*	(J + K − L)	($42,382)	($50,603)	($70,938)
N	New admissions[c]	(D/4)	225	288	438
O	Incremental inpatient income (loss)	(F × I × N)	$189,000	$235,750	$385,000
P	*Incremental financial impact of proposal*	(M + O)	$146,618	$185,147	$314,062
Q	Performance measure: new admissions	(N)	225	288	438

Other factors

Image: San Valens wants to maintain a positive image in the community as the hospital of choice for all patients, regardless of ability to pay.

Growth: San Valens wants to grow its inpatient services with unmet demand; the hospital is currently operating below full bed capacity.

Political: San Valens does not want to lose its geriatrics program nor its renowned director; as a bonus, Parkland patients reimburse well.

[a]*Note*: This exhibit provides details of the summary budget found in Exhibit 10-6. The details for each of the three practices, respectively, can be found in Exhibits 10-7b through 10-7d. LOS = length of stay, RVU = relative value unit.

[b]See Exhibit 10-6 and Exhibit 10-7e.

[c]Each new admission consumes 4 RUVs of service.

Exhibit 10–7b   Zero-based budget package for Crown Colony

Package: Salary, benefits, capital, and space needs
Organization: Hospitalist practice
Purpose: To provide inpatient care services for the Crown Colony patients
Method: Hospital will need an additional 0.5 FTEs of provider coverage to meet the demands of Crown Colony. This can probably be accommodated by more per diem assistance and by providing current physicians the opportunity to earn additional income by working extra shifts at the per diem rate.

Consequences of not approving this package: Crown Colony, as evidenced by its reimbursement rate, predominantly serves a working class, blue-collar community on the north side of the city, with slightly more Medicaid/Self-Pay patients than Westover. By not choosing this practice, San Valens could be seen as favoring communities who would best help the bottom line, rather than being a full provider of services for the entire region. There is no evidence of other competition for these patients, but there would be an image problem for the hospital of ignoring them.

	Assumptions		Crown Colony
	Practice Profile		
A	Number of primary care physicians		6
B	Proportion Medicare patients		46%
C	Proportion Medicaid/Self-Pay patients		10%
	Volume Projections		
D	Annual initial service RVUs		900
E	Annual follow-up service RVUs		2,900
F	Average LOS per admission, days		4.2
	Financials		
G	Incremental practice costs	(Ex 10-7e)	$162,082
H	Average reimbursement per RVU		$31.50
I	Average facility profit per inpatient day		$200
	Calculations		
J	Annual initial service revenues	(D × H)	$28,350
K	Annual follow-up service revenues	(E × H)	$91,350
L	Incremental practice costs per year	(G)	$162,082
M	*Incremental hospitalist group income (loss)*	(J + K − L)	($42,382)
N	New admissions[a]	(D / 4)	225
O	Incremental inpatient income (loss)	(F × I × N)	$189,000
P	*Incremental financial impact of proposal*	(M + O)	$146,618
Q	Performance measure: new admissions	(N)	225

[a] Each new admission consumes 4 RUVs of service.

Exhibit 10–7c   Zero-based budget package for Westover Family Practice

Package: Salary, benefits, capital, and space needs
Organization: Hospitalist practice
Purpose: To provide inpatient care services for the Westover Family Practice patients
Method: Hospital will need an additional 0.7 FTEs of provider coverage to meet the demands of Westover. This coverage cannot be accommodated by per diem or additional shift work alone. The hospital would have to hire another full-time physician to accommodate the workload, which would increase costs by $85,000 over what is projected.
Consequences of not approving this package: Westover Family Practice is ideally situated in an area with minimal competition for its services owing to a single bridge that discourages patients from traveling elsewhere for their primary care needs. Westover hopes to add two more physicians and three nurse practitioners over the next two years to grow its practice and ward off potential competitors. Ultimately, this would create more demand for the hospital, but San Valens would be overstaffed initially by budgeting for 1 physician FTE rather than 0.7, and there is no guarantee if or when Westover would expand.

	Assumptions		Westover Family Practice
	Practice Profile		
A	Number of primary care physicians		8
B	Proportion Medicare patients		51%
C	Proportion Medicaid/Self-Pay patients		6%
	Volume Projections		
D	Annual initial service RVUs		1,500
E	Annual follow-up service RVUs		3,600
F	Average LOS per admission, days		4.1
	Financials		
G	Incremental practice costs	(Ex 10-7e)	$202,603
H	Average reimbursement per RVU		$32.00
I	Average facility profit per inpatient day		$200
	Calculations		
J	Annual initial service revenues	(D × H)	$36,800
K	Annual follow-up service revenues	(E × H)	$115,200
L	Incremental practice costs per year	(G)	$202,603
M	*Incremental hospitalist group income (loss)*	(J + K − L)	($50,603)
N	New admissions[a]	(D / 4)	228
O	Incremental inpatient income (loss)	(F × I × N)	$235,750
P	*Incremental financial impact of proposal*	(M + O)	$185,147
Q	Performance measure: new admissions	(N)	288

[a] Each new admission consumes 4 RUVs of service

Exhibit 10–7d Zero-based budget package for Parkland Affiliates

Package: Salary, benefits, capital, and space needs
Organization: Hospitalist practice
Purpose: To provide inpatient care services for the Parkland Affiliates patients
Method: Hospital will need an additional 1.1 FTEs of provider coverage to meet the demands of Parkland Affiliates. This coverage would require hiring a full-time physician immediately and relying on additional per diem support to accommodate the expected demand.

Consequences of not approving this package: Parkland Affiliates serves a sizeable community of well-reimbursing elderly patients who have been vocal about their desires to be able to use San Valens services. In addition, San Valens has a reputable geriatric program, but the medical director of the program has become frustrated with limited referrals of late and has threatened to build his program elsewhere unless the hospital makes a concerted effort to generate more business. He also travels to Parkland Affiliates twice per month to see patients with unique medical issues and has established close ties with all of their physicians.

	Assumptions		Parkland Affiliates
	Practice Profile		
A	Number of primary care physicians		11
B	Proportion Medicare patients		79%
C	Proportion Medicaid/Self-Pay patients		4%
	Volume Projections		
D	Annual initial service RVUs		1,750
E	Annual follow-up service RVUs		6,000
F	Average LOS per admission, days		4.4
	Financials		
G	Incremental practice costs	(Ex 10-7e)	$330,563
H	Average reimbursement per RVU		$33.50
I	Average facility profit per inpatient day		$200
	Calculations		
J	Annual initial service revenues	(D × H)	$58,625
K	Annual follow-up service revenues	(E × H)	$201,000
L	Incremental practice costs per year	(G)	$330,563
M	*Incremental hospitalist group income (loss)*	(J + K − L)	($70,938)
N	New admissions[a]	(D / 4)	438
O	Incremental inpatient income (loss)	(F × I × N)	$385,000
P	*Incremental financial impact of proposal*	(M + O)	$314,062
Q	Performance measure: new admissions	(N)	438

[a] Each new admission consumes 4 RUVs of service.

Exhibit 10–7e   Calculation of salaries for all three practices

Basic Data:

Direct annual expenses per 1.0 hospitalist FTE:

Salaries and Benefits	Cost
Salary	$200,000
Malpractice insurance	$12,000
Health and dental insurances	$17,000
LTD/Life/AD&D insurances	$1,800
CME	$3,000
6% matching 401K	$12,000
Licenses/fees/dues	$2,400
Total direct costs	$248,200
Overhead costs as percentage of direct costs 22%	$54,604
T Total costs per 1.0 new hospitalist FTEs	$302,804

Practice Name	A Total Service RVUs[a]	B Hours/RVU (Given)	C Hours Needed (A × B)	D FTE Hours/Year (Given)	E Hospitalist Efficiency (Given)	F FTEs Needed (C/(D × E))	G Cost to Hire FTE[c] (F × T)	H Performance Measure[b] (Admissions)
Crown Colony	3,800	0.25	950	2,040	87%	0.5	$162,082	225
Westover Family Practice	4,750	0.25	1,188	2,040	87%	0.7	$202,603	288
Parkland Affiliates	7,750	0.25	1,938	2,040	87%	1.1	$330,563	438

[a] From Exhibit 10-7a, rows (D + E).
[b] From Exhibit 10-7a, row N: the number of projected new admissions is the performance target for each practice.
[c] Differences due to rounding.

Concluding Remarks about Zero-based Budgeting   Zero-based budgeting was introduced and broadly used in the mid-1960s, but it soon dropped out of favor, primarily because it was such a laborious process. Many organizations felt that too much time was being spent preparing and reviewing budget packages when in fact major changes rarely occurred. There are some signs, though, that zero-based budgeting is reemerging as health care organizations face an increasingly competitive environment, seek to implement new revenue enhancement and cost avoidance activities, and try to capture new market niches.

Budget Detail Based on the amount of detail they contain, budgets can be classified into three categories: line-item, program, and performance. A *line-item budget* has the least detail, merely listing revenues and expenses by category, such as labor, travel, and supplies. A line-item budget for the comprehensive level of care for the San Valens Hospital is shown in Exhibit 10–6.

A *program budget* not only contains the line items but also lists them by program. Exhibit 10–6 shows how the line-item budget for the three physician practices would look as a program budget by providing detail about the three practices, which if chosen singly or in combinations would provide incremental revenues.

Finally, a *performance budget* lists revenue and expenses by line item for each program or service but adds performance measure. Exhibit 10–6 compares the level of detail shown in line-item, program, and performance budgets. Exhibit 10–7a provides additional detail to support the summary zero-based budget in Exhibit 10–6.

Although virtually all organizations have annual budgets, increasingly each is part of a *multiyear budget*. Rather than forecast revenues and expenses for just one year, organizations are finding it necessary to use multiyear budgets to forecast three to five years in advance. Because conditions change, many organizations use *rolling budgets*, which are regularly updated and extended multiyear forecasts. For example, the budget submitted for 20X1 would cover the years 20X1 through 20X5. When the 20X2 budget is prepared, it will cover the years 20X2 through 20X6. In this way, the budget is always forecasting five years ahead. Some organizations "roll forward" their budgets more often than every year, updating their multiyear forecasts on a semiannual or even quarterly basis.

Single-year and multiyear budgets vary by the time horizon they forecast, whereas static and flexible budgets vary on the basis of volume projections. *Static budgets* forecast for a single level of activity, and *flexible budgets* forecast revenues and expenses for various levels of activities. For example, whereas a static budget in an ambulatory care setting might forecast revenues and expenses for 15,000 visits, a flexible budget would forecast revenues and expenses for a range of visits between 14,000 and 16,000 visits. The use of flexible budgets is an important tool for controlling expenses and is discussed in detail in Chapter Eleven.

Budget Modifications In most health care organizations, criteria are established beyond which managers must request permission to make changes to their budgets. The criteria are usually set as dollar amounts or a need to move funds from one category to another (or both). For example, an administrator may be able to move amounts under $1,000 within a category (such as labor) without needing higher approval but

---

Line-item Budget
The least detailed budget, showing only revenues and expenses by category, such as labor or supplies.

Program Budget
An extension of the line-item budget that shows revenues and expenses by program or service lines.

Performance Budget
An extension of the program budget that also lays out performance objectives.

Multiyear Budget
A budget that is forecast multiple years out, rather than just for the upcoming year.

Rolling Budget
A multiyear budget that is updated more frequently than annually, such as semiannually or quarterly.

Static Budget
A budget that uses a single or fixed level of activity.

Flexible Budget
A budget that accommodates a range or multiple levels of activities.

not from one category to another (such as from labor to equipment). Particularly dramatic examples of the need for budget revisions often occur during nursing shortages, when hospitals have to continually ask their boards to approve increases in nursing salaries or contract labor in the middle of the year.

TYPES OF BUDGETS

Although the term *the budget* is often used as if there were only one budget, most health care organizations develop four interrelated budgets: a statistics budget, an operating budget, a cash budget, and a capital budget. An overview of the relationship among these budgets is presented in Exhibit 10–8.

Statistics Budget

The first budget to develop is the statistics budget. The *statistics budget* identifies the amount of services that will be provided, usually listed by payor type, as in Exhibit 10–9.

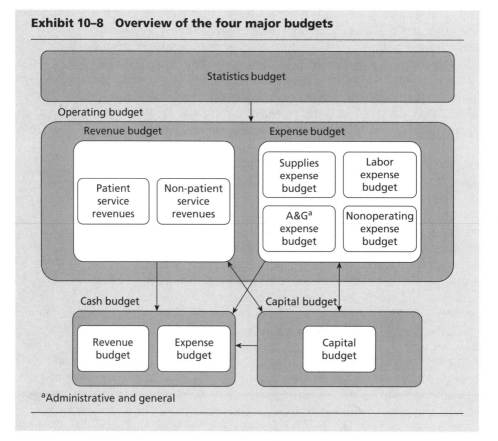

Exhibit 10–8   Overview of the four major budgets

Statistics budget

Operating budget

Revenue budget

Patient service revenues

Non-patient service revenues

Expense budget

Supplies expense budget

Labor expense budget

A&G[a] expense budget

Nonoperating expense budget

Cash budget

Revenue budget

Expense budget

Capital budget

Capital budget

[a]Administrative and general

Exhibit 10–9 Statistics budget for ZMG Hospitalist Practice (in RVUs)

Insurance Category	Jan	Feb	Mar	Apr	May	Jun	Jul	Aug	Sep	Oct	Nov	Dec	Total
Commercial	4,730	4,420	4,768	4,428	4,232	4,342	4,440	4,568	4,398	4,652	4,472	4,918	54,368
Medicare	7,360	6,872	7,412	6,888	6,588	6,758	6,902	7,108	6,840	7,238	6,960	7,648	84,574
Medicaid/Self-Pay	1,050	982	1,060	982	940	968	988	1,018	978	1,032	992	1,092	12,082
Total	13,140	12,274	13,240	12,298	11,760	12,068	12,330	12,694	12,216	12,922	12,424	13,658	151,024

- The *commercial payor* category includes a wide variety of nongovernmental entities that pay on behalf of the patient, including insurance companies, PPOs, and HMOs. These organizations usually pay a prenegotiated portion of full charges, though the amount of discount may vary considerably among payors and among procedures.

- *Medicare* is a governmental program that pays on behalf of those older than sixty-five, patients younger than sixty-five with certain disabilities, and patients with end-stage renal disease. Medicare Part A covers hospital stays, Medicare Part B covers physician and outpatient care, and Medicare Part D covers prescriptions. Within these categories, Medicare is usually a price setter. That is, it determines what it will pay for and how much it will pay.

- *Medicaid/Self-Pay* includes two types of payors that are often grouped together into a single category. Medicaid is a governmental program in which the federal government and state governments pay on behalf of certain low-income individuals and families who fit into an eligibility group that is recognized by federal and state law. Eligibility varies considerably from state to state. Medicaid typically pays considerably less than the other two categories of payors. The Self-Pay category comprises those who pay for their own care, as opposed to the other categories in which others, called *third parties*, pay on behalf of the patient. In some cases, though an individual may be covered by a third party, the patient may still have responsibility for part of the bill through copays and deductibles, as discussed in Chapter Thirteen.

Statistics Budget
The first budget to be prepared; one of the four major types of budgets. It identifies the amount of services that will be provided, typically categorized by payor type.

Exhibit 10–9 presents the statistics budget for ZMG Hospitalist Practice, a group practice that staffs hospitals with physician internists whose specialty is focused on inpatient care in the hospital setting. As discussed in more detail below, the statistics in this budget are stated in terms of relative value units (RVUs), which weight each type of encounter by the relative amount of resources it consumes. In the case of hospitalists, there are two main types of encounters: admissions and follow-up care (which includes discharges), with admissions consuming approximately twice the resources, mainly time, as a follow-up encounter.

Operating Budget

The *operating budget* (see Exhibit 10–10) is actually a combination of two budgets developed using the accrual basis of accounting: the revenue budget and the expense budget. Some organizations, especially those with relatively small non-operating items such as parking lot and gift shop revenues and expenses, include their nonoperating budget with their operating budget.

Operating Budget
One of the four major types of budgets, it comprises the revenue budget and the expense budget. The bottom line for this budget is net income.

The *revenue budget* is a forecast of the operating revenues that will be earned during the budget period (see Exhibit 10–10, rows A through E). It has two components: net patient revenues (row C) and nonpatient revenues (row D). The *expense budget* lists all operating and nonoperating

Exhibit 10-10 Operating budget for ZMG Hospitalist Practice

	Jan	Feb	Mar	Apr	May	Jun	Jul	Aug	Sep	Oct	Nov	Dec	Total
Revenues													
A Gross patient service revenues	$689,850	$644,385	$695,100	$645,645	$617,400	$633,570	$647,325	$666,435	$641,340	$678,405	$652,260	$717,045	$7,928,760
B − Deductions & allowances	267,810	250,170	269,870	250,632	239,695	246,031	251,337	258,786	249,004	263,356	253,206	278,369	3,078,266
C Net patient service revenues	422,040	394,215	425,230	395,013	377,705	387,539	395,988	407,649	392,336	415,049	399,054	438,676	4,850,494
D Nonpatient revenues	1,182	1,238	903	901	903	901	903	903	901	903	901	903	11,440
E Net revenues	423,221	395,453	426,133	395,914	378,608	388,440	396,891	408,552	393,237	415,952	399,955	439,578	4,861,934
Expenses													
Labor	443,250	469,866	458,866	455,510	455,510	455,979	464,413	464,413	464,413	464,413	465,413	495,494	5,557,539
Administrative and general	26,713	26,432	26,740	27,030	26,852	26,945	27,223	27,333	27,174	27,395	27,228	27,618	324,684
F Operating expenses	469,963	496,298	485,606	482,541	482,363	482,925	491,635	491,746	491,586	491,807	492,641	523,112	5,882,223
G Nonoperating expenses	1,300	1,750	1,750	1,750	1,300	1,300	1,300	1,300	1,300	1,300	1,300	1,300	16,950
H Total expenses	471,263	498,048	487,356	484,291	483,663	484,225	492,935	493,046	492,886	493,107	493,941	524,412	5,899,173
I Excess of revenues over expenses	($48,042)	($102,595)	($61,223)	($88,377)	($105,055)	($95,785)	($96,044)	($84,494)	($99,649)	($77,155)	($93,986)	($84,834)	($1,037,239)

Revenue Budget
A subset of the operating budget that is a forecast of the operating revenues that will be earned during the current budget period.

Expense Budget
A subset of the operating budget that is a forecast of the operating expenses that will be incurred during the current budget period.

expenses that are expected to be incurred during the budget period (see Exhibit 10–10, rows F and G). Perspectives 10–4 and 10–5 illustrate some of the major concerns health care organizations face with one part of the expense budget, labor.

Whether an item is classified as operating or nonoperating is subject to interpretation by each organization. Although this matter has received considerable attention over the years by both the accounting and health care financial management professions, there remains a lack of standardization among health care organizations in classifying specific line items.

> **Caution:** Throughout this chapter, the numbers in the exhibits may be slightly different from those computed on a calculator and between exhibits due to the internal rounding rules used in the computer program on which the examples are based.

Cash Budget

Whereas the operating budget describes the expected revenues and the related resource flows, the *cash budget* (see Exhibit 10–11) represents the organization's cash inflows

Perspective 10–4   Salary Cuts, Layoffs Planned at Beaumont

Executives at Beaumont Hospitals are taking salary cuts of 4 percent to 10 percent as part of a turnaround plan that includes cutting 500 jobs and slowing down construction projects at the Royal Oak, Michigan-based system.

Up to 165 people are facing layoffs, though some of them could find different jobs in the system. About 200 jobs have already been eliminated through attrition, and officials expect to cut another 135 that will voluntarily open up in coming months among the system's 18,000-person payroll, spokesman Bob Ortlieb said.

. . . The system is only the latest to announce triple-digit layoffs. This week, 868-bed MetroHealth Medical Center, Cleveland, announced 112 job cuts, and 367-bed St. John's Regional Medical Center, Joplin, Missouri, announced 160. News outlets reported several thousand job cuts at hospitals across the country in October and November, despite a November 7 Bureau of Labor Statistics report showing steady growth in health care employment for the tenth straight month in October.

Source: Carelson, J. 2008 (Nov. 18). Salary cuts, layoffs planned at Beaumont. Modern Healthcare.com. © 2008 Crain Communications, Inc.

Perspective 10–5   Potential Shortage of 500,000 Nurses Seen by 2025

The nursing workforce may face a deficit of 285,000 registered nurses by 2020, with the shortage growing to 500,000 by 2025 if there is no letup in demand, according to a national study released at a news conference in Washington.

A shortage of this magnitude could cripple health care quality, access, and safety for millions of patients, said Peter Buerhaus, director of the Center for Interdisciplinary Health Workforce Studies at Vanderbilt University Medical Center in Nashville and co-author of *The Future of the Nursing Workforce in the United States: Data, Trends and Implications*.

Compounding this problem is the fact that many nurses are among the 78 million baby boomers who will reach age 65 over the next two decades, Buerhaus said. Currently, the average age of a nurse is 43.7 years, but by 2012, the projection is most registered nurses will be over age 50, he said.

Source: Lubell, J. 2008 (May 6). Potential shortage of 500,000 nurses seen by 2025. Modern Healthcare.com. © 2008 Crain Communications, Inc.

and outflows. The bottom line in the operating budget is the net income for the period; the bottom line in the cash budget is the amount of cash available at the end of the period, Exhibit 10–11, row O. In addition to showing cash inflows and outflows, the cash budget also details when it is necessary to borrow to cover cash shortages and when excess funds are available to invest.

Key Point *The operating budget is developed using the accrual basis of accounting. Cash inflows and outflows of each line item must be estimated to convert the operating budget to the cash budget.*

Capital Budget

The *capital budget* (see Exhibit 10–12) summarizes the anticipated major purchases for the year. Capital budgets in outpatient facilities may be fairly small, but those for large systems with inpatient facilities may contain millions of dollars' worth of items.

Pro Forma Financial Statements and Ratios

Based on the information contained in these budgets, together with a small amount of additional information, an organization can develop pro forma financial statements.

Cash Budget
One of the four major types of budgets, it displays all of the organization's projected cash inflows and outflows. The bottom line for this budget is the amount of cash available at the end of the period.

Capital Budget
One of the four major types of budgets, it summarizes the anticipated major purchases for the year.

Exhibit 10–11 Cash budget for ZMG Hospitalist Practice

		Jan	Feb	Mar	Apr	May	Jun	Jul	Aug	Sep	Oct	Nov	Dec	Summary
A	Beginning balance	$200,000	$100,000	$100,000	$100,000	$100,000	$100,000	$100,000	$100,000	$100,000	$100,000	$100,000	$100,000	$200,000
B	Net revenues	435,415	419,574	412,877	412,293	396,637	387,755	390,940	397,694	399,805	402,469	406,315	414,088	4,875,862
C	Net expenditures	(454,405)	(481,471)	(510,071)	(469,634)	(467,184)	(503,653)	(477,510)	(478,310)	(512,310)	(476,310)	(477,310)	(545,392)	(5,853,563)
D	Cash avail before borrowing	181,011	38,103	2,806	42,659	29,452	(15,898)	13,430	19,384	(12,506)	26,159	29,004	(31,304)	322,299
E	Cash requirement	100,000	100,000	100,000	100,000	100,000	100,000	100,000	100,000	100,000	100,000	100,000	100,000	100,000
F	Cash excess (shortage)	81,011	(61,897)	(97,194)	(57,341)	(70,548)	(115,898)	(86,570)	(80,616)	(112,506)	(73,841)	(70,996)	(131,304)	(877,701)
G	Transfer excess to ST investments	(81,011)	–	–	–	–	–	–	–	–	–	–	–	(81,011)
H	Remaining deficit	–	(61,897)	(97,194)	(57,341)	(70,548)	(115,898)	(86,570)	(80,616)	(112,506)	(73,841)	(70,996)	(131,304)	(958,711)
I	Transfer from ST investment	0	61,897	74,544	10	10	10	10	10	10	10	10	10	136,531
J	Remaining deficit	0	0	(22,650)	(57,331)	(70,538)	(115,888)	(86,560)	(80,606)	(112,496)	(73,831)	(70,986)	(131,294)	(822,181)
K	Transfer from LT investment	0	0	113	59	58	59	58	59	59	58	59	58	641
L	Remaining deficit	0	0	(22,537)	(57,272)	(70,480)	(115,829)	(86,503)	(80,547)	(112,436)	(73,774)	(70,926)	(131,237)	(821,540)
M	Subsidy required	0	0	22,537	57,272	70,480	115,829	86,503	80,547	112,436	73,774	70,926	131,237	821,540
N	Total of transfers and subsidies	(81,011)	61,897	97,194	57,341	70,548	115,898	86,570	80,616	112,506	73,841	70,996	131,304	877,701
O	Ending balance	$100,000	$100,000	$100,000	$100,000	$100,000	$100,000	$100,000	$100,000	$100,000	$100,000	$100,000	$100,000	$100,000

Exhibit 10–12   Capital budget for ZMG Hospitalist Practice

	Purchase Price	Life, Years	Residual Value	Depreciation Base	Monthly Depreciation	Date of Purchase	Debt Financing	Financed from Cash
Anticipated purchases for 20X2:								
Computer network	$25,000	5	$500	$24,500	$408	Apr 20X2	100%	0%
HVAC upgrade	$12,000	8	$750	$11,250	$117	Jul 20X2	90%	10%
Total	$37,000							

Pro forma financial statements are prepared to show what the organization's regular financial statements will look like if all budgets are met exactly as planned. The regular financial statements are prepared after the accounting period ends and present the actual results of the organization's activities during the period. As an example of the relationship between the budgets and financial statements, ZMG Hospitalist Practice's operating budget (see Exhibit 10–10) could serve as its statement of operations, with only a few modifications in format. Developing the balance sheet and statement of cash flows is not as straightforward, but it can be done with only a small amount of additional information.

Once the pro forma financial statements have been developed, they can be subjected to ratio analysis just as with regular financial statements. This process is reversed in strategic financial planning, where the organization first identifies its goals in terms of the various categories of ratios (liquidity, profitability, capitalization, and activity) and then develops its budgets, over time, to meet the targets it has set for itself.

AN EXTENDED EXAMPLE OF HOW TO DEVELOP A BUDGET

This section shows how to develop the numbers in a budget, using ZMG Hospitalist Practice as an example. The term *a budget* really is shorthand for four interrelated budgets: the statistics, operating, cash, and capital budgets.

Statistics Budget

The statistics budget is created in three steps: develop an overall volume projection, categorize volume projection by payor and encounter type, and convert encounters to weighted encounters.

- *Develop overall volume projection.* A common approach to forecasting volume is to begin with the previous year's actual results and make adjustments for anticipated changes. In the example, the ZMG Hospitalist Practice makes the relatively gross assumption of 5 percent overall and monthly growth compared with the current year (Exhibit 10–13a). Although this approach is common, to the extent that major variations can be expected, a more refined month-by-month projection would help make the budget a better planning tool.

- *Categorize volume projections by payor and encounter type.* As eventually the amount of revenue earned by these encounters must be estimated, the next step is to further subdivide the number of encounters just developed by the type of payor and type of encounter. This is done by multiplying the number of encounters developed in Exhibit 10–13a by the payor and service mix information in Exhibit 10–13b, which reflects ZMG's payor mix by type of encounter based on their experience over the past several years. The ZMG practice uses three major categories of payors: commercial insurance, Medicare, and Medicaid/Self-Pay, and categorizes their encounters into two types, admissions and follow-up encounters. The result is the estimate of encounters by payor and type of encounter (Exhibit 10–13c).

Exhibit 10–13a   Calculation of number of encounters by payor type for the coming year

	Jan	Feb	Mar	Apr	May	Jun	Jul	Aug	Sep	Oct	Nov	Dec	Total
Total encounters for 20X1[a]	5,007	4,676	5,044	4,686	4,480	4,596	4,697	4,833	4,653	4,923	4,734	5,202	57,531
Projected growth	5%	5%	5%	5%	5%	5%	5%	5%	5%	5%	5%	5%	5%
Total encounters for 20X2	5,257	4,910	5,296	4,920	4,704	4,826	4,932	5,075	4,886	5,169	4,971	5,462	60,408

[a]From internal records of the organization.

Exhibit 10–13b   Distribution of encounters by payor and encounter type[a]

	Commercial	Medicare	Medicaid/ Self-Pay	Total
Admissions	9%	14%	2%	25%
Follow-up	27%	42%	6%	75%
Total	36%	56%	8%	100%

[a] From internal records of the organization.

Exhibit 10–13c Distribution of encounters by payor and type[a]

	Jan	Feb	Mar	Apr	May	Jun	Jul	Aug	Sep	Oct	Nov	Dec	Total
Commercial													
Admissions	473	442	477	443	423	434	444	457	440	465	447	492	5,437
Follow-up	1,419	1,326	1,430	1,328	1,270	1,303	1,332	1,370	1,319	1,396	1,342	1,475	16,310
Total	1,892	1,768	1,907	1,771	1,693	1,737	1,776	1,827	1,759	1,861	1,789	1,967	21,747
Medicare													
Admissions	736	687	741	689	659	676	690	711	684	724	696	765	8,458
Follow-up	2,208	2,062	2,224	2,066	1,976	2,027	2,071	2,132	2,052	2,171	2,088	2,294	25,371
Total	2,944	2,749	2,965	2,755	2,635	2,703	2,761	2,843	2,736	2,895	2,784	3,059	33,829
Medicaid/Self-Pay													
Admissions	105	98	106	98	94	97	99	102	98	103	99	109	1,208
Follow-up	315	295	318	295	282	290	296	305	293	310	298	328	3,625
Total	420	393	424	393	376	387	395	407	391	413	397	437	4,833
Total encounters	5,256	4,910	5,296	4,919	4,704	4,827	4,932	5,077	4,886	5,169	4,970	5,463	60,409

[a]Computed by multiplying the projected encounters in Exhibit 10-13a by the appropriate cell in Exhibit 10-13b, rounded to the nearest whole number. See Exhibit 10-13d for greater detail. Slight differences between Exhibit 10-13a and this exhibit are due to rounding.

Relative Value Units (RVUs)
A standardized weighting applied to services that reflects the amount of resource consumption to provide that service. A service assigned two RVUs consumes twice the resources as does a service assigned one RVU.

■ *Convert encounters to weighted encounters.* As admissions and follow-up encounters require different amounts of time, to determine staffing needs, it is necessary to convert these encounters into *weighted encounters*, commonly called *relative value units* (*RVUs*). Admissions encounters, when the hospitalist first encounters and examines the patient, take about an hour, whereas follow-up encounters take about a half hour each. Using 15 minutes as a basic unit of measurement for an RVU (that is, 1 RVU equals 15 minutes of work), admission encounters take approximately 4 RVUs and follow-up encounters take about 2 RVUs (Exhibit 10–13d). Multiplying the number of encounters by payor and type of encounter (Exhibit 10–13c) by the relative values of each type of encounter (Exhibit 10–13d), calculates the number of weighted encounters by payor and type of encounter (Exhibit 10–13e), Exhibit 10–13f shows how January's number of weighted encounters by payor and type of encounter (Exhibit 10–13e) were derived.

Operating Budget

As noted earlier, the operating budget (see Exhibit 10–10) comprises two budgets developed using the accrual basis of accounting: the revenue budget and the expense budget. Development of each of these budgets for ZMG Hospitalist Practice follows.

Gross charges
The amount that an organization would bill its patients if they all paid full charges.

Revenue Budget

The revenue budget has two primary parts: net patient revenues and nonpatient revenues.

Net charges
The amount that an organization bills its patients after accounting for discounts and allowances.

Net Patient Revenues As discussed in Chapter Two, there is a difference between gross charges and net charges. *Gross charges* are the amount the organization would bill if everyone paid full charges. *Net charges* are the amount the organization may bill after taking into account all discounts and allowances (except bad debt). Discounts and allowances include such items as contractual agreements between the health care provider and the payor, charity care, and sliding fee schedules.

Exhibit 10–13d   Relative value weights for admissions and follow-up encounters

Type of Visit	Weight
Admissions	4.00
Follow-up	2.00

Exhibit 10–13e Weighted encounters by payor and type[a]

	Jan	Feb	Mar	Apr	May	Jun	Jul	Aug	Sep	Oct	Nov	Dec	Total
Commercial													
Admissions	1,892	1,768	1,908	1,772	1,692	1,736	1,776	1,828	1,760	1,860	1,788	1,968	21,748
Follow-up	2,838	2,652	2,860	2,656	2,540	2,606	2,664	2,740	2,638	2,792	2,684	2,950	32,620
Total	4,730	4,420	4,768	4,428	4,232	4,342	4,440	4,568	4,398	4,652	4,472	4,918	54,368
Medicare													
Admissions	2,944	2,748	2,964	2,756	2,636	2,704	2,760	2,844	2,736	2,896	2,784	3,060	33,832
Follow-up	4,416	4,124	4,448	4,132	3,952	4,054	4,142	4,264	4,104	4,342	4,176	4,588	50,742
Total	7,360	6,872	7,412	6,888	6,588	6,758	6,902	7,108	6,840	7,238	6,960	7,648	84,574
Medicaid/Self-Pay													
Admissions	420	392	424	392	376	388	396	408	392	412	396	436	4,832
Follow-up	630	590	636	590	564	580	592	610	586	620	596	656	7,250
Total	1,050	982	1,060	982	940	968	988	1,018	978	1,032	992	1,092	12,082
Total	13,140	12,274	13,240	12,298	11,760	12,068	12,330	12,694	12,216	12,922	12,424	13,658	151,024

[a] Computed by multiplying the projected encounters by type and payor in Exhibit 10-13c by the RVUs (4 for admissions, 2 for follow-up) in Exhibit 10-13d, rounded to the nearest whole number.

Exhibit 10–13f   Illustration of how weighted encounters by payor type (Exhibit 10–13e) were developed

	Percentage of Encounters[a]	Encounters[b]	Weights[c]	Weighted Encounters[d]
January's Encounters:		5,257		
Commercial				
Admissions	9%	473	4.00	1,892
Follow-up	27%	1,419	2.00	2,838
Total	36%	1,892		4,730
Medicare				
Admissions	14%	736	4.00	2,944
Follow-up	42%	2,208	2.00	4,416
Total	56%	2,944		7,360
Medicaid/Self-Pay				
Admissions	2%	105	4.00	420
Follow-up	6%	315	2.00	630
	8%	420		1,050
Total[e]	100%	5,256		13,140

[a] Percentage of encounters can be found in Exhibit 10-13b.
[b] January's encounters can be found in Exhibit 10-13a. The remaining encounters are calculated by multiplying January's encounters by the corresponding percentage of encounters. The results correspond to those found in Exhibit 10-13c.
[c] Original weights can be found in Exhibit 10-13d.
[d] Weighted encounters are calculated by multiplying encounters by their weights. The results correspond to those in Exhibit 10-13e.
[e] Slight differences are due to rounding.

Exhibit 10–14a illustrates how the $422,040 net patient revenues for January in the operating budget were determined (Exhibit 10–10).

■ First, gross patient revenues were calculated by multiplying the number of weighted encounters for each payor by the charge for each weighted encounter, $52.50.

■ Next, the amount of allowances and discounts is calculated by multiplying the gross patient revenue for each payor times the discount percentage for that payor. Based on historical experience, the discount percentage is different for each category: 30 percent, 40 percent, and 70 percent for Commercial, Medicare, and

Exhibit 10–14a Illustration of how January's net patient service revenues in the ZMG Hospitalist Practice's operating budget (Exhibit 10–10) were developed

	A	B	C	D	E	F
			Gross Patient			Net Patient
	Weighted		Service	Discount		Service
	Encounters	Fees	Revenues	Percentage	Discount	Revenues
	(a)	(b)	(A × B)	(b)	(c)	(D × E)
Commercial						
Admissions	1,892	$52.50	$99,330			
Follow-up	2,838	$52.50	$148,995			
Total	4,730		$248,325	30%	$74,498	$173,828
Medicare						
Admissions	2,944	$52.50	$154,560			
Follow-up	4,416	$52.50	$231,840			
Total	7,360		$386,400	40%	$154,560	$231,840
Medicaid/Self-pay						
Admissions	420	$52.50	$22,050			
Follow-up	630	$52.50	$33,075			
Total	1,050		$55,125	70%	$38,588	$16,538
Charity care				1%	$165	
Total	13,140		$689,850		$267,810	$422,040

a Exhibit 10-13d.

b New information.

c The discount is computed by multiplying the total of gross charges for each payor by the discount percentage. In the case of Medicaid/Self-Pay, 1% of Medicaid/Self-Pay net revenues is considered charity care; therefore, this additional discount is computed by multiplying Medicaid/Self-Pay net patient service revenues by 1%.

Medicaid/Self-Pay, respectively. Also note that in the last category, Medicaid or Self-Pay, that the 1 percent charity care allowance is treated the same as an additional discount but on the remaining net patient service revenue balance after the initial discount is taken.

■ Finally, net patient revenues are calculated by subtracting the discount for each payor from its gross patient revenues.

Caution: In this situation, gross charges and gross revenues are used interchangeably.

Non-Patient Revenues In addition to patient service revenues, most organizations also have non-patient revenues. In the case of ZMG Hospitalist Practice, the non-patient revenues are interest and consulting fees. The estimate of interest earned is developed on a separate schedule related to the cash budget (not shown here). The estimate of consulting fees is based on a review of the organization's plans for this service. The calculation of the $11,440 of non-patient revenues in the operating budget (see Exhibit 10–10, Total column) is shown in Exhibit 10–14b, Total column.

Expense Budget

The second part of the operating budget (see Exhibit 10–10, rows F through H) is the expense budget. The expense budget itself is made up of three other budgets: the labor budget, supplies budget, and administrative and general budget (see Exhibit 10–15).

Exhibit 10–14b   Forecast of non-patient revenues for ZMG Hospitalist Practice[a]

	Jan	Feb	Mar	Apr	May	Jun	Jul	Aug	Sep	Oct	Nov	Dec	Total
Interest	$348	$405	$69	$68	$69	$68	$69	$69	$68	$69	$68	$69	$1,440
Consulting	833	833	833	833	833	833	833	833	833	833	833	833	10,000
Total	$1,182	$1,238	$903	$901	$903	$901	$903	$903	$901	$903	$901	$903	$11,440

[a]From internal records of the organization.

Exhibit 10–15   Overview of the operating expense budget

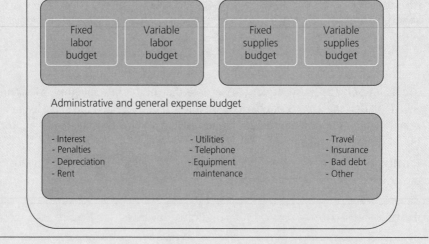

Labor Budget Note that the first item listed under expenses in the operating budget (Exhibit 10–10) is labor because it consumes the largest amount of the organization's resources. The amount listed for labor expense is developed in the *labor budget* (see Exhibit 10–16a), which itself is composed of two budgets: the fixed labor budget and the variable labor budget. The *fixed labor budget* forecasts the costs of salaried personnel; the *variable labor budget* accounts for additional labor costs, which vary as additional part-time personnel or overtime hours are needed. Development of ZMG Hospitalist Practice's labor budget follows.

The fixed labor budget (Exhibit 10–16b) consists solely of salaries (Exhibit 10–16c) and benefits (Exhibit 10–16d), usually presented by position or position category. An example of how the Physician I amounts in the labor budget are calculated for February is presented in Exhibits 10–16e and 10–16f. Note that ZMG Hospitalist Practice budgets by position, not individual.

Variable Labor Budget The second component of the labor budget is the variable labor budget (Exhibit 10–17a), which accounts for wages of nonsalaried employees and overtime. Health care organizations are increasingly turning to part-time employees because they can meet flexible demands and may cost less, often because benefits do not need to be paid to these workers. In the case of ZMG Hospitalist Practice, the variable labor budget can be found in the row titled "temporary wages."

Because the number of part-time and overtime hours per month vary depending on the overall workload, it is not necessary to develop this budget by position as was done for the fixed labor budget. Instead, this budget is developed by (1) estimating how many RVUs will be covered by full-time staff; (2) determining the required RVUs to provide service, based on demand; (3) determining the number of RVUs that cannot be covered by existing staff; (4) determining the number of hours it will take to cover the uncovered RVUs; and (5) determining the cost to hire staff to cover the uncovered RVU demand. In this example, it is assumed that all noncovered hours are filled with temporary staff, which are called *locum tenens*. There is no overtime.

1. The estimate of how many RVUs *will* be covered by full-time staff is shown in Exhibit 10–17b, row A. The development of these estimates involves making a considerable number of estimates, as shown in Exhibit 10–17c, which gives an example of how the RVU capacity for January's estimates were made.

2. The estimate of the required RVUs to provide service based on demand (Exhibit 10–17b, row B) comes directly from the bottom line of the statistics budget (Exhibit 10–9, Total).

3. To determine the number of RVUs that cannot be covered by existing staff (Exhibit 10–17b, row C), the RVU demand (step 2) is subtracted from the RVU capacity of the staff (step 1). If demand is higher than capacity, then temporary staff must be hired. (Remember in this example that there is no overtime.)

4. To determine the cost of hiring temporary staff (step 5), it is first necessary to convert the uncovered RVUs (step 3) to their hour equivalent (Exhibit 10–17b, row F).

Labor Budget
A subset of the expense budget, this budget is composed of the fixed labor budget and the variable labor budget.

Fixed Labor Budget
A subset of the labor budget that forecasts the cost of salaried personnel.

Variable Labor Budget
A subset of the labor budget that forecasts nonsalary labor costs, such as part-time employees and overtime hours.

Exhibit 10–16a The labor budget[a]

	Jan	Feb	Mar	Apr	May	Jun	Jul	Aug	Sep	Oct	Nov	Dec	Total
Fixed salaries	$383,333	$393,958	$393,958	$393,958	$393,958	$394,333	$401,667	$401,667	$401,667	$401,667	$402,500	$402,500	$4,765,167
Fixed benefits	59,917	61,552	61,552	61,552	61,552	61,646	62,746	62,746	62,746	62,746	62,913	62,913	744,579
Subtotal	443,250	455,510	455,510	455,510	455,510	455,979	464,413	464,413	464,413	464,413	465,413	465,413	5,509,746
Temporary wages		14,356	3,356									18,370	36,081
Bonus[b]												11,712	11,712
Total	$443,250	$469,866	$458,866	$455,510	$455,510	$455,979	$464,413	$464,413	$464,413	$464,413	$465,413	$495,494	$5,557,539

[a] This table illustrates how the Labor line item in the operating budget (Exhibit 10-10) was developed.
[b] As bonuses typically might be in the range of 10-20% of base salary, the small amount noted here warrants further attention as to how the bonus program is being implemented.

Exhibit 10–16b The fixed labor budget[a]

Position	Jan	Feb	Mar	Apr	May	Jun	Jul	Aug	Sep	Oct	Nov	Dec	Total
Physician I	$230,000	$241,500	$241,500	$241,500	$241,500	$241,500	$241,500	$241,500	$241,500	$241,500	$241,500	$241,500	$2,886,500
Physician II	168,667	168,667	168,667	168,667	168,667	168,667	177,100	177,100	177,100	177,100	177,100	177,100	2,074,600
Physician's Assistant	10,000	10,000	10,000	10,000	10,000	10,000	10,000	10,000	10,000	10,000	10,500	10,500	121,000
Nurse Practitioner	10,000	10,000	10,000	10,000	10,000	10,000	10,000	10,000	10,000	10,000	10,500	10,500	121,000
Administrative Director	10,000	10,500	10,500	10,500	10,500	10,500	10,500	10,500	10,500	10,500	10,500	10,500	125,500
Office Staff I	5,208	5,469	5,469	5,469	5,469	5,469	5,469	5,469	5,469	5,469	5,469	5,469	65,365
Office Staff II	9,375	9,375	9,375	9,375	9,375	9,844	9,844	9,844	9,844	9,844	9,844	9,844	115,781
Total	$443,250	$455,510	$455,510	$455,510	$455,510	$455,979	$464,413	$464,413	$464,413	$464,413	$465,413	$465,413	$5,509,746

[a] The totals appearing here are made up of a fixed salary component (Exhibit 10-16c) and benefits (Exhibit 10-16d).

Exhibit 10–16c Salaries schedule for the fixed labor budget

Position	Jan	Feb	Mar	Apr	May	Jun	Jul	Aug	Sep	Oct	Nov	Dec	Total
Physician I	$200,000	$210,000	$210,000	$210,000	$210,000	$210,000	$210,000	$210,000	$210,000	$210,000	$210,000	$210,000	$2,510,000
Physician II	146,667	146,667	146,667	146,667	146,667	146,667	154,000	154,000	154,000	154,000	154,000	154,000	1,804,000
Physician Assistant	8,333	8,333	8,333	8,333	8,333	8,333	8,333	8,333	8,333	8,333	8,750	8,750	100,833
Nurse Practitioner	8,333	8,333	8,333	8,333	8,750	8,750	8,750	8,750	8,750	8,750	8,750	8,750	100,833
Administrative Director	8,333	8,750	8,750	8,750	8,750	8,750	8,750	8,750	8,750	8,750	8,750	8,750	104,583
Office Staff I	4,167	4,375	4,375	4,375	4,375	4,375	4,375	4,375	4,375	4,375	4,375	4,375	52,292
Office Staff II	7,500	7,500	7,500	7,500	7,500	7,875	7,875	7,875	7,875	7,875	7,875	7,875	92,625
Total	$383,333	$393,958	$393,958	$393,958	$393,958	$394,333	$401,667	$401,667	$401,667	$401,667	$402,500	$402,500	$4,765,167

Exhibit 10–16d Benefits schedule for the fixed labor budget

Position	Jan	Feb	Mar	Apr	May	Jun	Jul	Aug	Sep	Oct	Nov	Dec	Total
Physician I	$30,000	$31,500	$31,500	$31,500	$31,500	$31,500	$31,500	$31,500	$31,500	$31,500	$31,500	$31,500	$376,500
Physician II	22,000	22,000	22,000	22,000	22,000	22,000	23,100	23,100	23,100	23,100	23,100	23,100	270,600
Physician's Assistant	1,667	1,667	1,667	1,667	1,667	1,667	1,667	1,667	1,667	1,667	1,750	1,750	20,167
Nurse Practitioner	1,667	1,667	1,667	1,667	1,667	1,667	1,750	1,750	1,750	1,750	1,750	1,750	20,167
Administrative Director	1,667	1,750	1,750	1,750	1,750	1,750	1,750	1,750	1,750	1,750	1,750	1,750	20,917
Office Staff I	1,042	1,094	1,094	1,094	1,094	1,094	1,094	1,094	1,094	1,094	1,094	1,094	13,073
Office Staff II	1,875	1,875	1,875	1,875	1,875	1,969	1,969	1,969	1,969	1,969	1,969	1,969	23,156
Total	$59,917	$61,552	$61,552	$61,552	$61,552	$61,646	$62,746	$62,746	$62,746	$62,746	$62,913	$62,913	$744,579

Exhibit 10–16e   Data used to construct ZMG Hospitalist Practice's fixed labor salaries and benefits[a]

	Number of FTEs	Average Salary	Base Salary	Benefit Percent	Date of Next Raise	Percent Raise
Physician I	12	$200,000	$2,400,000	15%	Feb-02	5%
Physician II	8	220,000	1,760,000	15%	Jul-02	5%
Physician's Assistant	1	100,000	100,000	20%	Nov-02	5%
Nurse Practitioner	1	100,000	100,000	20%	Nov-02	5%
Administrative Director	1	100,000	100,000	20%	Feb-02	5%
Office Staff I	1	50,000	50,000	25%	Feb-02	5%
Office Staff II	3	30,000	90,000	25%	Jun-02	5%

[a]All salaries and wages are paid twice monthly in equal amounts. The second payment is made on the last day of each month.

Exhibit 10–16f   How February's salaries and benefits for physician I category in Exhibits 10–16b through 10–16d were developed

	Item	Source	Annual Amount
A	Annual base salary/month	(Exhibit 10–16e)	$200,000
B	Raise	(Exhibit 10–16e)	5%
C	Salary after raise	(A × (1 + B))	$210,000
D	Benefits percentage	(Exhibit 10–16e)	15%
E	Benefits after raise	(C × D)	$31,500
F	Salary and benefits	(C + E)	$241,500

In calculating the hourly equivalent, estimates were made of both the number of hours that it takes for staff to "do" an RVU if they worked at 100 percent efficiency and the actual efficiency it is expected that they will work. In this example, the staff is assumed to be working at 87 percent efficiency (Exhibit 10–17b, row E). Assumptions like this are often made to take into account such factors as bottlenecks, delays, difficult cases, meetings, and the like.

Exhibit 10–17a   The variable labor budget

Position	Jan	Feb	Mar	Apr	May	Jun	Jul	Aug	Sep	Oct	Nov	Dec	Total
Variable staffing[a]	$0	$14,356	$3,356	$0	$0	$0	$0	$0	$0	$0	$0	$18,370	$36,081

[a]From Exhibit 10-17b, row H. Variable staff for ZMG Hospitalist Practice all *locum tenens*.

5.   Once the number of temporary staff hours is determined (step 4), finding the cost of those staff is straightforward (Exhibit 10–17b, row H). The number of temporary staff hours needed is multiplied by the cost per hour (Exhibit 10–17b, rows F and G).

Supplies Budget

Although some organizations have major supplies costs, this is not the case with ZMG Hospitalist Practice, which groups its supplies costs under "Other" in the administrative and general expense budget (Exhibits 10–18a and 10–18b). Organizations that have supplies costs may have a fixed supplies budget and a variable supplies budget. The *fixed supplies budget* covers items such as office supplies, which do not vary with the number of patients seen. The *variable supplies budget* includes those items that do vary with the activities. In a clinical setting, these would include items that vary with RVUs, such as disposable syringes, disposable gloves, and x-ray film. While the fixed supplies budget may be a constant amount each month, the variable supplies budget is likely to change monthly, as the number of RVUs changes.

Fixed Supplies Budget
A subset of the supplies budget that covers items that do not vary with volume.

Variable Supplies Budget
A subset of the supplies budget that includes items that vary with volume.

Often health care organizations want to make sure both that they do not run out of supplies in any month and that they begin the next month with a supply inventory. Thus, for any month, in addition to the supplies they start with (beginning inventory), they must estimate both the cost of the supplies they are going to use (cost of goods used) and the amount of supplies they will need to have on hand at the end of the month (ending inventory), which incidentally, becomes the opening inventory for the next month. The cost of goods used will appear as an expense on the statement of operations whereas the ending inventory will appear on the balance sheet as a current asset. The relationship among these is shown by the formula:

Opening Inventory + Purchases − Cost of Goods Used = Ending Inventory

Exhibit 10–17b Calculation of the variable labor budget

Position	Jan	Feb	Mar	Apr	May	Jun	Jul	Aug	Sep	Oct	Nov	Dec	Total
Physician I RVU capacity	7,235	6,535	7,235	7,002	7,235	7,002	7,235	7,235	7,002	7,235	7,002	7,235	85,190
Physician II RVU capacity	4,824	4,357	4,824	4,668	4,824	4,668	4,824	4,824	4,668	4,824	4,668	4,824	56,794
Physician Assistant RVU capacity	544	491	544	526	544	526	544	544	526	544	526	544	6,403
Nurse Practitioner RVU capacity	544	491	544	526	544	526	544	544	526	544	526	544	6,403
A Total RVU productive capacity	13,147	11,874	13,147	12,722	13,147	12,722	13,147	13,147	12,722	13,147	12,722	13,147	154,790
B Required RVUs based on demand	13,140	12,274	13,240	12,298	11,760	12,068	12,330	12,694	12,216	12,922	12,424	13,658	151,024
C Surplus (deficit): required RVUs vs. capacity	7	(400)	(93)	424	1,387	654	817	453	506	225	298	(511)	3,766
D Staffing RVUs per hour @ 100% efficiency	4	4	4	4	4	4	4	4	4	4	4	4	
E Actual efficiency	87%	87%	87%	87%	87%	87%	87%	87%	87%	87%	87%	87%	
F Additional hours needed based on uncovered RVUs	0	115	27	0	0	0	0	0	0	0	0	147	289
G Locum tenens MD, PA, and NP avg. hourly rate	$125	$125	$125	$125	$125	$125	$125	$125	$125	$125	$125	$125	$125
H Variable staffing (locum tenens) cost[a]	$0	$14,356	$3,356	$0	$0	$0	$0	$0	$0	$0	$0	$18,370	$36,081

[a] If additional hourly staffing is needed as shown by a deficit in row C, the formula is F × G. Otherwise, there is surplus capacity, and no extra hourly (*locum tenens*) staff is needed.

Exhibit 10–17c   Calculation of RVU productivity capacity in January

	(Givens):		
	Physician Productivity		
A	Number of Physician I	12	
B	Number of Physician II	8	
C	Shifts per year per full-time physician	204	
D	Hours per shift per physician	10	
E	Minutes per RVU	15	
F	RVUs per hour	4	
G	Physician efficiency	87%	
H	Days in this month	31	
	PA/NP Productivity		
I	Number Physician Assistants	1	
J	Number Nurse Practitioners	1	
K	Shifts per year per full-time PA or NP[a]	230	
L	Hours per day per PA or NP	8	
M	RVUs per hour	4	
N	PA or NP productivity	87%	
O	Days in this month	31	

	Calculations		Physician I	Physician II	Total
P	Number	(A) and (B)	12	8	
Q	RVUs per physician per year (365 days)	$(C \times D \times F \times G)$	7,099	7,099	
R	RVUs per day per physician	(Q/365)	19.4	19.4	
S	Days in this month	(H)	31	31	
T	RVU capacity this month	$(P \times R \times S)$	7,235	4,824	12,059

			Physician's Assistants	Nurse Practitioners	
U	Number	(I) and (J)	1	1	
V	RVUs per PA or NP per year	$(K \times L \times M \times N)$	6,403	6,403	
W	RVUs per day per PA or NP	(V/365)	17.5	17.5	
X	Days in this month	(O)	31	31	
Y	RVU capacity this month	$(U \times W \times X)$	544	544	1,088
Z	Total RVU capacity this month	(T + Y)			13,147

[a] Assumes 3 weeks of vacation, 1 week of sick leave, and 2 weeks of holidays.

An example of the calculations would look like this:

Beginning inventory	$5,154	Amount in ending inventory from the month before
Purchases	32,900	Amount of supplies necessary to deliver services this month and still have sufficient ending inventory
Goods available	38,054	Beginning inventory + purchases
Cost of goods used	−32,680	Amount of supplies necessary to deliver services this month
Ending inventory	$5,374	The desired amount of inventory to begin the next month; often is a percentage of next month's estimated cost of supplies used

Key point   *The reason that cost of goods used is used in the supplies budget rather than the cost of goods purchased is that accrual accounting is being used.*

Administrative and General Expense Budget

The last part of the expense section of the operating budget (Exhibit 10–10) is administrative and general (A & G) expenses, which are developed in the general and administrative budget (see Exhibit 10–18a). They comprise the day-to-day expenses that are not contained in the labor or supplies budgets. The assumptions for the A & G expenses for ZMG Hospitalist Practice are listed in Exhibit 10–18b. Incidentally, some organizations will consider interest and penalties as nonoperating expenses.

Cash Budget

As discussed in detail in Chapter Five, the cash budget is developed by determining when payments will be received from others and when payments will be made by the organization. Because it draws on information from the other budgets, the cash budget is the last budget to be developed.

The cash budget (Exhibit 10–11) is organized into two sections. The first section determines how much cash is available before borrowing; the second section compares the cash available with the cash required and then determines if cash will be needed from other sources (when there is a shortfall) or if cash will be invested (when there is an excess of cash).

To determine cash available, the cash inflows (revenues) are added, and outflows (expenditures) are subtracted from the beginning balance (Exhibit 10–11, rows A, B, C, and D).

The method to determine these inflows and outflows was discussed in Chapter Five, which shows how accrual data are converted into cash. Here we illustrate it by showing what happens to January's net income from commercial payors. As noted in

Exhibit 10–18a   Administrative and general expense budget

	Jan	Feb	Mar	Apr	May	Jun	Jul	Aug	Sep	Oct	Nov	Dec	Total
Interest	$137	$134	$131	$316	$311	$306	$382	$376	$369	$363	$357	$350	$3,533
Depreciation	456	456	456	864	864	864	981	981	981	981	981	981	9,846
Utilities	1,000	1,000	1,000	1,000	1,000	1,000	1,000	1,000	1,000	1,000	1,000	1,000	12,000
Rent	2,500	2,500	2,500	2,500	2,500	2,500	2,500	2,500	2,500	2,500	2,500	2,500	30,000
Cleaning	500	500	500	500	500	500	500	500	500	500	500	500	6,000
Other (phone, supplies, etc.)	600	600	600	600	600	600	600	600	600	600	600	600	7,200
Travel	5,000	5,000	5,000	5,000	5,000	5,000	5,000	5,000	5,000	5,000	5,000	5,000	60,000
Insurance	12,000	12,000	12,000	12,000	12,000	12,000	12,000	12,000	12,000	12,000	12,000	12,000	144,000
Equipment maintenance	300	300	300	300	300	300	300	300	300	300	300	300	3,600
Bad debt expense	4,220	3,942	4,252	3,950	3,777	3,875	3,960	4,076	3,923	4,150	3,991	4,387	48,505
Subtotal	26,713	26,432	26,740	27,030	26,852	26,945	27,223	27,333	27,174	27,395	27,228	27,618	324,684
Add: Nonoperating expenses	1,300	1,750	1,750	1,750	1,300	1,300	1,300	1,300	1,300	1,300	1,300	1,300	16,950
Total expenses	$28,013	$28,182	$28,490	$28,780	$28,152	$28,245	$28,523	$28,633	$28,474	$28,695	$28,528	$28,918	$341,634

Exhibit 10–18b Information used to construct the administrative and general expense budget

Item	Amount	Occurrence and Payment
Interest	Varies	Calculated on an amortization schedule[a]
Depreciation	Varies	Calculated on a depreciation schedule[a]
Utilities	$1,000	Per month, payable each month
Rent	$2,500	Per month, payable on the first day of each month
Cleaning	$500	Per month, payable in advance every three months
Other (phone, supplies, etc.)	$600	Per month, payable each month
Travel	$5,000	Per month, payable each month
Insurance	$12,000	Per month, payable each month
Equipment maintenance	$300	Per month, payable in advance every March
Bad debt	Varies	4% of charge-based and 3% of cost-based net patient revenues

[a]Not included; assume the number as a given for this example.

Exhibit 10–14a, ZMG Hospitalist Practice earned $173,828 in January on its Commercial Pay patients. Under the assumption that 28 percent will be collected in January, 45 percent in February, 14 percent in March, and 10 percent in April and that the remaining 3 percent will be written off, the cash inflow pattern is shown in Exhibit 10–19.

The second part of the cash budget (Exhibit 10–11) determines whether the organization has sufficient cash to begin the next month. ZMG Hospitalist Practice has decided that it should begin each month with $100,000 cash on hand (Exhibit 10–11, row E). If it does not have $100,000 (Exhibit 10–11, rows I through K), it would either have to obtain such funds from its own short-term or long-term investments (perhaps with some penalty for early withdrawal) or else borrow the funds from outside the organization (Exhibit 10–11, row M). Fortunately, ZMG Hospitalist Practice does not find itself in such a position in January, so it invests the excess $81,801 in short-term investments (Exhibit 10–11, row G). Exhibit 10–19 illustrates how January's net patient service revenues in Exhibit 10–14a would be converted into cash flows.

Capital Budget

The capital budget was initially presented in Exhibit 10–12. Although the budget for ZMG Hospitalist Practice is relatively small, large organizations may have capital budgets totaling millions of dollars. The items that appear on the capital budget are likely to have been part of a much larger list of requests that various departments submitted.

Exhibit 10–19 Converting accrual information into cash flows: ZMG Hospitalist Practice's revenues for January

January's Net Revenues Using the Accrual Basis of Accounting: Commercial Patients' Amount Collected in:	Percentage to Be Received by Month	Cash Inflow by Month[a]
January	28%	$48,672
February	45%	78,222
March	14%	24,336
April	10%	17,383
Written off	3%	5,215
Total	100%	$173,828

[a] Differences due to rounding.

The capital budget presented in Exhibit 10–12 lists financial information only. The term *capital budget* is also used to refer to the process of requesting large-dollar items. In many organizations, considerable information is requested in addition to summary financial figures to justify a capital investment. Such information is not limited to the revenue and expense projections discussed in Chapter Seven but also includes potential impact on patients, clinical staff, the organization as a whole, and the community.

Key point *The term capital budget is sometimes used to refer to not only summary information about the item being purchased but also potential financial impacts (see Chapter Seven) and impact on patients, clinical staff, the organization as a whole, and the community.*

SUMMARY

The budget is one of the most important documents of a health care organization and is the central document of the planning-and-control cycle. It identifies the revenues and resources that are needed for an organization to achieve its goals and objectives and allows the organization to monitor the actual revenues generated and its use of resources against what was planned.

The planning-and-control cycle has four major components: strategic planning, planning, implementing, and controlling. The purpose of strategic planning is to identify the organization's mission and strategy in order to position the organization for the future. A primary activity of the strategic planning process is an assessment of the organization's external and internal environments. The organization also develops specific tactical and operational plans that identify short-term goals and objectives in marketing or production, control, and financing the organization.

Five key dimensions along which organizations vary in regard to budgeting are participation, budget models, budget detail, budget forecasts, and budget modifications. Participation in the budgeting process varies from authoritarian to participative. The authoritarian approach is often called top-down budgeting because the budget is essentially dictated to the rest of the organization. In the participatory approach, the roles and responsibilities of the budgeting process are diffused throughout the organization. Advantages of the participatory approach include developing a shared understanding of the goals and objectives of the organization, developing cooperation and coordination, clarifying roles and responsibilities, motivating staff, and bringing about cost awareness. Its disadvantages are loss of control and excessive use of time and resources.

There are two budget models: incremental-decremental budgeting and zero-based budgeting. The incremental-decremental approach begins with what exists and gives a slight increase, no change, or a slight decrease to various line items, programs, or departments. Zero-based budgeting continually questions both the need for each program and its level of funding. In zero-based budgeting, each budgeting unit provides both an overall justification for its program and a series of requests to show what the program would look like at various levels of funding.

Based on the amount of detail they contain, budgets can be classified into three categories: line-item, program, and performance. A line-item budget has the least detail and merely lists revenues and expenses by category. A program budget not only lists the line items but also lists them by program. A performance budget lists not only line items and programs but also the performance goals that each program is expected to attain.

Because environmental conditions change, many organizations use rolling budgets, which are multiyear forecasts regularly updated and extended. Single-year and multiyear budgets vary by the time horizon they forecast; static and flexible budgets vary on the basis of volume projections. Static budgets forecast for a single level of activity; flexible budgets forecast revenues and expenses for various levels of activities.

Most health care organizations actually develop four interrelated budgets: a statistics budget, an operating budget, a cash budget, and a capital budget. The statistics budget identifies the amount of services that will be provided, usually by payor type.

The operating budget is a combination of two budgets developed using the accrual basis of accounting: the revenue budget and the expense budget. The revenue budget is a forecast of the operating revenues that will be earned during the budget period. It consists of net patient revenues and non-patient revenues. The expense budget lists all operating expenses that are expected to be incurred during the budget period, both fixed and variable.

The cash budget represents the organization's cash inflows and outflows. The bottom line of the cash budget is the amount of cash available at the end of the period. In addition to showing cash inflows and outflows, the cash budget also details when it is necessary to borrow when there are cash shortages and when excess funds can be invested.

The capital budget summarizes large purchases to be made during the year over a specified dollar amount. Capital budgets for outpatient facilities may be fairly small; those from large systems with inpatient facilities may contain millions of dollars' worth of items.

Based on the information contained in these budgets, plus small amounts of additional information, the organization develops pro forma financial statements. Pro forma financial statements are prepared before the accounting period and present what the organization's financial statements will look like if all budgets are met exactly as planned. Once the pro forma financial statements have been developed, they can be subjected to ratio analysis just as with regular financial statements.

KEY TERMS

a. Authoritarian approach
b. Capital budget
c. Cash budget
d. Controlling activities
e. Expense budget
f. Fixed labor budget
g. Fixed supplies budget
h. Flexible budget
i. Gross charges
j. Incremental-decremental approach
k. Labor budget
l. Line-item budget
m. Mission statement
n. Multiyear budget
o. Net charges
p. Operating budget

q. Participatory approach
r. Performance budget
s. Planning
t. Program budget
u. Relative value units (RVUs)
v. Revenue budget
w. Rolling budget
x. Short-term plans
y. Static budget
z. Statistics budget
aa. Strategic planning
bb. Top-down-bottom-up approach
cc. Top-down budgeting
dd. Variable labor budget
ee. Variable supplies budget
ff. Zero-based budgeting (ZBB)

KEY EQUATION

Opening Inventory + Purchases − Cost of Goods Used = Ending Inventory

QUESTIONS AND PROBLEMS

1. **Definitions.** Define the key terms above.

2. What is the purpose of the budget? Why are requests for budget revisions necessary? When should a formal request for a budget revision be submitted?

3. What are the major components of the planning-and-control cycle?

4. Discuss the role of strategic planning in the budgeting process. How does it differ from short-term planning?

5. What are the advantages and disadvantages of the participatory approach to budgeting?

6. What are the four major budgets of a health care organization? Briefly discuss each.

7. What is the difference between a line-item, program, and performance budget?

8. Using Exhibit 10–6 as an example, construct line-item, program, and performance budgets for a service or program in a health care organization.

9. **The statistics budget: forecasting encounters.** Instead of its current forecast, ZMG Hospitalist Practice estimates that it will not obtain a major HMO contract, and its encounters for July through December are expected to rise by only 0.5 percent a month from the previous year. Assuming these are the only changes to Exhibit 10–13a, prepare a new forecast of the number of encounters that will be made by commercial patients during the whole year.

10. **The statistics budget: forecasting encounters.** Instead of its current forecast, ZMG Hospitalist Practice estimates that its Medicare encounters will increase by 4 percent a month from January through June. In July it will obtain a major contract, and its encounters from July through December will go up by 10 percent a month. Assuming these are the only changes to Exhibit 10–13a, prepare a new forecast of the number of encounters that will be made by Medicare patients during the whole year.

11. **The statistics budget: RVU-weighted encounters.** What are RVU-weighted encounters? Why is it necessary to weight encounters by their intensity level?

12. **The statistics budget: changing intensity.** How would the estimate of Medicaid/Self-Pay encounters change if ZMG Hospitalist Practice estimated that its Medicaid/Self-Pay admissions comprised 1 percent of the encounters and the Medicaid/Self-Pay follow-up encounters comprised 7 percent of the encounters instead of the distribution of visits by intensity shown in Exhibit 10–13b?

13. **The statistics budget: changing RVU weight.** How would the estimate of commercial weighted encounters change (Exhibit 10-13e) if ZMG Hospitalist Practice estimated that its admissions had a relative value weight of 3.00 and the follow-up visits had a relative value weight of 1.50 (Exhibit 10–13d)?

14. **The statistics budget: changing RVU weight.** How would the estimate of Medicare weighted encounters change (Exhibit 10-13e) if ZMG Hospitalist Practice

estimated that its admissions had a relative value weight of 4.50 and the follow-up visits had a relative value weight of 2.75 (Exhibit 10–13d)?

15. **The revenue budget: calculating gross revenues.** Calculate ZMG Hospitalist Practice's Medicare January, February, and March gross revenues if the fee for an admission is $120 and the fee for a follow-up encounter is $60 (Exhibits 10–13e and 10–14a).

16. **The revenue budget: calculating gross revenues.** Calculate ZMG Hospitalist Practice's commercial January, February, and March gross revenues if the fee for an admission is $150 and the fee for a follow-up encounter is $65 (Exhibits 10–13e and 10–14a).

17. **The revenue budget: gross and net charges.** What is the difference between gross charges and net charges?

18. **The revenue budget: calculating net revenues.** Calculate ZMG Hospitalist Practice's Medicare January, February, and March net revenues if the fee for an admission is $50 and the fee for a follow-up encounter is $70. Medicare receives a 40 percent discount. (Exhibits 10–13e and 10–14a).

19. **The revenue budget: calculating net revenues.** Calculate ZMG Hospitalist Practice's Medicaid/Self-Pay January, February, and March net revenues if the fee for an admission is $50 and the fee for a follow-up encounter is $70. Medicaid receives a 70 percent discount. (Exhibits 10–13e and 10–14a).

20. **The labor budget: fixed and variable labor.** What is the difference between a fixed and a variable labor budget?

21. **The labor budget: calculating the fixed labor budget.** Instead of the raises stated in Exhibit 10–16e, assume that all benefits are 13 percent and all raises are 7 percent and calculate the fixed labor budget for January, February, and March. Assume that all the other assumptions in the exhibit remain the same. Explain why some salaries and benefits change from month to month and others do not.

22. **The labor budget: calculating the fixed labor budget.** Instead of the benefits stated in Exhibit 10–16e, assume that all benefits are 20 percent and all raises are 5 percent and calculate the fixed labor budget for January, February, and March. Assume that all the other assumptions in the exhibit remain the same. Explain why some salaries and benefits change from month to month and others do not.

23. **The labor budget: variable labor.** In the variable labor budget, why is it necessary to determine how many RVUs can be handled by full-time employees?

24. **The variable labor budget: direct and indirect time.** In the variable labor budget, why is it necessary to consider efficiency? (Exhibit 10–17).

25. **The variable labor budget: efficiency.** If the assumed efficiency of the clinicians changed to 80 percent, what would be the productive capacity for January? (Exhibit 10–17c).

26. **The variable labor budget: efficiency.** If the assumed efficiency of the clinicians changed to 90 percent, what would be the productive capacity for January (Exhibit 10–17c)?

11

RESPONSIBILITY ACCOUNTING

LEARNING OBJECTIVES

- Define decentralization and identify its major advantages and disadvantages
- Identify the major types of responsibility centers found in health care organizations and describe their characteristics
- Explain the relationship of responsibility, authority, and accountability in the performance measurement of responsibility centers
- Compute volume and rate variances for revenues
- Compute volume and cost variances for expenses

Health care organizations have become increasingly complex over the past quarter century. One of the major changes is decentralization, which presents interesting problems when measuring financial performance. Whereas Chapter Four dealt with measuring the financial performance of the organization as a whole, this chapter identifies the types of organizational units *within* a health care organization and measures their financial performance. These units may be as large as subsidiaries or as small as departments. This chapter begins with a discussion of decentralization and then discusses the types of responsibility centers that exist in decentralized organizations. Next, the concepts of responsibility, authority, and accountability are explored. Finally, questions of how to measure the performance of responsibility centers are addressed.

DECENTRALIZATION

Decentralization is the degree of dispersion of responsibility within an organization. Decentralization can evolve out of working arrangements or may be more formally prescribed in an organization's policies, procedures, and organizational structure. There are various advantages and disadvantages to decentralization, and each organization has to decide what level of decentralization is in its best interest.

Decentralization
The degree of dispersion of responsibility within a health care organization.

Advantages of Decentralization

Selected advantages and disadvantages of decentralization are presented in Exhibit 11–1. The advantages (in no particular order) include time, information relevance, quality, speed, talent, and motivation and allegiance.

Time From the point of view of central management, a major advantage of decentralization is an increase in time available to devote to other tasks. Ideally, decentralization

Exhibit 11–1 Selected advantages and disadvantages of decentralization

Advantages	Disadvantages
Time	Loss of control
Information relevance	Decreased goal congruence
Quality	Increased need for coordination
Speed	and formal communication
Talent	Lack of managerial talent
Motivation and allegiance	

should relieve the central office of day-to-day operational decision making, instead allowing it to concentrate more on tactical and strategic-level concerns.

Information Relevance By spreading the responsibility for decision making within the organization, the organization moves more toward a "need-to-know" environment where information is filtered at each level, and only the information needed for decision-making at higher levels is passed on.

Quality Those closer to a problem may be better suited to understand the specifics of the problem and be more responsive to the local context, thus leading to higher-quality decisions.

Speed Decentralized decision making allows those closest to the problem to respond more quickly by shortening six time-consuming steps in communication. The person who identifies the problem must

- *Communicate* the problem *up* the organization
- To those who must *receive* it. Then they
- *Become* aware of it,
- *Decide* a course of action, and
- *Communicate* their response *down* through the organization,
- Where it is ultimately *received* by the person authorized to *respond*.

Talent A health care organization must ensure that it is developing the management capability to allow it to reach its objectives. Although occasionally it may want to look outside the organization for "new blood," this process can become expensive, intrusive, and time-consuming. It can also be demoralizing to those within the organization. Decentralization helps to draw on and develop the expertise of existing staff.

Motivation and Allegiance By delegating responsibility to others, a health care organization can develop increased motivation and allegiance. Increased involvement in the planning, implementation, and control process encourages buy-in by the staff, who may then experience an increased sense of ownership, belonging, and pride in their work.

Disadvantages of Decentralization

In considering what degree of decentralization to have, a health care organization has to balance the advantages of decentralization with its disadvantages, which include:

- Loss of control
- Decreased goal congruence

- Increased need for coordination and formal communication
- Lack of managerial talent

Loss of Control By spreading responsibility throughout the organization, upper management loses direct control. For administrators who have an authoritarian style and for organizations that need top-level management's expertise, this can be a significant problem. The specific ramifications of loss of control also appear in the other disadvantages of decentralization, which are all highly interrelated.

Decreased Goal Congruence To the extent that responsibility is decentralized within the organization, organizational units tend to develop their own goals. To avoid this, considerable effort must be exerted to ensure that each division or unit is making consistent decisions that support the organization's strategic plan and are in the best interest of the organization as a whole, not just the division.

Increased Need for Coordination and Formal Communication If responsibility is decentralized within the organization, there is an increased need to coordinate efforts among the various units and divisions. This results in the need for more formal communications, meetings, policies, and procedures.

Lack of Managerial Talent If an organization decentralizes and does not have the talent available at lower levels to manage the new responsibilities, as a whole it could suffer greatly. This particular problem was all too common during the early stages of managed care development in the United States. Because no one in the organization had previous experience running managed care organizations, organizations placed people with experience running other health care entities in charge.

TYPES OF RESPONSIBILITY CENTERS

Responsibility Center
An organizational unit that has been formally given the responsibility to carry out one or more tasks, to achieve one or more outcomes, or both.

When responsibility is formally decentralized into organizational units, rather than informally to specific individuals, these units are called responsibility centers. A *responsibility center* is an organizational unit that has been formally given the responsibility to carry out one or more tasks or to achieve one or more outcomes (or both). The four most common types of responsibility centers in health care are service centers, cost centers, profit centers, and investment centers (see Exhibit 11–2).

Service Centers

Service centers, the most basic type of responsibility center, are primarily responsible for ensuring that services are provided to a population in a manner that meets the volume and quality requirements of the organization. Because service centers have no

Exhibit 11–2   The four main types of responsibility centers and their main areas of responsibility

	Type of Responsibility Center			
Areas of Responsibility	Service Centers	Cost Centers	Profit Centers	Investment Centers
Providing services	☒	☒	☒	☒
Controlling costs		☒	☒	☒
Generating profits			☒	☒
Making investments				☒

budgetary control, their main responsibilities revolve around scheduling, directing, and monitoring the staff and providing direct patient care. Although service centers use resources and thus affect costs, the actual budgetary control rests at a higher level in the organization. It is not unusual for nursing units to find themselves defined as service centers. They are responsible for patient care, but the budget is kept at the next higher level in the organization. Patient admitting and patient transportation are also often defined as service centers.

Service Centers
Organizational units that are primarily responsible for ensuring that health care-related services are provided to a population in a manner that meets the volume and quality requirements of the organization. They have no direct budgetary control.

Cost Centers

Cost centers, the most common type of responsibility center in health care organizations, are responsible for providing services and controlling their costs. Ideally, they should be integrally involved in the planning, budgeting, and control process, for they are primarily responsible for resource utilization within the organization. Because payment often cannot be *directly* tied to specific services under both flat-fee (i.e., DRG) and capitated payment systems, a large number of responsibility centers are categorized as cost centers rather than profit centers.

Cost Centers
Organizational units responsible for producing products or providing services and controlling their costs.

Types of cost centers in health care organizations include: production cost centers, clinical cost centers, and administrative cost centers. *Production cost centers* develop or sell products (or both). Certain laboratory and pharmacy activities fall in this category. *Clinical cost centers* are responsible for providing health care-related services to clients, patients, or enrollees. Examples include nursing and physical therapy. *Administrative cost centers* support the clinical cost centers and the organization as a whole. Included in this category are general administration, the business office, information services, quality control, admitting, medical records, and housekeeping. Administrative cost centers are often considered the *infrastructure* of the organization. As with

Production Cost Centers
Cost centers that are responsible for producing or selling products (or both).

Clinical Cost Centers
Cost centers that are responsible for providing health care-related services to clients, patients, or enrollees.

Administrative Cost Centers
Cost centers that support clinical cost centers and the organization as a whole. They are often considered the *infrastructure* of the organization.

nursing, units that may be classified as cost centers in one organization may be considered service centers in another.

Profit Centers

Although many *profit centers* are responsible for service-related activities, all profit centers are responsible for controlling their costs and earning revenues. In some cases, the costs may be larger than the revenue they generate. For example, a pediatric screening program in a health department, which has to be offered, might be charged with earning sufficient revenues to cover just half of its $100,000 cost. Thus, although the pediatric screening program is considered a profit center by the health department, the amount of profit in this case is actually a loss of $50,000. There are three types of profit centers in health care organizations: traditional profit centers, capitated profit centers, and administrative profit centers.

Profit Centers
Organizational units responsible for controlling costs and earning revenues.

Traditional Profit Centers *Traditional profit centers* are primarily responsible for making a profit selling goods or services. Traditional profit centers have proliferated recently. On the clinical side, much of this growth can be traced back to the emergence of product-line management in health care in the later part of the twentieth century. Common product (or service) lines include cardiology, women's and children's services, and oncology. Traditional profit centers profit through a combination of markups on service and controlling costs in fee-for-service situations, as well as by controlling costs in flat-fee arrangements such as the DRG payment system.

Traditional Profit Centers
Organizational units responsible for earning a profit by providing health care services. Revenues are earned either on a fee-for-service or a flat fee basis. Examples include cardiology, women's and children's services, and oncology.

Capitated Profit Centers *Capitated profit centers* earn revenues by agreeing to take care of defined health care needs of a population for a per-member fee, often regardless of the amount of services needed by any particular patient. Such organizations are commonly called HMOs, PPOs, or managed care organizations. Interestingly enough, many managed care organizations purchase services from traditional profit centers. For example, an HMO may purchase its cardiology services from one health network and many of its oncology services from a different hospital system. Because it receives a set amount to cover the health care needs of a population, providers receiving capitation have considerable incentive to control costs through efficiency (the most service for any level of cost), economy (low costs), and prevention.

Capitated Profit Centers
Organizational units responsible for earning a profit by agreeing to take care of defined health care needs of a population for a per-member fee (which is not directly tied to services). Examples include HMOs, PPOs, and various managed care organizations.

Administrative Profit Centers There are two types of *administrative profit centers*: those that sell inside the organization and those that—although they do not deliver health services—are responsible for generating new revenues from outside the organization. Examples of administrative profit centers that *may* be required to sell their services inside the organization, as opposed to having their costs absorbed as overhead, are legal services, computer services, and management engineering. The prices for these services that are charged internally to other organizational units are called *transfer prices*.

The setting of transfer prices is a delicate matter, and if they are set too high there are several possible negative consequences. They may encourage potential users to buy these services outside the organization. If internal units (i.e., departments, subsidiary organizations) must use these resources, then they may suboptimize their use to cut costs or use the services but be unhappy about it (causing morale problems).

Examples of administrative profit centers that are responsible for generating new revenues from outside the organization include development offices (whose primary function is to encourage donations and contributions to the organization) and field representatives for HMOs and PPOs, whose primary responsibility is to sign up markets for the organization. Other primary examples would be food services, gift shops, parking decks, and motel services. Incidentally, although their effects on profit are difficult to identify, marketing, advertising, and public relations may be considered administrative profit centers in some organizations (others may consider them cost centers).

Administrative Profit Centers
Organizational units that do not provide health care-related services but are responsible for their profit. There are two types: those who sell their services internally, and those whose primary responsibility is to bring revenues into the organization.

Transfer Prices
The prices for products or services that are charged internally to other organizational units.

Investment Centers

In addition to having all the responsibilities of a traditional profit center, *investment centers* are responsible for making a certain return on investment. For example, where a profit center might be content with a simple $100,000 profit, an investment center might find this unacceptable if it does not provide the desired return on investment. An example of this is shown in Exhibit 11–3, where a surgicenter earns $100,000 in profit,

---

Exhibit 11–3   An example evaluating an investment on its profit and return

A	Investment in new Surgicenter	(Given)	$1,000,000
B	Desired return on investment (ROI)[a]	(Given)	15%
C	Desired ROI in dollars[a]	(A × B)	$150,000
	Actual results:		
D	Net revenues	(Given)	$500,000
E	Expenses	(Given)	$400,000
F	Net income	(D – E)	$100,000
G	ROI	(F / A)	10%

Conclusion: Although the Surgicenter made a profit of $100,000, it did not meet the desired ROI of 15% the first year.

[a] Per year.

Perspective 11–1   Physicians Examine Deals

Physicians are angling to buy stakes in two struggling Midwest hospitals, believing that physician investment and management paired with not-for-profit health care partners can get better results.

An entrepreneurial family physician is leading an effort to restructure 167-bed Deaconess Hospital in Cincinnati as a for-profit joint venture with the hospital's not-for-profit parent, and a Rochester Hills, Michigan, urologist. The deal hinges on significant investment by six-hospital McLaren Health Care Corp . . .

The combination of physicians holding a financial stake in the hospital and having a greater voice in how it's run, Barber said, should yield a financial turnaround because it will "create a place where they feel more comfortable and do more work there because of that." . . .

In Michigan, North Oakland Medical Centers has been struggling badly. The hospital suffered an operating loss of $13.4 million in 2007 and had just eighteen days' cash on hand at the end of the year, according to Standard & Poor. The hospital missed a payment in March on $38 million in bonds issued under a lease agreement with the city of Pontiac. The Pontiac City Council on June 26 agreed to sell the hospital property to Oakland Physicians Medical Center, a limited liability corporation formed by a consortium of physicians led by urologist Anil Kumar . . .

Kumar said that the physicians are willing to invest as much as $6 million toward the total cost of the transaction, which he believes may be in the ballpark of $11 million, with $3 million owed to the Pontiac Hospital Finance Authority—which the cash-strapped city created to issue bonds for the hospital—and $6 million for the hospital's equipment and licenses . . .

Kumar said that he and his partners have studied North Oakland Medical Center's numbers and determined a modest increase in volume can make the hospital profitable, blaming the hospital's predicament on lax administration, low morale, and union rules standing in the way of employee accountability. The deal is expected to go forward after the hospital files for bankruptcy, probably in the next couple of weeks, Kumar said.

Source: Blesch, G. 2008 (Aug. 4). Modern Healthcare.com. © 2008 Crain Communications, Inc., 360 N Michigan Avenue, Chicago, IL 60601.

but this is an insufficient amount of revenue to earn a required 15 percent return per year on investment. Perspective 11–1 provides an example of physicians purchasing a hospital in hopes of earning a return.

Investment centers have proliferated in the past few decades and include all investor-owned health care entities that require their operating units to make a certain return. However, not all investment centers are investor-owned, for many not-for-profit health care organizations require various responsibility centers to make a certain return. It is not the ownership status that makes a responsibility center an investment center, it is the requirement that it make a certain return.

Investment Centers Organizational units that have all the responsibilities of a traditional profit center and are responsible for return on investment.

MEASURING THE PERFORMANCE OF RESPONSIBILITY CENTERS

The previous section categorized the different types of responsibility centers in terms of their increasing level of financial responsibility. However, measuring the performance of responsibility centers rests on the assumption that a responsibility center be held accountable only for those things over which it has control. Thus, responsibility is only one of three major attributes of a responsibility center. The other two are authority and accountability (see Exhibit 11–4).

Responsibility, Authority, and Accountability

The relationship among responsibility, authority, and accountability is straightforward. Ideally, managers should be given the *authority* to carry out their *responsibilities*. To the extent that this occurs, managers should expect to be held *accountable* for the performance of their responsibility centers (see Perspective 11–2.)

Responsibility Duties and obligations of responsibility center.

Authority Power to carry out a given responsibility.

Responsibility refers to the duties and obligations of a responsibility center, *authority* is the power to carry them out, and *accountability* is the extent to which there are consequences positive and/or negative, attached to carrying out responsibilities. Exhibit 11–4 shows that these three attributes do not always coincide, and discrepancies can lead to problems and frustrations.

Accountability The extent to which there are consequences attached to carrying out responsibilities.

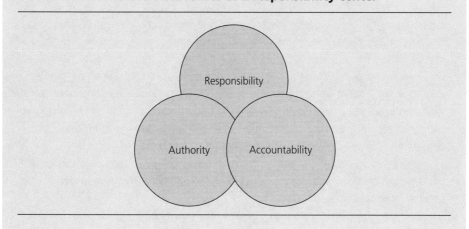

Exhibit 11–4   The basic attributes of a responsibility center

Perspective 11–2   The Calculus of Incentive Pay

Academic health centers, or AHCs, are complex organizations with multiple—and sometimes competing—goals and missions. The challenge for any AHC leader is to find the synergies that unify all stakeholders around common performance goals. An incentive compensation program can be a useful tool in aligning and galvanizing leadership to achieve unifying performance goals.

Before we go on to discuss how we measure success, let's look at what we mean by unifying performance goals. They include

- Overall mission and strategy. If there are varying or competing missions, are there any common themes?
- Quality and service. How well is the AHC serving its community and employees, supporting its academic and research mission and affecting healthcare?
- Financial viability. What is the financial health of the AHC? How do its individual operations contribute to its overall financial health?

As a necessary precursor to mission and strategic success, leaders must be able to define, measure, and track leadership performance goals in a consistent and timely manner. Board-level reporting of performance results that influence leadership compensation decisions are also important, especially in light of new Internal Revenue Service Form 990 disclosure requirements and governance reforms calling for greater transparency.

The board should have a solid understanding of the performance goals and expectations that affect leadership compensation decisions. Greater disclosure of performance results can also help educate the community and regulators about the AHC's achievements.

Academic center leaders should also be held accountable for performance decisions that affect not only their areas of operations but also the whole AHC. Effective operations management and planning processes are critical for leadership to work together on high-impact goals. This sometimes demands coordination between separate AHC boards, chief executive officers, and management teams. However, this should not be a barrier to developing an incentive compensation program that coordinates common performance goals, thus helping to weave disparate organizations together.

The use of incentive compensation among AHCs has increased significantly over the past decade. Most mid-sized to large AHCs now provide some form of incentive compensation to their clinical enterprise executive teams. However, incentive compensation in purely academic environments is much less prevalent.

While annual incentives are the most common programs, long-term incentive plans (i.e., three to five years) have gained some acceptance among larger AHCs with broad change strategies . . .

A September 2004 study by the University HealthSystem Consortium and Computer Science Corp. tends to buttress the validity of these notions. The AHCs

Perspective 11–2   (*Continued*)

identified in the study as high-performing organizations "achieve high performance through an operating philosophy and techniques that mobilize the entire organization (chairs, faculty, executive team, employees) to optimize overall medical center performance rather than the performance of individual entities, departments, or missions, and engage chairs and faculty in the identification, evaluation, and approval of changes."

Incentive compensation has been successful in many cases in helping AHCs develop consensus regarding the most important leadership performance priorities for a given time period; align leadership on key performance goals and targets related to these priorities; focus efforts and resources on achievement of performance goals and targets; and enhance effective communications and "buy-in" for performance goals, targets, and results.

There are a number of design characteristics that directly contribute to incentive compensation effectiveness:

- Narrowing the number of performance criteria to critical organizational mission and strategic priorities
- Including nonfinancial performance criteria (i.e., quality, service, resource management, human resources, education quality, and research productivity)
- Blending both organizational and individual performance goals specific to the responsibility areas of each eligible leader
- Defining measurable and realistic—but challenging—performance goals and providing consistent and timely reporting of results
- Ensuring that participants believe that they can influence the achievement of defined performance goals.
- Communicating progress, especially in the performance areas that require improvement. There are a number of steps that an academic medical center can take to develop an effective incentive compensation program:
  - Define the purpose of the incentive compensation program
  - Define who will be responsible for oversight of the program
  - Define the performance measurement period
  - Determine eligible participants for the plan
  - Determine award opportunities
  - Determine objective performance measures and goals, both AHC-wide and individual, covering a spectrum of performance
  - Establish minimum thresholds of performance for funding
  - Determine how qualitative performance or board/CEO discretion should play a role in determining awards

Source: Hefner, D., and Hastings, K. 2008 (July 28). Modern Healthcare.com © 2008 Crain Communications, Inc. Performance Measures.

Although responsibility centers should be held accountable for both financial and nonfinancial performance, this discussion is limited to an introduction to financial performance measures. Exhibit 11–5 shows that cost, profit, and investment centers, respectively, are held accountable for increasing levels of financial responsibility (note that service centers have no *direct* financial responsibilities). *Budget variances* are the most universal measure of financial performance internally.

Exhibit 11–5   Typical measures used to evaluate the financial performance of responsibility centers

Performance Measures	Type of center			
	Service Centers	Cost Centers	Profit Centers	Investment Centers
Budget variances				
Volume variances	☒	☒	☒	☒
Cost variances		☒	☒	☒
Acuity variances		☒	☒	☒
Revenue variances			☒	☒
Liquidity ratios				
Current ratio			☒	☒
Quick ratio			☒	☒
Days cash on hand			☒	☒
Activity ratios				
Asset turnover			☒	☒
Receivable turnover			☒	☒
Payables turnover			☒	☒
Capitalization ratios				
Debt to equity			☒	☒
Times interest earned			☒	☒
Debt service coverage			☒	☒
Profitability ratios				
Profit			☒	☒
Operating margin			☒	☒
Return on equity				☒
Return on assets				☒

BUDGET VARIANCES

A *budget variance* is the difference between what was budgeted and what actually occurred. Exhibit 11–6 shows an example of an ambulatory care clinic nonlabor budget that originally budgeted 1,000 visits during the month but actually provided 1,200 visits. Their expected net income was $35,000, and their actual net income was $47,000. Although it is tempting to assume that the $12,000 increase in net income was due to changes in the number of visits, often more than one factor is responsible for budget variances. The rest of this section presents an approach to systematically explain why a budget variance occurs.

As shown in Exhibit 11–7, it is common for health care organizations to separate their total budget variance (variance in net income) into the portion due to changes in revenue and the portion due to changes in expenses. The revenue variance is then broken down into the portion attributable to volume and the portion attributable to rate differences. The expense variance is subdivided into the portion due to volume and the part due to other factors. This model will now be used to explain the net income variance of $12,000 in Exhibit 11–6.

Budget Variance
The difference between what was planned (budgeted) and what was achieved (actual).

Revenue Variances

In Exhibit 11–6, both the number of visits and the revenues earned from them increased beyond what was budgeted. This resulted in a positive revenue variance of $17,000. This is called a *favorable* variance because more income was received than was budgeted. Using just this information, it is tempting to conclude that the increase in revenues was due to the increase in employees covered. In fact, a variance analysis of the change in revenues shows that this is only partly the case.

Step 1. Develop the Flexible Budget Estimate for Revenues In addition to the budgeted estimate and actual results, a variance analysis involves one more piece of

---

Exhibit 11–6 Revenue and expense variance information for an ambulatory care clinic

		Budgeted	Actual	Variance	
A	Visits	1,000	1,200	200	
B	Revenues	$100,000	$117,000	$17,000	Favorable
C	Expenses	$65,000	$70,000	$5,000	Unfavorable
D	Net income	$35,000	$47,000	$12,000	Favorable

Exhibit 11–7   Common variances used by health care organizations

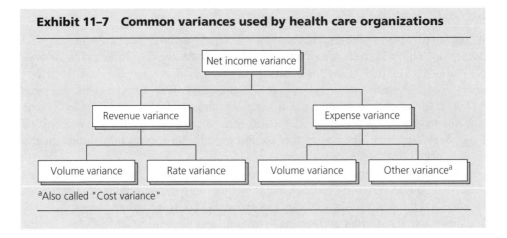

^aAlso called "Cost variance"

Flexible Budget
A budget that accommodates a range or multiple levels of activities.

information, called a flexible budget estimate. The *flexible budget esti-mate* adjusts for the actual volume being different from what was planned. The flexible budget estimate is what would have been bud-geted had the actual volume been known ahead of time. Determining the flexible budget estimate involves two steps: calculating the budgeted rate and then using this number to determine how much would have been budgeted had the actual volume been known.

Step 1A. Determine the Budgeted Revenue per Unit The budgeted revenues are $100.00 per visit. This is determined by dividing budgeted revenues, $100,000, by the budgeted number of visits, 1,000 (see Exhibit 11–8, Step 1A).

Step 1B. Develop the Flexible Budget Estimate The flexible budget estimate is the budgeted revenue per visit multiplied by the actual volume ($100.00 per visit ×1,200 visits = $120,000). This is the amount that would have been budgeted for revenues had it been known when the original budget was made that the actual volume would be 1,200 rather than 1,000 visits (see Exhibit 11–8, Step 1B).

A flexible budget estimates the revenues, expenses, or both over a range of vol-umes to forecast what the revenues and expenses would be at various levels. For example, by multiplying the $100.00 revenue per visit by a range of visits from 1,000 through 1,400, the clinic could develop a range of revenue estimates at selected levels (see Exhibit 11–8, rows D through F).

Both the range of volume estimates and the gap between each estimate are open to judgment. However, the range should include both the budgeted and actual volumes. Using this approach, the clinic just as easily could have estimated the results for a range of 800 to 1,500 using steps of 500. Either way, at 1,200 visits the budget esti-mate would have been $120,000.

Exhibit 11–8   Analysis of a revenue variance by volume and rate components

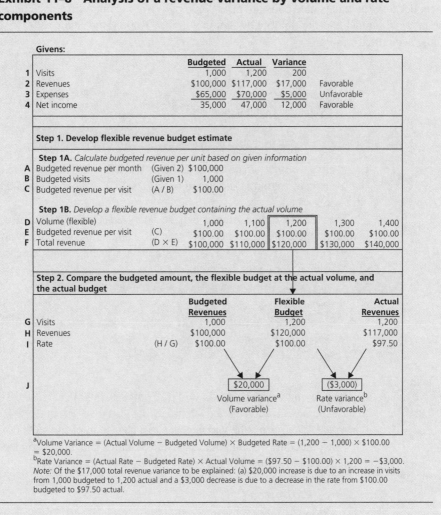

^aVolume Variance = (Actual Volume − Budgeted Volume) × Budgeted Rate = (1,200 − 1,000) × $100.00 = $20,000.
^bRate Variance = (Actual Rate − Budgeted Rate) × Actual Volume = ($97.50 − $100.00) × 1,200 = −$3,000.
Note: Of the $17,000 total revenue variance to be explained: (a) $20,000 increase is due to an increase in visits from 1,000 budgeted to 1,200 actual and a $3,000 decrease is due to a decrease in the rate from $100.00 budgeted to $97.50 actual.

Step 2. Calculate the Revenue Variance Due to Changes in Volume and Rate
This step begins by laying out, side by side, the three revenue budget figures: budgeted amount, flexible budget, and actual revenues (see Exhibit 11–8, rows G through I).

All that remains is to compare these three figures. The difference between the original budget, $100,000, and the flexible budget, $120,000, shows how much of the revenue variance is due to volume: $20,000 (Exhibit 11–8, row J). The difference between the flexible budget, $120,000, and actual results, $117,000, is the amount of the revenue variance that is due to a change in rate: −$3,000.

These differences can also be derived a different way. Looking at the volume variance, because the rate is held constant at $100.00 per visit, the only difference between the original budget and the flexible budget is volume (1,000 rather than 1,200 visits). Thus, using the formula:

Revenue Volume Variance
The portion of total variance in revenues due to the actual volume being either higher or lower than the budgeted volume. It is the difference between the revenues forecast in the original budget and those in the flexible budget. It can be computed using the formula: (actual volume – budgeted volume) × budgeted rate.

> Revenue Volume Variance = (Actual Volume – Budgeted Volume) × Budgeted Rate

the *revenue volume variance* is $20,000 [(1,200 – 1,000) × $100.00]. That is, because volume increased by 200 at $100.00 per visit, $20,000 extra was earned.

The –$3,000 rate variance can be analyzed similarly. Because the flexible budgeted revenue per visit was $100.00 and the actual revenue is $97.50 per visit ($117,000/120,000), there has been a rate decrease of $2.50 per visit. Using the formula:

> Revenue Rate Variance = (Actual Rate – Budgeted Rate) × Actual Volume

Revenue Rate Variance
The amount of the total revenue variance that occurs because the actual average rate varies from the one originally budgeted. It is the difference between the revenues forecast in the flexible budget and those actually earned. It can be calculated using the formula: (actual rate – budgeted rate) × actual volume.

the *revenue rate variance* is –$3,000 [($97.50 – $100.00) × 1,200]. Thus, because the organization earned $2.50 less per visit than was budgeted, and it provided 1,200 visits, the variance due to a change in rate is –$3,000.

The procedure to calculate revenue volume and rate variances is summarized in Exhibit 11–9.

Expense Variances

This section explains why the ambulatory clinic was $5,000 over its budgeted expenses ($65,000 – $70,000). As shown in Exhibit 11–10, analyzing expense variances is similar to analyzing revenue variances.

Step 1. Identify the Amount of Variance Due to Fixed Costs Although variable costs are directly affected by volume, fixed costs should not be. There are a number of reasons why fixed costs might have been incurred beyond what was budgeted. For example, there may be additional depreciation taken on the purchase of new equipment, unanticipated raises given, or new employees hired. (Consider that perhaps volume went beyond the relevant range into a higher "step" of step-fixed costs.) This example assumes that fixed expenses increased because additional equipment had to be leased for $1,000 per month.

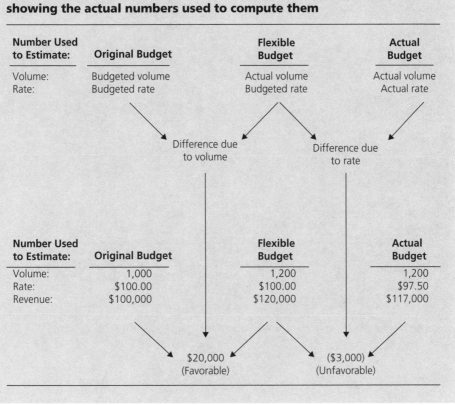

Exhibit 11–9 Derivation of the revenue volume and rate variances, showing the actual numbers used to compute them

Number Used to Estimate:	Original Budget	Flexible Budget	Actual Budget
Volume:	Budgeted volume	Actual volume	Actual volume
Rate:	Budgeted rate	Budgeted rate	Actual rate

Difference due to volume

Difference due to rate

Number Used to Estimate:	Original Budget	Flexible Budget	Actual Budget
Volume:	1,000	1,200	1,200
Rate:	$100.00	$100.00	$97.50
Revenue:	$100,000	$120,000	$117,000

$20,000 (Favorable)

($3,000) (Unfavorable)

Original expense variance (Exhibit 11–6, row C)	$5,000
Amount explained by fixed expenses (Exhibit 11–10, row B)	$1,000
Amount of expense variance still unexplained	$4,000

This explains $1,000 of the $5,000 expense variance. The following steps explain the remaining $4,000 unfavorable expense variance due to variable expenses.

Step 2. Develop a Flexible Expense Budget This step involves developing a flexible budget to determine how much would have been budgeted had it been known at the time the budget was prepared that the actual number of visits would be 1,200 and not 1,000.

Step 2A. Determine the Budgeted Cost per Unit The budgeted cost per unit in the example is calculated by dividing the $65,000 in budgeted expenses by the

Exhibit 11–10   Breaking down the expense variance into fixed, volume, and cost variances

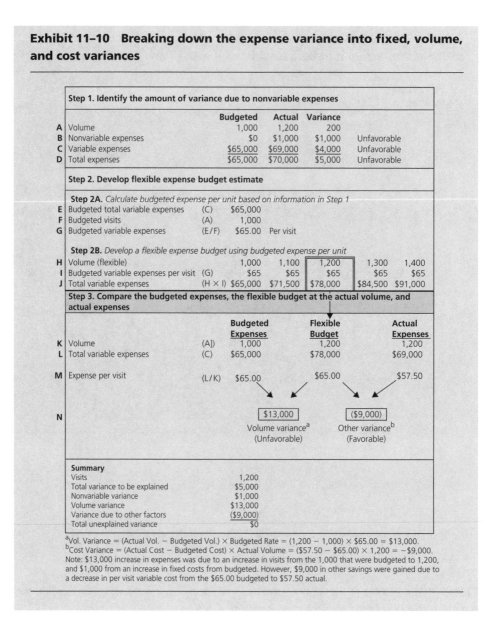

Step 1. Identify the amount of variance due to nonvariable expenses

		Budgeted	Actual	Variance	
A	Volume	1,000	1,200	200	
B	Nonvariable expenses	$0	$1,000	$1,000	Unfavorable
C	Variable expenses	$65,000	$69,000	$4,000	Unfavorable
D	Total expenses	$65,000	$70,000	$5,000	Unfavorable

Step 2. Develop flexible expense budget estimate

Step 2A. *Calculate budgeted expense per unit based on information in Step 1*

E	Budgeted total variable expenses	(C)	$65,000	
F	Budgeted visits	(A)	1,000	
G	Budgeted variable expenses	(E/F)	$65.00	Per visit

Step 2B. *Develop a flexible expense budget using budgeted expense per unit*

H	Volume (flexible)		1,000	1,100	1,200	1,300	1,400
I	Budgeted variable expenses per visit	(G)	$65	$65	$65	$65	$65
J	Total variable expenses	(H × I)	$65,000	$71,500	$78,000	$84,500	$91,000

Step 3. Compare the budgeted expenses, the flexible budget at the actual volume, and actual expenses

			Budgeted Expenses	Flexible Budget	Actual Expenses
K	Volume	(A])	1,000	1,200	1,200
L	Total variable expenses	(C)	$65,000	$78,000	$69,000
M	Expense per visit	(L/K)	$65.00	$65.00	$57.50

N

$13,000
Volume variance[a]
(Unfavorable)

($9,000)
Other variance[b]
(Favorable)

Summary	
Visits	1,200
Total variance to be explained	$5,000
Nonvariable variance	$1,000
Volume variance	$13,000
Variance due to other factors	($9,000)
Total unexplained variance	$0

[a]Vol. Variance = (Actual Vol. − Budgeted Vol.) × Budgeted Rate = (1,200 − 1,000) × $65.00 = $13,000.
[b]Cost Variance = (Actual Cost − Budgeted Cost) × Actual Volume = ($57.50 − $65.00) × 1,200 = −$9,000.
Note: $13,000 increase in expenses was due to an increase in visits from the 1,000 that were budgeted to 1,200, and $1,000 from an increase in fixed costs from budgeted. However, $9,000 in other savings were gained due to a decrease in per visit variable cost from the $65.00 budgeted to $57.50 actual.

1,000 budgeted visits (see Exhibit 11–10, Step 2A, rows E and F). Thus, the budgeted cost per visit is $65.00 (see Exhibit 11–10, Step 2A, row G).

Step 2B. Develop the Flexible Budget Estimate The flexible expense budget estimate is the budgeted cost per unit multiplied by the actual volume ($65.00 × 1,200 = $78,000). This is the amount that would have been budgeted for expenses had it been known when the original budget was made that the actual volume would be 1,200 rather than 1,000 visits (see Exhibit 11–10, Step 2B, rows H through J).

Step 3. Calculate the Expense Variance Due to Changes in Volume and Other Factors As in Step 2 of the revenue variance analysis presented earlier (Exhibit 11–8), this step begins by laying out side by side the three expense budget figures: budgeted, flexible, and actual expenses. From Exhibit 11–10, Step 3, the difference between the original budget, $65,000, and the flexible budget, $78,000, is the amount of the variance due to volume, $13,000 (rows L and N). The difference between the flexible budget and the actual results ($78,000 – $69,000 = –$9,000) is due to a change in costs per unit (also rows L and N). Note that this is a cost saving and is therefore considered *favorable*. Variable costs actually decreased from what was expected.

As with the revenue variances, expense variances can also be derived a different way. In regard to the volume variance, because the cost per unit is held constant ($65 per visit), the only difference between the original budget and the flexible budget is volume (1,200 rather than 1,000 visits). Thus, using the formula:

> Expense Volume Variance = (Actual Volume – Budgeted Volume) × Budgeted Cost per Unit

Expense Volume Variance
The portion of total variance in expenses that is due to the actual volume being either higher or lower than the budgeted volume. It is the difference between the expenses forecast in the original budget and those in the flexible budget. It can be computed using the formula: (actual volume – budgeted volume) × budgeted cost per unit.

the *expense volume variance* is $13,000 [(1,200 – 1,000) × $65.00]. This is because there were 200 more visits than budgeted at a cost of $100 per visit. The expense volume variance is the portion of total variance in variable expenses that is due to the actual volume being either higher or lower than the budgeted volume. It is the difference between the expenses forecast in the original budget and those in the flexible budget. It can be computed using the following formula: (actual volume – budgeted volume) × budgeted cost per unit.

The $9,000 savings shown in the remaining variance, called a cost variance, can be analyzed similarly. Because the flexible budgeted cost per

Key Point *In the formula for expense volume variance, the sign of the answer is crucial. A negative answer indicates a decrease in volume, but this is considered a* favorable variance *because it leads to a decrease in costs. A positive answer indicates an increase in volume, and this is considered an* unfavorable variance *because it leads to an increase in costs.*

Expense Cost Variance
The amount of the variable expense variance that occurs because the actual cost per unit varies from that originally budgeted. It is the difference between the variable expenses forecast in the flexible budget and those actually incurred. It can be calculated by the formula: (actual cost per unit – budgeted cost per unit) × actual volume.

visit was $65.00 and the actual cost per visit is $57.50 ($69,000 / 1,200), there is a decrease in the cost per visit of $7.50. Using the formula:

> Expense Cost Variance = (Actual Cost per Unit – Budgeted Cost per Unit) × Actual Volume

the *expense cost variance* is –$9,000. Thus, because the organization spent $7.50 less per visit than had been budgeted, and it provided 1,200 visits, the variance due to a change in cost per visit is –$9,000 (–$7.50 × 1,200). The procedure to calculate expense volume and cost variances is summarized in Exhibit 11–11.

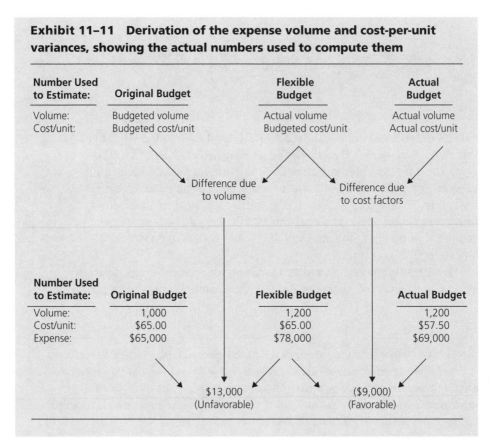

Exhibit 11–11 Derivation of the expense volume and cost-per-unit variances, showing the actual numbers used to compute them

Number Used to Estimate:	Original Budget	Flexible Budget	Actual Budget
Volume:	Budgeted volume	Actual volume	Actual volume
Cost/unit:	Budgeted cost/unit	Budgeted cost/unit	Actual cost/unit

Difference due to volume   Difference due to cost factors

Number Used to Estimate:	Original Budget	Flexible Budget	Actual Budget
Volume:	1,000	1,200	1,200
Cost/unit:	$65.00	$65.00	$57.50
Expense:	$65,000	$78,000	$69,000

$13,000 (Unfavorable)   ($9,000) (Favorable)

Although the amount of the cost variance was calculated, the reason for it is unclear. The cost variance could be due to a variety of factors, including changes in quality, case mix, intensity of services, efficiency, and wages. Although it is possible to decompose the cost variance into other variances, that methodology is beyond the scope of this text.

Summary of the Example When considering both revenues and expenses, the total variance was $12,000. Of this, a change in volume resulted in increased revenues of $20,000 and increased costs of $13,000. On the other hand, the change in rate from $100.00 to $97.50 decreased revenue by $33,000, and the change in cost per unit from $65.00 to $57.50 accounted for $9,000 in savings from what was budgeted. In addition, an additional fixed cost was incurred by leasing equipment at $1,000 per month.

Increase in visits from 1,000 to 1,200 (revenues)	$20,000
Increase in visits from 1,000 to 1,200 (expenses)	(13,000)
Decrease in rates from $100.00 to $97.50 per visit	(3,000)
Decrease in cost per visit from $65.00 to $57.50 per visit	9,000
Increase in fixed costs by hiring a contract RN	(1,000)
Total variance explained	$ 12,000

Key point *In the formula for expense cost variance, the sign of the answer is crucial. A negative answer indicates a decrease in variable cost per unit, but this is considered a* favorable variance *because it leads to decreased costs. A positive answer indicates an increase in variable cost per unit, but this is considered an* unfavorable variance *because it leads to increased costs.*

Beyond Variances

Budget variances are usually associated with the operating budget, which focuses on short-term *revenue attainment* (earning the amount of revenue budgeted) and *cost containment* (not spending more than budgeted). A more long-term focus is necessary to effect major efficiencies in the organization. Measures must be implemented to promote

Revenue Attainment
Earning the amount of revenue budget.

Cost Containment
Not spending more than is budgeted in the expense budget.

Revenue Enhancement
Finding supplemental
sources of revenue.

revenue enhancement (finding new sources of revenue) and *cost avoidance* (finding new ways to operate the business that eliminate certain classes of costs) in the long term. For instance, just-in-time (JIT) inventory methods deliver supplies "automatically" to the organization as needed, and they avoid many of the traditional costs of ordering, storing, and keeping track of inventories that flow through health care organizations. If only a short-term focus were used, the initial costs might discourage an administrator from installing such a system; however, long-term measures might encourage such a decision.

Cost Avoidance
Finding new ways to run
a business that eliminate
certain classes of costs.

Other Financial Performance Measures

Although budget variances are the most-used financial measure, various ratios are increasingly being used as financial performance measures for profit and investment centers. Although the use of these indicators is basically the same for profit centers and investment centers as it is for the organization as a whole, some complications arise when using these measures to judge the financial performance of divisions within the organization. The most common are:

- They may promote a lack of goal congruence; that is, they may encourage the organizational unit to make decisions that are in its own best interest but not in the best interest of the organization as a whole.

- They may introduce complicated measurement problems. For instance, when two organizational units share the same assets, it is difficult to partition the assets between the two units to calculate such measures as return on assets.

- They may promote short-term thinking.

Compensation Systems The responsibility, accountability, and authority components of responsibility accounting systems do not operate in isolation and may be highly intertwined with the employee compensation system. Although these systems can be extremely complex, they can be thought of as falling into three major categories: salary-based, at-risk, and mixed (see Exhibit 11–12 and Perspective 11–2).

Salary-Based Compensation System As the name implies, the fundamental attribute of a salary-based compensation system is that employees receive a guaranteed salary. Salaried employees know what they will get paid, and employers know what their salary expense will be over a given period of time. Such payments are based on employees "doing their job," and as such, provide no financial incentives to reward individual performance and promote group and organizational goals. They may not provide rewards because it is felt they are not necessary or the structure or infrastructure is not there to support them.

Exhibit 11–12   Major employee compensation models

Model	Major Attribute	Key Advantages	Key Disadvantages
Salary-based	Guaranteed salary	Income predictability	No financial incentives to reward individual performance and promote organizational goals
At-risk	Amount of compensation based totally on meeting performance goals	Financial incentives to reward individual performance and promote organizational goals	Income is not necessarily predictable and may be contingent on non-controllable forces
Mixed	Only a portion of salary is guaranteed and remainder based on meeting performance goals	Combines a level of salary predictability with rewards for performance	Depending on base and at risk distribution, may have the disadvantages of both systems

At-Risk Compensation System   In a full at-risk system, compensation is based totally on achieving certain targets, called performance goals. A major advantage of at-risk systems are that they financially reward performance and, if structured appropriately, can incent not only individual and group performance but participation as well in activities that help the organization as a whole (e.g., help other departments achieve their goals, serve on committees). A major disadvantage of total at-risk systems is that revenues of participants are uncertain, as are a portion of the expenses of the organization. This can be especially problematic to the extent that non-controllable forces (e.g., the economy) interfere with performance.

Mixed Compensation System   In a mixed system, a portion of compensation is at risk. If well designed, a system can provide for a base of certainty for part of compensation, yet still provide performance incentives. However, if not well structured, it may have the disadvantages of each (see Exhibit 11–12).

Compensation System Design   In designing compensation systems, a number of factors should be considered, including the goals of the system, which can generally be categorized into productivity and quality, financial viability, and general characteristics. In addressing each of these areas, both employers and employees have relatively specific concerns, which are presented in Exhibit 11–13.

Exhibit 11–13   Key goals of major employee compensation models

Model	Productivity and Quality	Financial Viability	Basic Characteristics of the Incentive System
Key employer concerns	Promotes **mission**-related goals	Promotes **margin**-related goals	Ease of implementation
Key employee concerns	Promotes personal work-life balance goals	Promotes financial goals	Fair, ease of understanding, ease of participating and consistently applied
Focus of incentives	Productivity and quality	Revenue generation, resource use, and profitability	Sufficiently motivating to each party's goals

SUMMARY

A growing trend in the structure of health care organizations is decentralization, which presents some interesting problems in the measurement of financial performance of organizational units. Decentralization is the degree of dispersion of responsibility within an organization.

The advantages of decentralization include time, information relevance, quality, speed, talent, and motivation and allegiance. The disadvantages include loss of control, decreased goal congruence, increased need for coordination and formal communication, and lack of managerial talent.

A responsibility center is an organizational unit that has been formally designated with the responsibility to carry out one or more tasks or to achieve one or more outcomes. There are four major types of responsibility centers:

- Service centers are responsible for ensuring that health care-related services are provided to a population in a manner that meets the volume and quality requirements of the organization. They have no direct budgetary control.

- Cost centers are responsible for providing services and controlling their costs. They are the primary level in the organization with direct budget control. The three types of cost centers in health care organizations are production, clinical, and administrative cost centers. Production cost centers develop and/or sell products. Clinical cost centers provide health care-related services to clients, patients, or enrollees. Administrative cost centers provide support to the clinical cost centers and the organization as a whole. Often included in this category are general administration, the business office, information services, admitting, medical records, and housekeeping.

- Profit centers are responsible for controlling costs and earning revenues. The three types of profit centers are traditional profit centers, capitated profit centers, and administrative profit centers.
- Investment centers are responsible for attaining a return on investment.

The relationship between responsibility, accountability, and authority is straightforward. Ideally, managers should be given the authority to carry out their responsibilities. To the extent that this occurs, managers are held accountable for the performance of their responsibility centers. Responsibility refers to the duties and obligations of a responsibility center; authority is the power to carry out a given responsibility; and accountability means there are consequences, both positive and/or negative, attached to carrying out responsibilities.

Cost, profit, and investment centers, respectively, are held accountable for increasing levels of financial responsibility. (Service centers have no direct financial responsibilities.) Budget variances are the most universal measure of financial performance. A budget variance is the difference between what was budgeted and what actually occurred. It is common for health care organizations to separate their total budget variance (variance in net income) into revenue variances and expense variances. The revenue variance is broken down into volume and rate variances. The expense variance is separated into volume variance and other factors.

The revenue volume variance is the portion of total variance in revenues due to the actual volume being either higher or lower than the budgeted volume. It is the difference between the revenues forecast in the original budget and those in the flexible budget. It can be computed using the following formula: (actual volume – budgeted volume) $\times$ budgeted rate. The rate variance is the amount of the total revenue variance that occurs because the actual average rate received varies from that originally budgeted. It is the difference between the revenues forecast in the flexible budget and those actually earned. It can be calculated using the formula: (actual rate – budgeted rate) $\times$ actual volume.

The expense volume variance is the portion of total variance in variable expenses due to the actual volume being either higher or lower than the budgeted volume. It is the difference between the expenses forecast in the original budget and those in the flexible budget. It can be computed using the following formula: (actual volume – budgeted volume) $\times$ budgeted cost per unit.

The expense cost variance is the amount of the variable expense variance that occurs because the actual cost per visit varies from that originally budgeted. It is the difference between the variable expenses forecast in the flexible budget and those actually incurred. It can be calculated by the formula: (actual cost per unit – budgeted cost per unit) $\times$ actual volume. The cost variance could be due to a variety of factors, including changes in quality, case mix, intensity of service, efficiency, and wages.

In addition to variances, which tend to focus on operational concerns, organizations may also be concerned with longer-term goals of revenue enhancement and cost avoidance. To attain operational as well as strategic goals, employers may often use financial and nonfinancial ratios and may use compensation systems designed to achieve various goals.

KEY TERMS

a. Accountability
b. Administrative cost centers
c. Administrative profit centers
d. Authority
e. Budget variance
f. Capitated profit centers
g. Clinical cost centers
h. Cost avoidance
i. Cost centers
j. Cost containment
k. Decentralization
l. Expense cost variance
m. Expense volume variance

n. Flexible budget
o. Investment centers
p. Production cost center
q. Profit centers
r. Responsibility
s. Responsibility center
t. Revenue attainment
u. Revenue enhancement
v. Revenue rate variance
w. Revenue volume variance
x. Service centers
y. Traditional profit centers
z. Transfer price

KEY EQUATIONS

Expense Cost Variance = (Actual Cost per Unit − Budgeted Cost per Unit) × Actual Volume

Expense Volume Variance = (Actual Volume − Budgeted Volume) × Budgeted Cost per Unit

Revenue Rate Variance = (Actual Rate − Budgeted Rate) × Actual Volume

Revenue Volume Variance = (Actual Volume − Budgeted Volume) × Budgeted Rate

QUESTIONS AND PROBLEMS

1. **Definitions.** Define the terms above.

2. **Advantages of decentralization.** List and discuss the advantages associated with decentralization.

3. **Disadvantages of decentralization.** List and discuss the disadvantages of decentralization.

4. **Types of responsibility centers.** Describe the four types of responsibility centers, including the characteristics of each.

5. **Responsibility centers.**

   a. What is the most common type of responsibility center?

   b. What is the most basic type of responsibility center?

6. **Identifying responsibility centers.** Identify each responsibility center below as either a service center, cost center (clinical or administrative), profit center (capitated or administrative), or investment center. Explain your choices:

   a. Radiology department that must control its own costs.

   b. Admitting department of a hospital.

   c. HMO.

   d. Stand-alone outpatient clinic that must earn a 10 percent ROI.

   e. Volunteer department with no budget.

   f. Development office.

7. **The relationship among accountability, responsibility, and authority.** What is the relationship of accountability, responsibility, and authority with respect to a responsibility center?

8. **Transfer prices.** What are transfer prices? Discuss their major disadvantages.

9. **Performance measures.** What is the most commonly used financial performance measure?

10. **Performance measures.** Name two financial measures used to judge the performance of investment centers that are not used to measure the financial performance of profit centers.

11. **Performance measures.** What are major disadvantages of using traditional performance measures?

12. **Variance analysis.** What does the term *variance analysis* mean when applied to financial performance of health care organizations?

13. **Budget variances.** What are the most common types of budget variances used in health care organizations?

14. **Cost variances.** What can account for cost variances?

15. **ROI for an investment center.** An outpatient clinic invests $2,300,000. The desired ROI is 12 percent. In the first year, revenues are $750,000 and expenses are $370,000. Does the clinic meet its ROI requirement that year?

16. **ROI for an investment center.** A new cardiac catheterization lab was constructed at Havea Heart Hospital. The investment for the lab was $450,000 in equipment costs and $50,000 in renovation costs. A desired return on investment is 12 percent. Once the lab was constructed, 5,000 patients were served in the first year and were charged $340 for each procedure. The annual fixed cost for the catheterization lab is $1,000,000, and the variable cost is $129 per procedure. What is the catheterization lab's profit? Did this profit meet its desired ROI?

17. **Detailed variance analysis.** The following are planned and actual revenues for Cutting Edge Surgery Center. Because they are one of four surgery centers in the community, the administrator is concerned with his rates in relation to those of his competitors.

	Planned	**Actual**
Surgical volume	1,500	1,700
Gift shop revenues	$15,000	$17,000
Surgery revenues	$500,500	$750,750
Parking revenues	$15,000	$17,000

a. Determine the total variance between the planned and actual budgets.

b. Determine the service-related revenues and calculate service-related variance still unexplained.

c. Prepare a flexible budget estimate. Present side by side the budget, flexible budget estimate, and actual surgical revenue (and related volumes).

d. Determine what variance is due to change in volume and what variance is due to change in rates.

e. Determine the volume variance and rate variance based on per unit rates.

18. **Detailed variance analysis.** The administrator of Break-a-Leg Hospital is aware of the need to keep his costs down because he just negotiated a new capitated arrangement with a large insurance company. The following are selected planned and actual expenses for the previous month.

	Planned	**Actual**
Patient days	24,000	23,000
Pharmacy	$100,000	$140,000
Miscellaneous supplies	$56,000	$67,500
Fixed overhead costs	$708,000	$780,000

a. Determine the total variance associated with the planned and actual expenses.

b. Calculate the amount of service-related variance.

c. Prepare a flexible expense estimate for variable costs. Compare budget, flexible budget, and actual (show related volumes).

d. Determine what variance is due to change in volume and what variance is due to change in rates.

e. Determine the volume variance and rate variance based on per unit rates.

19. **Detailed variance analysis.** A dermatology clinic expects to contract with an HMO for an estimated 80,000 enrollees. The HMO expects 1 in 4 of its enrolled members to use the dermatology services per month. At the end of the year, the dermatology clinic's business manager looked at her monthly figures and saw that the number of enrolled members had increased by 5 percent over the budgeted amount and that 1 in 3 of the total HMO members had used the dermatology services per month. Net monthly revenues of the dermatology clinic were budgeted at $260,000 but were actually $450,000. Monthly expenses for the clinic were budgeted at $200,000 but were actually $270,000.

a. Prepare a monthly revenue and expense variance report for the clinic.

b. Are these variances favorable or unfavorable? Why?

12

PROVIDER COST-FINDING METHODS

LEARNING OBJECTIVES

- Identify three methods for estimating costs
- Calculate costs using the step-down method
- Calculate costs using activity-based costing
- Understand the major advantages and disadvantages of activity-based costing

Cost Object
Anything for which costs are being estimated, such as a population, a test, a visit, a patient, or a patient day.

Finding the costs to serve various populations (e.g., the elderly, Medicare patients, rehabilitation patients), to produce various goods and services, and to work with various payors (e.g., Medicaid, insurance companies) is an important activity for most health care providers. A *cost object* is anything for which costs are being estimated, such as a population, a test, a visit, a patient, or a patient day. This chapter discusses the three most commonly used approaches to find costs for various cost objects: the cost-to-charge ratio, the step-down method, and activity-based costing.

COST-TO-CHARGE RATIO

Cost-to-Charge Ratio
A method to estimate costs that assumes that they are a certain percentage of charges (or reimbursements).

Historically, the *cost-to-charge ratio, CCR,* is one of the most common methods used by dentists and physicians to estimate costs. It is based on an assumed relationship of costs to charges, usually determined by industry norms or special studies. CCR begins with charges (or reimbursement) and assumes that costs are a certain percentage of this amount. For example, a group planning a dental office might use the rule of thumb that all nondirect labor expenses amounted to 22 percent of charges.

The main advantage of this approach is simplicity. The disadvantages include:

- Though the ratio used may be typical for the industry or a segment of the industry, it may not apply well to any particular organization

- If the ratio were determined by a study, to the extent that volume or service mix deviates from the figures used in the study, the CCR may become inaccurate

- To the extent that the fixed or variable cost composition has changed, the ratio may provide an inaccurate measurement

- To the extent that an overall ratio is used for all procedures, the CCR may underestimate or overestimate the cost of individual procedures.

Although the CCR is relatively simple to implement, more complex health care organizations usually use a step-down or an activity-based costing approach, either of which is commonly thought to be more accurate.

Step-Down Method
A cost-finding method based on allocating costs that are not directly paid for to products or services to which payment is attached. The method derives its name from the stair-step pattern that results from allocating costs.

STEP-DOWN METHOD

The *step-down method* is a cost-finding method based on allocating costs that are not directly paid for to products or services that are. The example in Exhibit 12–1 shows three responsibility centers to which payment is not attached (utilities, administration, and laboratory) and three to which revenues are attached (walk-in services, pediatric services,

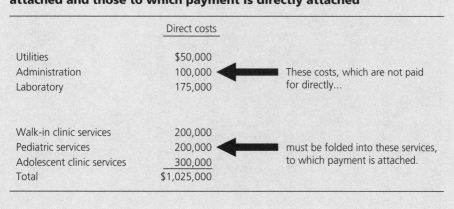

Exhibit 12–1   Example of costs for which payment is not directly attached and those to which payment is directly attached

	Direct costs	
Utilities	$50,000	
Administration	100,000	These costs, which are not paid for directly...
Laboratory	175,000	
Walk-in clinic services	200,000	
Pediatric services	200,000	must be folded into these services, to which payment is attached.
Adolescent clinic services	300,000	
Total	$1,025,000	

and adolescent services). The goal of the step-down method is to allocate the costs of the support centers (utilities, administration, and laboratory) fairly among each of the three patient services. The full step-down allocation is shown in Exhibit 12–2.

There are four steps to allocate the costs of nondirectly paid-for costs to services for which payment is attached:

- Determine an allocation base and compile basic statistics.
- Convert basic statistics for the step-down approach.
- Calculate allocation percentages.
- Allocate costs from the support centers to each of the centers below it (thus the "down" in "step-down").

These steps will now be followed to allocate utilities, administration, and laboratory costs, respectively.

Allocating Utilities

An *allocation base* is an item used to allocate costs, based on its relationship to why the costs occurred. Some common allocation bases are listed in Exhibit 12–3. The better the cause-and-effect relationship between why the cost occurred and the allocation basis, the more accurate the cost allocation. Because of their causal relationship to costs, allocation bases are also called *cost drivers* (discussed in more detail below). A common base to allocate utilities is square footage, on the assumption that actual utility usage is proportional to the size of the space a service occupies.

Exhibit 12–4 highlights those parts of Exhibit 12–2 relevant to allocating utilities. Because administration occupies 1,000 of the 10,000 square

Allocation Base
A statistic (e.g., square feet, number of full-time employees) used to allocate costs, based on its relationship to why the costs occurred.

Exhibit 12-2 The step-down method of allocating costs

| | Step 1: Compile Basic Statistics | | | Step 2: Compute Converted Statistics | | |
| | A | B | C | D | E | F |
	Square Feet	Direct Costs	Lab Tests	Square Feet	Direct Costs	Lab Tests
Utilities		$50,000				
Administration	1,000	$100,000		1,000		
Laboratory	2,000	$175,000		2,000	$175,000	
Walk-in services	2,000	$200,000	250	2,000	$200,000	250
Pediatric services	2,500	$200,000	450	2,500	$200,000	450
Adolescent services	2,500	$300,000	300	2,500	$300,000	300
Total	10,000	$1,025,000	1,000	10,000	$875,000	1,000

| | Step 3: Compute Allocation % | | | |
| | G | H | I | J |
	Utilities (Square Feet)	Administration (Direct Costs)	Laboratory (Tests)	Direct Costs
Utilities				$50,000
Administration	10%			$100,000
Laboratory	20%	20.0%		$175,000
Walk-in services	20%	22.9%	25%	$200,000
Pediatric services	25%	22.9%	45%	$200,000
Adolescent services	25%	34.3%	30%	$300,000
Total	100%	100%	100%	$1,025,000

| | Step 4: Allocate Costs[a] | | | |
| | K | L | M | N |
	Utilities	Administration	Laboratory	Total
Utilities	($50,000)			
Administration	$5,000	($105,000)		
Laboratory	$10,000	$21,000	($206,000)	
Walk-in services	$10,000	$24,000	$51,500	$285,500
Pediatric services	$12,500	$24,000	$92,700	$329,200
Adolescent services	$12,500	$36,000	$61,800	$410,300
Total	$0	$0	$0	$1,025,000

[a] Differences are due to rounding.

Exhibit 12–3 Some common allocation bases

Costs to Be Allocated	Allocation Basis
Billing office	Number of bills
General administration	Direct costs of department
	Number of FTEs[a]
Laboratory[b]	Weighted average costs of tests
	Number of tests
Medical records	Number of records "pulled"
Nursing[b]	Nursing hours
	Acuity-weighted hours
Purchasing	Number of purchase orders
Rent, utilities, cleaning	Square Feet

[a] Full-time-equivalent employees.
[b] Laboratory and nursing are frequently charged directly to patients, rather than being allocated.

feet of the facility (see Exhibit 12–4, columns A and D), it is allocated 10 percent (column G) of the $50,000 direct cost of utilities, which is $5,000 (column K). Similarly, because the laboratory and the walk-in services each occupy 2,000 of the 10,000 square feet (columns A and D), each is allocated 20 percent (column G), which is $10,000 (column K). Finally, because the pediatric and adolescent services each occupy 2,500 square feet (columns A and D), each is allocated 25 percent (column G), which is $12,500 (column K).

Allocating Administrative Costs

Exhibit 12–5 highlights those parts of Exhibit 12–2 relevant to allocating administrative costs. Note that instead of allocating just the $100,000 in direct administrative costs that were there at the beginning of the allocation (column J), $105,000 is allocated from Administration, $100,000 in direct administrative costs, and an additional $5,000 that has been allocated to Administration from Utilities.

The allocation base used to allocate administration is direct costs (see Exhibit 12–5, column E), based on the assumption that administrative costs are incurred by each of the other responsibility centers in the same proportion as are their direct costs. Another allocation base sometimes used to allocate administrative costs is the number of FTEs (full-time-equivalent employees) in each responsibility center. This assumes that administrative costs are incurred in proportion to the number of employees working in each responsibility center.

Exhibit 12–4 Steps in the step-down process relevant to the allocation of utility costs

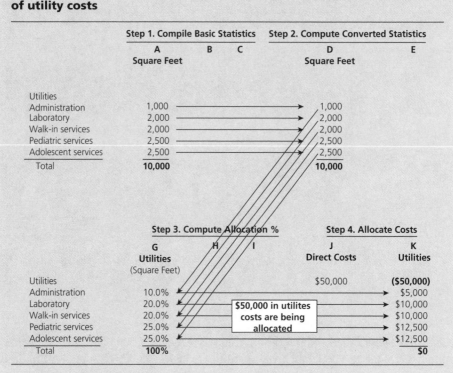

Although the procedure here is similar to allocating utilities, there is one major difference. Note that in column B of Exhibit 12–5, there is $1,025,000 in direct costs, including $50,000 in utilities and $100,000 in administrative direct costs, whereas in column E there is only $875,000 in direct costs because utilities and administrative direct costs have been omitted. This is done for two reasons: First, by convention, the step-down allocation method always proceeds downward from one responsibility center to those below it. Thus, no administrative costs are allocated (upward) to utilities. Therefore, the $50,000 in utilities cost is excluded (column E) when determining the proportional share of administration to be allocated on the basis of direct costs. Second, because administration is fully allocated to the services below it, it cannot give any of its cost to itself. Therefore, in using direct costs as the basis to determine what percentage of the administrative costs being allocated go to the services below it, the $100,000 in administrative direct costs are omitted (column E).

Without the $150,000 of utilities and administration, there is $875,000 in direct costs over which to allocate administration. Laboratory has $175,000 in direct costs (column E), and thus it receives $175,000/$875,000 or 20 percent (column H) of the

Exhibit 12–5 Steps in the step-down process relevant to the allocation of administrative costs

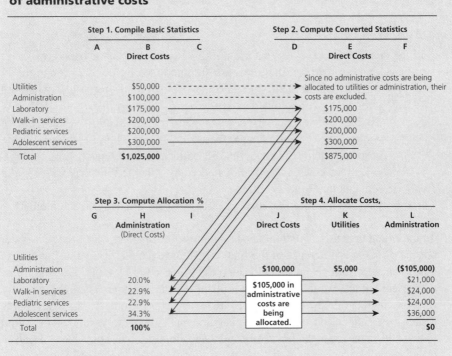

$105,000 in administration being allocated, which is $21,000 (column L). The walk-in services clinic has $200,000 of direct costs (column E), so it receives $200,000/$875,000 or 22.9 percent (column H) of the $105,000 in administrative costs being allocated, which is $24,000 (column L). The remaining administrative costs are allocated to the pediatric and adolescent services in a similar manner (column L).

Allocating Laboratory Costs

The only costs that have not yet been allocated are those of the laboratory. Note that in Exhibit 12–2, instead of the original $175,000 in direct laboratory costs, $206,000 is being allocated (column M). This is because in addition to its own direct costs, laboratory also includes $10,000 in costs allocated from utilities and $21,000 in costs allocated from administration.

Laboratory costs are allocated on the basis of lab tests under the assumption that the fair share of the laboratory costs due to each of the three services is in proportion to the number of tests each service ordered (see Exhibit 12–2, column C). Using lab tests as a basis, the walk-in services clinic is allocated 25 percent (column I) of the $206,000 (column M), which is $51,500 (column M). The pediatric services and the adolescent services clinics are allocated 45 percent and 30 percent, respectively (column I) of the $206,000 (column M), which are $92,700 and $61,800, respectively (column M).

Fully Allocated Cost

After all the costs of the services that are not directly paid for have been allocated to those services that are paid for, the totals are summed (see Exhibit 12–2, column N).

Fully Allocated Cost
The cost of a cost object that includes both its direct costs and all other costs allocated to it.

Rather than the $200,000 it costs to deliver walk-in services when only direct costs are considered, the *fully allocated costs* are $285,500. Similarly, pediatric services changed from $200,000 to $329,200, and adolescent services changed from $300,000 to $410,300 when allocated costs are included. Thus, the fully allocated cost reflects both the original direct costs and all allocated costs, but the total cost, $1,025,000, remains the same as before.

The following are final comments regarding the step-down allocation method:

- To the extent they use a different allocation basis, the *order* in which the services are allocated makes a difference in the final costs. For example, if administration were placed ahead of utilities in the allocation order, the costs of walk-in, pediatric, and adolescent services would be different from those in the example. There are two some-times conflicting rules of thumb to help choose a reasonable order: first, rank-order the centers being allocated from highest dollar amount to lowest dollar amount (according to this rule, in the example, laboratory and then administration should have been listed ahead of utilities); or second, list the centers from highest to lowest in an order that reflects the number of other centers they affect. It was for this reason that the centers were ordered as they were in the example, with laboratory being last.

- The *allocation basis* used to allocate costs makes a difference in the final costs. If the number of FTEs instead of direct dollars were the allocation basis for administration, and there was a low correlation between the two, then the costs of walk-in, pediatric, and adolescent services would be different.

- The number of centers to which costs are allocated makes a difference. For example, if there were four services instead of three, then the costs allocated to the original three services (walk-in, pediatric, and adolescent) would be different (probably less).

- Although the step-down method is the most widely used because of its legacy from Medicare, there are several other related methods available to providers to calculate costs. These are the direct method, the double apportionment method, and the reciprocal method. Because they are used relatively infrequently, they are not discussed here.

- The step-down method is useful for pricing and reimbursement-related decisions but is less useful for controling costs. There are other methods, including activity-based costing, that are better for cost control.

Most inpatient facilities use the step-down method to report their Medicare costs. As shown in Perspective 12–1, there is more to finding costs than just the cost allocation method, one key point being that the costs being reported are allowable. Perspective 12–2 illustrates problems that may arise in using a cost report as the basis for calculating a cost-to-charge ratio.

ACTIVITY-BASED COSTING

Although the step-down method of cost allocation is widely used to find the cost of services for pricing and reimbursement purposes, a newer cost-finding method, called

---

Perspective 12–1 Duke Hospital Overstated Wage Data, OIG Says

Duke University Hospital overstated wage data by $9.3 million in its 2006 Medicare cost report, potentially causing overpayments to all of the hospitals in its statistical area, [Health and Human Services] inspector general's office concluded in audit findings posted May 6.

The 789-bed hospital in Durham, North Carolina, has agreed to work with its Medicare intermediary to correct the data in its public-use file, which the inspector general's office found would distort the area's wage index for fiscal 2009.

According to the report (www.oig.hhs.gov/oas/reports/region1/10700511.pdf), more than half the erroneous sum reported in its Medicare Part A wage data was explained by misreported fringe benefits, primarily tuition reimbursement for employees' family members who were not active employees of the hospital. Another portion, which Duke disputed in its response to the government, represents costs of services provided by nurse practitioners and clinical social workers generally covered under Part B.

Further mistakes led the hospital to omit 52,000 hours associated with the wage data reported. Together, the errors resulted in an average hourly wage rate of $31.51, which was 2 percent higher than the inspector general's office concluded it should have been.

"We were pleased to be able to work with the OIG to correct certain elements of our wage index data before those data were used in the fiscal year 2009 prospective payment system," Stuart Smith, Duke University Health System's assistant vice president for reimbursement, said in a written statement.

Source: Blesch, G. 2008 (May 7). Modern Healthcare.com. © 2008 Crain Communications, Inc., 360 N Michigan Avenue, Chicago, IL 60601.

Perspective 12–2   Cost-to-Charge Ratio Based on Faulty Data

Objective

Our objective was to determine whether Georgia's method of computing inpatient hospital cost outlier payments effectively limited outlier payments to high-cost cases.

Summary of Findings

Georgia's method of computing inpatient hospital cost outlier payments did not effectively limit outlier payments to high-cost cases. Instead of applying a current cost-to-charge ratio (costs divided by charges) to current billed charges from July 1998 through December 2002, the state agency applied an outdated cost-to-charge ratio to current billed charges, thus increasing cost outlier payments.

The calculation of inpatient cost outlier payments includes applying the cost-to-charge ratio to current billed charges. During the audit period, actual cost-to-charge ratios steadily declined as current billed charges increased, which should have resulted in lower outlier payments. However, except for making an adjustment in 2002, the state agency kept outlier payments artificially high by not updating cost-to-charge ratios at a pace commensurate with increasing hospital charges. The state agency relied on historical cost-to-charge ratios because its state plan amendments required the use of audited cost report data to calculate cost-to-charge ratios. Audited cost reports typically run about four years behind the current year. Thus, the state agency relied on outdated cost-to-charge ratios in determining outlier payments.

If the state agency continues to use outdated cost-to-charge ratios, it is likely that cost outlier payments will continue to increase as hospitals increase charges faster than costs. Had the state agency applied current cost-to-charge ratios to convert billed charges to costs, it could have saved approximately $22.7 million in cost outlier payments between 1998 and 2002 at the three hospitals reviewed. We believe that additional savings exist at other hospitals.

Recommendation

We recommend that the state agency amend its Medicaid State plan to require that the data for calculating cost-to-charge ratios be based on submitted cost reports instead of audited cost reports.

Source: 2006 (May). Office of Audit Services, Office of the Inspector General, Department of Health and Human Services Review of Medicaid's Cost Outlier Payments, OIG Report A-04-0400009.

activity-based costing (ABC), is receiving increased attention by health care providers. ABC is based on the paradigm that activities consume resources and products consume activities (see Exhibit 12–6). Therefore, if activities or processes are controlled, then costs will be controlled. Similarly, if the resources an activity uses can be measured, a more accurate picture of the actual costs of services can be found, as compared with traditional cost allocation.

Activity-Based Costing
A method to estimate costs of a service or product by measuring the costs of the activities it takes to produce that service or product.

Traditional cost allocation is called a top-down approach because it begins with all costs and allocates them downward into various services for which payment will be received (see Exhibit 12–7a). ABC, on the other hand, is called a bottom-up approach because it finds the cost of each service at the lowest level, the point at which resources are used, and aggregates them upward into products (see Exhibit 12–7b).

For example, in Exhibit 12–8, the service "Normal Delivery" comprises three intermediate products (or processes): prenatal visit, labor and delivery, and postpartum care.

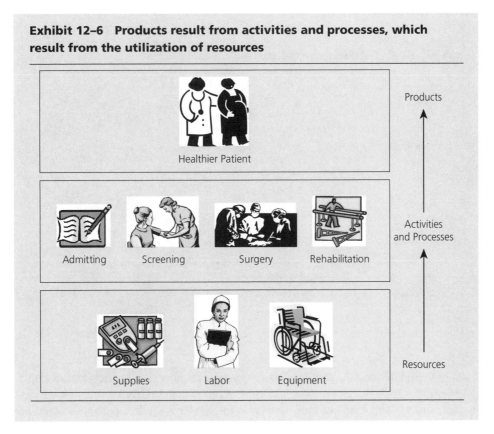

Exhibit 12–6   Products result from activities and processes, which result from the utilization of resources

Healthier Patient — Products

Admitting   Screening   Surgery   Rehabilitation — Activities and Processes

Supplies   Labor   Equipment — Resources

Exhibit 12–7a   Traditional costing

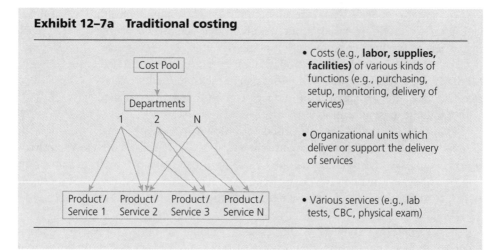

Exhibit 12–7b   Activity-based costing

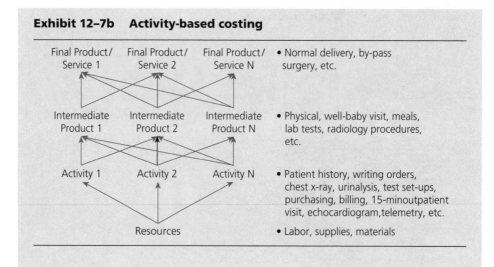

Each of these intermediate products encompasses a number of activities. For example, the prenatal visit includes urinalysis, complete blood count (CBC), vital signs, recent history, and so forth. Each of these activities might also include a portion of what are usually considered indirect costs, such as those associated with ordering supplies, medical records, or financial counseling.

Exhibit 12–8 Examples of intermediate products and activities for a normal delivery

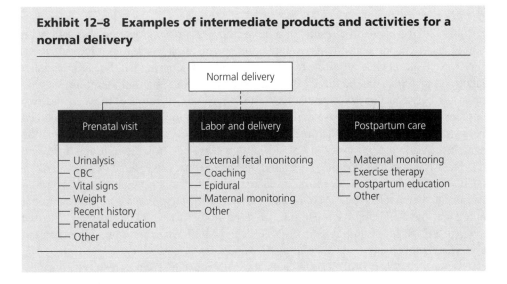

Costing Terminology

Before continuing, it is important to understand three key terms: direct costs, indirect costs, and cost drivers. *Direct costs* are costs (e.g., nursing costs) that an organization can trace to a particular cost object (e.g., a patient). *Indirect costs* are costs that an organization is not able to directly trace to a particular cost object. For example, many health care organizations have great difficulty tracing to a particular patient or service such items as the cost of the billing clerk, rent, or information systems. Thus, a cost is not direct or indirect by its nature but by the ability of the organization to trace it to a cost object.

An important difference between traditional cost allocation and ABC is how each handles indirect costs. Traditional cost allocation methods usually deal with indirect costs by allocating them to cost objects using relatively gross cause-and-effect relationships. ABC attempts to overcome this problem by more directly tracing costs to their cost objects or finding more precise cost drivers. *Cost drivers* are things that cause a change in the cost of an activity.

For example, under traditional step-down costing, purchasing costs might be bundled with other administrative costs and allocated to a service based on the relative size of its budget. Under ABC it is more likely that the costs of purchasing would be allocated to that service more precisely on the basis of the number of purchase orders emanating from that service or even more precisely by measuring the number of minutes spent processing purchase orders from that department.

Direct Costs
Costs that can be traced to a particular cost object.

Indirect Costs
Costs that cannot be traced to a particular cost object. Common indirect costs include billing, rent, utilities, information services, and overhead. Typically, these costs are allocated to cost objects according to an accepted methodology (e.g., step-down method).

Cost Driver
That which causes a change in the cost of an activity.

An Example

Exhibit 12–9 compares the results of a more traditional cost allocation approach with that of an ABC approach. In this example, the organization is offering three outpatient services: an initial visit, a routine regular visit, and an intensive visit. It is assumed that labor and materials can be directly traced to each type of visit, and therefore, they do not vary between the two approaches. Thus, the main difference between the two approaches (as is often the case in practice) is the allocation of overhead. As explained below, the traditional approach uses a single cost driver, visits, and thus assigns the same overhead cost per visit, $17.50, to all three services (row 3, columns A, B, and C). The ABC approach, on the other hand, uses three cost drivers and derives an overhead cost per visit of $28.88 for an initial visit, $13.65 for a regular visit, and $16.33 for an intensive visit (row 3, columns D, E, and F). Thus, relative to the traditional approach, the ABC approach estimates overhead cost to be $11.38 higher than the average $17.50 for an initial visit, and $3.85 and $1.17 lower for a regular and intensive visit, respectively (row 3, columns G, H, and I).

When spread across all 10,000 visits, these unit cost differences result in considerably different estimates of the total cost for each type of visit. Using the $17.50 estimate for overhead costs for each visit, the conventional method estimates the total costs of an initial, regular, and intensive visit to be, respectively, $130,000, $237,500, and $307,500 (row 8, columns A, B, and C). On the other hand, the ABC approach estimates the total cost of initial, regular, and intensive visits to be, respectively, $152,750, $218,250, and $304,000 (row 8, columns D, E, and F). Thus, the ABC approach estimates that the initial visit cost as $22,750 more than what was estimated using a conventional approach and the regular and intensive visits costs as $19,250 and $3,500 less, respectively, than the conventional approach's estimate (row 8, columns G, H, and I). Such differences can be highly significant when making decisions. In the case of the initial visits, the cost estimate differed by more than 17 percent ($22,750/$130,000 = 0.175). Exhibit 12–10 illustrates more closely how the numbers in Exhibit 12–9 were derived.

In Exhibit 12–10, the total overhead cost is $175,000 (row 4, column D). Under the conventional method, it is assumed that all overhead costs are driven by visits. Thus, the $175,000 in overhead is divided by the 10,000 visits made during the year to calculate the average cost per visit for each type of visit, $17.50 (row 4, columns E, F, G, and H).

Rather than assuming that overhead costs are driven solely by the number of visits, the ABC approach assumes multiple cost drivers. In this case, the ABC approach breaks down overhead costs into four categories and looks more closely at what may be driving the $175,000 overhead cost. The four categories are the intake process, medical records, billing, and other (see rows 6 through 9). The intake process occurs when background information is gathered and an account is set up for each new patient. It is assumed that these costs occur each time a new-patient visit occurs; thus, the cost driver is a new-patient visit (row 6, column J). Assuming that the total salaries and benefits of all the employees engaged in this process are $17,500 (row 6, column I)

Exhibit 12-9 A comparison of the results of using a conventional versus an ABC approach to costing three services

Conventional Cost Method
Visit Type

	A Initial	B Regular	C Intensive
Per visit costs			
1 Direct materials (etc.)	$2.50	$3.00	$10.00
2 Direct labor	$45.00	$27.00	$75.00
3 Estimated overhead	$17.50	$17.50	$17.50
4 Total cost / visit	$65.00	$47.50	$102.50
Total visit costs			
5 Direct materials (etc.)	$5,000	$15,000	$30,000
6 Direct labor	$90,000	$135,000	$225,000
7 Estimated overhead	$35,000	$87,500	$52,500
8 Total costs	$130,000	$237,500	$307,500

Activity Based Costing
Visit Type

	D Initial	E Regular	F Intensive
Per visit costs			
1 Direct materials (etc.)	$2.50	$3.00	$10.00
2 Direct labor	$45.00	$27.00	$75.00
3 Estimated overhead	$28.88	$13.65	$16.33
4 Total cost / visit	$76.38	$43.65	$101.33
Total visit costs			
5 Direct materials (etc.)	$5,000	$15,000	$30,000
6 Direct labor	$90,000	$135,000	$225,000
7 Estimated overhead	$57,750	$68,250	$49,000
8 Total costs	$152,750	$218,250	$304,000

Difference in Cost Estimates (ABC – Traditional)
Visit Type

	G Initial	H Regular	I Intensive
Per visit costs			
1 Direct materials (etc.)	$0.00	$0.00	$0.00
2 Direct labor	$0.00	$0.00	$0.00
3 Estimated overhead	$11.38	($3.85)	($1.17)
4 Total cost / visit	$11.38	($3.85)	($1.17)
Total visit costs			
5 Direct materials (etc.)	$0.00	$0.00	$0.00
6 Direct labor	$0.00	$0.00	$0.00
7 Estimated overhead	$22,750	($19,250)	($3,500)
8 Total costs	$22,750	($19,250)	($3,500)

Exhibit 12–10 A comparison of a conventional and an ABC approach to costing three services

Givens: overall percentages and totals

	GA	GB	GC	GD	GE	GF	GG
		Visit Type		Row	Overhead		Annual
	Initial	Regular	Intensive	Total	Total	Total	Hours
Number of visits	20%	50%	30%	100%		10,000	
Number of new visits	80%	10%	10%	100%		2,500	
Direct materials (etc.)	10%	30%	60%	100%		$50,000	
Direct labor	20%	30%	50%	100%		$450,000	
Intake / referral	70%	10%	20%	100%	10%		2,040
Medical records	30%	40%	30%	100%	10%		2,040
Billing	50%	20%	30%	100%	20%		4,080
Other	33%	33%	33%	100%	60%		
Total overhead					100%	$175,000	

	Basic Data: Total Cost by Visit Type				Calculation of Cost / Unit by Visit Type			
	A	B	C	D	E	F	G	H
	Initial	Regular	Intensive	Total				Cost / Unit
	(Given)	(Given)	(Given)	(A+B+C)	Initial	Regular	Intensive	Formula:
1 Number of visits	2,000	5,000	3,000	10,000				
2 Direct materials (etc.)	$5,000	$15,000	$30,000	$50,000	$2.50	$3.00	$10.00	(Row 2 / Row1)
3 Direct labor	$90,000	$135,000	$225,000	$450,000	$45.00	$27.00	$75.00	(Row 3 / Row1)
4 Estimated overhead (total is a given)				$175,000	$17.50	$17.50	$17.50	(D4 / D1)
5 Cost / visit: conventional method					$65.00	$47.50	$102.50	(Sum: Rows 2–4)

Basic data and calculation of unit costs using a conventional approach

Exhibit 12–10 (Continued)

1) Annual projections of overhead costs by activity and cost driver; 2) Unit cost calculations for these overhead activities

Cost and Cost Driver Information

	Activity	I Cost (Given)	J Driver (Given)	K Units (Given)		L Unit Cost (I / K)	
6	Intake	$17,500	New visits	2,500	New visits	$7.00	Per new visit
7	Medical records	$17,500	Hours spent	2,040	Hours	$8.58	Per hour
8	Billing	$35,000	Hours spent	4,080	Hours	$8.58	Per hour
9	Other	$105,000	Visits	10,000	Visits	$10.50	Per visit
10	Total	$175,000					

3) Basic data: actual annual operating results of cost drivers to be used in assigning ABC overhead cost

Visit type

		M Initial (Given)	N Regular (Given)	O Intensive (Given)	P Total (M+N+O)
11	New visits	2,000	250	250	2,500
12	Medical records	612	816	612	2,040
13	Billing	2,040	816	1,224	4,080
14	Other	2,000	5,000	3,000	10,000

Additional basic data

(Continued)

515

Exhibit 12–10   A comparison of a conventional and an ABC approach to costing three services (*Continued*)

Calculation of total and per vist overhead costs using ABC

		Q	R	S	T	U
			Visit Type			
		Initial	Regular	Intensive	Total	Formula
15	New visits	$14,000	$1,750	$1,750	$17,500	(L6 × Row 11)
16	Medical records	$5,250	$7,000	$5,250	$17,500	(L7 × Row 12)
17	Billing	$17,500	$7,000	$10,500	$35,000	(L8 × Row 13)
18	Other	$21,000	$52,500	$31,500	$105,000	(L9 × Row 14)
19	Total	$57,750	$68,250	$49,000	$175,000	(Sum: Rows 15–18)
20	Per visit	$28.88	$13.65	$16.33	$17.50	(Row 19 / Row 1)

Unit cost estimates using ABC

ABC		V	W	X	Y
			Visit Type		
		Initial	Regular	Intensive	Formula
21	Direct materials	$2.50	$3.00	$10.00	(Row 2, Cols. E,F,G)
22	Direct labor	$45.00	$27.00	$75.00	(Row 3, Cols. E,F,G)
23	Overhead	$28.88	$13.65	$16.33	(Row 20)
24	Total using ABC	$76.38	$43.65	$101.33	(Sum: Rows 21–23)

Derivation of unit costs using an ABC approach

Exhibit 12-10 (Continued)

Comparison of unit costs: ABC vs. conventional

		Visit Type			
	Z Initial	AA Regular	AB Intensive	AC	AD Formula
25 Total conventional	$65.00	$47.50	$102.50		(Row 5, Cols. E,F,G)
26 Amount ABC estimate is more (less) than conventional	$11.38	($3.85)	($1.17)		(Row 24 – Row 25)

Comparison of total costs: ABC vs. conventional

		Visit Type		Total	
	AE Initial	AF Regular	AG Intensive	AH (AE+AF+AG)	AI Formula
Activity based costing method					
27 Number of visits	2,000	5,000	3,000	10,000	(Row 1)
28 Direct materials	$5,000	$15,000	$30,000	$50,000	(Row 2)
29 Direct labor	$90,000	$135,000	$225,000	$450,000	(Row 3)
30 Overhead	$57,750	$68,250	$49,000	$175,000	(Row 27 × Row 23)
31 **Total ABC**	$152,750	$218,250	$304,000	$675,000	(Sum: Rows 28–30)
Conventional method					
32 Direct materials	$5,000	$15,000	$30,000	$50,000	(Row 2)
33 Direct labor	$90,000	$135,000	$225,000	$450,000	(Row 3)
34 Overhead	$35,000	$87,500	$52,500	$175,000	(Row 27 × Row 5, E,F,G)
35 **Total conventional**	$130,000	$237,500	$307,500	$675,000	(Sum: Rows 32–34)
36 Amount ABC estimate is more (less) than conventional	**$22,750**	**($19,250)**	**($3,500)**	**$0**	(Row 31 – Row 35)

Comparison of total costs and unit costs: ABC vs. conventional

517

and there are 2,500 visits a year (row 6, column K), the intake process costs the organization $7.00 ($17,500 /$2,500) for each new patient (row 6, column L). Because there were 2,000 new patients making initial visits, 250 new patients each making a regular visit (referrals) and 250 patients making an intensive visit (row 11, columns M, N, O, and P), it costs $14,000 for the intake process for these new patients ($7.00/patient × 2,000 new patients) and $1,750 each ($7.00/patient × 250 patients) for regular and intensive visits, respectively (row 15, columns Q, R, S, T, and U).

The second category, medical records, refers to the process of coding and charting the visit onto the medical records (row 7). Because it is assumed that these costs are driven by the time spent coding and charting, the cost driver is hours spent (row 7, column J). Because the salary and benefit costs associated with medical records are $17,500 and there are 2,040 hours devoted to this activity, the cost per hour is $8.58 (row 7, columns I, J, K, and L). The medical records staff estimates that it spent 30 percent, 40 percent, and 30 percent of its time with initial, regular, and intensive visit records, respectively. This equates to 612, 816, and 612 hours for each of the respective types of visits (row 12, columns M, N, O, and P). At $8.58 per hour, the initial visits medical record cost is $5,250 ($8.58/hour × 612 hours) whereas the regular and intensive visit medical record costs are $7,000 ($8.58/hour × 816 hours) and $5,250 ($8.58/hour × 612 hours), respectively (row 16, columns Q, R, S, T, and U).

The billing costs and other costs are derived in a similar manner to those just discussed. When this process is completed, the estimated total overhead cost of initial visits is $57,750, and those of regular and intensive visits are $68,250 and $49,000, respectively (row 19, columns Q, R, and S). Dividing these numbers by the number of visits in their respective categories (rows 1, 19, and 20) results in the per visit cost estimates of $28.88 ($57,750 / 2,000 visits) for initial visits, $13.65 ($68,250 / 5,000 visits) for regular visits, and $16.33 ($49,000 / 3,000 visits) for intensive visits. As can be seen, these numbers are different from the $17.50 overhead cost per visit estimated using the conventional approach.

The various parts are now in place to compare costs using a conventional approach and an ABC approach. Under the ABC approach, the per visit costs for an initial, regular, and intensive visit, respectively, are $76.38, $43.65, and $101.33 (row 24, columns V, W, and X). Under the conventional method, they are $65.00, $47.50, and $102.50, respectively, for these same types of visits (row 25, columns Z, AA, and AB). Thus, on a comparative basis, the ABC approach estimates that the cost of an initial visit is $11.38 higher than that calculated using the conventional approach, and the costs of a regular and intensive visit are $3.85 and $1.17, respectively, lower (row 26, columns Z, AA, and AB).

The differences between the cost per visit estimates using ABC and a conventional approach are totally due to how the overhead is handled. The conventional approach used a single cost driver, total visits, to derive a $17.50 per visit overhead rate (row 4, columns E, F, and G). As stated above, the ABC approach decomposed overhead into four separate categories of activities. It then determined the unit cost of each type of activity based on what was driving these costs. Thus, the ABC approach more closely matched the actual usage of resources by each type of visit.

The importance of having the more accurate cost estimates from ABC cannot be overemphasized. For example, assume that the practice decided to charge $70.00 per visit for initial visits thinking its costs were $65.00, as derived by the conventional method, but they were really $76.38 (as shown by using ABC). They would be pricing at a loss, when they thought they were making a profit.

 Caution: Though more precise, ABC costs are still average costs. As noted in chapter 9, incremental costs should be used in make/buy-type decisions.

There are a number of other differences between the traditional step-down and ABC methods, but a discussion of these is beyond the scope of this text. However, in many cases these two methods are likely to yield vastly different estimates of cost. Although the step-down method is relatively inexpensive to implement and may provide an adequate estimate in some cases, those using ABC feel it provides several advantages, including increased accuracy and insights on how to control processes and, thus, costs. In the future, the management of most health care facilities will be faced with weighing the relatively low costs of the step-down method against the added costs, greater precision, and cost-control of ABC. In an increasingly cost-driven health care system, it is likely that ABC will gain greater prominence.

SUMMARY

Because they are assuming more risk, providers must be able to measure their costs accurately. Providers generally use one of three approaches: the cost-to-charge ratio, the step-down method, or activity-based costing. The step-down method finds costs by allocating those costs that are not directly paid for into products or services to which payment is attached. It is a top-down approach because it begins with all costs and allocates them downward into various services for which payment will be received. As a result of methodological idiosyncrasies, those performing a step-down cost finding must pay considerable attention to the order of allocation, the allocation basis, and the number of cost centers. The step-down method is useful for pricing and reimbursement-related decisions but should not be used to control costs.

Activity-based costing not only finds costs but also helps to control them. ABC is a bottom-up approach because it finds the cost of each service at the point at which resources are used and then aggregates them upward into products. ABC is based on the paradigm that activities consume resources and processes consume activities. Therefore, because the use of resources is what causes cost (by definition), if activities or processes are controlled, then costs will be controlled. Similarly, if the resource use of an activity can be measured, then a more accurate picture of the actual costs of services can be determined.

KEY TERMS

a. Activity-based costing
b. Allocation base
c. Cost drivers
d. Cost object
e. Cost-to-charge ratio

f. Direct costs
g. Fully allocated costs
h. Indirect costs
i. Step-down method

QUESTIONS AND PROBLEMS

1. **Definitions.** Define the terms above.

2. **Cost-to-charge ratio.** What is the basic concept of the cost-to-charge ratio method of estimating costs? Give an example.

3. **Cost-to-charge ratio.** Discuss the four major concerns of using the cost-to-charge ratio method.

4. **Step-down method.** Discuss how the step-down method of cost allocation derives its name.

5. **Cost allocation and cost drivers.** What is the relationship between the concepts *cost allocation basis* as used in the step-down method and *cost driver* as used in ABC?

6. **Fully allocated costs.** What is the difference between a cost object's direct cost and its fully allocated cost? Give an example.

7. **Step-down method.** Identify and discuss four points that must be considered when using the step-down method of cost allocation.

8. **ABC and step-down methods.** What are the advantages and disadvantages of ABC relative to the step-down method of cost allocation?

9. **Activity-based costing.** In Exhibit 12–10, suppose that instead of 2,000, 5,000, and 3,000 visits for an initial, regular, and intensive visit, respectively, the number of visits was 3,000, 5,000, and 2,000. Assume that the intake, new visits, medical records, and billing costs do not change in number or distribution.

    a. Would there be a change in the overhead cost *per visit* of an initial visit using either the conventional or ABC methods?

    b. Would there be a change in the *total* overhead cost of initial visits using either the conventional or ABC methods?

10. **Activity-based costing.** In Exhibit 12–10, suppose that instead of 2,000, 5,000, and 3,000 visits for an initial, regular, and intensive visit, respectively, the number of visits was 2,500, 6,000, and 1,500. Assume that the intake, new visits, medical records, and billing costs do not change in number or distribution.

a. Would there be a change in the overhead cost *per visit* of an initial visit using either the conventional or ABC methods?

b. Would there be a change in the *total* overhead cost of initial visits using either the conventional or ABC methods?

11. **Cost allocation.** Use the information in Exhibit 12–11 to answer these questions.

a. David Paul, the new administrator for the surgical clinic, was trying to figure out how to allocate his indirect expenses. His staff was complaining that the current method of taking a percentage of revenues was unfair. He decided to try to allocate utilities based on square footage for each department, to allocate administration based on direct costs, and to allocate laboratory based on tests. What would the results be?

b. Kathleen Aceti, the nurse manager of the cystoscopy suite, was given approval to add more space to her current area by converting 500 square feet of administrative space into another cystoscopy bay. What will her new fully allocated expenses be? (Assume that there are no new additional costs incurred by adding the 500 square feet.)

c. Mara Kelsey, the manager of the endoscopy suite, was concerned about adding more space. She contends that if the two units were combined, fewer staff would be needed, and direct costs could be reduced by $50,000 ($25,000 in each unit). She also feels that the Day-Op area is underutilized, and that 500 square feet could be used by a combined unit when excess capacity was needed. Assuming that the 500 square feet was to be allocated equally between the endoscopy and cystoscopy suites, what would the total allocated costs for each of these two services be under this scenario?

12. **Cost Allocation.** Use the information in Exhibit 12–12 to answer these questions.

a. David Paul, the new administrator for the surgical clinic, was trying to figure out how to allocate his indirect expenses. He decided to try to allocate utilities based on square footage of each department, to allocate administration based on direct costs, and to allocate laboratory based on tests. How would indirect costs be distributed as a result?

b. Nick Zeeman, the director of laboratories, was given approval to add 250 square feet of space to the lab by expanding into the Day-Op suite, which lost the space. What will his new fully allocated expenses be? (Assume that there are no new additional costs incurred by adding the 250 square feet.)

c. Callie Zev, the manager of the endoscopy suite, was concerned about adding more space to cystoscopy. She contends that if the two units were combined, fewer staff would be needed, and direct costs could be reduced by $40,000 ($20,000 in each unit). She also feels that the Day-Op area is underutilized

Exhibit 12–11 Basic statistics for cost allocation in a surgery clinic used in Problem 11

	A Square Feet	B Direct Costs	C Lab Tests
Utilities		$200,000	
Administration	2,000	$500,000	
Laboratory	2,000	$625,000	
Day-Op suite	3,000	$1,400,000	4,000
Cystoscopy	1,500	$350,000	500
Endoscopy	1,500	$300,000	500
Total	10,000	$3,375,000	5,000

Exhibit 12–12 Basic statistics for cost allocation in a surgery clinic used in Problem 12

	Square Feet	Direct Costs	Lab Tests
Utilities		$100,000	
Administration	1,500	$400,000	
Laboratory	3,000	$725,000	
Day-Op suite	4,500	$1,200,000	4,000
Cystoscopy	2,500	$400,000	500
Endoscopy	3,000	$350,000	500
Total	14,500	$3,175,000	5,000

and that 200 square feet could be used by a combined unit when excess capacity was needed. Assuming that the 200 square feet were to be allocated equally between the endoscopy and cystoscopy suites, what would the total allocated costs for each of these two services be under this scenario?

13. **Traditional and activity-based costing.** Use the information in Exhibit 12–13 to answer these questions.

a. What is the *per unit* cost of an initial, regular, and intensive visit using the conventional and ABC approaches?

b. What is the *total cost* of initial, regular, and intensive visits using the conventional and ABC approaches?

Exhibit 12–13 Data for cost allocation in Problem 13

Total Cost by Visit Type

Basic Data

		A Initial Given	B Regular Given	C Intensive Given	D Total A+B+C
1	Number of visits	5,000	10,000	5,000	20,000
2	Direct materials (etc.)	$21,000	$14,000	$35,000	$70,000
3	Direct labor	$80,000	$80,000	$240,000	$400,000
4	Estimated overhead [total is a given]				$150,000
5	Cost/visit: conventional method				

1) Basic data: annual projections of overhead costs by activity

Cost Driver Information

	Activity	I Cost Given	J Driver Given	K Units Given	
6	Intake	$22,500	New Visits	2,500	New visits
7	Medical records	$22,500	Time Spent	2,040	Hours
8	Billing	$45,000	Time Spent	4,080	Hours
9	Other	$60,000	Visits	20,000	Visits
10	Total	$150,000			

2) Basic data: actual annual operating results of cost drivers to be used to assign abc overhead cost

Visit Type

		M Initial Given	N Regular Given	O Intensive Given	P Total M+N+O
11	New visits	1,500	750	250	2,500
12	Medical records	204	612	1,224	2,040
13	Billing	2,040	816	1,224	4,080
14	Other	5,000	10,000	5,000	20,000

Exhibit 12–14 Data for cost allocation in Problem 14

Basic data and calculation of unit costs using a conventional approach

Total Cost by Visit Type

	A	B	C	D
		Basic data		
	Initial	Regular	Intensive	Total
	Given	Given	Given	A+B+C
1 Number of visits	3,000	7,500	4,500	15,000
2 Direct materials (etc.)	$5,000	$10,000	$35,000	$50,000
3 Direct labor	$52,500	$70,000	$227,500	$350,000
4 Estimated overhead total is a given				$125,000
5 Cost / visit: conventional method				

Additional basic data

1) Basic data: annual projections of overhead costs by activity

Cost Driver Information

	I	J	K	
Activity	Cost	Driver	Units	
	Given	Given	Given	
6 Intake	$25,000	New visits	1,000	New visits
7 Medical records	$25,000	Time spent	2,040	Hours
8 Billing	$37,500	Time spent	4,080	Hours
9 Other	$37,500	Visits	15,000	Visits
10 Total	$125,000			

2) Basic data: actual annual operating results of cost drivers to be used to assign ABC overhead cost

Visit Type

	M	N	O	P
	Initial	Regular	Intensive	Total
	Given	Given	Given	M+N+O
11 New visits	800	100	100	1,000
12 Medical records	612	816	612	2,040
13 Billing	2,040	816	1,224	4,080
14 Other	3,000	7,500	4,500	15,000

14. **Traditional and activity-based costing.** Use the information in Exhibit 12–14 to answer these questions.

    a. What is the *per unit* cost of an initial, regular, and intensive visit using the conventional and ABC approaches?

    b. What is the total cost of initial, regular, and intensive visits using the conventional and ABC approaches?

13

PROVIDER PAYMENT SYSTEMS

LEARNING OBJECTIVES

- Identify the history, theory, and characteristics of the major types of payment systems
- Identify the tactics payors and providers use to reduce their financial risk
- Determine the cost per member per month for specific procedures
- Understand the new wave of innovations in health care payment systems

This chapter provides an introduction to the development of the *health care payment system* in the United States and some of the basic methods used to determine health care payments. The evolution of the payment system will be emphasized in light of the ongoing public policy debate about the roles, responsibilities, and effects of the payment system on various stakeholders, including:

- Patients
- Providers—including physicians, institutional providers, and ancillary providers (e.g., physical therapists, laboratories, hospices, and home care providers)
- Employers
- Payor—including various levels of government agencies and managed care organizations
- Regulators—including governmental and private agencies (e.g., the Joint Commission on Accreditation of Healthcare Organizations and the National Committee for Quality Assurance)

Simply put, this debate has been over "Who gets paid?" "How much?" "By whom?" "For what types of services?" and "With what consequence?"

All health care systems attempt to balance cost, quality, and access. Over the years, each of these three facets has received more or less emphasis in the U.S. health care system as various stakeholders have asked and attempted to answer such questions as: "For the cost, are we getting sufficient quality and access?" (see Perspective 13–1) and "What would it cost to provide better quality care to the uninsured and underinsured?" Although this debate continues, it largely focuses on the roles of governmental entities, *payors*, and providers, not individual consumers (see Exhibit 13-1). Meanwhile, health care providers are on the front line every day, trying to balance their missions and their margins, walking a fine line between the art of healing, the science of medicine, and the business of health care.

Payor
An entity that is responsible for paying for the services of a health care provider; typically this is an insurance company or a government agency.

 Key Point   *By convention, the terms* payor *and* payer *are used interchangeably.*

To truly understand the current health care payment system, it is important to have insight into how it has evolved (see Exhibit 13–2).

Before the late 1920s and early 1930s, health care was funded primarily by patients. The growth of the country's population, however, brought additional costs in the form of more doctors and more health care facilities. The burden of paying for health care shifted to employers and later to government. A summary of key events in this evolution follows, ending with some future trends.

Exhibit 13–1   Key elements in the debate undergirding the U.S. health care payment system

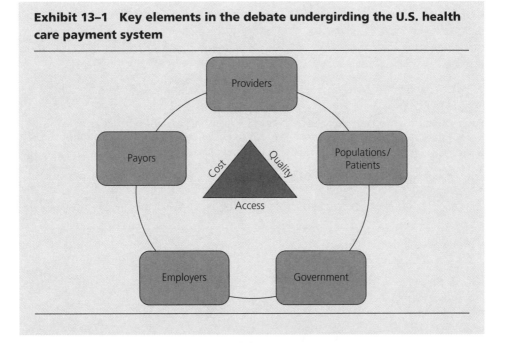

Perspective 13–1   How Does the United States Rank in Health Care Quality and Access?

In comparing the U.S. health care system with those of five other developed countries—Australia, Canada, Germany, New Zealand, the United Kingdom—the U.S. health care system ranks last or next-to-last on five dimensions of a high-performance health system: quality, access, efficiency, equity, and healthy lives. The United States does rank first on provision and receipt of preventive care; however, it has low scores on chronic care management and safe, coordinated, and patient-centered care. The reason why other countries have higher scores is because they are further along than the United States in using information technology and a team approach to manage chronic conditions and coordinate care. Information systems in countries like Germany, New Zealand, and the United Kingdom enhance the ability of physicians to identify and monitor patients with chronic conditions. A lack of universal health insurance coverage may be a contributing factor behind the United States' poor performance on access. However, it spends over $6,100 per capita, whereas Great Britain and New Zealand spend $2,500 and $2,080 per capita, respectively.

Source: Davis, K., Schoen, C., Schoenbaum, S. C., Doty, M. M., Holmgren, A. L., Kriss, J. L., and Shea, K. K. 2007 (May 15). Mirror, mirror on the wall: an international update on the comparative performance of American health care. *Commonwealth Fund*, vol. 59.

Caution: The topic of payment system-related issues in the United States is extremely complicated and ever-changing, and this chapter provides only a basic introduction. The following sites are recommended for more details and updates:

- The Centers for Medicare and Medicaid Services: http://www.cms.hhs.gov/default.asp?
- Agency for Healthcare Research and Quality: http://www.ahrq.gov
- The Kaiser Family Foundations: http://www.kff.org
- PriceWaterhouseCoopers: Health Research Institute: http://healthcare.pwc.com
- Medpac: http://www.medpac.gov/
- American Health Systems Annual Survey: http://www.aha.org/aha/research-and-trends/health-and-hospital-trends/2007.html (updated annually)

Exhibit 13–2   Key events in the evolution of the health care payment system in the United States

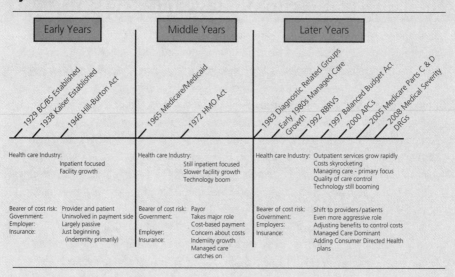

THE EARLY YEARS OF PAYMENT SYSTEM, 1929 TO 1964

Defining events	Industry trends
• BC/BS established 1929 • Kaiser established 1930s • Hill-Burton hospital construction act 1946	• Advent of indemnity insurance • Rapid growth of hospitals (inpatient focus) • Employers largely passive

The payment system during this period was largely a combination of *charge-based, fee-for-service,* and *employer-based indemnity insurance.* Typically, regardless of the extent of employer involvement in the payment for health services (whether the employer paid a portion, all, or none of the charges for the services), the provider was the *price-setter.* Despite the massive amount of government funding created for facility development, there was relatively little federal or state government involvement as payors.

Charge-Based
A method of payment that is based on the charge of the provider.

Blue Cross and Blue Shield Established

In 1929, Justin Ford Kimball, an official at Baylor University in Dallas, introduced a plan to guarantee schoolteachers twenty-one days of hospital care for $6 per year. Other groups of employees in the area soon joined the plan, known as the Baylor Plan, and the idea attracted national attention. By 1939 the Blue Cross symbol was officially adopted by a commission of the American Hospital Association (AHA) as the national emblem for plans like the Baylor Plan that met certain guidelines.

Fee-for-Service
A method of reimbursement based on payment for services rendered, with a specific fee correlated to each specific service. An insurance company, the patient, or a government program such as Medicare or Medicaid (discussed later) may make payment.

 Key Point *A detailed history of Blue Cross-Blue Shield can be found at:*
http://www.bcbs.com/about/history

Blue Cross and Blue Shield (BC-BS) plans were attractive to both consumers and providers. They guaranteed that payment would be made for covered services (such as twenty-one days in the hospital). All covered individuals paid their *premium* based on a *community rating,* and payment was made directly to the hospital. In terms common today: a *third party* (the payor, BC-BS in this case) would pay *the second party* (the provider, hospitals in this case) on behalf of *the first party* (the patient).

As a result of wage freezes (due primarily to the United States' involvement in World War II), labor forces resorted to bargaining for

Indemnity Insurance
A plan that reimburses physicians for services performed or beneficiaries for medical expenses incurred. Typically, the employer, patient, or both pay a monthly premium to the plan for a predetermined set of health care benefits.

Price Setter
The entity that controls the amount paid for a health care service.

Premium
A monthly payment made by a person, an employer, or both to an insurer that makes one eligible for a defined level of health care for a given period of time.

Community Rating
A rating method used by indemnity and HMO insurers that guarantees that there will be equivalent amounts collected from members of a specific group without regard to demographics such as age, sex, size of covered group, and industry type.

The First Party
Typically, the patient in a health care encounter.

The Second Party
Typically, the provider (hospital or physician) in a health care encounter.

The Third Party
Typically, the payor (insurance company or government agency) in a health care encounter.

more benefits, including better health care coverage. It was at this time that private, for-profit, insurance companies began to be major competitors with BC-BS plans. It was during this period (the late 1930s) that the Kaiser Health Plan began. The Kaiser Engineering Company provided a health care benefit for its employees who were involved in the construction of the Grand Coulee Dam and the Los Angeles Aqueduct by providing physician services in a company-sponsored clinic and hospital services at local hospitals.

Along with the existence of few other prepaid health care plans, the Kaiser plan grew throughout the 1940s and 1950s, expanding beyond the realm of its own employees and becoming the prototypical staff model *health maintenance organization*. In the Kaiser plan, physicians were salaried, patients received care in a controlled environment, and all services (except hospital services) were provided in a single facility. HMOs are addressed in greater detail later in this chapter.

With the population boom after World War II, and with the continued industrialization of the United States, a great need arose for the development of adequate health care facilities—in particular, hospital beds and support facilities. The Hill-Burton Act of 1946 provided government-supported grants to build and upgrade hospitals.

Before 1946, the U.S hospital system had evolved with great disparities in facilities and accessibility. With about one-third of the country's counties without a hospital and many of the existing facilities of substandard quality, the intent of this legislation was to fund development in geographic areas that were without health care facilities. During the period between 1947 and 1975 (the end of Hill-Burton expenditures), almost seven thousand hospitals received assistance, with many rural areas gaining access to hospital care for the first time.

THE MIDDLE YEARS OF PAYMENT SYSTEM, 1965 TO 1983

Defining Events	Industry Trends
• Medicare/Medicaid established • HMO Act	• Indemnity insurance growth • Managed care catching on • Technology boom on the horizon • Cost risk shifts to payor • Employers concerned about costs

During the middle years, governments became heavily involved as payors through two new programs (Medicare and Medicaid), employers played a relatively passive role, there was a trend toward trying to manage care, and a movement away from the provider as a price-setter.

Because of the influence of the government as a payor, the late 1960s and 1970s represented a plateau in the evolution of payment systems. Medical costs, while still rising during this period, were relatively manageable. Although employers were concerned about cost, they continued to pay for rich health care benefits. Technology was beginning to boom but had not yet advanced to the point where it materially affected the cost of providing or paying for services. Indemnity insurance dominated, and providers were generally satisfied with the payment systems employed during this time. For the most part, payment systems revolved around cost-based and charge-based methods, an overview of which can be found in Appendix H.

Increasing Concerns about Costs and Access

Although the Hill-Burton Act improved access by catalyzing the construction of new hospitals, paying for the care provided at these new and improved facilities (and new technology associated with them) was becoming increasingly expensive. While being employed was one way to access health care coverage, there was a growing concern about the ability to pay for care by the unemployed, the underinsured (perhaps self-employed or employed by an employer not offering an insurance benefit, for example), the poor, the young, the elderly, and the disabled. Thus, much of the national debate focused on the issue of access to care.

Medicare and Medicaid

The government's role in the payment of health care, which to this point had been passive (both on a federal and a state-specific basis), changed dramatically in the mid-1960s with President Lyndon Johnson's administration. The formation of a "Medical Care" Program (Medicare), established largely to help pay for care of those aged sixty-five years and older, and the creation of a companion "Medical Aid" program (Medicaid), designed to provide assistance to the medically indigent and those with certain categories of disabilities, marked the beginning of a new era in U.S. health care (see Exhibit 13–3).

CMS
The Center for Medicare and Medicaid Services. The acronym is pronounced: "sims." See *HCFA*.

The governmental department that now oversees Medicare and Medicaid is known as the *Center for Medicare and Medicaid Services (CMS)*. Until 2001, it was called the Health Care Financing Administration or *HCFA*.

Key Point *History of Medicare: Much of our current payment system is driven by the government's role in the payment system. A more detailed history can be found on the CMS site at: http://www.cms.hhs.gov/history.*

Exhibit 13–3 Medicare and Medicaid entitlement programs

	Medicare	Medicaid
Who pays for program?	Federal tax on income	Federal and state tax on income (Feds pay larger share based on state's per capita income)
Who is covered?	People aged 65 and older Some people with disabilities under age 65 People with end-stage renal disease	People with disabilities The poor Needy women and children
How many are covered?	1980: 28.5 million 1990: 34.2 million 2000: 39 million 2007: 41 million 2025: 62 million (projected)	1981: 20.2 million 1990: 23.9 million 2000: 33.6 million 2005: 45.6 million
Expenditures	1980: $36 billion 1990: $108 billion 2000: $221 billion 2007: $431 billion	1980: $24.7 billion 1990: $71.2 billion 2000: $205 billion 2006: $314 billion

Source: Kaiser Family Foundation Web page: http.www.kff.org, Medicaid Data Sources: http://www.cms.hhs.gov/MedicaidDataSourcesGenInfo/Downloads/mmcer06.pdf, and Medicare: http://www.cms.hhs.gov/MedicareEnRpts/Downloads/Trends00-04.pdf.

HCFA
The Health Care Financing Administration: The U.S. government's department that oversaw the provision of and payment for health care provided under its entitlement programs (Medicare, Medicaid) until 2001.

At its inception, Medicare paid hospitals based on the hospital's costs, using *cost-based reimbursement* paid on a *retrospective* basis. At the end of a period after care was provided (typically, at the end of a year), the hospital would submit a report, the *Medicare Cost Report*, detailing all of the costs associated with the provision of Medicare services throughout that period. The government, in turn, would scrutinize the costs being claimed and would allow or disallow costs on the basis of standards.

Also during this period, the HMO Act of 1972 was passed under the administration of President Richard Nixon. This had a major impact on *managing care* in later years by empowering the staff model HMO (discussed later) to become a common system practiced outside of the mainstream medical society. The act allowed certain competitive advantages for qualifying HMOs, but these generally languished and became more interested in cost containment.

THE LATER YEARS OF PAYMENT SYSTEM, 1984 TO PRESENT

Defining Events	Industry Trends
• Diagnosis Related Groups	• Managed care is dominant theme
• RBRVS	• Government taking more aggressive role
• Balanced Budget Act of 1997	• Flat fee payment systems for all providers of care
• APCs	• Costs shift back to provider
• Medicare Modernization Act of 2003	• Technology booming
• Pay for Performance (P4P)	• Employers adjusting benefits to control costs
• Medicare –Severity DRGs	• Consumer initiatives (Health Savings Account)

Health care infrastructure and technology grew exponentially over the early and middle years of the modern health care era. Programs such as *Medicare* and *Medicaid*, which were originally designed to fill relatively small gaps in access, felt the brunt of this growth. Because of this, the government was experiencing unexpected difficulties trying to pay for the benefits it had created. Under the Balanced Budget Act of 1997 (BBA 1997), Congress made drastic cuts to Medicare inpatient payments and gave its beneficiaries the option to receive care through a private health plan. Employers as well were growing increasingly concerned about cost containment as health care costs and employee health benefits began to eat into corporate profits. Other payors were also experiencing difficulties in matching the premiums they were receiving with the payments they were making to providers. This set the stage for a change of the locus of risk from payors to providers. As the economy improved in the late 1990s, corporations improved their benefits to employees and allowed insurers to provide less restrictive forms of care. In 2003 Congress passed the Medicare Modernization Act, which allowed prescription drug coverage to its beneficiaries, known as Medicare Part D. In addition, the law enhanced the compensation for health plans that allowed Medicare beneficiaries the option to enroll in a private health plan instead of the traditional fee-for-service Medicare program. These health plans were called Medicare Advantage (MA) plans and offered more benefits than the traditional Medicare program, known as Medicare Part C. These Medicare health plans were being paid 13 percent more than regular coverage, and as of 2008, Congress was considering legislation to reduce their payments.

Medicare
A nationwide, federally financed health insurance program for people aged sixty-five and older. It also covers certain people younger than sixty-five who are disabled or have chronic kidney (end-stage renal) disease. Medicare Part A is the hospital inpatient insurance program; Part B covers physician and outpatient services. Part C allows beneficiaries to receive benefits through private health plans, and Part D covers prescription drug benefit plans.

Medicaid
A federally mandated program operated and partially funded by individual states (in conjunction with the federal government) to provide medical benefits to certain low-income people. The state, under broad federal guidelines, determines what benefits are covered, who is eligible, and how much providers will be paid.

Prospective Payment System
A payment method that establishes rates, prices, or budgets before services are rendered and costs are incurred. Providers retain or absorb at least a portion of the difference between established revenues and actual costs.

Cost-Based Reimbursement
Using the provider's cost of providing services (i.e., supplies, staff salaries, space costs, etc.) as the basis for reimbursement.

Retrospective Payment
Method for reimbursing a provider after the service has been delivered.

Managed Care
Any of a number of arrangements designed to control health care costs through monitoring, prescribing, or proscribing the provision of health care to a patient or population.

Diagnosis-Related Groups

It was at this point that the government changed its reimbursement method for Medicare from a cost-based payment system to a *prospective payment system*, commonly known as the diagnosis-related groups (DRG) system. Prospective payment shifts the risk from payor to provider. In this system, the provider is paid a predetermined flat amount for an inpatient admission. If the provider's costs are below that flat amount, the hospital retains the difference. However, they are at risk for the amount of their costs to exceed the payment they receive. Therefore, it becomes extremely important for the hospital to understand and control its costs while maintaining appropriate levels of access and quality.

Under DRGs, the government's payment to providers of inpatient services for Medicare recipients is based on a *flat rate* (see below) for all services rendered in each of the diagnosis-based categories. Each DRG serves to group clinically similar services in a way that accounts for predicted resource consumption. Each of these predetermined groupings is then assigned a DRG payment. DRGs were initially intended to account for case mix, or the acuity of services required in caring for a patient. For example, an inpatient stay involving neurosurgery and an intensive care recovery will be paid a higher rate than one involving a normal obstetric delivery. However, in fiscal year 2008, CMS replaced 538 DRGs with 745 new Medicare Severity-adjusted DRGs (MS-DRGs). The purpose of this adjustment was to develop a more equitable payment system with respect to the condition of the patient and to avoid incentives to select healthier patients whose medical condition did not warrant a higher payment. The MS-DRG system revamps and expands the list of complications and comorbidities to include major illnesses that utilize more resources. It also requires quality reporting and will no longer pay for the cost of certain preventable conditions.

The Medicare inpatient payment is derived by a series of adjustments to a standard base payment rate. For fiscal year 2008, the operating base rate was $4,964. This base rate is adjusted by a wage index to account for geographic differences in labor costs. For qualifying hospitals, other adjustments such as disproportionate share for treating low-income patients and for medical education can also be made to the payment. Medicare assigns a weight for each of the 745 DRGs to account for the cost of a case compared with the average costs of all cases. For example, a relatively simple procedure or diagnosis, a medical stay driven by a skin disorder might be slightly lower, at 1.75, and a heart transplant requiring extensive resources might be weighted at 23.67 (see Exhibit 13–4). A hospital's payment is unaffected by the length of stay; it is expected that some patients will stay longer than others, and hospitals will offset the higher costs of a longer stay with the lower costs of a reduced stay. CMS annually updates both the DRG weights and the geographic adjustments.

Exhibit 13–4   Examples of diagnosis-related groups

DRG	Description	Relative Weight	Geographic Adjustment[a]	Average Payment per Weighted Unit	Total DRG Payment
592	Skin ulcers with MCC[b]	1.7515	0.97	$4,964	$8,434
175	Pulmonary embolism with MCC[b]	1.5796	0.97	$4,964	$7,606
1	Heart transplant	23.6701	0.97	$4,964	$113,973

[a] Geographic adjustment varies by area.
[b] MCC = major complications and comorbidity
Source: CMS Web page http://www.cms.hhs.gov/AcuteInpatientPPS/

Flat Fee Systems

These efforts by the government defined the third era of payment systems: "the later years" and the entry of many payors into the world of flat fee payment that were part of payer contracts to hospitals as well as physician practices and outpatient care centers. These fixed payment rates are discussed below for each provider type.

Flat Fees for Hospitals *Flat fee* systems in general pay a predefined amount for a unit of service. The fee may be established by the payor alone or as a result of negotiations between the payor and provider. As with cost-based systems, the units of service paid for vary widely and include the following:

- Per procedure
- Per inpatient day
- Per admission
- Per discharge
- Per diagnosis

By paying a flat fee, the payor is limiting its liability. By accepting a flat fee, the provider is accepting the risk that it can offer the service for less than the payment. If a provider cannot offer a service for less than it is paid, it has several alternatives: absorb the cost, transfer the cost to another payor, improve efficiency, or drop the service (or all of these).

Flat Fee: A predefined amount of money paid to a provider for a unit of service.

DRGs
A patient classification scheme used by Medicare that clusters patients into categories on the basis of patients' illnesses, diseases, and medical problems. These classifications are then used to pay providers a set amount based on the diagnosis-related group in which the patient has been classified.

MS-DRGs
Medicare severity-adjusted DRGs; CMS's DRG-based payment system that replaced the DRG payment system. It was designed to better correlate payments with patient severity.

RBRVS
Resource-based relative value system, a system of paying physicians based on the relative value of the services rendered.

RVU
Relative value unit.

Flat Fees for Physicians For professional (i.e., physician) services, the corresponding system is the resource-based relative value system *(RBRVS)*, which was developed by the government in 1992. This system assigns a relative value to every one of more than seven thousand professional services (including pathology-laboratory and radiology) and establishes a flat fee for those services based on their relative weight compared with a standard relative value unit *(RVU)* of 1.00.

RBRVS *Two helpful discussions of RBRVS can be found at the site for the American Medical Association: http://www.ama-assn.org/ama/pub/category/16391.html and the American Academy of Pediatrics: http://www.aap.org/visit/codingrbrvs.htm*

MS-DRGs *To find out more about MS-DRGs, see the CMS Web site http://www.cms.hhs.gov/apps/media/fact_sheets.asp and type in the keyword box "inpatient payment 2009" which will provide information about: "Medicare Policy Changes for the Fiscal Year (FY) 2009 Hospital Inpatient Prospective Payment System."*

Flat Fees for Outpatient Care The ambulatory payment classification (APC) system is an outpatient prospective payment system that was implemented in 2000 by the government in accordance with the Balanced Budget Act of 1997. This legislation was enacted to reduce and stabilize the amount of reimbursement hospitals receive for outpatient care and to shift the financial risk of care to the hospital. The development of this system came in response to the exponential growth of the cost and the volume of outpatient medicine. With the stringent DRGs in place and improved technology that could not have been fully anticipated, an unexpected result was that hospitals converted many procedures from inpatient to outpatient (including free-standing ambulatory surgical centers).

Key Point *For additional information regarding APCs, go to http://www.cms.hhs.gov/hospitaloutpatientPPS*

As seen in Exhibit 13–5, more patients are receiving their care on an outpatient basis than with hospital admission. It was this rise in outpatient visits, driving up outpatient expenses, that resulted in the development and implementation of the *APCs*. Although APCs primarily apply to hospital outpatient services, they have no relationship with professional fees to physicians.

Exhibit 13-5   Cumulative change in the percentage increase in hospital admissions and outpatient visits, 1998–2006

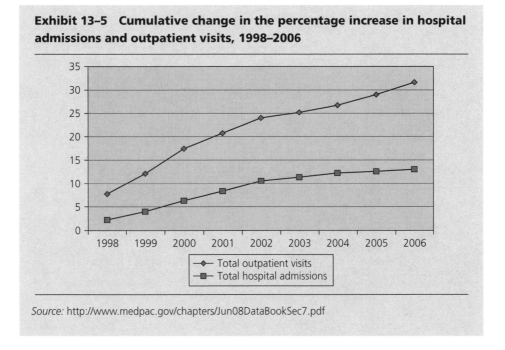

Source: http://www.medpac.gov/chapters/Jun08DataBookSec7.pdf

The total number of APCs is over 800. Each APC represents a bundle of services that are similar in clinical intensity, resource utilization, and cost. APC payments apply to outpatient surgery, outpatient clinics, emergency department services, and observation services. APC payments also account for services related to outpatient testing (such as radiology, nuclear medicine imaging) and therapies (such as certain drugs, intravenous infusion therapies, and blood products). The payment is determined by multiplying a standard conversion factor, which is adjusted for labor wage differences, across geographic locations by the relative weight assigned to the APC. The relative weight measures the resources consumed in providing the specific service and is based on the median cost for the service. For example, APC 332, which is for a CT scan of the brain, has a relative weight of 3.04. Multiplying the conversion factor of $63.39 by 3.04 yields a final payment for this service of $193.96.

APC
A fixed-fee payment system instituted by CMS to shift the financial risk of care to the provider in the provision of outpatient services to Medicare recipients. APCs primarily apply to hospital outpatient services.

As a safety measure, Medicare created an additional formula designed to guarantee slow growth in APC reimbursement levels. On a going-forward basis, it was determined that the APCs would be increased annually by a percentage that would be 1 percent less than the medical cost inflation factor specific to outpatient services. As an example, if the overall medical cost index for all services related to outpatient care was 4.5 percent, then the APCs would be adjusted by 3.5 percent.

Other Payors Follow Suit Health care was so expensive that domestic employers complained they were spending a disproportionate amount on health care compared

Exhibit 13–6   National healthcare expenditures as a percent of GDP, 2000 to 2017 estimated

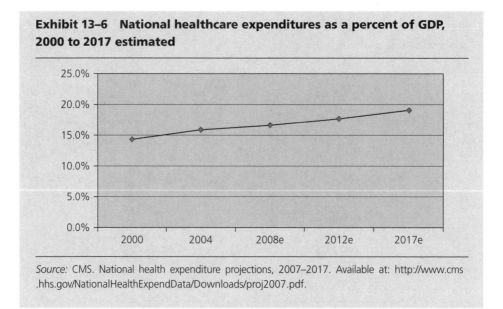

Source: CMS. National health expenditure projections, 2007–2017. Available at: http://www.cms .hhs.gov/NationalHealthExpendData/Downloads/proj2007.pdf.

with their peer employers in other nations. Many U.S. companies found it difficult to compete when the cost of their products had to be artificially inflated to cover the monies spent on health care. In 2004, health care expenditures were 15.9 percent of the gross domestic product (GDP) and are projected to grow to 19.6 percent of GDP by 2017 (see Exhibit 13–6).

Although some employers tried to organize in coalitions to leverage their buying power and gain economies of scale in health care purchasing, this movement never caught on nationally. The overall complaint against the fee-for-service medicine facing employers was that service providers have inherent incentives to perform more surgeries, hold patients in the hospital longer, and (arguably) even provide services that are not medically necessary.

Following the lead of the government and its cost-containment efforts, its use of prospective payment on both inpatient and outpatient services, many commercial payors adopted the same methodologies. Again, the use of these methods limited the ability of the provider to a set dollar amount per inpatient stay or outpatient case. The use of prospective payment also provided greater predictability of medical expenditures for payors.

MANAGED CARE AND RISK SHARING

During this period, the changing dynamic between payors and providers was driven by a desire to shift the financial risk from the payors (who traditionally held it) to the providers. The payment methods became increasingly creative and complex as payors and providers became focused on "managing care" and cost-containment. This managed care concept created an entire industry devoted to controlling the expenditure of health care dollars.

A number of managed care organizations were publicly traded, and earnings pressures from Wall Street and demands from employers to keep fees under control drove many managed care organizations to walk a fine line between an overriding concern for patient "member" care and the larger issues of profit and loss. America developed a love-hate relationship with managed care organizations. When President Bill Clinton proposed a radical overhaul of the U.S. health care system through a government-led "managed competition" system, there was a strong reaction to limit government involvement from a broad range of stakeholders in the health care system, including employers, employees, providers, and managed care companies. By the mid-1990s managed care, which had held considerable promise for controlling costs while maintaining quality, became fixed in the public's mind as a system that limited the quality of and access to care for the sake of financial gain.

Despite all of the public outcry against restriction of provider choice and access, and for all of the public distaste for some of the stringent medical management mechanisms that came into being, the fact is that in the early 1990s, medical costs plateaued in the United States for the first time in many years. However, improvement in the economy and the pressure to retain workers forced employers to negotiate less restrictive managed care plans. Under these plans, employees no longer required prior approval by their primary care physician to directly access specialists. However, by early 2000, employers had to pay higher premiums to implement these less restrictive health plans (see Perspective 13–2). By 2008, many employees were faced with considerably higher copayments and deductibles, if they were covered by their employer at all.

Perspective 13–2   Rising Private Health Insurance Premiums and the Effects on Wage Increases for Employees

Private health insurance premiums experienced a dramatic decline in the 1990s as a result of restrictive managed care plans. However, employee pushback resulted in more open access to providers, and as a result, employers were paying a higher premium. From 1999 to 2008, cumulative healthcare premiums rose by 119% while the growth in workers wages grew cumulatively over the same period by only 34%. This outcome suggests that employers are forgoing wage increases to pay for these higher health insurance premiums.

Source: Kaiser Family Foundation. 2009 (March). Trends and Costs in Health Care Spending. Available at: http://www.kff.org/insurance/

Overview of Managed Care

The predominance of managed care in the later years catalyzed the evolution of many payment schemes. The term *managed care* is often used as if it were referring to a specific type of care and payment arrangement. In fact, the term is used to describe a wide variety of options, with HMOs, preferred provider organizations *(PPOs)*, and point of service (POS) plans being the three dominant managed care models. They are arranged in Exhibit 13–7 according to the degree that they manage the care-giving process and share risks between payors and providers and are discussed in turn below.

Perhaps the easiest way to understand the structures and payment methods of managed care is to contrast them with typical fee-for-service models of care. As discussed previously, the fee-for-service arrangement is most commonly characterized by independent providers who are paid "reasonable charges" for providing "necessary" services to patients who make an unrestricted choice to go to them.

PPOs The PPO is a network of independent providers approved in advance by the payor to provide a specific service or range of services at *predetermined* (usually discounted) *rates*. It is based on some restriction of access and utilization in return for a discount.

HMOs *HMO* is a term used to describe a specific type of company or insurer that offers medical care to a covered population. There are two general types of HMOs: the *group model HMO* (consisting of a loose affiliation of providers that acts as an entity and contracts to cover the health care needs of a covered population) and a *staff model HMO* (whereby the providers are actually employed by the HMO) where patients receive care in controlled or owned facilities (e.g., Kaiser Permanente plans).

Predetermined Rates
A set fee paid to a provider for an inpatient episode of care.

Health Maintenance Organization (HMO)
A legal corporation that offers health insurance and medical care. HMOs typically offer a range of health care services at a fixed price. Two types of HMOs are staff model and group model.

Staff Model HMO
An HMO that owns its clinics and employs its doctors.

Group Model HMO
An HMO that contracts with medical groups for services.

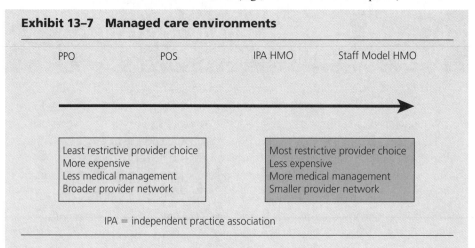

Exhibit 13–7   Managed care environments

PPO   POS   IPA HMO   Staff Model HMO

Least restrictive provider choice
More expensive
Less medical management
Broader provider network

Most restrictive provider choice
Less expensive
More medical management
Smaller provider network

IPA = independent practice association

POS A *POS* arrangement is a hybrid between an HMO and a PPO. Although patients are encouraged to see *participating providers* to receive their most financially favorable benefit, at the point of service, they may see a nonparticipating provider, though usually at some additional cost or reduced benefit.

Methods of Managed Care Payments

The following methods of payment are used in various ways by the entities described above to help manage care and share risk.

Steerage

Steerage is one of a variety of straightforward, market-driven techniques designed to increase or maintain market share. To increase volume (and thus reduce fixed costs per unit), providers give payors a discount in exchange for the payors' agreeing to employ mechanisms that direct patients to the participating provider. An example of steerage is the "center of excellence" designation used by insurers. Typically in this situation, a provider has distinguished itself as a high-quality provider of one or more services. This is most often accomplished by meeting or exceeding predetermined criteria established by a payor. Once a provider is chosen as a "center of excellence" by a payor, the payor agrees to *steer* those in need of the services covered to the provider. Providers also implement strict benefit differentials to ensure that their population utilizes participating providers who have joined the managed care organization's network. If a patient uses a participating provider, the copayments and benefits might be avoidable, whereas if a nonparticipating provider is used, the benefits might be greatly reduced or there may even be no benefits whatsoever. To help ensure that patients are steered in a certain direction, providers and insurers look to the beginning of the health care continuum: the patient's primary physician.

Many providers, including hospitals, integrated networks, HMOs, and PPOs, purchase or affiliate with primary care physician providers to make sure that a patient stays within their system. These providers are known as *gatekeepers*. The gatekeepers control both the level of care and who provides it. If a patient seeks care outside the network for anything other than an emergency, there is usually a penalty in the form of a hefty copayment or total denial of payment.

The *members*, then, have a real financial incentive to stay within a network of participating providers, and subsequently, the participating providers get the volume increases promised as a benefit of being in the managed care organization's network. In exchange for the added volume, the provider gives the payor a *discount*. Depending on the competition,

POS
A hybrid between an HMO and a PPO in which patients are given the incentive to see providers participating in a defined network but may see non-network providers, though usually at some additional cost.

PPO
A network of independent providers preselected by the payor to provide a specific service or range of services at predetermined (usually discounted) rates to the payor's covered members.

Participating Provider
A provider who has contracted with the health plan to provide medical services to covered members at predetermined rates.

Steerage
An arrangement in which an entity (often an employer or payor) receives a discount for agreeing to recommend patients to a provider.

Primary Care Provider
A physician (typically a family medicine, internal medicine, pediatric, and sometimes an obstetrics-gynecology provider) who is the primary caregiver of a patient.

Gatekeepers
Providers (typically the primary care provider) who must preapprove care received by a patient, such as a visit to a specialist. Gatekeepers are used in most POS and HMO plans.

discounts can range from 5 percent to 40 percent of normal charges. Although 40 percent seems like an enormous discount, many providers feel that if their variable costs are being met, then the additional volume is worth the discount. Steerage, discounts, and allowances have been only partially successful in bringing down costs to employers.

Copayments and Deductibles

One of the simplest methods of risk sharing is through copayments and deductibles, where patients absorb some of the cost of service provision. With *copayments*, members covered by a plan are required to pay part of the cost of the service. For instance, if the fee for an office visit is $90, the patient may have to pay $25, and the insurance pays the remainder of the allowable reimbursement, up to the remaining $65. With *deductibles*, the person covered is responsible for paying a certain base amount before coverage begins. For instance, a patient may be required to pay for the first $500 of service before the third party pays any of the bill. Exhibit 13–8 shows an example of a health care plan that uses copayments and deductibles.

Two risk-reducing outcomes occur as a result of copayments and deductibles: insurers do not have to pay the portion of the bill that the copayment and deductible

Exhibit 13–8   Example of employee benefits using copayments and deductibles

Service	Plan Coverage		Employee Responsibility	
	Participating Provider	Nonparticipating Provider	Participating Provider	Nonparticipating Provider
MD office visit	100% after copayment	70% after copayment	$25 copayment per visit	$35 copayment per visit
Emergency room visit	100%	100%	Subject to plan approval	Subject to plan approval
Inpatient stay	100% after deductible	70% after deductible	$200 deductible per stay; $1,000 maximum per year	$200 deductible per stay; $1,000 maximum per year
Prescription drugs	100% after copayment	70% after deductible	$20 copayment per prescription	$30 copayment per prescription

amounts cover, and copayments and deductibles are designed to encourage people to seek less care (especially in the common tiered copayment schedule, where a primary care visit may cost $25, a specialty visit is $35, and an emergency room or urgent care copayment is $50). The copays and deductibles are generally low enough to be affordable if care is really needed but high enough to make people think twice before seeking unnecessary care, and they generally make people consider whether they are seeking care in the most appropriate location.

Copayment
Requiring the patient to pay part of the health care bill. These payments are used to prevent overutilization of services.

Deductibles
When the patient covered is responsible for paying a certain base amount before coverage begins.

Per Diem

Another method of payment is a *per diem* ("per day") rate, which is similar to case rates. A payor negotiates an amount that it will pay for one day of care, which includes all hospital charges associated with the inpatient day (including nursing care, surgeries, medications, etc.). The day of care can be defined in several ways. Certainly a day in an intensive care unit (ICU) is more expensive than a day on a regular unit. Therefore, the per diem rate for the ICU might be $1,700 and for the regular unit might be $1,000. For a patient who spends seven days in the hospital, two in the ICU and five on the regular unit, the payment would be

$$
\begin{array}{rl}
2 \text{ Days @ } \$1,700 & = \$3,400 \\
+\ 5 \text{ Days @ } \$1,000 & = \underline{\$5,000} \\
\textbf{Total} & = \$8,400
\end{array}
$$

To reduce their financial risk under per diems, payors place limits on length of stay. They may even put limits within the length of stay. For example, in the seven-day stay, the insurer may say (based on its analysis of the situation compared with its national statistics) that a total of seven days is fine, but it may only allow one day in the ICU, not two. Typically per diems favor the managed care organization, which has control over the number of days allowed as a benefit, even if it does not necessarily have the ability to discharge the patient.

Per Diem
An amount a payor will pay for one day of care, which includes all hospital charges associated with the inpatient day (including nursing care, surgeries, medications, etc.).

Another way that insurers attempt to manage their risk is to encourage outpatient treatment, only approving hospital admission for the sickest of patients. As the level of acuity rises, so do the expenses associated with care. This can be a troubling aspect of per diems from providers' perspective. They are concerned that though a rate will be negotiated on a wide variety of patient types, only the sickest and most complicated cases will end up at their hospital. Thus, their costs will rise above the per diem.

Case Rates

Another form of managing care and sharing risk is to negotiate a rate that is all-inclusive of everything that the hospital provides during the entire inpatient stay. In this instance, the insurer and the provider agree to a fixed rate, which limits the liability of the payor and shifts some of the financial risk to the provider. This negotiated rate is known as a *case rate*. For example, a hospital might agree to accept $30,000 for a patient who needs a coronary artery bypass graft (CABG). Of particular concern to providers when considering case rates is the complicated case, referred to as an *outlier* or, informally, a "train wreck," that ends up costing far more than the negotiated rate. Providers are taking a big risk if they are guaranteed only $30,000 for a given procedure, but unusual complications of the case cost in the hundreds of thousands of dollars.

The benefit to providers is that if the case is of lower severity or the patient experiences a shorter stay than expected, then the case rate may well be in excess of costs and sometimes even in excess of charges. Although this is uncommon, providers often have a false sense of confidence that they can manage the care of patients to such a level that they will "win" in the case-rate scenario. What they fail to realize often is that once the financial risk for the provision of health care services is handed from the payor to the provider, the payor may have no real incentive to assist in the medical management of the patient. In fact, every penny the managed care organization spends on administration by helping the hospital is really a penny of annual profit lost. It is easy to see why hospitals have become increasingly shy about contracting with this method unless they are certain that they have the medical management protocol in place to allow them to benefit.

One method providers use to limit the exposure that comes with the possibility that charges will go far beyond negotiated rates is to negotiate a level of charges over which the hospital is no longer totally liable, called a *stop-loss* limit. For example, in the case just described, a hospital and insurer might agree that $50,000 is the maximum amount for which the provider is totally liable (see Exhibit 13–9). If a patient's charges exceed $50,000, the insurer will pay the provider for charges over this amount. Many times insurers and providers share this risk by negotiating a discount, for example 20 percent, off the excess charges. Continuing with the CABG example, if a patient incurs a total of $75,000 on a CABG case (Row A), this is a stop-loss case. The insurer pays the provider $30,000 (Row B, the negotiated case rate) plus 80 percent of the charges over the $50,000 stop-loss or $20,000 [0.80 × ($75,000 − $50,000) Rows C, D]. This stop-loss reduces the loss to the provider from $45,000 (Row C: $75,000 cost − $30,000 negotiated payment) to $25,000 (Row G: $75,000 cost − $30,000 negotiated payment − $20,000 stop-loss payment). Risk is shared between the provider and the insurer.

Capitation

In capitation, the basic premise is that a provider agrees in advance to cover the health care needs of a defined population for a set amount (often *per member per month* [PMPM] or per member per year [PMPY]), which is prepaid to the provider. The gamble for the provider, of course, is that the cost of the medical expenditures provided to the HMO member will be less than the capitated payment amount prepaid to the

Exhibit 13–9 Example of a stop-loss implementation

A	Total charges		$75,000
B	Negotiated case rate payment		30,000
C	Balance	A − B	45,000
D	Amount over stop-loss ($50,000)	A − $50,000	25,000
E	Additional payment from insurer	0.8 × D	20,000
F	Total insurance payment	B + E	50,000
G	Remaining balance (amount for which the provider is at risk)	A − B − E	$25,000

provider, in which case the provider is able to retain the difference. The philosophy is that this payment system will encourage prudent medical management and preventive care, which will prevent more expensive inpatient care in the future, for example.

Inherent in capitation, however, is that the very act of providing services in any form causes the provider to incur a cost that would not have been incurred if the service had not been provided. In short, there is a perverse incentive in the short run to provide a minimum level of care or *not* to provide care at all: to withhold care, to settle for a less expensive but less effective course of treatment or to create obstacles for patients in being able to access care (only having appointments available weeks or months in advance so as to discourage unnecessary utilization). In the instance of hospitals, patients have allegedly been discharged prematurely or, again, have not received a more expensive course of treatment when a cheaper "band-aid" approach would suffice. In short, although capitation was initially intended to force a new level of fiscal accountability on providers—really forcing them to understand the costs of medical care and use only the most cost-effective treatments—it has become a controversial payment form because of the temptation it presents to focus more on the short-term financial aspects of medical care than on patient care itself.

Premium Rate-Setting Methods The methods for deriving the premiums used by managed care companies (i.e., HMOs) for capitation are complicated because accurate actuarial information is absolutely critical to pricing the coverage appropriately. There are two basic methods that payors use when developing premiums: community rating and *experience rating*. The obvious difference is that community rating evaluates the health risk of a population as a whole, whereas experience rating focuses on assessing the potential medical expenditures of individuals and then aggregates them into a group premium.

Capitation
A method of payment in which the provider is paid a fixed amount, over a set period of time, usually a month or a year, for each person served no matter what the actual number or nature of services delivered.

Per Member Per Month (PMPM)
Generally used by HMOs and their medical providers as an indicator of revenue, expenses, or utilization of services per member per one-month period.

Experience Rating
The method of setting premium rates based on the actual health care costs of a group or groups.

Managed care organizations attempt to know as much information as possible about the covered population to develop reliable predictions of how much health care will be utilized. For example, the cost to cover the hospital care required for colon and rectal cancer can be predicted if enough is known about the covered population. Information such as the number of men (particularly white men because the incidence is higher among this group), fifty-plus age group size (incidence increases over age fifty), general diet of the population (higher fat content causes higher incidence), and income level (income is a predictor of diet) can all provide valuable predictive input. Once a predicted number of potential cases is determined and a potential length of stay estimated, the potential cases are multiplied by the average length of stay, yielding the total number of expected hospital days. The insurer then seeks the lowest price it can find for this number of inpatient days. It often uses all the tools described in this chapter to obtain this rate, such as promising steerage and contracting via per diems, case rates, or both.

For example, assume a payor covers 100,000 lives. After studying all the detailed demographic data (age, gender, etc.), it is determined that 19.1 individuals from this population could be diagnosed with colon or rectal cancer in a given year. The current treatment for this illness requires an average stay in the hospital of 6.5 days. Thus, the payor must be prepared to cover 124 days of hospital care (19.1 cases at 6.5 days per case). If the payor can negotiate a rate with providers of $1,000 per day, the total cost will be approximately $124,000 for the year. Taking this amount and dividing it by the number of covered lives (100,000) gives a figure of $1.24 per year or $0.103 per month that it must charge its members to cover this health care need. To cover its administrative costs and desired profit, the payor may add an additional 15 percent (ranges between 15 and 25 percent) to the $0.103, creating a final figure of $0.12 PMPM (see Exhibit 13–10).

This method can be repeated for all covered health care needs to create the final monthly premium. All events resulting in health care costs such as the number of strokes, heart attacks, accidents, mental illnesses, and kidney failures must be accurately predicted and their costs analyzed to create a viable premium. The premium amount will obviously vary based on services covered and the size and demographics of the covered population. It is also dependent on the provider climate.

When rating various groups, payors may also consider such things as the types of industry, applying conversion factors to account for potential differences in health care expenditures. For example, covering a group of twenty-five men who are in an accounting firm will probably result in fewer claims related to industrial accidents than covering a construction crew of twenty-five men. Likewise, groups with women in the twenty-five-to-forty age group might be expected to have more pregnancies and subsequent well-child checkups than would a group of older adults. Competition is also a factor that forces premiums to be lower. For example, a West Coast premium, where competition among HMOs for lives is fierce and competition between providers for patients is tight, might be under $100 PMPM whereas a premium in an area where few

Conversion Factor
Actuarial-based formulas developed to adjust rates allowing for differences in population demographics.

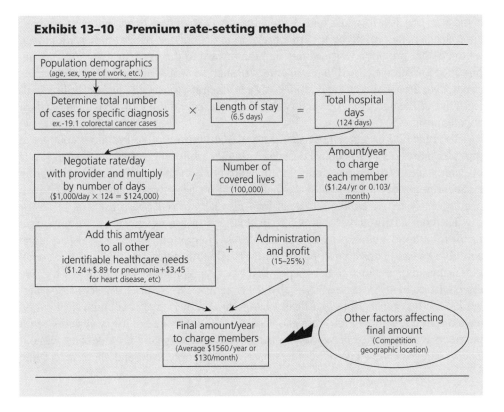

Exhibit 13–10   Premium rate-setting method

Population demographics
(age, sex, type of work, etc.)

Determine total number of cases for specific diagnosis
ex.-19.1 colorectal cancer cases
× Length of stay (6.5 days) = Total hospital days (124 days)

Negotiate rate/day with provider and multiply by number of days
($1,000/day × 124 = $124,000)
/ Number of covered lives (100,000) = Amount/year to charge each member ($1.24/yr or 0.103/month)

Add this amt/year to all other identifiable healthcare needs
($1.24+$.89 for pneumonia+$3.45 for heart disease, etc)
+ Administration and profit (15–25%)

Final amount/year to charge members
(Average $1560/year or $130/month)

Other factors affecting final amount
(Competition geographic location)

HMO options are available for employees and benefit coverage levels are richer might exceed $130 PMPM.

Percentage of Premium Capitation   To regain some of the control lost to insurers, in the early to mid-1990s, a prominent trend was for providers to accept a *percentage of the managed care premium* to provide all of the care needed by that patient population. For example, if an insurer charges its members a monthly premium of $130, the provider may say, "If you pay me 80 percent of that premium ($104), I will provide everything your patient needs." Although this saves both the provider and the payor from having to negotiate for every service the provider offers, it does, however, place the financial burden of supplying all the health care needs directly on the provider. This is similar to the case rates described earlier because it pays a fixed price for a service. In this instance, however, it is much more global, in that the provider is not simply accepting the risk for providing an entire episode of care but rather is responsible for the financial risk associated with the patient's medical experience for a predetermined period for covered services (generally, one-month increments for a year).

The advantage to the provider is that he or she has an ongoing cash flow from a pool of people who may or may not need health care. Again, this creates an incentive for the provider to prevent illness and reduce the odds that a patient will need to seek a more expensive form of care in the future. One of the disadvantages of these approaches is that often, by the time prevention occurs, the patient may have moved on to another provider, thus diminishing the reward to the initial provider for having provided preventive care. If a payor agrees to such an arrangement, it typically retains about 15 to 20 percent of the premium for administrative services such as billing, collections, utilization review, quality assurance, credentialing of providers, and of course, profit.

To enter into an agreement such as a global percentage-of-premium contract, a provider must be able to control costs and provide a full range of services at all levels of care. The provider must control either through ownership or affiliation anything a patient might need. Exhibit 13–11 lists several services that should be offered by a health care system to enable it to enter into this realm of risk-sharing.

The complexity and global nature of this type of arrangement was an important factor for a trend among providers in the 1990s: integration. Within a brief period, an entirely new set of acronyms sprang to life: PHOs (physician-hospital organizations), POs (physician organizations), super PHOs (an aggregation of PHOs on a more regional basis), IDSs (integrated delivery systems), PSNs (provider-sponsored networks), and so forth. Both "vertically integrated delivery systems" with health systems offering womb-to-tomb care and "horizontally integrated delivery systems" with providers owning broad networks of primary and specialty care providers throughout a service region were born. Providers became more organized and eager to provide

Exhibit 13–11   Selected services offered by an integrated health care system

Primary Care	Secondary Care	Tertiary Care	Quaternary Care	Ancillary Services
General practitioners	Community hospitals	Trauma centers	Transplant centers	Home health
Nurse practitioners	Birthing centers	Intensive care units	Burn centers	Nursing homes
Physician assistants	Emergency services	Specialty physicians	Emergency air transport	Hospice care
Urgent care centers	Ambulance services			Dental plans
				Prescription plans
				Hotel accommodations

a complete scope of services, partially in response to the need to be able to survive and compete in this changing environment.

Other Forms of Capitation In the global percentage of premium capitation scenarios like the ones described above, a large hospital or health system is most often the holder of the risk (because hospitals and health systems typically are the only providers to have enough solvency to be able to cover the downside risk if the overall medical expenditures exceed the capitation revenues). However, often working beneath the surface of such global arrangements are smaller, more specialized versions of capitation. Global professional (physician) capitation, primary care or specialty care capitation, and ancillary capitation are some examples. In all these formats, the basic premise is the same: capitation is simply a prepayment of healthcare, with the provider being at risk for medical expenditures that exceed the amount prepaid based on anticipated expenditures. Physician capitation has some nuances, however, due to the many variations that exist.

In single-provider primary care capitation, the primary care gatekeeper physician (whether a family medicine, internal medicine, or pediatric physician) will receive a set amount for a fixed population and will have to provide all primary care services. Depending on how the contract is negotiated between the primary care provider and the payor, the capitated amount may also include all or some specialty services for the fixed population, which the primary care physician must subsequently pay. This payment may be on a fee-for-service or *subcapitated basis* with the specialist receiving either a fixed amount (e.g., \$2 PMPM) or a variable amount (e.g., 4 percent of the professional capitation) to provide a subset of professional services such as orthopedic services.

Often multiprovider capitation agreements are structured on the same premise, except that a global amount will be allotted to the mult-provider group, and all professional (nonhospital, nonancillary) care must be paid from that single pool. The individual providers within that group determine the most equitable way to divide the pool of dollars, which takes the payor out of the equation in terms of this subdivision of professional money but which often creates tensions and confusion among physicians who are trying to standardize the values of services. In this case, negotiations must occur between the primary care and specialty care physicians as a whole, in order to establish two smaller budgets within the professional capitation amount. Tensions can flare even more when the specialists themselves have to determine how to weight the value of the services they provide. Is glaucoma surgery more "valuable" than setting a broken bone? How much more difficult or simple is back surgery than urologic surgery?

One method that providers have employed to equitably divide the specialty portion of the professional capitation amount is through a *zero-based budget*, which is based on dividing the entire medical budget through a sliding scale of RVUs. The sliding scale is intended to equalize disparities between the ever-subjective assessment of how difficult

Subcapitation
Where the primary care physician pays a portion of the total capitated dollars received to another provider (i.e., specialist).

Zero-Based Budget (Capitation)
Dividing the entire amount of capitation (the "budget") among all the providers, essentially leaving nothing or "zero" at the end of every accounting period.

Contact Capitation
A method of capitation whereby each specialty has its own capitation pool, and uses of services by a physician only affects that physician's compensation, not the whole specialty network's compensation.

one procedure is compared with another (particularly when attempting to compare two procedures or services that are dissimilar in nature, such as the back and urologic surgeries mentioned above). In such a scenario, monies are distributed retrospectively based on the number or "work units" that each physician has provided (with the RVUs simply taken from the RBRVS scale discussed earlier), so that each physician is rewarded commensurate with the number of RVUs provided.

A similar technique known as *contact capitation* creates a pool of funds for each specialty. These funds are then divided among the physicians in that specialty based on the number of contacts that the individual specialist receives during a specific period of time (e.g., a month, six months, or a year), with one contact being awarded during that time period for each specialty referral from a primary care physician. The specialty care physician is then responsible for that patient for the time period. Contact capitation, while interesting and effective in theory, has not been employed on a large scale because of the effort required to monitor the comparative performance of the physicians within the group. Despite the administrative burden, zero-based budgets and contact capitation are indicative of the types of techniques being explored as providers seek more uniform and more equitable ways to be compensated for care (see Exhibit 13–12 for an example of a global capitation model).

Exhibit 13–12   Global capitation model

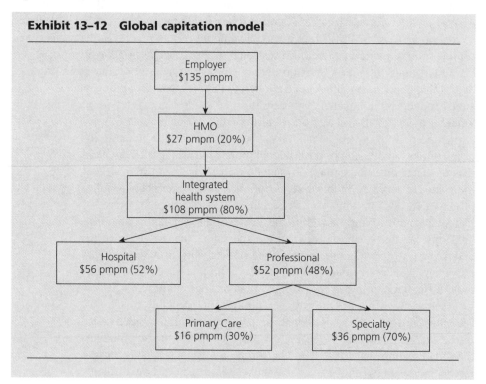

Despite its early success and popularity, capitation as a payment method has come under severe scrutiny by all parties and in the media in the past few years. Although some had predicted it would become *the* managed care payment system, its use as the dominant method of payment for managed care in the future is uncertain. There is actually a shift underway of risk back toward the payors. Many of the current negotiations between payors and providers have returned to the methods of old such as "percentage discounts." Providers have seemed to reach their saturation point with risk and are turning away business associated with capitation-type arrangements.

EVOLVING ISSUES

Payment systems will continue to evolve in reaction to external forces, such as pressure of disclosing quality-of-care information connecting it with payment pricing and consumer choice in health care and demands for health care reform. Hospitals generate more than half of their patient revenues from Medicare and Medicaid. Policymakers expect declining payment rates for Medicare and Medicaid to slow the growth of government spending as a result of declining federal and state economies. Recently, Medicare and other payors have pressured health care providers to accept a linkage between quality-of-care criteria and payment levels. Two areas that link quality with payment are "pay for performance" measures and "pay for reporting" measures. The underlying forces for reporting these quality data and linking them to payment were to provide reliable and valid data so health care consumers can make informed decisions in selecting a hospital based on quality and price and to create an incentive for hospitals to report these data.

Pay for Reporting

Under the Medicare Modernization Act of 2003, CMS hospitals created an incentive to report on ten medical conditions or incur a 0.4 percentage point reduction in their annual payment updates. The reporting measures include quality data measuring hospital performance and patient satisfaction coupled with payment information.

 Quality Information online *CMS in conjunction with Hospital Quality Alliance has established the Hospital Compare Web site, which allows for comparison among hospitals on quality measures: http://www.hospitalcompare .hhs.gov.*

The specific quality measures include surgical care improvement, patient assessment of the provider, and hospital outcome of care measures that predict mortality or death rates and relate to several medical conditions: heart attack, heart failure and pneumonia, children's asthma. These measures provide information to patients on how effective a hospital is in the provision of care. For example, for the care for heart attack patients, the hospitals are requested to report the following information:

- Percentage of heart attack patients given aspirin at arrival
- Percentage of heart attack patients given aspirin at discharge
- Percentage of heart attack patients given a beta blocker at discharge.

The care measures for surgical infection prevention include the percentage of surgery patients who received preventive antibiotic(s) one hour before incision and the percentage of surgery patients who received treatment to prevent blood clots within 24 hours before or after selected surgeries to prevent blood clots.

The hospital outcome of care, which is measured by risk-adjusted mortality rate, measures the results of care. Using Medicare claims data, CMS uses a statistical model to predict a risk-adjusted mortality or death rate during the hospital stay and within thirty days of hospital admission for heart attack or heart failure or pneumonia. Deaths due to patient treatment in the hospital and the possibility that hospitals discharge their patients too soon are why death rate data are collected thirty days within hospital admission. Because patients do not have the same risk of death, the mortality rate is also adjusted for the impact of risk factors that are unique to the patient—such as age, severity of illness(es), and other medical problems—that can place some patients at greater risk of dying than others. Perspective 13–3 gives an example of how one hospital's mortality rate for pneumonia compares with a nationwide average.

Perspective 13–3   Hospital's Outcome for Care by Risk-Adjusted Mortality Rates for Pneumonia

Hospitalized pneumonia patients who were treated at St. Mark's Hospital in Utah had the state's lowest projected mortality rate in the thirty days after their admission. The reported risk-adjusted mortality rate was 8.9 percent for pneumonia patients treated between July 2006 and June 2007. In contrast, the U.S. national rate was 11.4 percent. For all Utah hospitals, mortality rates for heart attack, heart failure, and pneumonia patients were in line with national rates.

The director of respiratory care and neurodiagnostic services claims that the lower death rate may have resulted from the hospital's aggressive implementation of the "ventilator bundle," which includes keeping patients' head elevated, their mouth free of secretions, and their stomach acid neutralized. In addition, a hospital pulmonologist believes that good communication and teamwork among the key caregivers of radiologists, pulmonologists, nurses, hospitalists, and infectious disease physicians contributed to the lower rate.

Source: McCann, S., and Rosetta, L. 2008 (Aug. 21). Utah's lowest pneumonia mortality rate at St. Mark's: Data from all Utah hospitals in line with national statistics. *Salt Lake Tribune*; available at: http://www.sltrib.com/news/ci_10260269.

Finally, questions related to patients' assessments of their hospital stay include measures of nurse and physician communication with the patient, such as did nurses and physicians treat you with courtesy? and did nurses and physicians listen and explain things to you? Other questions relate to the cleanliness and quietness of the rooms, the explanation of medicines and recovery at home, and the overall rating of the hospital. The hospital comparison Web site from the U.S. Department of Health and Human Services provides further explanation of this information along with reporting data for all acute care hospitals in the United States. Hospitals also evaluate themselves with patient-satisfaction surveys such as Press Ganey, which provide comparative benchmarking results.

Pay for Performance

In 2003 CMS, in conjunction with Premier Inc., also implemented a voluntary program that compensated hospitals that received high scores for quality-of-care measures. Approximately 280 hospitals across the United States participated in this program. Hospitals were scored on quality-of-care measures for inpatient care related to heart attacks, heart failure, pneumonia, CABG, and hip and knee replacement. For heart attacks, hospitals were scored on whether they provided the patient with aspirin on arrival and for patients who were smokers whether they provided adult smoking cessation counseling or advising. Within each clinical condition, measures were aggregated into a composite score.

Pay-for-Performance Information *A main source of information about various aspects of pay-for-performance is the Agency for Health Care Research and Quality, a government agency in the Department of Health and Human Services: http://www.ahrq.gov. Another excellent site regarding quality related to Medicaid is: http://www.cms.hhs.gov/MedicaidSCHIPQualprac.*

Under each medical condition, hospitals with scores within the top 50th percentile were listed as "top performers." If a hospital was listed in the top 10th percentile for a given clinical condition, it received a 2 percent bonus to its DRG payment. Hospitals in the 20th percentile for a given clinical condition received a 1 percent payment added to its DRG payment. In 2007 hospitals within the demonstration project that scored below the bottom 90th percentile hospitals had their DRG payment reduced by 1 percent, and hospitals scoring at the 100th percentile would have their DRG payment reduced by 2 percent.

MEDICAL ERRORS

To make hospitals accountable for medical errors and improve quality of care for its patients, Medicare, along with commercial health plans (Blue Cross, Wellpoint, Cigna, etc.) will no longer pay for medical errors that are clearly preventable as well as serious medical mistakes. In the case of Medicare, they will stop payment for eight medical conditions during a hospital stay, including the following:

- Leaving sponges or needles in the body during surgery
- Using the wrong blood type
- Air embolisms
- Catheter-associated infections from urinary tract
- Vascular care
- Surgical site infections
- Bed ulcers
- Hospital-acquired injuries during a hospital stay such as broken bones sustained from falls.

CONSUMER CHOICE IN HEALTH CARE

Health Savings Accounts The employee sets aside funds to pay for qualified medically related expenses such as copayments and deductibles from inpatient stays, outpatient and physician visits, prescription drugs, eyewear, dental visits, and the like. The dollars are placed in a bank account, and the employee can withdraw these funds tax-free to pay for qualifying medical expenses. In addition, the consumer can carry over these funds from year to year and allow them to not only accrue but earn interest on these accounts.

Health Reimbursement Accounts The employer sets asides dollars for the employee to pay for qualified medical expenses. In contrast to health savings accounts, the contributed funds cannot earn interest and they are not portable; however, they can be carried over from year to year.

Higher health insurance premiums are causing corporations who previously offered traditional health insurance to their employees to either stop providing traditional health insurance for their employees or to offer them high-deductible health plans. Another reason for offering high-deductible plans is that consumers can decide how to use their medical dollars and in turn shop around for less costly medical care as well as reduce their consumption of health care. With a high-deductible health plan, employers pay lower premiums to the health plan for insurance coverage for serious illnesses or injuries. One type of health plan may offer a deductible of around $1,200 for individual coverage and $2,400 for family coverage. Because they are high-deductible plans, employees may be required to set aside funds to pay for deductibles and any other copayments or noncovered medical expenses, such as prescription drugs, dental visits, or eyewear. This type of account is called a *health savings account* and allows consumers to make tax-free withdrawals to pay for qualified medical expenses that are not covered by their health plan. These accounts can earn interest on the balance and can be carried over from year to year without any dollar limit. In addition, they are portable in that if the employee changes jobs, he or she can keep these dollars.

Another type of insurance product is called a *health reimbursement arrangements*, whereby the employer sets aside a certain dollar amount each time period for employees to cover their out-of-pocket medical expenses, such as copayments, deductibles, drugs, and other health care-related expenses not covered by the employer's health plan. Unlike health savings accounts, health reimbursement accounts do not allow one to earn interest on these funds, and they are not portable; however, employees can carry over their balances from year to year.

Key Point *Additional information about medical savings accounts can be found at http://www.cms.hhs.gov/MSA.*

INFORMATION TECHNOLOGY

The business of health care continues to evolve as providers, payors, and employers seek solutions to questions that have never previously been posed. While the introduction of new technology addresses some of these issues, it also raises new ones and often calls into question presumptions that were previously accepted as true. Nowhere is this clearer than in one of the growing fields in health care that offers astounding possibilities for the future: the area commonly known as *health care informatics* or information technology (IT) (see Perspective 13–4).

Where employers and providers once thought health care data were an inessential by-product of simple claims payment, today there is a strong, even urgent, need for information that is timely, informative, and in a usable format. Throughout the health

Perspective 13–4   Capital Budgeting for Information Technology

From November 2007 through February 2008, *Modern Healthcare* surveyed 145 hospitals about their capital spending and allocation for information technology (IT). They reported that 36 percent of the hospitals spent more than 21 percent of their budget over the past three years on IT while 64 percent spent 20 percent or less. The median spending range for IT was between 11 percent and 20 percent of their capital budget. In terms of future IT spending, there was a complete reversal. In the next three years, they found that 71 percent of the hospitals would spend less than 20 percent, whereas only 29 percent of the hospitals would spend more than 21 percent. However, one respondent noted that budget numbers may vary across hospitals because IT purchases for radiology departments, such as picture archiving and communication systems (PACS), are excluded from the IT department budgets of some hospitals. The surveyed hospitals list below their top three priority IT purchases:

57.9 percent indicated electronic health records
45.5 percent indicated inpatient clinical IT systems
36.6 percent indicated ambulatory clinical IT systems

Other IT capital purchases include communications links to physicians (29.7 percent), physician practice management systems (25 percent), and PACS (15.9 percent).

Source: Conn, J. 2008 (Feb. 25). Still taking small steps. Sticking with the basics. *Modern Healthcare,* S1, S4, respectively.

care industry, there is a constant need and desire to push the borders into areas that have never been explored before. The information services arena has evolved from an accounting-based, relatively basic means of analyzing charge and payment data to an integral part of modern health care delivery and payment.

Early efforts focused on how components of the delivery system (physicians, hospitals, etc.) performed and interacted financially with one another. Retrospective analysis of this sort depended on analyzing postpayment claims data, understanding where the health care dollar was spent, and comparing that with national and regional benchmarks of what the financial performance should have been, based on industry norms.

This was the next significant step beyond simply understanding cost structures and whether charges were appropriate for specific procedures and in the marketplace. Particularly with providers and payors, the need for this sort of intricate information was critical to their ability to implement successful medical management programs and, ultimately then, to their financial success. An entire sector of IT and health care informatics companies has grown to meet this need.

The level of complexity and sophistication of information available to providers, payors, and employers is evolving quickly. New forms and formats of information are emerging to predict what *might* happen with the clinical and financial experiences of a population. In some of the new information technologies being developed and refined, the relationship between past and present medical data on a patient-specific level can even be used to prospectively assess the medical risk of a group population, information that was completely unavailable even two or three years ago.

Although hospitals continue to invest in health care technology, they are confronted with trying to measuring the financial returns from this capital investment. Perspective 13–5 provides an example of how one hospital justified its investment in IT.

Perspective 13–5   Financial Benefits from IT

Investment in IT is considered a driving factor for improving patient care; the critical question asked by CEO, CFO, and board members is whether hospitals achieve a financial return from their IT investments. The inability to measure and account for financial benefits from IT investments has led some hospital managers to avoid making these types of capital investments that can provide for more efficient, higher-quality care while improving patient and provider satisfaction.

One health care system that decided to make this decision is Banner Health, which implemented an IT system at its newest hospital, Banner Estrella Medical Center in Phoenix, Arizona. By investing in IT and receiving input from physicians, pharmacists, nurses, informaticists, and other clinicians, the hospital designed new work flows and established evidence-based order sets. The improved IT design and standard order sets were implemented across departmental functions such as care management, clinical

Perspective 13–5   (*Continued*)

documentation, computerized provider order entry (CPOE), nursing orders management, and medication administration and scheduling, as well as processes in departments such as health information management, emergency services, obstetrics, pediatrics, pharmacy, and surgery. This IT investment resulted in a $2.6 million cost savings by greater retention in nurses, which lowered recruiting, hiring, and training of new nurses; reduced accounts receivable bills by one day, which resulted in faster payment; decreased the incidence of adverse drug events, length of stay, pharmacy costs, and overtime expenses for nurses as a result of improving their efficiency in charting and shifting tasks; and reduced forms costs because information was digitized.

Source: Hensing, J., Dahlen, D., Warden, M., Norman, J. V., Wilson, B. C., and Kisiel, S. 2008 (Feb. 1. Measuring the benefits of IT-enabled care transformation. *Healthcare Financial Management*, 62(2).

SUMMARY

Health care services have grown along with the growth in the American population. Different payment methods have been tried to find a reasonable balance among costs, quality, and access. Health care payment in the United States has remained a "living experiment" from the early days of private, cash-based exchange through the middle and later years where commercial and government payors were involved in a massive exercise of trial-and-error while testing different payment methods and structures of care delivery.

Various systems include charge-based payment, where providers receive payment based on actual charges and payors bear the risk; cost-based payment, where providers are paid based on the cost of providing services and payors still bear the risk; and finally, flat fee systems where the provider is paid a predetermined amount and the providers bear the risk.

There has also been a growth in the types of health care payors. Indemnity companies, governmental payors, and finally managed care organizations have all played major roles in trying to balance cost, quality, and access. Discounts, steerage, per diems, case rates, community or experience rating, benchmarking, managed care, and capitation are all examples of these methods.

After nearly one hundred years of experimentation, we have learned that balancing cost, quality, and access is an ongoing process and will be influenced in the future by the trends discussed in the first chapter of this text.

KEY TERMS

a.	Allowable costs	dd.	MD
b.	APCs	ee.	Members
c.	Capitation	ff.	MS-DRGs
d.	Case rates	gg.	Participating provider
e.	Charge-based	hh.	Payor
f.	CMS	ii.	Per diem
g.	Community rating	jj.	Per member per month (PMPM)
h.	Contact capitation	kk.	Predetermined rates
i.	Conversion factor	ll.	Preferred provider organization (PPO)
j.	Copayment		
k.	Cost-based reimbursement	mm.	Premium
l.	Cost-shifting	nn.	Premiums
m.	Deductibles	oo.	Price setter
n.	Diagnosis-related groups (DRGs)	pp.	Primary care provider
o.	Discounts	qq.	Point-of-service plan (POS)
p.	Experience rating	rr.	Prospective payment system (PPS)
q.	Fee-for-service		
r.	Financial requirements	ss.	Retrospective payment
s.	Flat fee	tt.	Resource-based relative value system (RBRVS)
t.	Gatekeeper		
u.	Group model HMO	uu.	RVU
v.	Health Care Financing Administration (HCFA)	vv.	Staff model HMO
		ww.	Steerage
w.	Health maintenance organization (HMO)	xx.	Stop-loss
		yy.	Subcapitation
x.	Health savings accounts	zz.	The first party
y.	Health reimbursement accounts	aaa.	The second party
z.	Indemnity insurance	bbb.	The third party
aa.	Managed care	ccc.	Usual, customary, and reasonable charges
bb.	Medicaid		
cc.	Medicare	ddd.	Zero-based budget (capitation)

QUESTIONS AND PROBLEMS

1. Define the key terms listed above.

2. What were the major events and trends that defined the early, middle, and later periods of the U.S. health care system? In each period describe:

   a. The major events and trends.

   b. The price setter.

   c. The predominant method of payment and the unit to which payment is attached.

3. What was the driving force behind the development of Blue Cross and Blue Shield?

4. Name the units of service on which cost-based payers may pay providers.

5. What drove the development of Medicare? Who is covered under Medicare?

6. What drove the development of Medicaid? Who is covered under Medicaid?

7. Who pays for the Medicare and Medicaid programs?

8. How do copayments and deductibles reduce risk?

9. Why do providers desire "steerage?"

10. What do providers fear most under a case-rate model?

11. What are some methods insurers use to limit their risk under per diem arrangements?

12. Who bears the risk under a flat rate system? Why?

13. What factors determine what a flat rate payment to a provider should be?

14. Why was the DRG system developed?

15. What are APCs? Why were they developed?

16. Why do HMOs use prevention and case management?

17. How do HMOs determine their premiums?

18. If an HMO covered 150,000 lives, expected twenty-five myocardial infarctions (MIs) to occur each year within the covered lives, would expect a length of stay of 4.5 days for each MI, and had to pay an average of $950 per day for each day the MI patient was in the hospital, what would the PMPM cost to the HMO be? What would have to be charged to the patient or employer if the HMO had administrative costs equaling 10 percent of its costs and it wanted a profit margin of 7 percent?

19. Given the same scenario as in question 18, what if the HMO's shareholders demanded a 9 percent profit margin? What would the premium be in this case?

20. In question 19, what if the employer or patient refused to pay the new premium? What would the HMO offer to pay the hospital for an inpatient day? (Hint: Try lowering the per diem rate until the PMPM charge with a 9 percent profit margin equals the PMPM charge with the 7 percent in Problem 18.)

21. What if in question 20 the hospital refused to take the new rate, the employer refused to pay the new premium, and the employer decided to take its employees (10,000) to another HMO? Also, suppose these departing employees-members represented six percent of the total MI cases. What would the new PMPM premium be for the 140,000 remaining members? (Hint: revert back to question 18 information, except for changes in employees and MI cases.)

22. Who bears the financial risk in a capitated payment system?

23. Name and describe four different types of capitation.

24. Why would a provider be willing to accept a global capitation payment?

QUESTIONS FROM APPENDIX H

1. What are four factors to consider when developing charges in a charge-based system?

2. What charge method primarily uses the market price to establish a charge?

3. What charge method relies on the case mix, volume, and financial requirements of the institution?

4. What is the difference between determining charges on an average-cost basis and a weighted-cost basis?

5. What are the steps in determining weighted-average costs?

6. Describe the two margin-based approaches to developing charges.

7. Compare and contrast health savings accounts with health reimbursement accounts.

APPENDIX H

COST-BASED PAYMENT SYSTEMS

REASONABLE AND ALLOWABLE COSTS

In establishing cost-based payment systems, the natural tension that exists between providers and payors revolves around five issues: reasonableness, case mix, service mix, staff mix, and efficiency.

- *Reasonableness* issues are concerned with the cost of one provider versus others. In this regard, payors often set boundaries to establish what is usual, customary, and reasonable. For instance, a payor may pay only up to 85 percent of the cost of a procedure, based on an analysis of a profile of all providers who have submitted cost reports.

- *Case mix* issues revolve around patient eligibility. For instance, although a hospital incurs legitimate costs in treating a patient who has a deviated septum, a payor may decide not to pay for this surgery because the patient failed to receive all necessary preadmission certification. Similarly, if a health department treats a pregnant woman who resides outside its county, the county's prenatal care program may not pay for the treatment because the patient was outside the location eligibility guidelines.

- *Service mix* issues focus on the appropriateness of care. For instance, in treating stroke patients, the provider may feel that recreational therapy is an important part of treatment. Though it may be, the payor may not pay for this service because it does not consider it a necessary service within its guidelines.

- *Staff mix* issues pertain to the appropriateness of who provides service. In the mental health field, for example, although a payor may agree that a patient needs psychological services, it might not pay for care provided by a pastoral counselor who is not a licensed psychologist.

- *Efficiency* issues address questions of the appropriateness of the cost of service per unit rendered. A hospital with a low volume may have high unit costs or a radiology center with old equipment may have to take several x-rays just to get one good one. In such instances, although the payor may agree to pay for some level of the service, it will not pay for what it feels are inefficiencies.

Cost-Shifting
Charging one group of patients more to make up for underpayment by others. Most commonly, charging some privately insured patients more to make up for underpayment by Medicaid or Medicare.

Under any of these five conditions, if the payor denies payment and the service has already been rendered, the provider has two choices: absorb the cost, or transfer the cost to another payor. This latter technique is called *cost-shifting* or *cross-subsidization*. Under this system, "over"-reimbursement or reimbursement in excess of total costs is used for one service to cover the costs associated with "under"-reimbursement of another service where reimbursement is less than total costs. This technique has been one of the major reasons for a rise in the number of alternatives to cost-based systems.

UNIT-BASED PAYMENT SYSTEMS

Two key issues that arise in cost-based payment systems are "What is the unit of service to which payments are attached?" and "What are reasonable and allowable costs?" There are a variety of units on which cost-based payors pay providers, including:

Allowable Costs
Costs that are allowable under the principles of reimbursement by government (Medicaid, Medicare) and other payors.

- Per procedure
- Per inpatient day
- Per admission
- Per discharge
- Per diagnosis

Unfortunately for many providers, there is little consistency among third parties with respect to the unit of service on which payment is made. It is not unusual for a single provider to receive payments from Medicare on the basis of DRGs, from private insurance companies on the basis of reasonable charges, and from managed care organizations in the form of capitation. Although it is relatively straightforward to have a cost-finding system that establishes the costs for any one of these payment schemes, it takes a complicated information system to find costs along several of these bases at once.

CHARGE-BASED SYSTEMS

A charge-based system is based in large part on the assumption that a provider is entitled to a reasonable return for its efforts. It relies heavily on the market to ensure that profits are not excessive. Although it would seem that charge-based payment systems are "reactionary" in nature from the payor perspective (because it is the providers who establish the charges on the front-end and seemingly dictate the level of payment), the dynamic is not that simple. What follows is the reasoning that underlies the establishment of provider charges.

In setting charges, a provider must consider a wide range of costs that must be covered. These fall into the same categories discussed in the working capital chapter (operations, opportunities, contingencies, and return on investment). Together, these comprise the organization's *financial requirements*.

- *Operations.* This category includes covering all operating costs, now and into the future. That is, charges must cover costs associated with supplies, equipment, labor, and working capital; have sufficient margin to ensure that staff remains current; and keep technology and facilities sufficiently up-to-date.
- *Opportunities.* Providers must build into their charges a reasonable markup so they can take advantage of opportunities to hold on to or expand existing markets, serve new markets, or exit existing markets.

- *Contingencies.* The changing health care environment presents not only various opportunities but also various unforeseen events such as evolving payment systems, labor shortages, and uncovered catastrophic events. Therefore, charges must build in a reasonable margin for such contingencies that siphon off the organization's capital.

- *Return on investment.* For for-profit providers, charges must also sufficiently compensate the organization and its owners for an investment.

Financial Requirements For health care providers, this is a combination of issues related to operations, opportunities, contingencies, and return on investment.

Although all these methods have been employed, they all share a common concern from the point of view of payors: are they reasonable? Two ways of dealing with this problem have been to limit payments only to that part of charge considered reasonable or to employ another basis of payment altogether.

HISTORICAL, MARKET, OR PAYOR METHOD

The *historical, market, or payor method* is extremely simple: charges are established by a combination of what the organization has traditionally charged, what similar organizations charge, and what payors will pay. This approach to establishing charges is only loosely related to costs, but it is widely used, especially in ambulatory care settings.

WEIGHTED-AVERAGE METHOD

The *weighted-average method* sets charges as a function of the number and type of procedures an organization performs and the financial requirements of the organization. For instance, assume a small health care clinic expects 10,000 visits and anticipates having $1,000,000 in financial requirements next year (see Exhibit H–1). If visit type is ignored, the clinic could set its price by charging the same price for each visit, $100 ($1,000,000 / 10,000). However, charging each visit an average price of $100 overlooks questions of equity. Because each visit does not consume the same resources, some patients would pay more than their fair share while others would pay less.

An alternative to charging each visit the same amount is to take into account the type of visit and to weight these visits by the relative amount of resources they consume. This is accomplished through the following steps:

- Step 1: Categorize visits by resource consumption. Exhibit H–1 assumes there are three types of visits: brief, routine, and complex. It further assumes that 60 percent (6,000) of the 10,000 visits are brief, 30 percent (3,000) routine, and 10 percent (1,000) complex.

- Step 2: Convert visits by category into weighted visit units by category. Exhibit H–1 also assumes that routine visits consume twice the resources, and complex visits consume four times the resources as brief visits. Because the 3,000 routine visits consume twice the resources as brief visits, they count the same as if

Exhibit H–1 Selected services offered by an integrated health care system

	Givens					
A	Number of procedures	a	10,000			
B	Financial requirements	b	$1,000,000			
C	Average charge per visit	B/A	$100			

	D Type of visit	a	**Brief**	**Routine**	**Complex**	**Total**
E	% Distribution of visit by type	a	60%	30%	10%	100%
F	Relative weight of visit by type	a	1	2	4	
G	Number of visits	A × E	6,000	3,000	1,000	10,000
H	Number of weighted visits	F × G	6,000	6,000	4,000	16,000
I	Charge per weighted visit	c	$62.50	$62.50	$62.50	$62.50
J	Total charges	H × I	$375,000	$375,000	$250,000	$1,000,000
K	Charges using average charge	C × G	$600,000	$300,000	$100,000	$1,000,000
L	Overcharge or undercharge compared with weighted average charge	J − K	($225,000)	$75,000	$150,000	$0

a Given.
b Includes all financial requirements of the organization, not just ongoing operating costs.
c [B]/total number of weighted visits (16,000) in row H.

they were 6,000 brief visits (row H: 3,000 × 2). Similarly, because the complex visits consume four times the resources as a brief visit, the actual 1,000 complex visits count as if they were 4,000 brief visits (1,000 × 4). Thus, the actual 10,000 undifferentiated visits become 16,000 weighted visit units (6,000 brief + 6,000 routine + 4,000 complex visits, row H).

■ Step 3: Determine charge per weighted visit unit and apply charges to categories. Rather than spreading the $1,000,000 in financial requirements over 10,000 visits and charging $100, the $1,000,000 now can be spread over 16,000 weighted visit units and the charge reduced to $62.50 ($1,000,000 / 16,000) per weighted visit unit. For instance, although there are 3,000 routine visits, they equal 6,000 weighted visits. At $62.50 each, they will raise $375,000 (row J).

Note in row L that there is a considerable difference between charging the average price ($100) for all visits and charging by taking into account the amount of resources used. By weighting for resource consumption, those making a brief visit pay $225,000 less, and those making routine and complex visits pay, respectively, $75,000 and $150,000 more than they would under the undifferentiated system. Some would argue that this is more equitable. This is the logic Medicare used to establish the RBRVS system currently in use in ambulatory care reimbursement along with APCs.

MARGIN APPROACHES

There are two margin-based approaches to setting charges: cost plus and coverage. The *cost-plus approach* starts with cost and adds a margin for profit. For instance, assume a free-standing radiology center desires to make a 10 percent profit over and above its cost. If it has determined that the cost of performing a certain radiological procedure is $125, then it adds a 10 percent surcharge of $12.50, creating a final charge of $137.50. The cost-plus approach is most often used with ancillary services such as radiology, pharmacy, and laboratory services.

The *coverage approach* essentially sets charges using a break-even type of formula. Once the organization's cost structure, desired profit, and projected volume are known, charges can be set. Notice in Exhibit H–2 that the charge changes with volume. If the organization thought that 5,000 visits could be expected, it would establish a charge of $48 per visit, whereas if volume were forecast at 7,500 visits, it would establish a charge of $39 per visit.

Exhibit H–2   Illustration of the coverage approach to setting charges

A Variable cost per unit $20

B	C	D	E	F	G	H	I
				Direct	Direct		
		Total	Financial	Fixed	Variable	Other	Desired
Volume	Charge	Charges	Requirements	Costs	Costs	Costs	Profit
(Given)	(D/B)	(E)	(F+G+H+I)	(Given)	(A × B)	(Given)	(Given)
5,000	$48	$240,000	$240,000	$100,000	$100,000	$20,000	$20,000
5,500	$45	$247,500	$250,000	$100,000	$110,000	$20,000	$20,000
6,000	$43	$258,000	$260,000	$100,000	$120,000	$20,000	$20,000
6,500	$42	$273,000	$270,000	$100,000	$130,000	$20,000	$20,000
7,000	$40	$280,000	$280,000	$100,000	$140,000	$20,000	$20,000
7,500	$39	$292,500	$290,000	$100,000	$150,000	$20,000	$20,000
8,000	$38	$304,000	$300,000	$100,000	$160,000	$20,000	$20,000
8,500	$36	$306,000	$310,000	$100,000	$170,000	$20,000	$20,000
9,000	$36	$324,000	$320,000	$100,000	$180,000	$20,000	$20,000
9,500	$35	$332,500	$330,000	$100,000	$190,000	$20,000	$20,000
10,000	$34	$340,000	$340,000	$100,000	$200,000	$20,000	$20,000

GLOSSARY

Accountability Sanctions, both positive and negative, attached to carrying out responsibilities.

Accrual basis of accounting An accounting method that tracks the flow of resources and the revenues those resources helped to generate. It tracks revenues when earned and resources when used, regardless of the flow of cash in or out of the organization. This is the standard method in use today.

Accumulated depreciation The total amount of depreciation taken on an asset since it was put into use.

Activity-based costing A method of estimating costs of a service or product by estimating the costs of the activities it takes to produce that service or product.

Administrative cost centers Cost centers that support clinical cost centers and the organization as a whole. They are often considered the infrastructure of an organization.

Administrative profit centers Organizational units that do not provide health care-related services but are responsible for their profit. There are two types: those that sell their services internally and those whose primary responsibility is to bring revenues into the organization.

Aging schedule A table that shows the percentage of receivables being collected in each month.

Allocation base A statistic (e.g., square feet, number of full-time employees) used to allocate costs, based on its assumed relationship to why the costs occurred.

Allowable costs Costs that are allowable under the principles of reimbursement of government (Medicaid, Medicare) and other payors.

Ambulatory procedure classifications (APCs) Enacted by the federal government in 2000, a prospective payment system for hospital outpatient services, similar to DRGs, that reimburses a fixed amount for a bundled set of services.

Amortization (1) The allocation of the acquisition cost of debt to the period that it benefits. (2) The gradual process of paying off debt through a series of equal periodic payments. Each payment covers a portion of the principal plus current interest. The periodic payments are equal over the lifetime of the loan, but the proportion going toward the principal gradually increases. The amount of a payment can be determined by using the formula to calculate the present value of an annuity.

Annuity A series of equal payments made or received at regular time intervals.

Annuity due A series of equal annuity payments made or received at the beginning of each period.

APC A flat-fee payment system instituted by the government to control the payment for outpatient services provided to Medicare recipients; see *ambulatory procedure classifications*.

Asset mix The amount of working capital an organization keeps on hand relative to its potential working capital obligations.

Assets Resources that an organization owns, typically recorded at their original costs.

Authoritarian approach Budgeting and decision making that are done by relatively few people concentrated in the highest level of the organizational structure; opposite of the *participatory approach*.

Authority Power to carry out a given responsibility.

Avoidable fixed cost A fixed cost that is avoided if a particular alternative is chosen; *example:* full-time nursing costs saved if a service is closed.

Basic accounting equation Assets = liabilities + net assets.

Billing float Delay getting a bill to the patient or third-party payor (such as an insurance company). This includes the time to assemble the bill in-house as well as the time to send the bill to the correct person or place.

Bond A form of long-term financing whereby an issuer receives cash from a lender (an investor) and in return issues a promissory note (a "bond") agreeing to make principal or interest payments or both on specific dates.

Break-even analysis A technique to analyze the relationship among revenues, costs, and volume; also called "cost-volume-profit or CVP analysis."

Break-even point The point where total revenues equal total costs.

Budget variance The difference between what was planned (budgeted) and what was achieved (actual).

Cannibalization This occurs when a new service decreases the revenues from other established services or product lines; these are considered cash outflows.

Capital appreciation Occurs whenever an investment is worth more when it is sold than when it was purchased.

Capital budget One of the four major types of budgets, it summarizes the anticipated purchases for the year. Typically, to be included, all items in this budget must have a minimum purchase price, such as $500.

Capital investment decision Decisions involving major dollar investments that are expected to achieve long-term benefits for an organization.

Capital investments Large-dollar multiyear investments.

Capital lease A lease that lasts for an extended period of time, up to the life of the leased asset. This type of lease cannot be canceled without penalty, and at the end of the lease period, the lessee may have the option to purchase the asset; also called a *financial lease*.

Capitated profit centers Organizational units responsible for earning a profit by agreeing to take care of the health care needs of a population for a per-member fee (which is not directly tied to services); examples include *HMOs*, *PPOs*, and various managed care organizations.

Capitation (1) A system that pays providers a specific amount in advance to care for the health care needs of a population over a specific time period. Providers are usually paid on a per member per month (PMPM) basis. The provider then assumes the risk that the cost of caring for the population will not exceed the aggregate PMPM amount received. (2) A payment mechanism where the insurer prepays a health care provider an agreed-on amount per member that covers a designated set of services over a defined time. Typically, these payments are made on a PMPM basis. If there are no terms to the contrary, in return for the capitated payments, the provider agrees to bear all the risk for the costs of services provided. If the provider's costs are below the capitation, the provider can keep the difference. If the provider's costs are more than the capitation, the provider is at risk for the difference. (3) A method of payment in which the provider is paid a fixed amount over a set period, usually a month or a year for each person served no matter what the actual number or nature of services delivered.

Care mapping A process that specifies in advance the preferred treatment regimen for patients with particular diagnoses. This is also referred to as a "clinical pathway," "clinical protocol," or "practice guideline."

Case rate A rate that covers everything that a hospital provides during an entire inpatient stay.

Cash basis of accounting An accounting method that tracks when cash was received and when cash was expended, regardless of when services were provided or resources were used.

Cash budget One of the four major types of budgets, it displays all of the organization's projected cash inflows and outflows. The bottom line for this budget is the amount of cash available at the end of the period.

Charge based A method of payment that is based on the charge of the provider.

Charity care discounts Discounts from gross patients accounts receivable given to those who cannot pay their bills.

Clinical cost centers Cost centers that provide health care-related services to clients, patients, or enrollees.

CMS The Center for Medicare and Medicaid Services; the acronym is pronounced "sims."

Collateral (1) A tangible asset that is pledged as a promise to repay a loan. If the loan is not paid, the lending institution as a legal recourse may seize the pledged asset. (2) An asset with clear value (such as land or buildings) that is pledged against a loan to reduce risk to the lender. If the loan is not paid off satisfactorily, the lender has a legal claim to seize the pledged asset.

Collection float The time between when a bill is paid and the payment is deposited.

Commitment fee A percentage of the unused portion of a credit line that is charged to the potential borrower.

Common costs Costs that benefit a number of services and whose costs are shared by all; *examples*: rent, utilities, and billing; also called *joint costs*.

Community rating A rating method required of indemnity and HMO insurers that guarantees that there will be equivalent amounts collected from members of a specific group without regard to demographics such as age, sex, size of covered group, and industry type.

Compensating balance A designated dollar amount on deposit with a bank that a borrower is required to maintain.

Compliance The need to abide by governmental regulations, whether they be for the provision of care, billing, privacy, accounting standards, security, or the like.

Compound interest method A method of calculating interest on both the original principal and on all interest accumulated since the beginning of the investment time period.

Compounding Converting a present value into its future value, taking into account the time value of money; see *compound interest method*. It is the opposite of discounting.

Contact capitation A method of capitation whereby each specialty has its own capitation pool, and use of services by a physician affects only that physician's compensation, not the whole specialty network's compensation.

Contra-asset An asset that when increased decreases the value of a related asset on the books. Two primary examples are accumulated depreciation, which is the contra-asset to properties and equipment, and the allowance for uncollectibles, which is the contra-asset to accounts receivable.

Contribution margin per unit Per unit revenue minus per unit variable cost. If all other costs (fixed costs, overhead, etc.) remain the same, it is the amount of profit made on each additional unit produced.

Contribution margin rule If the contribution margin per unit is positive and no other additional costs will be incurred, then it is in the best financial interest of the organization to continue to provide additional units of that service, even if the organization is not fully covering all of its other costs.

Contribution margin, total Total revenues minus total variable costs.

Controlling activities Activities that provide guidance and feedback to keep the organization within its budget once it has been approved and is being implemented.

Conversion factor Actuarial-based formulas developed to adjust rates allowing for differences in population demographics.

Copayment Requiring the patient to pay part of the health care bill. These payments are used to prevent over-utilization of services.

Corporate compliance Mandated legislation and regulations bestowed on health care institutions to ensure fairness, accuracy, honesty, and quality in the provision of and billing for health care services.

Corporate compliance officer The individual (or department) responsible for knowing the corporate compliance rules and regulations and for ensuring that the organization strictly abides by them.

Cost avoidance The ability of an organization to find new ways to operate that eliminate certain classes of costs.

Cost-based reimbursement Using the provider's cost of providing services (supplies, staff salaries, space costs, etc.) as the basis for reimbursement.

Cost centers Organizational units responsible for providing services and controlling their costs.

Cost containment Not spending more than is budgeted in the expense budget.

Cost driver That which causes a change in the cost of an activity.

Cost object Anything for which a cost is being estimated, such as a population, a test, a visit, a patient, or a patient day.

Cost of capital The rate of return required to undertake a project; the cost of capital accounts for both the time value of money and risk; also called the *hurdle rate* or *discount rate*.

Cost-shifting When providers try to get one payor to pay for costs that have not been covered by another payor, a common example being a provider's trying to compensate for low Medicaid payments by increasing charges to a private insurer.

Cost-to-charge ratio (CCR) A method to estimate costs that assumes that costs are a certain percentage of charges (or reimbursements).

Current assets Assets that will be consumed (used up) within one year (or one time period).

Current liabilities Financial obligations due within one year (or one time period).

Decentralization The dispersion of responsibility within a health care organization.

Deductibles When the patient covered is responsible for paying a certain base amount before coverage begins.

Defensive medicine The tendency of health care practitioners to do more testing and to provide more care for patients than might otherwise be necessary and to protect themselves against potential litigation.

Depreciation A measure of how much a tangible asset (such as plant or equipment) has been used up or consumed.

Diagnosis-related groups (DRGs) A system to classify inpatients based on their diagnoses, used by both Medicare and private insurers. In the most pervasive system, there are approximately one thousand diagnostic categories.

Direct costs Costs (e.g., nursing costs) that an organization can trace to a particular cost object (e.g., a patient).

Disbursement float An organization's practice of delaying payment as long as possible to its creditors without causing ill will.

Discount When the market rate is higher than the coupon rate, a bond is said to be selling at a discount from its par value; see also *premium*.

Discount rate See *cost of capital*.

Discounted cash flows Cash flows that have been adjusted to account for the cost of capital.

Discounting Converting future cash flows into their present value taking into account the time value of money; it is the opposite of compounding.

Discounts A reduction in the charge for services.

Dividends Represents the portion of profit that an organization distributes to equity investors.

DRGs A patient classification scheme used by Medicare that clusters patients into categories on the basis of their illnesses, diseases, and medical problems. These classifications are then used to pay providers a set amount based on the *diagnosis-related group* in which the patient has been classified.

Effective interest rate The approximate annual interest rate incurred by not taking advantage of a supplier's discount offer to pay bills early.

Electronic health record (EHR) An online version of patient medical records that can include patient demographics, insurance information, dictations and notes, medication and immunization histories, ancillary test results, and so forth. Under strict security permissions, the information can be accessed either in-house or in private office settings; also called an *electronic medical record*.

Electronic medical record (EMR) See *electronic health record*.

Expansion decision Capital investment decision designed to increase the operational capability of a health care organization.

Expense budget A subset of the operating budget that is a forecast of the operating expenses that will be incurred during the current budget period.

Expense cost variance The amount of the variable expense variance that occurs because the actual cost per visit varies from that originally budgeted. It is the difference between the variable expenses forecast in the flexible budget and those actually incurred. It can be calculated by the formula: (actual cost per unit − budgeted cost per unit) × actual volume.

Expense volume variance The portion of total variance in variable expenses that is due to the actual volume being either higher or lower than the budgeted volume. It is the difference between the expenses forecast in the original budget and those in the flexible budget. It can be computed using the following formula: (actual volume − budgeted volume) × budgeted cost per unit.

Experience rating The method of setting premium rates based on the actual health care costs of a group or groups.

Factoring Selling accounts receivable at a discount, usually to a financial institution. The latter then assumes the role of trying to collect on the outstanding payment obligations.

Feasibility study A study that examines market and management factors that affect the issuer's ability to generate the necessary cash flows to meet principal and interest requirements.

Fee-for-service A method of reimbursement based on payment for services rendered, with a specific fee correlated to each specific service. An insurance company, the patient, or a government program such as Medicare or Medicaid (discussed later) may make payment.

Financial lease See *capital lease*.

Financial leverage The degree to which an organization is financed by long-term debt.

Financial requirements For health care providers, this is a combination of issues related to operations, opportunities, contingencies, and return on investment.

Financing mix How an organization chooses to finance its working capital needs.

First party Typically the patient in a health care encounter.

Fixed costs Costs that stay the same in total over the relevant range but change inversely on a per unit basis as activity changes.

Fixed income security A bond that pays fixed amounts of interest at regular periodic intervals, usually semiannually.

Fixed labor budget A subset of the labor budget that forecasts the cost of salaried personnel.

Fixed supplies budget A subset of the supplies budget that covers those items that do not vary by patient volume.

Flat fee A predefined amount of money paid to a provider for a unit of service.

Flexible budget A budget that accommodates a range or multiple levels of activities.

Float The time delay of the process of assembling a bill until depositing the payment in the bank and making subsequent payments to creditors.

Fully allocated cost The cost of an item that includes both its direct costs and all other costs allocated to it.

Fund balance A term used until 1996 for owners' equity by not-for-profit health care organizations. It was replaced with the present term, *net assets*, for nongovernmental not-for-profit organizations.

Future value (FV) What an amount invested today (or a series of payments made over time) will be worth at a given time in the future using the compound interest method, which accounts for the time value of money; see also *present value*.

Future value factor The factor used to compound a present amount to its future worth. It is the reciprocal of the present value factor and is calculated using the formula $(1 + i)^n$.

Future value factor of an annuity (FVFA) A factor that when multiplied by a stream of equal payments equals the future value of that stream; see also *present value factor of an annuity*.

Future value of an annuity What an equal series of payments will be worth at some future date using compound interest; see also *future value factor of an annuity* and *present value of an annuity*.

Future value of an annuity table Table of factors that shows the future value of equal flows at the end of each period, given a particular interest rate.

Future value table Table of factors that shows the future value of a single investment at a given interest rate.

Gatekeepers Providers (typically the *PCP*) who must preapprove care received by a patient, such as a visit to a specialist. Gatekeepers are utilized in most *POS* and *HMO* plans.

Global payments A system of paying providers whereby the fees for all providers (hospitals, physicians, home health care agencies) are included in a single negotiated amount. This is sometimes called "bundling" of services. In nonglobal payment systems, each provider is paid separately.

Goodwill An amount paid above and beyond the book value of an asset when it is sold, in part to offset the seller from potential lost future earnings from the asset had it not been sold.

Gross charges The amount that an organization would bill its patients if they all paid full charges; see *net charges*.

Group model HMO A health maintenance organization (HMO) that contracts with medical groups for services.

Group purchasing organizations (GPOs) Third-party entities that contract with multiple hospitals to offer materials cost savings by negotiating large-volume discounted contracts with vendors. In return for its services, the GPO retains a margin based on sales.

Health Care Financing Administration (HCFA) The U.S. government department that oversaw the provision of and payment for health care provided under its entitlement programs (Medicare, Medicaid) until 2001.

Health Insurance Portability and Accountability Act (HIPAA) A set of federal compliance regulations enacted in 1996 to ensure standardization of billing, privacy, and reporting as institutions enter a paperless age.

Health maintenance organization (HMO) A legal corporation that offers health insurance and medical care. HMOs typically offer a range of health care services at a fixed price; see *capitation*.

Hedging The art of offsetting high variable rate debt payments with returns from high-rate investments.

Horizontal analysis A method of analyzing financial statements that looks at the percentage change in a line item from one year to the next. It is computed by the formula (subsequent year – previous year)/previous year.

Hurdle rate See *required rate of return*.

Incremental cash flows Cash flows that occur solely as a result of a particular action such as undertaking a project.

Incremental costs Additional costs incurred solely as a result of an action or activity or a particular set of actions or activities.

Incremental-decremental approach A method of budgeting that starts with an existing budget to plan future budgets.

Indemnity insurance A plan that reimburses physicians for services performed or beneficiaries for medical expenses incurred. Typically, the employer, patient (or both) pays a monthly premium to the plan for a predetermined set of health care benefits.

Indirect costs Costs that an organization is not able to directly trace to a particular cost object. Common indirect costs include the cost of the billing clerk, rent, computer costs, and many so-called overhead costs.

Interest A payment to creditors who have loaned the organization funds or otherwise extended credit.

Internal rate of return The rate of return on an investment that makes the net present value equal to $0 after all cash flows have been discounted at the same rate. It is also the discount rate at which the discounted cash flows over the life of the project exactly equal the initial investment.

Internal rate of return method A method to evaluate the financial feasibility of an investment decision that compares the investment's rate of return with that return required by the organization.

Investment centers Organizational units that not only have all the responsibilities of a traditional profit center but also are responsible for making a certain return on investment.

Joint costs See *common costs*.

Labor budget A subset of the expense budget, it is composed of the fixed labor budget and the variable labor budget.

Lessee An entity that negotiates the use of another's asset via a lease.

Lessor An entity that owns an asset that is then leased out.

Letter of credit Offered through a bank, this can be used to enhance the creditworthiness of an institution and, hence, a bond's rating.

Liabilities The financial obligations (i.e., debts) of an organization.

Line-item budget The least-detailed budget, showing only revenues and expenses by category, such as labor or supplies.

Liquidity A measure of how quickly an asset can be converted into cash.

Lockbox A post office box located near a Federal Reserve Bank or branch, from which the bank will pick up and process checks quickly, but for a fee.

Managed care Any of a number of arrangements designed to control health care costs through monitoring, prescribing, or proscribing the provision of health care to a patient or population.

Market value What a bond would sell for in today's open market.

Medicaid A federally mandated program operated and partially funded by individual states (in conjunction with the federal government) to provide medical benefits to certain low-income people. The state, under broad federal guidelines, determines what benefits are covered, who is eligible, and how much providers will be paid.

Medical home A partnership between primary care providers (PCPs), the patients, and their families to deliver comprehensive care over the long term in a variety of settings.

Medical savings accounts A limited amount of money an employee can take as pretaxed income to pay for medically related items such as physician visits, pharmaceuticals, eyewear, dental visits, and the like. The pretax income is placed in an escrow account held by the employer. The employee must submit receipts for care received to get reimbursed.

Medical tourism Patients who travel to foreign countries to obtain normally expensive medical services at a steep discount. Even including a family escort, who get the added benefit of foreign travel, the total cost is less than what it would be at home.

Medicare A nationwide federally financed health insurance program for people aged sixty-five and older. It also covers certain people younger than sixty-five who are disabled or have chronic kidney (end-stage renal) disease. Medicare Part A is the hospital insurance program; Part B covers physicians' services. Created by the 1965 amendment to the Social Security Act.

Medicare Part D Prescription drug coverage for Medicare enrollees, begun in 2006, that offsets some of the out-of-pocket costs for medications. Enrollees pay an additional monthly premium for this supplemental benefit.

Members People who are covered by a health care plan. Typically the member or the employer of the member (or both) pays a premium to the plan for the privilege of being covered.

Mission statement A statement that guides the organization by identifying the unique attributes of the organization, why it exists, and what it hopes to achieve. Some organizations divide these attributes between a vision and a mission statement.

Multiyear budget A budget that is forecast multiple years out, rather than just for the upcoming year.

Net assets In not-for-profit organizations, the difference between assets and liabilities (assets minus liabilities).

Net charges The amount that an organization bills its patients after accounting for discounts and allowances; see *gross charges*.

Net income Excess of revenues over expenses.

Net present value (NPV) The present value of future cash flows related to an investment net (less) the cost of the initial investment. It represents the difference between the initial amount paid for an investment and the future cash inflows that the investment will bring in, after adjusting for the cost of capital.

Net present value method A method to evaluate the financial feasibility of an investment decision based solely on the resulting net present value. It uses a specific discount rate that may not be equal to the organization's required rate of return.

Net proceeds from a bond issuance Gross proceeds less the underwriter's and others' issuance fees.

Nonavoidable fixed costs A fixed cost that will remain even if a particular service is discontinued. *Example:* full-time nursing costs in an organization that will continue, even though one of several services is dropped.

Noncurrent assets The resources of the organization that will be used or consumed over periods longer than one year.

Noncurrent liabilities The financial obligations not due within one year.

Nonregular cash flows Cash flows that occur sporadically or on an irregular basis. A common nonregular cash flow is salvage value, receipt of funds following a one-time sale of an asset at the end of its useful life.

Notes to financial statements Additional key information written out in detail that is not presented in the body of the financial statement.

Operating budget One of the four major types of budgets, it comprises the revenue budget and the expense budget. The bottom line for this budget is net income.

Operating cash flows Cash flows that occur on a regular basis, oftentimes following implementation of a project; also called *regular cash flows*.

Operating income Income derived from an organization's main line of business.

Operating lease A lease that lasts shorter than the useful life of the leased asset, typically one year or less. This type of leasing arrangement can be canceled at any time without penalty, but there is no option to purchase the asset once the lease has expired.

Opportunity cost Proceeds lost by forgoing other opportunities.

Ordinary annuity A series of equal annuity payments made or received at the end of each period.

Outstanding bond issue A bond that trades in the marketplace.

Owner's equity In for-profit institutions, the difference between assets and liabilities (assets *minus* liabilities).

Par value The face value amount of a bond; it is the amount the bondholder is paid at maturity, and it does not include any coupon payments.

Participating provider A provider who has contracted with a health plan to provide medical services to covered members at predetermined rates.

Participatory approach A method of budgeting in which the roles and responsibilities of putting together a budget are diffused throughout the organization, typically originating at the department level. There are guidelines to follow, and approval must be secured by top management. It is opposite to the *authoritarian approach*.

Pay for performance (P4P) A recent alternative payment arrangement that bases partial reimbursement or creates additional reimbursement incentives for providers based on adherence to predefined standards for quality of care. Indicators include various patient outcomes and frequency and type of tests ordered and services performed.

Payback method A method to evaluate the feasibility of an investment by determining how long it would take until the initial investment is recovered, disregarding the time value of money.

Payor An entity that is responsible for paying for the services of a health care provider. Typically this is an insurance company or a government agency; commonly referred to as a *third party*.

Per diem An amount a payor will pay for one day of care, which includes all hospital charges associated with the inpatient day (including nursing care, surgeries, medications, etc.).

Per member per month (PMPM) Generally used by HMOs and their medical providers as an indicator of revenue, expenses, or utilization of services per member per one-month period.

Performance budget An extension of the program budget that also lays out performance objectives.

Perpetuity An annuity for an infinite period of time; also called a "perpetual annuity."

Planning The process of identifying goals, objectives, tasks, activities, and resources necessary to carry out the strategic plan of an organization over the next time period, typically one year.

Point of service (POS) A hybrid between a HMO and a PPO in which patients are given the incentive to see providers participating in a defined network but may see non-network providers, though usually at some additional cost.

Predetermined rates A set fee paid to a provider for an inpatient episode of care.

Preferred provider organization (PPO) A network of independent providers preselected by the payor to provide a specific service or range of services at predetermined (usually discounted) rates to the payor's covered members.

Premium A monthly payment made by a person, employer, or both to an insurer that makes one eligible for a defined level of health care for a given period of time.

Premium When the market rate is lower than the coupon rate, a bond is said to be selling at a premium; see also *discount*.

Present value (PV) The value today of a payment (or series of payments) to be received in the future, taking into account the cost of capital.

Present value factor The factor used to discount a future amount to its current worth. It is the reciprocal of the future value factor and is calculated using the formula $1/(1 + i)^n$.

Present value factor of an annuity (PVFA) A factor that when multiplied by a stream of equal payments equals the present value of that stream.

Present value of an annuity What a series of equal payments in the future is worth today, taking into account the time value of money.

Present value of an annuity table Table of factors that shows the worth today of equal flows at the end of each future period, given a particular interest rate.

Present value table Table of factors that shows what a single amount to be received in the future is worth today at a given interest rate.

Price setter The entity that controls the amount paid for a health care service.

Primary care provider (PCP) A physician (typically a family medicine, internal medicine, pediatric, and sometimes obstetrics and gynecology provider) who is the primary care giver of a patient.

Product margin Total contribution margin minus avoidable fixed costs: the amount that a service contributes to covering all other costs after it has covered costs that are there solely because the service is offered (its total variable cost and avoidable fixed costs) and would not be there if the service were dropped.

Product margin decision rule If a service's product margin is positive, the organization will be better off financially if it continues with the service, *ceteris paribus* ("all else being the same"). Conversely, if a service's product margin is negative, the organization will be better off financially if it discontinues the service, *ceteris paribus*.

Production cost centers Cost centers that are responsible for: producing or selling products.

Profit centers Organizational units responsible for controlling costs and earning revenues.

Program budget An extension of the line-item budget that shows revenues and expenses by program or service lines.

Prospective payment system (PPS) (1)The payment system used by Medicare to reimburse providers a predetermined amount. This system is commonly referred to as the PPS or DRG payment system. Several payment methods fall under the umbrella of PPS, including *DRGs* (inpatient admissions), *APCs* (outpatient visits); *RBRVS* (professional services); and RUGs (skilled nursing home care). (2) A payment method that establishes rates, prices, or budgets before services are rendered and costs are incurred. Providers retain or absorb at least a portion of the difference between established revenues and actual costs.

Ratio An expression of the relationship between two numbers as a single number.

RBRVS A system of paying physicians based on the relative value of the services rendered.

Red herring A preliminary official statement offered to prospective buyers of a bond by the underwriters to help determine a fair market price for the bond.

Regular cash flows See *operating cash flows*.

Relative value units (RVUs) A standardized weighting applied to services that reflects the amount of resource consumption to provide that service. A service assigned 2 RVUs consumes twice the resources as a service assigned 1 RVU.

Relevant range The range of activity over which *total fixed costs* or *per unit variable cost* does not vary.

Replacement decision Capital investment decision designed to replace older assets with newer ones.

Required market rate The market interest rate on similar-risk bonds.

Required rate of return An organization's minimally acceptable *internal rate of return* on any investment to justify an initial investment; also called *cost of capital* or *hurdle rate*.

Residual value See *salvage value*.

Resource-based relative value scale (RBRVS) See *RBRVS*.

Responsibility Duties and obligations of a responsibility center.

Responsibility center An organizational unit that has been formally given the responsibility to carry out one or more tasks or achieve one or more outcomes (or both).

Retail health care Generally preventive care walk-in medical services provided in a retail outlet, such as a pharmacy, by a licensed care provider.

Retained earnings A second type of benefit to an investor. These are in the form of the portion of the profits the organization keeps in-house to use in growth and support of its mission.

Retrospective payment Method for reimbursing a provider after the service has been delivered.

Revenue attainment Earning the amount of revenue budgeted.

Revenue budget A subset of the operating budget that is a forecast of the operating revenues that will be earned during the current budget period.

Revenue enhancement Finding supplemental sources of revenue.

Revenue rate variance The amount of the total revenue variance that occurs because the actual average rate charged varies from the one originally budgeted. It is the difference between the revenues forecast in the flexible budget and those actually earned. It can be calculated using the formula (actual rate – budgeted rate) $\times$ actual volume.

Revenue volume variance The portion of total variance in revenues due to the actual volume being either higher or lower than the budgeted volume. It is the difference between the revenues forecast in the original budget and those in the flexible budget. It can be computed using the formula: (actual volume – budgeted volume) $\times$ budgeted rate.

Risk pools A generally large population of individuals who are all simultaneously insured under the same arrangement, regardless of working status. Health care utilization—and therefore cost—is more stable for larger groups than it is for smaller groups, which makes larger groups' costs more predictable for insurers and thus less of a risk.

Rolling budget A multiyear budget that is updated more frequently than annually, such as semiannually or quarterly.

RVU See *relative value unit*.

Sale-leaseback arrangement A type of capital lease whereby an institution sells an owned asset and then simultaneously leases it back from the purchaser. The selling institution retains rights to use the asset but benefits from the immediate acquisition of cash from the sale.

Salvage value The amount of cash to be received when an asset is sold, usually at the end of its useful life; also called *terminal value*.

Sarbanes-Oxley Act Federal legislation designed to tighten accounting standards in financial reporting and that holds top executives personally liable as to the accuracy and fairness of their financial statements.

Scrap value See *salvage value*.

Second party Typically, the provider (hospital or physician) in a health care encounter.

Service centers Organizational units that are primarily responsible for ensuring that health care-related services are provided to a population in a manner that meets the volume and quality requirements of the organization. They have no direct budgetary control.

Shareholders' equity Another name for *owners' equity*.

Short-term plans Specific plans that identify an organization's short-term goals and objectives in more detail, primarily in regard to marketing or production, control, and financing the organization.

Simple interest method A method to calculate interest only on the original principal amount. The principal is the amount invested.

Sinking fund A fund into which monies are set aside each year to ensure that a bond can be liquidated at maturity.

Staff model HMO An HMO that owns its clinics and employs its physicians.

Stark Law Legislation enacted by CMS in 2005 to guard against providers' ordering self-referrals for Medicare or Medicaid patients directly to any settings in which they have a vested financial interest; also referred to as "anti-kickback" legislation.

Static budget A budget that uses a single or fixed level of activity.

Statistics budget The first budget to be prepared; one of the four major types of budgets; it identifies the amount of services that will be provided, typically categorized by payor type.

Step-down method A cost-finding method based on allocating costs that are not directly paid for to products or services to which payment is attached. The method derives its name from the stair-step pattern that results from allocating costs.

Step-fixed costs Costs that increase in total over wide, discrete steps.

Stop-loss A method providers use to limit the exposure that comes with the possibility that charges will go far beyond negotiated rates, a level of charges over which the provider is no longer totally liable.

Straight-line depreciation A method by which an asset is depreciated an equal amount each year until it reaches its salvage value at the end of its useful life.

Strategic decision Capital investment decision designed to increase a health care organization's strategic (long-term) position.

Strategic planning Identifying an organization's mission, goals, and strategy to best position itself for the future.

Subcapitation Where the primary care physician pays a portion of the total capitated dollars received to another provider (i.e., specialist).

Sunk costs Costs incurred in the past. They should not be included in NPV-type analyses.

Target costing Controlling costs or decreasing profit margins (or both) to meet or beat a predetermined price or reimbursement rate.

Tax shield An investment that reduces the amount of income tax that has to be paid, often because interest and depreciation expenses are tax deductible.

Term loan A loan typically issued by a bank that has a maturity of one to ten years.

Terminal value See *salvage value*.

Third party Typically the payor (insurance company or government agency) in a health care encounter.

Third-party payors Commonly referred to as third parties, these are organizations that pay on behalf of patients.

Time value of money The concept that a dollar received today is worth more than a dollar received in the future.

Top-down budgeting See *authoritarian approach*.

Top-down or bottom-up approach See *participatory approach*.

Traditional profit centers Organizational units responsible for earning a profit by providing health care services. Revenues are earned on either a fee-for-service or flat-fee basis. Examples include cardiology, women's and children's services, and oncology.

Trend analysis A type of horizontal analysis that looks at changes in line items compared with a base year. It is calculated [(any subsequent year – base year)/base year] $\times$ 100.

Transfer prices The prices for products or services that are charged internally to other organizational units.

Trustee An agent for bondholders who ensures that the health care facility is making timely principal and interest payments to the bondholders and complies with legal covenants of the bond.

Variable costs Costs that stay the same per unit but change directly in total with a change in activity over the relevant range: total variable cost = variable cost per unit $\times$ number of units of activity.

Variable labor budget A subset of the labor budget that forecasts nonsalary labor costs, such as part-time employees and overtime hours.

Variable supplies budget A subset of the supplies budget that includes items that vary based on the volume of patients seen.

Vertical analysis A method for analyzing financial statements that answers the general question: what percentage of one line item is another line item? Also called common-size analysis because it converts every line item to a percentage, thus allowing comparisons among the financial statements of different organizations.

Working capital strategy The amount of working capital that an organization determines it must keep available as a cushion to protect against unforeseen expenditures.

Yield to maturity The rate at which the market value of a bond is equal to the bond's present value of future coupon payments plus.

Zero-based budget (capitation) Dividing the entire amount of capitation (the "budget") among all the providers, essentially leaving nothing or "zero" left at the end of every accounting period.

Zero-based budgeting (ZBB) An approach to budgeting that continually questions both the need for existing programs and their level of funding as well as the need for new programs. Zero-based budgeting is often referred to as ZBB.

USEFUL WEB SITES

1. ***Agency for Healthcare Research and Quality (and P4P Guide)***

   Link: http://www.ahrq.gov (home page).

   P4P Guide: http://www.ahrq.gov/qual/p4pguide.pdf

   > Web site: a. It is a freely available resource. b. This site provides information on national health care quality measures and health care outcomes research. The pay-for-performance guide was created in 2006.

2. ***AHA Trend Data***

   Link: http://www.aha.org/aha/research-and-trends/trendwatch/2007chartbook.html or go to AHA Web site and click on Research and Trends, then Trendwatch, and 2007 Chartbook.

   > Web site: a. It is a freely available resource. b. These reports are released by the American Hospital Association annually. These data are compiled from various sources and provide information on health and hospital trends. Some of the other reports available here also provide insights into issues like workforce shortage, disaster preparedness, health care costs, and others.

3. ***AHA HIPAA Standards***

   Link: http://www.aha.org/aha/issues/HIPAA/resources.html or go to the AHA Web site and click on Issues, then HIPAA, and then Resources.

   > Web site: a. It is a freely available resource. b. HIPAA (The Health Insurance Portability and Accountability Act of 1996) has established new standards for the movement and use of health care information. This link provides information on transaction, privacy, and security: the three types of standards created by HIPAA.

4. ***American Hospital Directory***

   Link: http://www.ahd.com.

   > Web site: a. Some free information plus detailed information for paid subscribers. b. The AHD (American Hospital Directory) provides online data for over six thousand hospitals. Their database of information about hospitals is built from both public and private sources, including Medicare claims data, hospital cost reports, and other files obtained from the federal Centers for Medicare and Medicaid Services (CMS, formerly HCFA). The directory also includes AHA Annual Survey Data licensed from Health Forum, an American Hospital Association company. It makes available free hospital information

and state and national stats. However, greater detailed information is available for paid subscribers.

5. CMS Resource Base

Link: http://www.cms.hhs.gov/home/tools.asp or go to the CMS Web site and click on Tools.

Web site: a. Free resource center. b. CMS is the Centers for Medicare and Medicaid services established as a result of these programs being signed into law in 1965. Since 1965, a number of changes have been made to CMS programs. The link above is for the resource base made available by this center. Resources include Medicare and Medicaid information by provider type, information by special topics, and so forth.

6. CMS Statistics, Trends, and Reports

Link: http://www.cms.hhs.gov/home/rsds.asp or go to the CMS Web site and click on Research, Statistics, Data and Systems.

Link: http://www.cms.hhs.gov/CMSLeadership/09_Office_OACT.asp#TopOfPage (Office of the Actuary).

Link: http://www.cms.hhs.gov/NationalHealthExpendData (National Health Expenditure Data).

Web site: a. Free resource center. b. CMS is the Centers for Medicare and Medicaid services established as a result of these programs being signed into law in 1965. Since 1965, a number of changes have been made to CMS programs. The link above is for the research, statistics, trends, and reports made available freely by the CMS.

7. Healthcare Finance Group

Link: http://www.hfgusa.com.

Web site: a. The link above leads to the HFG home page. Healthcare Finance Group Inc. (HFG) is a specialty finance company investing exclusively in the health care industry. b. HFG's clients include acute care hospitals, skilled nursing facilities, home health agencies, large physician groups, pharmacy services, long-term acute care and rehab hospitals, and behavioral health and diagnostic imaging centers. They provide secured revolving lines of credit, term loans, real estate loans, and letters of credit from $5 million to $100 million to health care service providers who are their clients. Click on link to find out about available services.

8. Healthcare Financial Management Association (HFMA)

Link: http://www.hfma.org/library or go to HFMA Web site and click on Resource library.

Web site: a. Paid Web site. Free information is available only about HFMA. b. HFMA is considered a leader on top trends and issues facing the health care industry. It is a membership organization for health care financial management executives and leaders and currently consists of more than 34 000 members. Many different magazines are published by HFMA, and each of these is sold for different prices unless one becomes a member of HFMA, which requires an annual subscription fee.

9. *HealthLeaders Media*

Link: http://www.healthleadersmedia.com/index.cfm (home page).

Web site: A free site offering current stories and events in the areas of leadership, finance, technology, physicians, hospitals, health plans, marketing, quality, and also global and human resource issues. The site also offers access to magazines, e-newsletters, blogs, discussions, webcasts, statistics, and white papers.

10. *Hospital and Healthcare System Financial Statements from Bond Issues*

Link: Muni-OS (http://www.munios.com) (home page) and Electronic Municipal Market Access (http://www.emma.msrb.org).

Web site: The Muni-OS Web site requires registration, which is free. Both Web sites allow one to download the financial statements of hospitals and health care systems that have issued municipal bonds by downloading the "Official Statement" of the bond issue. It also provides detailed information about the bond issuance, specifically the amount of the issue, bond issuer, underwriter of the bond, and so forth. It also defines what the proceeds of the bond will be used for.

11. *Leapfrog Group*

Link: http://www.leapfroggroup.org/home (home page).

Web site: a. It is a freely available resource with an opportunity for paid membership with additional benefits. b. This organization aims to promote health care quality and safety and to make outcomes publicly available for consumer review. It offers provider benchmarking and rewards to hospitals with high-quality standards who encourage transparency in outcomes reporting.

12. *Managed Care Magazine*

Link: http://www.managedcaremag.com (home page).

Web site: Free, with an opportunity for free digital subscriptions. The site's articles cover the business of medicine as well as research articles on health care financing and delivery.

13. National Association of Health Underwriters

Link: http://www.nahu.org/consumer/guides.cfm or go to NAHU Web site and click on Consumer Information and then Guides.

Web site: a. Free consumer information and paid membership. b. NAHU provides free consumer information on any health insurance-related issue in the link provided above. One can also locate a health insurance agent to extract detailed information. To be a member of NAHU requires a membership fee.

14. National Association of Rural Health Clinics

Link: http://www.narhc.org/resources/resources.php or go to NARHC Web site and click on Resources.

Web site: a. Free resources plus a paid membership. b. NARHC is the only national organization dedicated exclusively to improving the delivery of quality, cost-effective health care in rural underserved areas through the Rural Health Clinics Program (RHC Program). NARHC is a vital link between health clinics and federal legislators and regulators as it brings the real-world experience of rural health clinic practice to policy making and policy makers. NARHC works with Congress and other federal agencies. To be a member of NARHC requires a membership fee. However, NARHC makes available some reports and information resources freely, which can be accessed via the link above. Most of the information related to RHCsis made freely available through this link.

15. New York Times

Link: http://nytimes.com (home page) or from the home page, go to news by industry.

Web site: Free of charge. It provides news by industry, such as health, business, and technology. Although all information is freely accessible, there is a charge to reproduce information for publication elsewhere.

16. North Carolina Healthcare Information and Communications Alliance (NCHICA)

Link: http://www.nchica.org (home page) and http://www.nchica.org/HIPAAResources/NPI.htm (resource link).

Web site: a. Partially free resources plus paid membership. Full-time students at accredited institutions of higher learning are charged $25 annually to become nonvoting members. b. The North Carolina Healthcare Information and Communications Alliance, Inc. (NCHICA) is a nationally recognized nonprofit organization. It is a consortium that serves as an open and effective forum for health information technology (HIT) initiatives in North Carolina. It is dedicated to improving health care through information technology and secure communications. It offers resources in HIPAA, privacy, (Electronic Data Interchange, and so forth.

17. Office of the Inspector General (OIG)

Link: http://www.oig.hhs.gov (home page).

Web site: a. It is a freely available resource. b. This office is responsible for monitoring health care programs under the Department of Health and Human Services and monitoring the health and well-being of the patient members served. The office does audits, investigations, and inspections of health care organizations to ensure strict accordance to federally mandated guidelines.

18. Henry J. Kaiser Family Foundation

Link: http://www.kff.org (Home page).

Web site: A nonpartisan organization that provides factual information free of charge for policy research and other means. The foundation does its own research, and it is not associated with Kaiser Permanente.

19. U.S. Department of Health and Human Services

Link: http://www.hhs.gov and from here, there are links to any area or agency of interest.

Web site: a. A free resource center. b. This is the link to the home page for this federal agency. From this link, we can access and search electronically available HHS information; we can also go directly to HHS agencies' (also referred to as Operating Divisions [OPDIVs]) home pages.

20. Wall Street Journal

Link: http://online.wsj.com/public/us (home page) or from the home page, go to news by industry.

Web site: This site provides news by industry. but it requires the user to become a subscriber to have online access to all the information provided in the *Wall Street Journal*. Student subscription is available for a subsidized rate of $29.95 for fifteen weeks. It provides business news and helps locate articles on health care finance.

INDEX

589